KAPLAN

MCAT®

General Chemistry Review

2027–2028

Edited by Alexander Stone Macnow, MD

ACKNOWLEDGMENTS

Editor-in-Chief, 2027–2028 Edition
M. Dominic Eggert

Contributing Editors, 2027–2028 Edition
Ae-Ri Kim, PhD; Elizabeth Minten, MD PhD; Gregory J. Riviello, MA; Christopher Vestuto

Prior Edition Editorial Staff: Elisabeth Fassas, MD MSc

Published by Kaplan North America, LLC
1515 West Cypress Creek Road
Fort Lauderdale, Florida 33309

Printed in India.

ISBN: 979-8-3497-0121-4

10 9 8 7 6 5 4 3 2 1

TABLE OF CONTENTS

THE *KAPLAN MCAT REVIEW* TEAM

Alexander Stone Macnow, MD
Editor-in-Chief

Áine Lorié, PhD
Editor

Derek Rusnak, MA
Editor

Mikhail Alexeeff
Kaplan MCAT Faculty

Laura L. Ambler
Kaplan MCAT Faculty

Krista L. Buckley, MD
Kaplan MCAT Faculty

Kristen L. Russell, ME
Editor

Pamela Willingham, MSW
Editor

Melinda Contreras, MS
Kaplan MCAT Faculty

Samantha Fallon
Kaplan MCAT Faculty

Jason R. Selzer
Kaplan MCAT Faculty

M. Dominic Eggert
Editor

Faculty Reviewers and Editors: Elmar R. Aliyev; James Burns; Jonathan Cornfield; Alisha Maureen Crowley; Nikolai Dorofeev, MD; Benjamin Downer, MS; Colin Doyle; Christopher Durland; Marilyn Engle; Eleni M. Eren; Raef Ali Fadel; Elizabeth Flagge; Adam Grey; Rohit Gupta, Jonathan Habermacher; Tyra Hall-Pogar, PhD; Justine Harkness, PhD; Scott Huff; Samer T. Ismail; Ae-Ri Kim, PhD; Elizabeth A. Kudlaty; Kelly Kyker-Snowman, MS; Ningfei Li; John P. Mahon; Brandon McKenzie; Matthew A. Meier; Nainika Nanda; Caroline Nkemdilim Opene; Kaitlyn E. Prenger; Uneeb Qureshi; Jason Selzer; Allison St. Clair; Bela G. Starkman, PhD; Chris Sun; Michael Paul Tomani, MS; Bonnie Wang; Ethan Weber; Lauren K. White; Nicholas M. White; Allison Ann Wilkes, MS; Kerranna Williamson, MBA; and Tony Yu.

Thanks to Kevin Anderson; Rebecca Anderson; Jeff Batzli; Jurre Blom; Hari Priya Chandran; Eric Chiu; James Coleman; Deepika Devan; Tim Eich; Samantha Fallon; Tyler Fara; Owen Farcy; Dan Frey; Robin Garmise; Rita Garthaffner; Joanna Graham; Allison Gudenau; Allison Harm; Beth Hoffberg; Aaron Lemon-Strauss; Keith Lubeley; Diane McGarvey; Leonard Mendoza; Petros Minasi; Elizabeth Minten, MD, PhD; Beena P V; John Polstein; Deeangelee Pooran-Kublall, MD, MPH; Andrea Repole; Rochelle Rothstein, MD; Larry Rudman; Tor Sanden; Srividhya Sankar; Sylvia Tidwell Scheuring; Carly Schnur; Aiswarya Sivanand; Todd Tedesco; Karin Tucker; Lee Weiss; Christina Wheeler; Kristen Workman; Amy Zarkos; and the countless others who made this project possible.

GETTING STARTED CHECKLIST

Getting Started Checklist

- [ ] Register for your free online assets: if you bought this book new as part of a set, scan the QR code on the front of the book set's slipcase and enter the unique code there; if you bought this book separately, instead go to **www.kaptest.com/booksonline**.
- [ ] Create a study calendar that ensures you complete content review and sufficient practice by Test Day!
- [ ] As you finish a chapter and the online practice for that chapter, check it off on the table of contents.
- [ ] Register to take the MCAT at **www.aamc.org/mcat.**
- [ ] Set aside time during your prep to make sure the rest of your application—personal statement, recommendations, and other materials—is ready to go!
- [ ] Take a moment to admire your completed checklist, then get back to the business of prepping for this exam!

PREFACE

And now it starts: your long, yet fruitful journey toward wearing a white coat. Proudly wearing that white coat, though, is hopefully only part of your motivation. You are reading this book because you want to be a healer.

If you're serious about going to medical school, then you are likely already familiar with the importance of the MCAT in medical school admissions. While the holistic review process puts additional weight on your experiences, extracurricular activities, and personal attributes, the fact remains: along with your GPA, your MCAT score remains one of the two most important components of your application portfolio—at least early in the admissions process. Each additional point you score on the MCAT pushes you in front of thousands of other students and makes you an even more attractive applicant. But the MCAT is not simply an obstacle to overcome; it is an opportunity to show schools that you will be a strong student and a future leader in medicine.

We at Kaplan take our jobs very seriously and aim to help students see success not only on the MCAT, but as future physicians. We work with our learning science experts to ensure that we're using the most up-to-date teaching techniques in our resources. Multiple members of our team hold advanced degrees in medicine or associated biomedical sciences, and are committed to the highest level of medical education. Kaplan has been working with the MCAT for over 50 years and our commitment to premed students is unflagging; in fact, Stanley Kaplan created this company when he had difficulty being accepted to medical school due to unfair quota systems that existed at the time.

We stand now at the beginning of a new era in medical education. As citizens of this 21st-century world of healthcare, we are charged with creating a patient-oriented, culturally competent, cost-conscious, universally available, technically advanced, and research-focused healthcare system, run by compassionate providers. Suffice it to say, this is no easy task. Problem-based learning, integrated curricula, and classes in interpersonal skills are some of the responses to this demand for an excellent workforce—a workforce of which you'll soon be a part.

We're thrilled that you've chosen us to help you on this journey. Please reach out to us to share your challenges, concerns, and successes. Together, we will shape the future of medicine in the United States and abroad; we look forward to helping you become the doctor you deserve to be.

Good luck!

Alexander Stone Macnow, MD
Editor-in-Chief
Department of Pathology and Laboratory Medicine
Hospital of the University of Pennsylvania

BA, Musicology—Boston University, 2008
MD—Perelman School of Medicine at the University of Pennsylvania, 2013

ABOUT THE MCAT

Anatomy of the MCAT

Here is a general overview of the structure of Test Day:

Section	Number of Questions	Time Allotted
Test-Day Certification		4 minutes
Tutorial (optional)		10 minutes
Chemical and Physical Foundations of Biological Systems	59	95 minutes
Break (optional)		10 minutes
Critical Analysis and Reasoning Skills (CARS)	53	90 minutes
Lunch Break (optional)		30 minutes
Biological and Biochemical Foundations of Living Systems	59	95 minutes
Break (optional)		10 minutes
Psychological, Social, and Biological Foundations of Behavior	59	95 minutes
Void Question		3 minutes
Satisfaction Survey (optional)		5 minutes

The structure of the four sections of the MCAT is shown below.

Chemical and Physical Foundations of Biological Systems	
Time	95 minutes
Format	• *59 questions* • *10 passages* • *44 questions are passage-based, and 15 are discrete (stand-alone) questions.* • *Score between 118 and 132*
What It Tests	• *Biochemistry: 25%* • *Biology: 5%* • *General Chemistry: 30%* • *Organic Chemistry: 15%* • *Physics: 25%*

Critical Analysis and Reasoning Skills (CARS)	
Time	90 minutes
Format	• *53 questions* • *9 passages* • *All questions are passage-based. There are no discrete (stand-alone) questions.* • *Score between 118 and 132*
What It Tests	Disciplines: • *Humanities: 50%* • *Social Sciences: 50%* Skills: • *Foundations of Comprehension: 30%* • *Reasoning Within the Text: 30%* • *Reasoning Beyond the Text: 40%*
Biological and Biochemical Foundations of Living Systems	
Time	95 minutes
Format	• *59 questions* • *10 passages* • *44 questions are passage-based, and 15 are discrete (stand-alone) questions.* • *Score between 118 and 132*
What It Tests	• *Biochemistry: 25%* • *Biology: 65%* • *General Chemistry: 5%* • *Organic Chemistry: 5%*
Psychological, Social, and Biological Foundations of Behavior	
Time	95 minutes
Format	• *59 questions* • *10 passages* • *44 questions are passage-based, and 15 are discrete (stand-alone) questions.* • *Score between 118 and 132*
What It Tests	• *Biology: 5%* • *Psychology: 65%* • *Sociology: 30%*
Total	
Testing Time	375 minutes (6 hours, 15 minutes)
Total Seat Time	447 minutes (7 hours, 27 minutes)
Questions	230
Score	472 to 528

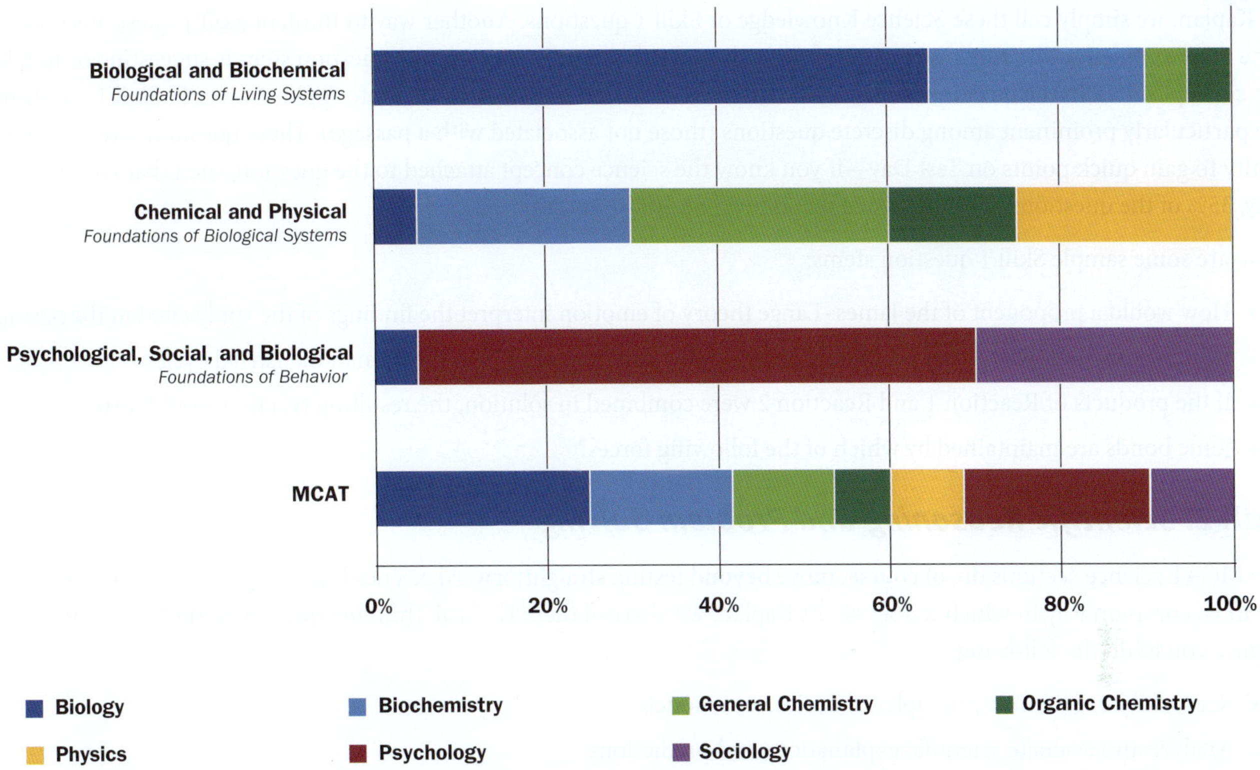

Scientific Inquiry and Reasoning Skills (SIRS)

The AAMC has defined four *Scientific Inquiry and Reasoning Skills* (SIRS) that will be tested in the three science sections of the MCAT:

1. *Knowledge of Scientific Concepts and Principles* (35% of questions)
2. *Scientific Reasoning and Problem-Solving* (45% of questions)
3. *Reasoning About the Design and Execution of Research* (10% of questions)
4. *Data-Based and Statistical Reasoning* (10% of questions)

Let's see how each one breaks down into more specific Test Day behaviors. Note that the bullet points of specific objectives for each of the SIRS are taken directly from the *Official Guide to the MCAT Exam*; the descriptions of what these behaviors mean and sample question stems, however, are written by Kaplan.

Skill 1: *Knowledge of Scientific Concepts and Principles*

This is probably the least surprising of the four SIRS; the testing of science knowledge is, after all, one of the signature qualities of the MCAT. Skill 1 questions will require you to do the following:

- Recognize correct scientific principles
- Identify the relationships among closely related concepts
- Identify the relationships between different representations of concepts (verbal, symbolic, graphic)
- Identify examples of observations that illustrate scientific principles
- Use mathematical equations to solve problems

At Kaplan, we simply call these Science Knowledge or Skill 1 questions. Another way to think of Skill 1 questions is as "one-step" problems. The single step is either to realize which scientific concept the question stem is suggesting or to take the concept stated in the question stem and identify which answer choice is an accurate application of it. Skill 1 questions are particularly prominent among discrete questions (those not associated with a passage). These questions are an opportunity to gain quick points on Test Day—if you know the science concept attached to the question, then that's it! On Test Day, 35% of the questions in each science section will be Skill 1 questions.

Here are some sample Skill 1 question stems:

- How would a proponent of the James–Lange theory of emotion interpret the findings of the study cited in the passage?
- Which of the following most accurately describes the function of FSH in the human menstrual cycle?
- If the products of Reaction 1 and Reaction 2 were combined in solution, the resulting reaction would form:
- Ionic bonds are maintained by which of the following forces?

Skill 2: *Scientific Reasoning and Problem-Solving*

The MCAT science sections do, of course, move beyond testing straightforward science knowledge; Skill 2 questions are the most common way in which it does so. At Kaplan, we also call these Critical Thinking questions. Skill 2 questions will require you to do the following:

- Reason about scientific principles, theories, and models
- Analyze and evaluate scientific explanations and predictions
- Evaluate arguments about causes and consequences
- Bring together theory, observations, and evidence to draw conclusions
- Recognize scientific findings that challenge or invalidate a scientific theory or model
- Determine and use scientific formulas to solve problems

Just as Skill 1 questions can be thought of as "one-step" problems, many Skill 2 questions are "two-step" problems, and more difficult Skill 2 questions may require three or more steps. These questions can require a wide spectrum of reasoning skills, including integration of multiple facts from a passage, combination of multiple science content areas, and prediction of an experiment's results. Skill 2 questions also tend to ask about science content without actually mentioning it by name. For example, a question might describe the results of one experiment and ask you to predict the results of a second experiment without actually telling you what underlying scientific principles are at work—part of the question's difficulty will be figuring out which principles to apply in order to get the correct answer. On Test Day, 45% of the questions in each science section will be Skill 2 questions.

Here are some sample Skill 2 question stems:

- Which of the following experimental conditions would most likely yield results similar to those in Figure 2?
- All of the following conclusions are supported by the information in the passage EXCEPT:
- The most likely cause of the anomalous results found by the experimenter is:
- An impact to a person's chest quickly reduces the volume of one of the lungs to 70% of its initial value while not allowing any air to escape from the mouth. By what percentage is the force of outward air pressure increased on a 2 cm^2 portion of the inner surface of the compressed lung?

Skill 3: *Reasoning About the Design and Execution of Research*

The MCAT is interested in your ability to critically appraise and analyze research, as this is an important day-to-day task of a physician. We call these questions Skill 3 or Experimental and Research Design questions for short. Skill 3 questions will require you to do the following:

- Identify the role of theory, past findings, and observations in scientific questioning
- Identify testable research questions and hypotheses
- Distinguish between samples and populations and distinguish results that support generalizations about populations
- Identify independent and dependent variables
- Reason about the features of research studies that suggest associations between variables or causal relationships between them (such as temporality and random assignment)
- Identify conclusions that are supported by research results
- Determine the implications of results for real-world situations
- Reason about ethical issues in scientific research

Over the years, the AAMC has received input from medical schools to require more practical research skills of MCAT test takers, and Skill 3 questions are the response to these demands. This skill is unique in that the outside knowledge you need to answer Skill 3 questions is not taught in any one undergraduate course; instead, the research design principles needed to answer these questions are learned gradually throughout your science classes and especially through any laboratory work you have completed. It should be noted that Skill 3 comprises 10% of the questions in each science section on Test Day.

Here are some sample Skill 3 question stems:

- What is the dependent variable in the study described in the passage?
- The major flaw in the method used to measure disease susceptibility in Experiment 1 is:
- Which of the following procedures is most important for the experimenters to follow in order for their study to maintain a proper, randomized sample of research subjects?
- A researcher would like to test the hypothesis that individuals who move to an urban area during adulthood are more likely to own a car than are those who have lived in an urban area since birth. Which of the following studies would best test this hypothesis?

Skill 4: *Data-Based and Statistical Reasoning*

Lastly, the science sections of the MCAT test your ability to analyze the visual and numerical results of experiments and studies. We call these Data and Statistical Analysis questions. Skill 4 questions will require you to do the following:

- Use, analyze, and interpret data in figures, graphs, and tables
- Evaluate whether representations make sense for particular scientific observations and data
- Use measures of central tendency (mean, median, and mode) and measures of dispersion (range, interquartile range, and standard deviation) to describe data
- Reason about random and systematic error

- Reason about statistical significance and uncertainty (interpreting statistical significance levels and interpreting a confidence interval)
- Use data to explain relationships between variables or make predictions
- Use data to answer research questions and draw conclusions

Skill 4 is included in the MCAT because physicians and researchers spend much of their time examining the results of their own studies and the studies of others, and it's very important for them to make legitimate conclusions and sound judgments based on that data. The MCAT tests Skill 4 on all three science sections with graphical representations of data (charts and bar graphs), as well as numerical ones (tables, lists, and results summarized in sentence or paragraph form). On Test Day, 10% of the questions in each science section will be Skill 4 questions.

Here are some sample Skill 4 question stems:

- According to the information in the passage, there is an inverse correlation between:
- What conclusion is best supported by the findings displayed in Figure 2?
- A medical test for a rare type of heavy metal poisoning returns a positive result for 98% of affected individuals and 13% of unaffected individuals. Which of the following types of error is most prevalent in this test?
- If a fourth trial of Experiment 1 was run and yielded a result of 54% compliance, which of the following would be true?

SIRS Summary

Discussing the SIRS tested on the MCAT is a daunting prospect given that the very nature of the skills tends to make the conversation rather abstract. Nevertheless, with enough practice, you'll be able to identify each of the four skills quickly, and you'll also be able to apply the proper strategies to solve those problems on Test Day. If you need a quick reference to remind you of the four SIRS, these guidelines may help:

Skill 1 (**Science Knowledge**) questions ask:

- Do you remember this science content?

Skill 2 (**Critical Thinking**) questions ask:

- Do you remember this science content? And if you do, could you please apply it to this novel situation?
- Could you answer this question that cleverly combines multiple content areas at the same time?

Skill 3 (**Experimental and Research Design**) questions ask:

- Let's forget about the science content for a while. Could you give some insight into the experimental or research methods involved in this situation?

Skill 4 (**Data and Statistical Analysis**) questions ask:

- Let's forget about the science content for a while. Could you accurately read some graphs and tables for a moment? Could you make some conclusions or extrapolations based on the information presented?

Critical Analysis and Reasoning Skills (CARS)

The *Critical Analysis and Reasoning Skills* (CARS) section of the MCAT tests three discrete families of textual reasoning skills; each of these families requires a higher level of reasoning than the last. Those three skills are as follows:

1. *Foundations of Comprehension* (30% of questions)
2. *Reasoning Within the Text* (30% of questions)
3. *Reasoning Beyond the Text* (40% of questions)

These three categories of skills are tested through nine humanities- and social sciences-themed passages, with approximately 5 to 7 questions per passage. Let's take a more in-depth look into these three types. Again, the bullet points of specific objectives for each of the CARS are taken directly from the *Official Guide to the MCAT Exam*; the descriptions of what these behaviors mean and sample question stems, however, are written by Kaplan.

Foundations of Comprehension

Questions in this category will ask for basic facts and simple inferences about the passage; the questions themselves will be similar to those seen on reading comprehension sections of other standardized exams like the SAT® and ACT®. *Foundations of Comprehension* questions will require you to do the following:

- Understand the basic components of the text
- Infer meaning from rhetorical devices, word choice, and text structure

This covers a wide range of question skills (Summarize Text, Recognize Opinion, Paraphrase Detail, and Interpret Meaning), but finding the correct answer to all *Foundations of Comprehension* questions will follow from a basic understanding of the passage and the point of view of its author (and occasionally that of other voices in the passage). Because these questions tend to avoid digging too deeply into the passage, Kaplan calls these *surface* questions.

Here are some sample *Foundations of Comprehension* question stems:

- **Summarize Text**—The author's primary thesis in this passage is:
- **Recognize Opinion**—Based on the information in the second paragraph, which of the following is the most accurate summary of the opinion held by Schubert's critics?
- **Paraphrase Detail**—According to the passage, which of the following is FALSE about literary reviews in the 1920s?
- **Interpret Meaning**—The word "obscure" (paragraph 3), when used in reference to the historian's actions, most nearly means:

Reasoning Within the Text

While *Foundations of Comprehension* questions will usually depend on interpreting a single piece of information in the passage or understanding the passage as a whole, *Reasoning Within the Text* questions require more thought because they will ask you to identify the purpose of a particular piece of information in the context of the passage, or ask how one piece of information relates to another. *Reasoning Within the Text* questions will require you to:

- Integrate different components of the text to draw relevant conclusions

In other words, questions in this type often ask either *How do these two details relate to one another?* or *What else must be true that the author didn't say?* The CARS section will also ask you to judge certain parts of the passage or even judge the author. These questions, which fall under the *Reasoning Within the Text* skill, can ask you to identify authorial bias, evaluate the credibility of cited sources, determine the logical soundness of an argument, identify the importance of a particular fact or statement in the context of the passage, or search for relevant evidence in the passage to support a given conclusion. This category, which Kaplan refers to as *deep* questions because of their tendency to venture into the deep reasoning of the passage, encompasses the following skills: Describe Purpose, Evaluate Reasoning, and Make Deduction.

Here are some sample *Reasoning Within the Text* question stems:

- **Describe Purpose**—The author's discussion of the effect of socioeconomic status on social mobility primarily serves which of the following functions?
- **Evaluate Reasoning**—Which of the following facts is used in the passage as the most prominent piece of evidence in favor of the author's conclusions?
- **Make Deduction**—In putting together the argument in the passage, the author most likely assumes:

Reasoning Beyond the Text

The distinguishing factor of *Reasoning Beyond the Text* questions is in the title of the category: the word *Beyond*. Questions of this type, which make up a larger share of the CARS section than questions from either of the other two types, will always introduce a completely new situation that was not present in the passage itself; these questions will ask you to determine how one influences the other. *Reasoning Beyond the Text* questions will require you to:

- Apply or extrapolate ideas from the passage to new contexts
- Assess the impact of introducing new factors, information, or conditions to ideas from the passage

Because they always introduce ideas not discussed in the passage, Kaplan refers to these as *new info* questions. They test the following skills: Anticipate Response, Predict Outcome/Explanation, Imagine Example/Analogy, and Strengthen/Weaken Argument.

Here are some sample *Reasoning Beyond the Text* question stems:

- **Anticipate Response**—If a document were located that demonstrated Berlioz intended to include a chorus of at least 700 in his *Grande Messe des Morts*, how would the author likely respond?
- **Imagine Example/Analogy**—Which of the following is the best example of a "virtuous rebellion," as it is defined in the passage?
- **Predict Outcome/Explanation**—Extending the author's discussion of ancient Greek history, a conflict between a democracy and an oligarchy would most likely result in:
- **Strengthen/Weaken Argument**—Which of the following sentences, if added to the end of the passage, would most WEAKEN the author's conclusions in the last paragraph?

CARS Summary

Through the *Foundations of Comprehension* category of skills, the CARS section tests many of the reading skills you have been building on since grade school, albeit in the context of very challenging doctorate-level passages. But through the two other categories (*Reasoning Within the Text* and *Reasoning Beyond the Text*), the MCAT demands that you understand the deep structure of passages and the arguments within them at an advanced level. And, of course, all of this is tested under very tight timing restrictions: only 102 seconds per question—and that doesn't even include the time spent reading the passages.

Here's a quick reference guide to the three categories and 11 skills tested in CARS:

Foundations of Comprehension skills:

- Interpret Meaning: Use context to determine what a word/phrase from the passage is intended to communicate.
- Recognize Opinion: Identify what the author or someone else feels about a passage idea based on word choice or other context clues.
- Paraphrase Detail: Recognize a specific piece of information that is stated or strongly implied at one location in the passage.
- Summarize Text: Articulate the main idea of the passage or of a part of it.

Reasoning Within the Text skills:

- Describe Purpose: Identify why the author wrote the passage or a part of it.
- Evaluate Reasoning: Characterize logical connections between ideas in the passage.
- Make Deduction: Infer a claim that follows from multiple parts of the passage, such as an assumption in an argument.

Reasoning Beyond the Text skills:

- Anticipate Response: Identify what the author or someone else would feel/say/do about a new situation based on its similarities to passage ideas.
- Predict Outcome/Explanation: Apply causal reasoning or another connection from the passage to a new situation.
- Strengthen/Weaken Argument: Characterize the logical relationship between a new claim and arguments from the passage.
- Imagine Example/Analogy: Identify new examples of categories defined in the passage or analogies of passage concepts.

Scoring

Each of the four sections of the MCAT is scored between 118 and 132, with the median at approximately 125. This means the total score ranges from 472 to 528, with the median at about 500. Why such peculiar numbers? The AAMC stresses that this scale emphasizes the importance of the central portion of the score distribution, where most students score (around 125 per section, or 500 total), rather than putting undue focus on the high end of the scale.

Note that there is no wrong answer penalty on the MCAT, so you should select an answer for every question—even if it is only a guess.

The AAMC has released the 2022–2024 correlation between scaled score and percentile, as shown on the following page. It should be noted that the percentile scale is adjusted and renormalized over time and thus can shift slightly from year to year. Percentile rank updates are released by the AAMC around May 1 of each year.

Total Score	Percentile	Total Score	Percentile
528	100	499	46
527	100	498	42
526	100	497	39
525	100	496	36
524	100	495	34
523	99	494	31
522	99	493	28
521	98	492	25
520	97	491	23
519	96	490	21
518	95	489	18
517	94	488	16
516	92	487	14
515	91	486	12
514	89	485	11
513	87	484	9
512	84	483	8
511	82	482	6
510	79	481	5
509	77	480	4
508	74	479	3
507	71	478	2
506	68	477	2
505	65	476	1
504	62	475	1
503	58	474	<1
502	55	473	<1
501	52	472	<1
500	49		

Source: AAMC. 2025. *Summary of MCAT Total and Section Scores.* Accessed October 2025. **https://students-residents.aamc.org/mcat-research-and-data/percentile-ranks-mcat-exam**

Further information on score reporting is included at the end of the next section (see *After Your Test*).

MCAT Policies and Procedures

We strongly encourage you to download the latest copy of *MCAT® Essentials*, available on the AAMC's website, to ensure that you have the latest information about registration and Test Day policies and procedures; this document is updated annually. A brief summary of some of the most important rules is provided here.

MCAT Registration

The only way to register for the MCAT is online. You can access AAMC's registration system at **www.aamc.org/mcat**.

The AAMC posts the schedule of testing, registration, and score release dates in the fall before the MCAT testing year, which runs from January into September. See the AAMC's website for the exact dates that registration opens each year. There is one standard registration fee, but the fee for changing your test date or test center increases the closer you get to your MCAT.

Fees and the Fee Assistance Program (FAP)

Payment for test registration must be made by American Express, Discover, MasterCard, or VISA. As described earlier, the fee for rescheduling your exam or changing your testing center increases as one approaches Test Day. In addition, it is not uncommon for test centers to fill up well in advance of the registration deadline. For these reasons, we recommend identifying your preferred Test Day as soon as possible and registering. There are ancillary benefits to having a set Test Day, as well: when you know the date you're working toward, you'll study harder and are less likely to keep pushing back the exam. The AAMC offers a Fee Assistance Program (FAP) for students with financial hardship to help reduce the cost of taking the MCAT, as well as for the American Medical College Application Service (AMCAS®) application. Further information on the FAP can be found at **www.aamc.org/students/applying/fap**.

Testing Security

On Test Day, you will be required to present a qualifying form of ID. Generally, a current driver's license or United States passport will be sufficient (consult the AAMC website for the full list of qualifying criteria). When registering, take care to spell your first and last names (middle names, suffixes, and prefixes are not required and will not be verified on Test Day) precisely the same as they appear on this ID; failure to provide this ID at the test center or differences in spelling between your registration and ID will be considered a "no-show," and you will not receive a refund for the exam.

During Test Day registration, other identity data collected may include: a digital palm vein scan, a Test Day photo, a digitization of your valid ID, and signatures. Some testing centers may use a metal detection wand to ensure that no prohibited items are brought into the testing room. Prohibited items include all electronic devices, including watches and timers, calculators, cell phones, and any and all forms of recording equipment; food, drinks (including water), and cigarettes or other smoking paraphernalia; hats and scarves (except for religious purposes); and books, notes, or other study materials. If you require a medical device, such as an insulin pump or pacemaker, you must apply for accommodated testing. During breaks, you are allowed access to food and drink, but not to electronic devices, including cell phones.

Testing centers are under video surveillance and the AAMC does not take potential violations of testing security lightly. The bottom line: *know the rules and don't break them.*

Accommodations

Students with disabilities or medical conditions can apply for accommodated testing. Documentation of the disability or condition is required, and requests may take two months—or more—to be approved. For this reason, it is recommended that you begin the process of applying for accommodated testing as early as possible. More information on applying for accommodated testing can be found at **www.aamc.org/students/applying/mcat/accommodations**.

After Your Test

When your MCAT is all over, no matter how you feel you did, be good to yourself when you leave the test center. Celebrate! Take a nap. Watch a movie. Get some exercise. Plan a trip or outing. Call up all of your neglected friends or message them on social media. Go out for snacks or drinks with people you like. Whatever you do, make sure that it has absolutely nothing to do with thinking too hard—you deserve some rest and relaxation.

Perhaps most importantly, do not discuss specific details about the test with anyone. For one, it is important to let go of the stress of Test Day, and reliving your exam only inhibits you from being able to do so. But more significantly, the Examinee Agreement you sign at the beginning of your exam specifically prohibits you from discussing or disclosing exam content. The AAMC is known to seek out individuals who violate this agreement and retains the right to prosecute these individuals at their discretion. This means that you should not, under any circumstances, discuss the exam in person or over the phone with other individuals—including us at Kaplan—or post information or questions about exam content to Facebook, Student Doctor Network, or other online social media. You are permitted to comment on your "general exam experience," including how you felt about the exam overall or an individual section, but this is a fine line. In summary: *if you're not certain whether you can discuss an aspect of the test or not, just don't do it!* Do not let a silly Facebook post stop you from becoming the doctor you deserve to be.

Scores are typically released approximately one month after Test Day. The release is staggered during the afternoon and evening, ending at 5 p.m. Eastern Standard Time. This means that not all examinees receive their scores at exactly the same time. Your score report will include a scaled score for each section between 118 and 132, as well as your total combined score between 472 and 528. These scores are given as confidence intervals. For each section, the confidence interval is approximately the given score ± 1; for the total score, it is approximately the given score ± 2. You will also be given the corresponding percentile rank for each of these section scores and the total score.

AAMC Contact Information

For further questions, contact the MCAT team at the Association of American Medical Colleges:

MCAT Resource Center
Association of American Medical Colleges
www.aamc.org/mcat
(202) 828-0600
www.aamc.org/contactmcat

HOW THIS BOOK WAS CREATED

The *Kaplan MCAT Review* project began shortly after the release of the *Preview Guide for the MCAT 2015 Exam*, 2nd edition. Through thorough analysis by our staff psychometricians, we were able to analyze the relative yield of the different topics on the MCAT, and we began constructing tables of contents for the books of the *Kaplan MCAT Review* series. A dedicated staff of 30 writers, 7 editors, and 32 proofreaders worked over 5,000 combined hours to produce these books. The format of the books was heavily influenced by weekly meetings with Kaplan's learning-science team.

In the years since this book was created, a number of opportunities for expansion and improvement have occurred. This edition is the product of our largest revision since the series' creation more than a decade ago.

To better accommodate students who prefer learning visually, our six science titles have added more than 500 new images and updated more than a hundred existing figures. All of these new images were chosen by an expert team of MCAT faculty members, led by veteran teachers and tutors with advanced science or medical degrees. Our objective with these new images was not to add visual flair but to enhance student learning outcomes. Toward that end, our team of medical illustrators partnered with our MCAT experts to ensure scientific accuracy and relevance for the exam.

On top of this extensive science image expansion, we completely rewrote *Critical Analysis and Reasoning Skills Review* based on what we've learned from more than ten years of helping students improve on the CARS section in our classrooms. In addition to this collective experience, internal data suggests that our new approach is more effective at helping students get higher CARS scores. Our streamlined and simplified CARS strategies accompany an extended focus on the critical thinking skills tested on the exam, best embodied by our new Skillbuilder activities that enable targeted skill practice in a lower pressure setting.

These books were submitted for publication in January 2026. For any updates after this date, please visit www.kaptest.com/retail-book-corrections-and-updates.

If you have any questions about the content presented here, email KaplanMCATfeedback@kaplan.com. For other questions not related to content, email booksupport@kaplan.com.

Each book has been vetted through at least ten rounds of review. To that end, the information presented in these books is true and accurate to the best of our knowledge. Still, your feedback helps us improve our prep materials. Please notify us of any inaccuracies or errors in the books by sending an email to KaplanMCATfeedback@kaplan.com.

USING THIS BOOK

Kaplan MCAT General Chemistry Review, and the other six books in the *Kaplan MCAT Review* series, bring the Kaplan classroom experience to you—right in your home, at your convenience. This book offers the same Kaplan content review, strategies, and practice that make Kaplan the #1 choice for MCAT prep.

This book is designed to help you review the general chemistry topics covered on the MCAT. Please understand that content review—no matter how thorough—is not sufficient preparation for the MCAT! The MCAT tests not only your science knowledge but also your critical reading, reasoning, and problem-solving skills. Do not assume that simply memorizing the contents of this book will earn you high scores on Test Day; to maximize your scores, you must also improve your reading and test-taking skills through MCAT-style questions and practice tests.

Learning Objectives

At the beginning of each section, you'll find a short list of objectives describing the skills covered within that section. Learning objectives for these texts were developed in conjunction with Kaplan's learning science team, and have been designed specifically to focus your attention on tasks and concepts that are likely to show up on your MCAT. These learning objectives will function as a means to guide your study, and indicate what information and relationships you should be focused on within each section. Before starting each section, read these learning objectives carefully. They will not only allow you to assess your existing familiarity with the content, but also provide a goal-oriented focus for your studying experience of the section.

MCAT Concept Checks

At the end of each section, you'll find a few open-ended questions that you can use to assess your mastery of the material. These MCAT Concept Checks were introduced after numerous conversations with Kaplan's learning science team. Research has demonstrated repeatedly that introspection and self-analysis improve mastery, retention, and recall of material. Complete these MCAT Concept Checks to ensure that you've got the key points from each section before moving on!

Science Mastery Assessments

At the beginning of each chapter, you'll find 15 concept-focused multiple-choice questions. These are designed to help you assess your understanding of the chapter before you begin reading the chapter. Using the guidance provided with the assessment, you can determine the best way to review each chapter based on your personal strengths and weaknesses. Most of the questions in the Science Mastery Assessments focus on the first of the *Scientific Inquiry and Reasoning Skills* (*Knowledge of Scientific Concepts and Principles*), although there are occasional questions that fall into the second or fourth SIRS *Scientific Reasoning and Problem-Solving* and *Data-Based and Statistical Reasoning*, respectively). You can complete each chapter's assessment in a testing interface in your online resources, where you'll also find a test-like passage set covering the same content you just studied to ensure you can also apply your knowledge the way the MCAT will expect you to!

Sidebars

The following is a guide to the five types of sidebars you'll find in *Kaplan MCAT General Chemistry Review:*

- **Bridge:** These sidebars create connections between science topics that appear in multiple chapters throughout the *Kaplan MCAT Review* series.
- **Key Concept:** These sidebars draw attention to the most important takeaways in a given topic, and they sometimes offer synopses or overviews of complex information. If you understand nothing else, make sure you grasp the Key Concepts for any given subject.
- **MCAT Expertise:** These sidebars point out how information may be tested on the MCAT or offer key strategy points and test-taking tips that you should apply on Test Day.
- **Mnemonic:** These sidebars present memory devices to help recall certain facts.
- **Real World:** These sidebars illustrate how a concept in the text relates to the practice of medicine or the world at large. While this is not information you need to know for Test Day, many of the topics in Real World sidebars are excellent examples of how a concept may appear in a passage or discrete (stand-alone) question on the MCAT.

What This Book Covers

The information presented in the *Kaplan MCAT Review* series covers everything listed on the official MCAT content lists. Every topic in these lists is covered in the same level of detail as is common to the undergraduate and postbaccalaureate classes that are considered prerequisites for the MCAT. Note that your premedical classes may include topics not discussed in these books, or they may go into more depth than these books do. Additional exposure to science content is never a bad thing, but all of the content knowledge you are expected to have walking in on Test Day is covered in these books.

Chapter profiles, on the first page of each chapter, represent a holistic look at the content within the chapter, and will include a pie chart as well as text information. The pie chart analysis is based directly on data released by the AAMC, and will give a rough estimate of the importance of the chapter in relation to the book as a whole. Further, the text portion of the Chapter Profiles includes which AAMC content categories are covered within the chapter. These are referenced directly from the AAMC MCAT exam content listing, available on the testmaker's website.

You'll also see High-Yield badges scattered throughout the sections of this book:

In This Chapter

1.1 Amino Acids Found in Proteins High Yield

LEARNING OBJECTIVES

After Chapter 1.1, you will be able to:

These badges represent the top 100 topics most tested by the AAMC. In other words, according to the testmaker and all our experience with their resources, a High-Yield badge means more questions on Test Day.

This book also contains a thorough glossary and index for easy navigation of the text.

In the end, this is your book, so write in the margins, draw diagrams, highlight the key points—do whatever is necessary to help you get that higher score. We look forward to working with you as you achieve your dreams and become the doctor you deserve to be!

Studying with This Book

In addition to providing you with the best practice questions and test strategies, Kaplan's team of learning scientists are dedicated to researching and testing the best methods for getting the most out of your study time. Here are their top four tips for improving retention:

Review multiple topics in one study session. This may seem counterintuitive—we're used to practicing one skill at a time in order to improve each skill. But research shows that weaving topics together leads to increased learning. Beyond that consideration, the MCAT often includes more than one topic in a single question. Studying in an integrated manner is the most effective way to prepare for this test.

Customize the content. Drawing attention to difficult or critical content can ensure you don't overlook it as you read and re-read sections. The best way to do this is to make it more visual—highlight, make tabs, use stickies, whatever works. We recommend highlighting only the most important or difficult sections of text. Selective highlighting of up to about 10% of text in a given chapter is great for emphasizing parts of the text, but over-highlighting can have the opposite effect.

Repeat topics over time. Many people try to memorize concepts by repeating them over and over again in succession. Our research shows that retention is improved by spacing out the repeats over time and mixing up the order in which you study content. For example, try reading chapters in a different order the second (or third!) time around. Revisit practice questions that you answered incorrectly in a new sequence. Perhaps information you reviewed more recently will help you better understand those questions and solutions you struggled with in the past.

Take a moment to reflect. When you finish reading a section for the first time, stop and think about what you just read. Jot down a few thoughts in the margins or in your notes about why the content is important or what topics came to mind when you read it. Associating learning with a memory is a fantastic way to retain information! This also works when answering questions. After answering a question, take a moment to think through each step you took to arrive at a solution. What led you to the answer you chose? Understanding the steps you took will help you make good decisions when answering future questions.

Online Resources

In addition to the resources located within this text, you also have online resources awaiting you. If you purchased this book as part of a 7-book set, scan the QR code that appears on your slipcase (the illustrated box that originally contained the books) and enter your unique access code, which appears on a sticker on the front of that slipcase. If you purchased this book separately, book-specific resources are available at **www.kaptest.com/booksonline**. Make sure to log on and take advantage of free practice and other resources!

Please note that access to the online resources is limited to the original owner of this book.

STUDYING FOR THE MCAT

The first year of medical school is a frenzied experience for most students. To meet the requirements of a rigorous work schedule, students either learn to prioritize their time or else fall hopelessly behind. It's no surprise, then, that the MCAT, the test specifically designed to predict success in medical school, is a high-speed, time-intensive test. The MCAT demands excellent time-management skills, endurance, and grace under pressure both during the test as well as while preparing for it. Having a solid plan of attack and sticking with it are key to giving you the confidence and structure you need to succeed.

Creating a Study Plan

The best time to create a study plan is at the beginning of your MCAT preparation. If you don't already use a calendar, you will want to start. You can purchase a planner, print out a free calendar from the Internet, use a built-in calendar or app on one of your smart devices, or keep track using an interactive online calendar. Pick the option that is most practical for you and that you are most likely to use consistently. If you purchased this book new as part of a set, your online resources come with a study plan to space out your readings, chapter quizzes, full-length practice tests, and other study materials (see the previous page for how to log on).

Once you have a calendar, you'll be able to start planning your study schedule with the following steps:

1. **Fill in your obligations and choose a day off.**

   Write in all your school, extracurricular, and work obligations first: class sessions, work shifts, and meetings that you must attend. Then add in your personal obligations: appointments, lunch dates, family and social time, etc. Making an appointment in your calendar for hanging out with friends or going to the movies may seem strange at first, but planning social activities in advance will help you achieve a balance between personal and professional obligations even as life gets busy. Having a happy balance allows you to be more focused and productive when it comes time to study, so stay well-rounded and don't neglect anything that is important to you.

   In addition to scheduling your personal and professional obligations, you should also plan your time off. Taking some time off is just as important as studying. Kaplan recommends taking at least one full day off per week, ideally from all your study obligations but at minimum from studying for the MCAT.

2. **Add in study blocks around your obligations.**

   Once you have established your calendar's framework, add in study blocks around your obligations, keeping your study schedule as consistent as possible across days and across weeks. Studying at the same time of day as your official test is ideal for promoting recall, but if that's not possible, then fit in study blocks wherever you can.

   To make your studying as efficient as possible, block out short, frequent periods of study time throughout the week. From a learning perspective, studying one hour per day for six days per week is much more valuable than studying for six hours all at once one day per week. Specifically, Kaplan recommends studying for no longer than three hours in one sitting. Within those three-hour blocks, also plan to take ten-minute breaks every hour. Use these breaks to get up from your seat, do some quick stretches, get a snack and drink, and clear your mind. Although ten minutes of break for every 50 minutes of studying may sound like a lot, these breaks will allow you to deal with distractions and rest your brain so that, during the 50-minute study blocks, you can remain fully engaged and completely focused.

3. **Add in your full-length practice tests.**

   Next, you'll want to add in full-length practice tests. You'll want to take one test very early in your prep and then spread your remaining full-length practice tests evenly between now and your test date. Staggering tests in this way allows you to form a baseline for comparison and to determine which areas to focus on right away, while also providing realistic feedback throughout your prep as to how you will perform on Test Day.

When planning your calendar, aim to finish your full-length practice tests and the majority of your studying by one week before Test Day, which will allow you to spend that final week completing a brief review of what you already know. In your online resources, you'll find a sample study calendar to use as a starting point. This sample calendar may include more focus than you need in some areas, and less in others, and it may not fit your timeline to Test Day. You will need to customize your study calendar to your needs using the steps above.

The total amount of time you spend studying each week will depend on your schedule, your personal prep needs, and your time to Test Day, but it is recommended that you spend somewhere in the range of 300–350 hours preparing before taking the official MCAT. One way you could break this down is to study for three hours per day, six days per week, for four months, but this is just one approach. You might study six days per week for more than three hours per day. You might study over a longer period of time if you don't have much time to study each week. No matter what your plan is, ensure you complete enough practice to feel completely comfortable with the MCAT and its content. A good sign you're ready for Test Day is when you begin to earn your goal score consistently in practice.

How to Study

The MCAT covers a large amount of material, so studying for Test Day can initially seem daunting. To combat this, we have some tips for how to take control of your studying and make the most of your time.

Goal Setting

To take control of the amount of content and practice required to do well on the MCAT, break the content down into specific goals for each week instead of attempting to approach the test as a whole. A goal of "I want to increase my overall score by 5 points" is too big, abstract, and difficult to measure on the small scale. More reasonable goals are "I will read two chapters each day this week." Goals like this are much less overwhelming and help break studying into manageable pieces.

Active Reading

As you go through this book, much of the information will be familiar to you. After all, you have probably seen most of the content before. However, be very careful: Familiarity with a subject does not necessarily translate to knowledge or mastery of that subject. Do not assume that if you recognize a concept you actually know it and can apply it quickly at an appropriate level. Don't just passively read this book. Instead, read actively. Highlighting can be an excellent tool, but use it sparingly: highlighting every sentence isn't active reading, it's coloring. Frequently stop and ask yourself questions while you read (e.g., *What is the main point? How does this fit into the overall scheme of things? Could I thoroughly explain this to someone else?*). By making connections and focusing on the grander scheme, not only will you ensure you know the essential content, but you also prepare yourself for the level of critical thinking required by the MCAT.

Focus on Areas of Greatest Opportunity

If you are limited by only having a minimal amount of time to prepare before Test Day, focus on your biggest areas of opportunity first. Areas of opportunity are topic areas that are highly tested and that you have not yet mastered. You likely won't have time to take detailed notes for every page of these books; instead, use your results from practice materials to determine which areas are your biggest opportunities and seek those out. After you've taken a full-length test, make sure you are using your performance report to best identify areas of opportunity. Skim over content matter for which you are already demonstrating proficiency, pausing to read more thoroughly when something looks unfamiliar or particularly difficult. Begin with the Science Mastery Assessment at the beginning of each chapter. If you can get all of those questions correct within a reasonable amount of time, you may be able to quickly skim through that chapter, but if the questions prove to be more difficult, then you may need to spend time reading the chapter or certain subsections of the chapter more thoroughly.

Practice, Review, and Tracking

Leave time to review your practice questions and full-length tests. You may be tempted, after practicing, to push ahead and cover new material as quickly as possible, but failing to schedule ample time for review will actually throw away your greatest opportunity to improve your performance. The brain rarely remembers anything it sees or does only once. When you carefully review the questions you've solved (and the explanations for them), the process of retrieving that information reopens and reinforces the connections you've built in your brain. This builds long-term retention and repeatable skill sets—exactly what you need to beat the MCAT!

One useful tool for making the most of your review is the How I'll Fix It (HIFI) sheet. You can create a HIFI sheet, such as the sample below, to track questions throughout your prep that you miss or have to guess on. For each such question, figure out why you missed it and supply at least one action step for how you can avoid similar mistakes in the future. As you move through your MCAT prep, adjust your study plan based on your available study time and the results of your review. Your strengths and weaknesses are likely to change over the course of your prep. Keep addressing the areas that are most important to your score, shifting your focus as those areas change.

Section	Q #	Topic or skill	Why I missed it	How I'll fix it
Chem/Phys	*42*	*Nuclear chem.*	*Confused electron absorption and emission*	*Reread Physics Chapter 9.2*
Chem/Phys	*47*	K_{eq}	*Didn't know right equation*	*Memorize equation for* K_{eq}
CARS	*2*	*Paraphrase Detail*	*Didn't read "not" in answer choice*	*Slow down when finding match*
CARS	*4*	*Make Deduction*	*Forgot to research answer*	*Reread passage and predict first*

Where to Study

One often-overlooked aspect of studying is the environment where the learning actually occurs. Although studying at home is many students' first choice, several problems can arise in this environment, chief of which are distractions. Studying can be a mentally draining process, so as time passes, these distractions become ever more tempting as escape routes. Although you may have considerable willpower, there's no reason to make staying focused harder than it needs to be. Instead of studying at home, head to a library, quiet coffee shop, or another new location whenever possible. This will eliminate many of the usual distractions and also promote efficient studying; instead of studying off and on at home over the course of an entire day, you can stay at the library for three hours of effective studying and enjoy the rest of the day off from the MCAT.

No matter where you study, make your practice as much like Test Day as possible. Just as is required during the official test, don't have snacks or chew gum during your study blocks. Turn off your music, television, and phone. Practice on the computer with your online resources to simulate the computer-based test environment. When completing practice questions, do your work on scratch paper or noteboard sheets rather than writing directly on any printed materials since you won't have that option on Test Day. Because memory is tied to all of your senses, the more test-like you can make your studying environment, the easier it will be on Test Day to recall the information you're putting in so much work to learn.

CHAPTER 1

ATOMIC STRUCTURE

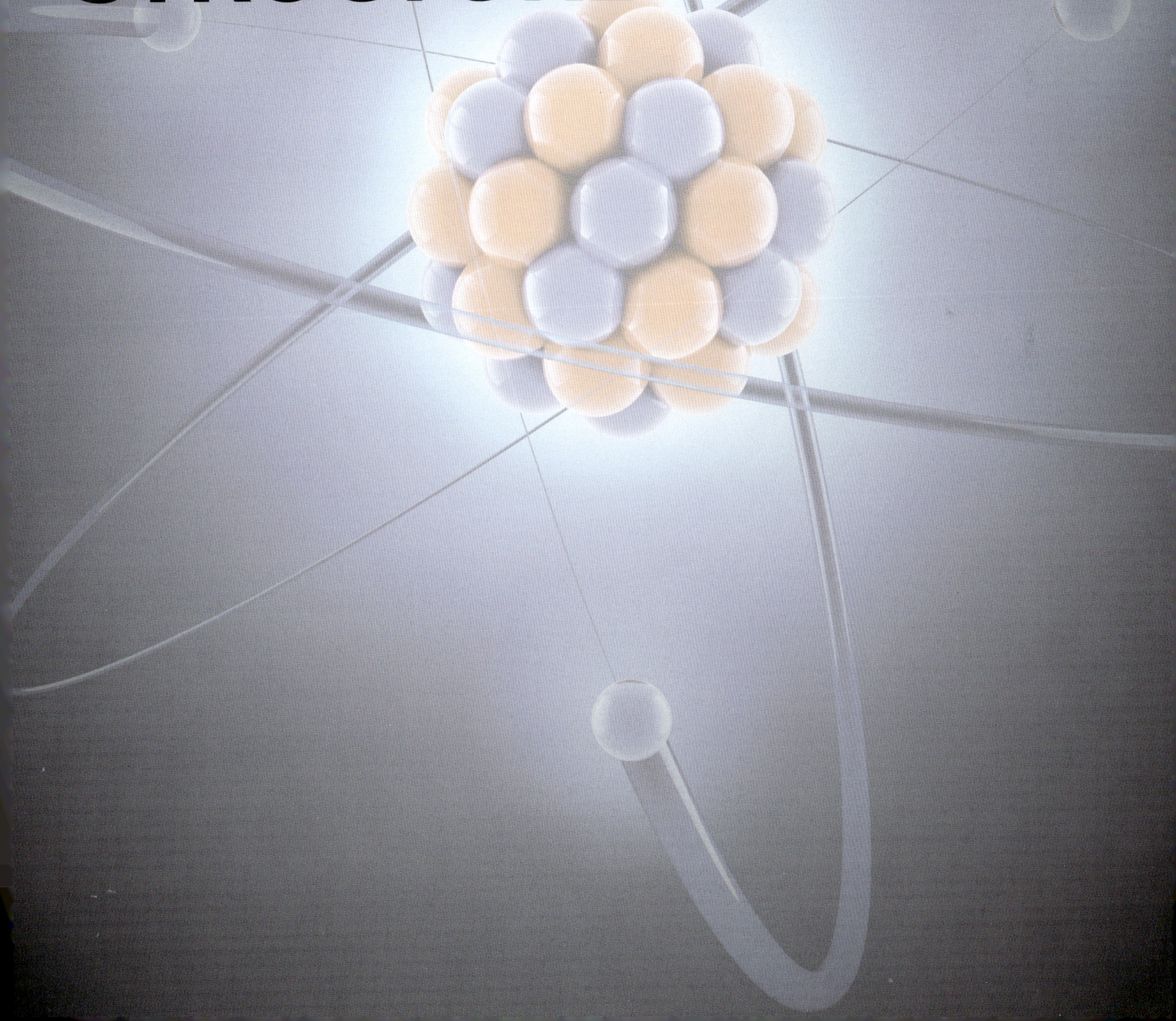

SCIENCE MASTERY ASSESSMENT

Every pre-med knows this feeling: there is so much content I have to know for the MCAT! How do I know what to do first or what's important?

While the high-yield badges throughout this book will help you identify the most important topics, this Science Mastery Assessment is another tool in your MCAT prep arsenal. This quiz (which can also be taken in your online resources) and the guidance below will help ensure that you are spending the appropriate amount of time on this chapter based on your personal strengths and weaknesses. Don't worry though—skipping something now does not mean you'll never study it. Later on in your prep, as you complete full-length tests, you'll uncover specific pieces of content that you need to review and can come back to these chapters as appropriate.

How to Use This Assessment

If you answer 0–7 questions correctly:

Spend about 1 hour to read this chapter in full and take limited notes throughout. Follow up by reviewing **all** quiz questions to ensure that you now understand how to solve each one.

If you answer 8–11 questions correctly:

Spend 20–40 minutes reviewing the quiz questions. Beginning with the questions you missed, read and take notes on the corresponding subchapters. For questions you answered correctly, ensure your thinking matches that of the explanation and you understand why each choice was correct or incorrect.

If you answer 12–15 questions correctly:

Spend less than 20 minutes reviewing all questions from the quiz. If you missed any, then include a quick read-through of the corresponding subchapters, or even just the relevant content within a subchapter, as part of your question review. For questions you answered correctly, ensure your thinking matches that of the explanation and review the Concept Summary at the end of the chapter.

1. Which of the following is the correct electron configuration for Zn^{2+}?
   - **A.** $1s^22s^22p^63s^23p^64s^03d^{10}$
   - **B.** $1s^22s^22p^63s^23p^64s^23d^8$
   - **C.** $1s^22s^22p^63s^23p^64s^23d^{10}$
   - **D.** $1s^22s^22p^63s^23p^64s^03d^8$

2. Which of the following quantum number sets is possible?
   - **A.** $n = 2; l = 2; m_l = 1; m_s = +\frac{1}{2}$
   - **B.** $n = 2; l = 1; m_l = -1; m_s = +\frac{1}{2}$
   - **C.** $n = 2; l = 0; m_l = -1; m_s = -\frac{1}{2}$
   - **D.** $n = 2; l = 0; m_l = 1; m_s = -\frac{1}{2}$

3. What is the maximum number of electrons allowed in a single atomic energy level in terms of the principal quantum number n ?
   - **A.** $2n$
   - **B.** $2n + 2$
   - **C.** $2n^2$
   - **D.** $2n^2 + 2$

4. Which of the following equations describes the maximum number of electrons that can fill a subshell?
   - **A.** $2l + 2$
   - **B.** $4l + 2$
   - **C.** $2l^2$
   - **D.** $2l^2 + 2$

5. Which of the following atoms only has paired electrons in its ground state?
   - **A.** Sodium
   - **B.** Iron
   - **C.** Cobalt
   - **D.** Helium

6. An electron returns from an excited state to its ground state, emitting a photon at $\lambda = 500$ nm. What would be the magnitude of the energy change if one mole of these photons were emitted? (Note: $h = 6.626 \times 10^{-34}$ J · s, $N_A = 6.02 \times 10^{23}$ mol^{-1})
   - **A.** 3.98×10^{-21} J
   - **B.** 3.98×10^{-19} J
   - **C.** 2.39×10^{3} J
   - **D.** 2.39×10^{5} J

7. Suppose an electron falls from $n = 4$ to its ground state, $n = 1$. Which of the following effects is most likely?
   - **A.** A photon is absorbed.
   - **B.** A photon is emitted.
   - **C.** The electron moves into a *p*-orbital.
   - **D.** The electron moves into a *d*-orbital.

8. Which of the following isotopes of carbon is LEAST likely to be found in nature?
   - **A.** ^{6}C
   - **B.** ^{12}C
   - **C.** ^{13}C
   - **D.** ^{14}C

9. Which of the following best explains the inability to measure position and momentum exactly and simultaneously according to the Heisenberg uncertainty principle?
   - **A.** Imprecision in the definition of the meter and kilogram
   - **B.** Limits on accuracy of existing scientific instruments
   - **C.** Error in one variable is increased by attempts to measure the other
   - **D.** Discrepancies between the masses of nuclei and of their component particles

10. Which of the following electronic transitions would result in the greatest gain in energy for a single hydrogen electron?

- **A.** An electron moves from $n = 6$ to $n = 2$.
- **B.** An electron moves from $n = 2$ to $n = 6$.
- **C.** An electron moves from $n = 3$ to $n = 4$.
- **D.** An electron moves from $n = 4$ to $n = 3$.

11. Suppose that an atom fills its orbitals as shown:

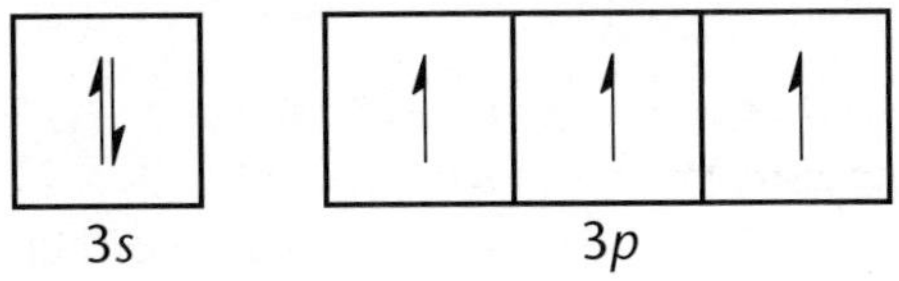

Such an electron configuration most clearly illustrates which of the following laws of atomic physics?

- **A.** Hund's rule
- **B.** Heisenberg uncertainty principle
- **C.** Bohr model
- **D.** Rutherford model

12. How many total electrons are in a ^{133}Cs cation?

- **A.** 54
- **B.** 55
- **C.** 78
- **D.** 132

13. The atomic weight of hydrogen is 1.008 amu. What is the percent composition of hydrogen by isotope, assuming that hydrogen's only isotopes are ^{1}H and ^{2}D?

- **A.** 92% H, 8% D
- **B.** 99.2% H, 0.8% D
- **C.** 99.92% H, 0.08% D
- **D.** 99.992% H, 0.008% D

14. Consider the two sets of quantum numbers shown in the table, which describe two different electrons in the same atom.

n	l	m_l	m_s
2	1	1	$+\frac{1}{2}$
3	1	−1	$+\frac{1}{2}$

Which of the following terms best describes these two electrons?

- **A.** Parallel
- **B.** Opposite
- **C.** Antiparallel
- **D.** Paired

15. Which of the following species is represented by the electron configuration $1s^22s^22p^63s^23p^64s^13d^5$?

I. Cr

II. Mn^+

III. Fe^{2+}

- **A.** I only
- **B.** I and II only
- **C.** II and III only
- **D.** I, II, and III

Answer Key

1. **A** (See section 1.1)
2. **B** (See section 1.4)
3. **C** (See section 1.4)
4. **B** (See section 1.4)
5. **D** (See section 1.4)
6. **D** (See section 1.3)
7. **B** (See section 1.1)
8. **A** (See section 1.2)
9. **C** (See section 1.4)
10. **B** (See section 1.3)
11. **A** (See section 1.3)
12. **A** (See section 1.1)
13. **B** (See section 1.2)
14. **A** (See section 1.4)
15. **B** (See section 1.1)

The relevant section of the chapter to review for each question is given in parentheses after the correct answer. Detailed explanations can be found at the end of the chapter.

CHAPTER 1

ATOMIC STRUCTURE

In This Chapter

CHAPTER PROFILE

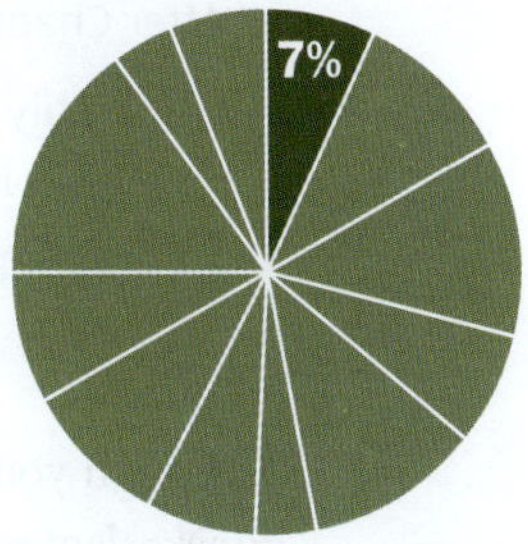

The content in this chapter should be relevant to about 7% of all questions about general chemistry on the MCAT.

This chapter covers material from the following AAMC content category:

4E: Atoms, nuclear decay, electronic structure, and atomic chemical behavior

Introduction

Chemistry is the investigation of the atoms and molecules that make up our bodies, our possessions, the food we eat, and the world around us. There are different branches of chemistry, three of which are tested directly on the MCAT: general (inorganic) chemistry, organic chemistry, and biochemistry. Ultimately, all investigations in chemistry are seeking to answer the questions that confront us in the form—the shape, structure, mode, and essence—of the physical world that surrounds us.

Many students feel similarly about general chemistry and physics: *But I'm premed,* they say. *Why do I need to know any of this? What good will this be when I'm a doctor? Do I only need to know this for the MCAT?* Recognize that to be an effective doctor, one must understand the physical building blocks that make up the human body. Pharmacologic treatment is based on chemistry; many diagnostic tests used every day detect changes in the chemistry of the body.

So, let's get down to the business of learning and remembering the principles of the physical world that help us understand what all this "stuff" is, how it works, and why it behaves the way it does—at both the molecular and macroscopic levels. In the process of reading through these chapters and applying your knowledge to practice questions, you'll prepare yourself for success not only on the *Chemical and Physical Foundations of Biological Systems* section of the MCAT but also in your future career as a physician.

This first chapter starts our review of general chemistry with a consideration of the fundamental unit of matter—the atom. First, we focus on the subatomic particles that make it up: protons, neutrons, and electrons. We will also review the Bohr and quantum mechanical models of the atom, with a particular focus on the similarities and differences between them.

MCAT EXPERTISE

The building blocks of the atom are also the building blocks of knowledge for the general chemistry concepts tested on the MCAT. By understanding these particles, we will be able to use that knowledge as the "nucleus" of understanding for all of general chemistry.

1.1 Subatomic Particles

LEARNING OBJECTIVES

After Chapter 1.1, you will be able to:

- Identify the subatomic particles most important for determining various traits of an atom, including charge, atomic number, and isotope
- Determine the number of protons, neutrons, and electrons within an isotope, such as ^{14}C

Although you may have encountered in your university-level chemistry classes such subatomic particles as *quarks*, *leptons*, and *gluons*, the MCAT's approach to atomic structure is much simpler. There are three subatomic particles that you must understand: protons, neutrons, and electrons.

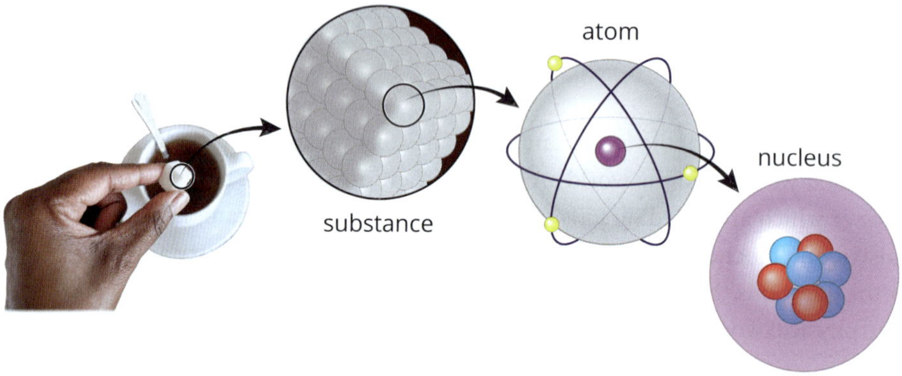

Figure 1.1 Matter: From Macroscopic to Microscopic

Protons

Protons are found in the **nucleus** of an atom, as shown in Figure 1.1. Each proton has an amount of charge equal to the fundamental unit of charge ($e = 1.6 \times 10^{-19}$ C), and we denote this fundamental unit of charge as "+1 *e*" or simply "+1" for the proton. Protons have a mass of approximately one **atomic mass unit** (**amu**). The **atomic number** (*Z*) of an element, as shown in Figure 1.2, is equal to the number of protons found in an atom of that element. As such, it acts as a unique identifier for each element because elements are defined by the number of protons they contain. For example, all atoms of oxygen contain eight protons; all atoms of gadolinium contain 64 protons. While all atoms of a given element have the same atomic number, they do not necessarily have the same mass—as we will see in our discussion of isotopes.

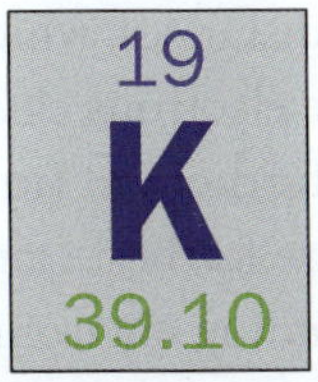

Figure 1.2 Potassium, from the Periodic Table
Potassium has the symbol K (Latin: kalium), atomic number 19, and atomic weight of approximately 39.1.

Neutrons

Neutrons, as the name implies, are neutral—they have no charge. A neutron's mass is only slightly larger than that of the proton, and together, the protons and the neutrons of the nucleus make up almost the entire mass of an atom. Every atom has a characteristic **mass number** (A), which is the sum of the protons and neutrons in the atom's nucleus. A given element can have a variable number of neutrons; thus, while atoms of the same element always have the same atomic number, they do not necessarily have the same mass number. Atoms that share an atomic number but have different mass numbers are known as **isotopes** of the element, as shown in Figure 1.3. For example, carbon ($Z = 6$) has three naturally occurring isotopes: ${}^{12}_{6}\text{C}$, with six protons and six neutrons; ${}^{13}_{6}\text{C}$, with six protons and seven neutrons; and ${}^{14}_{6}\text{C}$, with six protons and eight neutrons. The convention ${}^{A}_{Z}\text{X}$ is used to show both the atomic number (Z) and the mass number (A) of atom X.

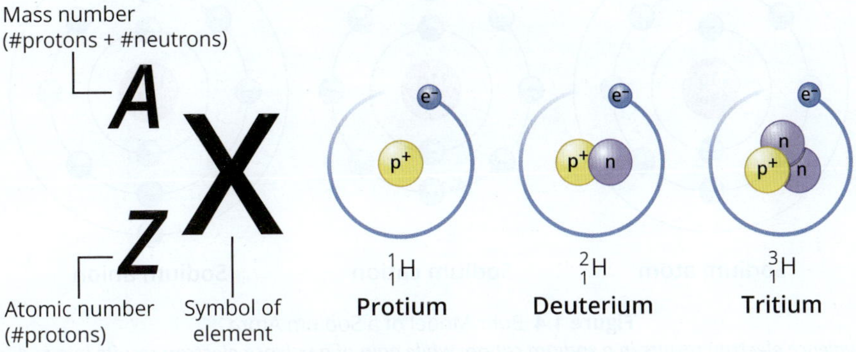

Figure 1.3 Isotopes of Hydrogen
Atoms of the same element have the same atomic number (Z = 1) but may have varying mass numbers (A = 1, 2, or 3).

Electrons

Electrons move through the space surrounding the nucleus and are associated with varying levels of energy. Each electron has a charge equal in magnitude to that of a proton, but with the opposite (negative) sign, denoted by "$-1\ e$" or simply "-1." The mass of an electron is approximately $\frac{1}{2000}$ that of a proton. Because subatomic particles' masses are so small, the electrostatic force of attraction between the unlike charges of the proton and electron is far greater than the gravitational force of attraction based on their respective masses.

Electrons move around the nucleus at varying distances, which correspond to varying levels of electrical potential energy. The electrons closer to the nucleus are at lower energy levels, while those that are further out (in higher **electron shells**) have higher energy. The electrons that are farthest from the nucleus have the strongest interactions with the surrounding environment and the weakest interactions with the nucleus. These electrons are called **valence electrons**; they are much more likely to become involved in bonds with other atoms because they experience the least electrostatic pull from their own nucleus. Generally speaking, the valence electrons determine the reactivity of an atom. As we will discuss in Chapter 3 of *MCAT General Chemistry Review*, the sharing or transferring of these valence electrons in bonds allows elements to fill their highest energy level to increase stability. In the neutral state, there are equal numbers of protons and electrons; losing electrons results in the atom gaining a positive charge, while gaining electrons results in the atom gaining a negative charge. Typically, only the valence electrons are lost (or gained) during ionization of atoms (shown with sodium in Figure 1.4) since they are least attracted to the nucleus. A positively charged atom is called a **cation**, and a negatively charged atom is called an **anion**.

BRIDGE

Valence electrons will be very important to us in both general and organic chemistry. Knowing how tightly held those electrons are will allow us to understand many of an atom's properties and how it interacts with other atoms, especially in bonding. Bonding is so important that it is discussed in Chapter 3 of both *MCAT General Chemistry Review* and *MCAT Organic Chemistry Review*.

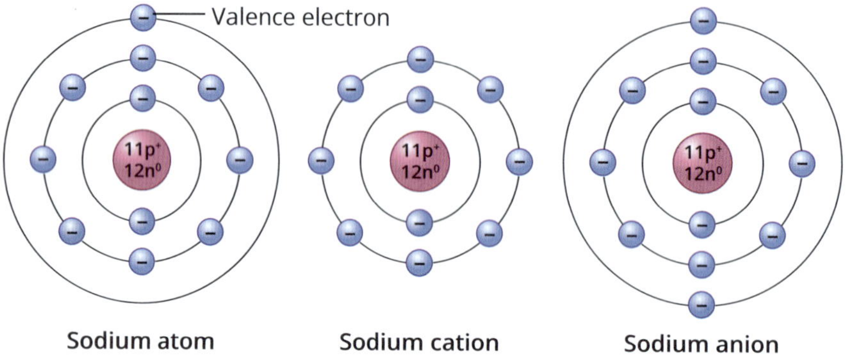

Figure 1.4 Bohr Model of a Sodium Atom
Loss of a valence electron results in a sodium cation, while gain of a valence electron results in a sodium anion. Sodium cations are far more common.

Some basic features of the three subatomic particles are shown in Table 1.1.

Subatomic Particle	Symbol	Relative Mass	Charge	Location
Proton	p, p^+, or ${}^1_1H$	1	+1	Nucleus
Neutron	n^0 or ${}^1_0n$	1	0	Nucleus
Electron	e^- or ${}^{\ 0}_{-1}e$	0	−1	Orbitals

Table 1.1 Subatomic Particles

Example: Determine the number of protons, neutrons, and electrons in a nickel-58 atom and in a nickel-60 +2 cation.

Solution: ^{58}Ni has an atomic number of 28 and a mass number of 58. Therefore, ^{58}Ni will have 28 protons, 28 electrons, and 58 – 28, or 30, neutrons.

$^{60}Ni^{2+}$ has the same number of protons as the neutral ^{58}Ni atom. However, $^{60}Ni^{2+}$ has a positive charge because it has lost two electrons; thus, Ni^{2+} will have 26 electrons. Also, the mass number is two units higher than for the ^{58}Ni atom, and this difference in mass must be due to two extra neutrons; thus, it has a total of 32 neutrons.

MCAT CONCEPT CHECK 1.1

Before you move on, assess your understanding of the material with these questions.

1. Which subatomic particle is the most important for determining each of the following properties of an atom?
   - Charge:

   ____

   - Atomic number:

   ____

   - Isotope:

   ____

2. In nuclear medicine, isotopes are created and used for various purposes; for instance, ^{18}O is created from ^{18}F. Determine the number of protons, neutrons, and electrons in each of these species.

Particle	Protons	Neutrons	Electrons
^{18}O			
^{18}F			

BRIDGE

Solutions to concept checks for a given chapter in *MCAT General Chemistry Review* can be found near the end of the chapter in which the concept check is located, following the Concept Summary for that chapter.

1.2 Atomic Mass vs. Atomic Weight

LEARNING OBJECTIVES

After Chapter 1.2, you will be able to:

- Describe atomic mass and atomic weight
- Recall the units of molar mass
- Predict the number of protons, neutrons, and electrons in a given isotope

There are a few different terms used by chemists to describe the heaviness of an element: atomic mass and mass number, which are essentially synonymous, and atomic weight. While the atomic weight is a constant for a given element and is reported in the periodic table, the atomic mass or mass number varies from one isotope to another. In this section, carefully compare and contrast the different definitions of these terms—because they are similar, they can be easy to mix up on the MCAT.

Atomic Mass

As we've seen, the mass of one proton is approximately one amu. The size of the atomic mass unit is defined as exactly $\frac{1}{12}$ the mass of the carbon-12 atom, approximately 1.66×10^{-24} g. Because the carbon-12 nucleus has six protons and six neutrons, an amu is approximately equal to the mass of a proton or a neutron. The difference in mass between protons and neutrons is extremely small; in fact, it is approximately equal to the mass of an electron.

The **atomic mass** of an atom (in amu) is nearly equal to its **mass number**, the sum of protons and neutrons (in reality, some mass is lost as binding energy, as discussed in Chapter 9 of *MCAT Physics and Math Review*). Atoms of the same element with varying mass numbers are called **isotopes** (from the Greek for "same place"). Isotopes differ in their number of neutrons and are referred to by the name of the element followed by the mass number; for example, carbon-12 or iodine-131. Only the three isotopes of hydrogen, shown in Figure 1.3, are given unique names: *protium* (Greek: "first") has one proton and an atomic mass of 1 amu; *deuterium* ("second") has one proton and one neutron and an atomic mass of 2 amu; *tritium* ("third") has one proton and two neutrons and an atomic mass of 3 amu. Because isotopes have the same number of protons and electrons, they generally exhibit similar chemical properties.

KEY CONCEPT

- Atomic number (Z) = number of protons
- Mass number (A) = number of protons + number of neutrons
- Number of protons = number of electrons (in a neutral atom)
- Electrons are not included in mass calculations because they are much smaller.

KEY CONCEPT

When an element has two or more isotopes, no one isotope will have a mass exactly equal to the element's atomic weight. Bromine, for example, is listed in the periodic table as having a mass of 79.9 amu. This is an average of the two naturally occurring isotopes, bromine-79 and bromine-81, which occur in almost equal proportions. There are no bromine atoms with an actual mass of 79.9 amu.

Atomic Weight

In nature, almost all elements exist as two or more isotopes, and these isotopes are usually present in the same proportions in any sample of a naturally occurring element. The weighted average of these different isotopes is referred to as the **atomic weight** and is the number reported on the periodic table. For example, chlorine has two main naturally occurring isotopes: chlorine-35 and chlorine-37. Chlorine-35 is about three times more abundant than chlorine-37; therefore, the atomic weight of chlorine is closer to 35 than 37. On the periodic table, it is listed as 35.5. Figure 1.5 illustrates the half-lives of the different isotopes of the elements; because half-life corresponds with stability, it also helps determine the relative proportions of these different isotopes.

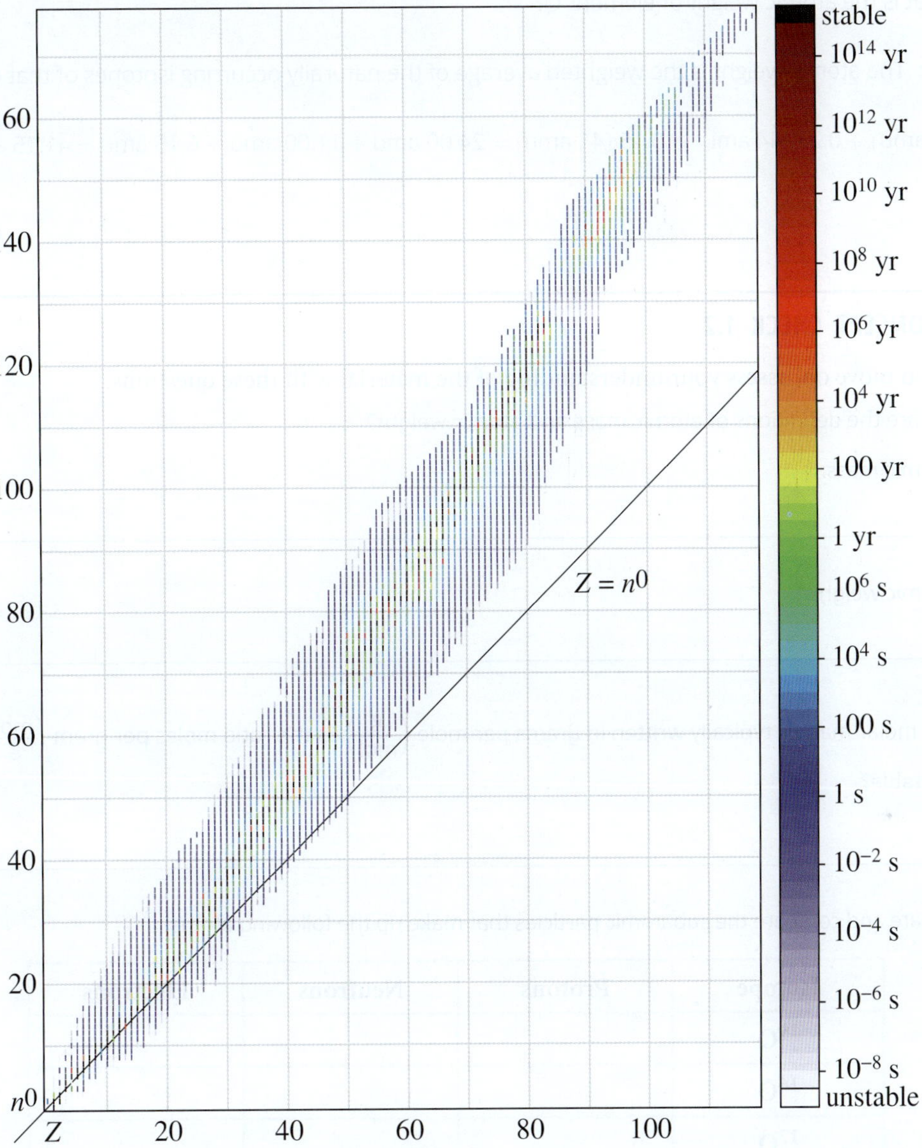

Figure 1.5 Half-Lives of the Different Isotopes of Elements
Half-life is a marker of stability; generally, longer-lasting isotopes are more abundant.

The utility of the atomic weight is that it represents both the mass of the "average" atom of that element, in amu, and the mass of one mole of the element, in grams. A mole is a number of "things" (atoms, ions, molecules) equal to **Avogadro's number,** $N_A = 6.02 \times 10^{23}$. For example, the atomic weight of carbon is 12.0 amu, which means that the average carbon atom has a mass of 12.0 amu (carbon-12 is *far* more abundant than carbon-13 or carbon-14), and 6.02×10^{23} carbon atoms have a combined mass of 12.0 grams.

MNEMONIC

Atomic **mass** is nearly synonymous with **mass** number. Atomic **weight** is a **weighted** average of naturally occurring isotopes of that element.

Example: Element Q consists of three different isotopes: A, B, and C. Isotope A has an atomic mass of 40 amu and accounts for 60 percent of naturally occurring Q. Isotope B has an atomic mass of 44 amu and accounts for 25 percent of Q. Finally, isotope C has an atomic mass of 41 amu and accounts for 15 percent of Q. What is the atomic weight of element Q?

Solution: The atomic weight is the weighted average of the naturally occurring isotopes of that element:

$$0.60\ (40\ \text{amu}) + 0.25\ (44\ \text{amu}) + 0.15\ (41\ \text{amu}) = 24.00\ \text{amu} + 11.00\ \text{amu} + 6.15\ \text{amu} = 41.15\ \text{amu}$$

MCAT CONCEPT CHECK 1.2

Before you move on, assess your understanding of the material with these questions.

1. What are the definitions of atomic mass and atomic weight?
   - Atomic mass:
   - Atomic weight:
2. While molar mass is typically written in grams per mole $\left(\frac{\text{g}}{\text{mol}}\right)$, is the ratio moles per gram $\left(\frac{\text{mol}}{\text{g}}\right)$ also acceptable?
3. Calculate and compare the subatomic particles that make up the following atoms.

Isotope	Protons	Neutrons	Electrons
^{19}O			
^{16}O			
^{17}O			
^{19}F			
^{16}F			
^{238}U			
^{240}U			

1.3 Rutherford, Planck, and Bohr High Yield

LEARNING OBJECTIVES

After Chapter 1.3, you will be able to:

- Calculate the energy of transition for a valence electron that jumps energy levels
- Calculate the wavelength of an emitted photon given the energy emitted by an electron
- Calculate the energy of a photon given its wavelength

In 1910, Ernest Rutherford provided experimental evidence that an atom has a dense, positively charged nucleus that accounts for only a small portion of the atom's volume. Eleven years earlier, Max Planck developed the first quantum theory, proposing that energy emitted as electromagnetic radiation from matter comes in discrete bundles called **quanta**. The **energy** of a quantum, he determined, is given by the **Planck relation**:

$$E = hf$$

Equation 1.1

where h is a proportionality constant known as **Planck's constant**, equal to 6.626×10^{-34} J · s, and f (sometimes designated by the Greek letter nu, ν) is the frequency of the radiation.

Bohr Model

In 1913, Danish physicist Niels Bohr used the work of Rutherford and Planck to develop his model of the electronic structure of the hydrogen atom. Starting from Rutherford's findings, Bohr assumed that the hydrogen atom consisted of a central proton around which an electron traveled in a circular orbit. He postulated that the centripetal force acting on the electron as it revolved around the nucleus was created by the electrostatic force between the positively charged proton and the negatively charged electron.

Bohr used Planck's quantum theory to correct certain assumptions that classical physics made about the pathways of electrons. Classical mechanics postulates that an object revolving in a circle, such as an electron, may assume an infinite number of values for its radius and velocity. The angular momentum ($L = mvr$) and kinetic energy $\left(K = \frac{1}{2}mv^2\right)$ of the object could therefore take on any value. However, by incorporating Planck's quantum theory into his model, Bohr placed restrictions on the possible values of the angular momentum. Bohr predicted that the possible values for the **angular momentum** of an electron orbiting a hydrogen nucleus could be given by:

$$L = \frac{nh}{2\pi}$$

Equation 1.2

where n is the principal quantum number, which can be any positive integer, and h is Planck's constant. Because the only variable is the principal quantum number, the angular momentum of an electron changes only in discrete amounts with respect to the principal quantum number. Note the similarities between quantized angular momentum and Planck's concept of quantized energy.

MCAT EXPERTISE

The "High-Yield" badge on this section indicates that the content is frequently tested on the MCAT.

BRIDGE

Recall from Chapter 8 of *MCAT Physics Review* that the speed of light (or any wave) can be calculated using $v = f\lambda$. The speed of light, c, is $3 \times 10^8 \frac{\text{m}}{\text{s}}$. This equation can be incorporated into the equation for quantum energy to provide different derivations.

MCAT EXPERTISE

When you see a formula in your review or on Test Day, focus on ratios and relationships. This simplifies our calculations to a conceptual understanding, which is usually enough to lead us to the right answer. Further, the MCAT tends to ask how changes in one variable may affect another variable, rather than a plug-and-chug application of complex equations.

Bohr then related the permitted angular momentum values to the **energy of the electron** to obtain:

$$E = -\frac{R_H}{n^2}$$

Equation 1.3

where R_H is the experimentally determined **Rydberg unit of energy**, equal to $2.18 \times 10^{-18} \frac{J}{\text{electron}}$. Therefore, like angular momentum, the energy of the electron changes in discrete amounts with respect to the quantum number. A value of zero energy was assigned to the state in which the proton and electron are separated completely, meaning that there is no attractive force between them. Therefore, the electron in any of its quantized states in the atom will have an attractive force toward the proton; this is represented by the negative sign in Equation 1.3. Ultimately, the only thing the energy equation is saying is that the energy of an electron increases—becomes less negative—the farther out from the nucleus that it is located (increasing n). This is an important point: while the magnitude of the fraction is getting smaller, the actual value it represents is getting larger (becoming less negative).

KEY CONCEPT

At first glance, it may not be clear that the energy (E) is directly proportional to the principal quantum number (n) in Equation 1.3. Take notice of the negative sign, which causes the values to approach zero from a more negative value as n increases (thereby increasing the energy). Negative signs are as important as a variable's location in a fraction when it comes to determining proportionality.

Think of the concept of quantized energy as being similar to the change in gravitational potential energy that you experience when you ascend or descend a flight of stairs. Unlike a ramp, on which you could take an infinite number of steps associated with a continuum of potential energy changes, a staircase only allows you certain changes in height and, as a result, allows only certain discrete (quantized) changes of potential energy. This is depicted in Figure 1.6.

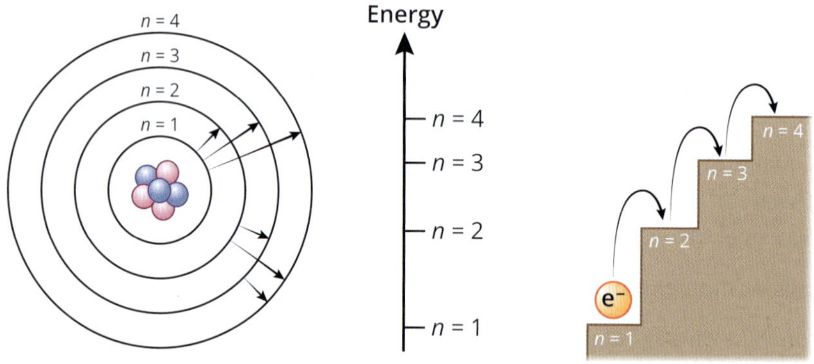

Figure 1.6 Quantized Energy Levels of an Electron

Bohr came to describe the structure of the hydrogen atom as a nucleus with one proton forming a dense core, around which a single electron revolved in a defined pathway (**orbit**) at a discrete energy value. If one could transfer an amount of energy exactly equal to the difference between one orbit and another, this could result in the electron "jumping" from one orbit to a higher energy one. These orbits had increasing radii, and the orbit with the smallest, lowest-energy radius was defined as the ground state ($n = 1$). More generally, the **ground state** of an atom is the state of lowest energy, in which all electrons are in the lowest possible orbitals. In Bohr's model, if the electron was promoted to an orbit with a larger radius (higher energy),

MCAT EXPERTISE

Note that all systems tend toward minimal energy; thus on the MCAT, atoms of any element will generally exist in the ground state unless subjected to extremely high temperatures or irradiation.

the atom was said to be in the excited state. In general, an atom is in an **excited state** when at least one electron has moved to a subshell of higher than normal energy (see Figure 1.7).

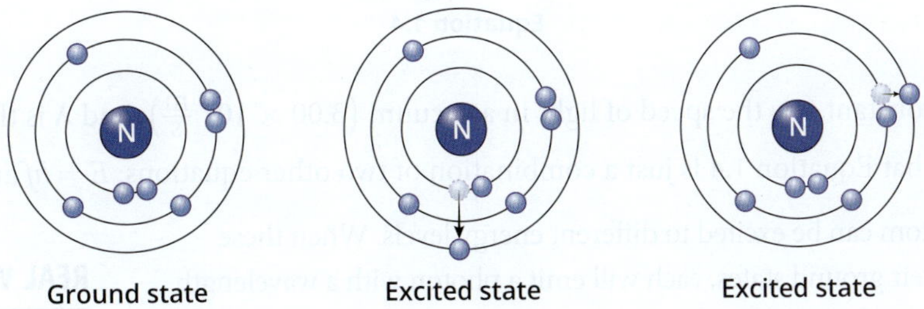

Figure 1.7 Excited States of a Nitrogen Atom (Bohr Model)
The transition from ground state to excited state can involve different electrons.

Bohr likened his model of the hydrogen atom to the planets orbiting the sun, in which each planet traveled along a roughly circular pathway at set distances—and energy values—from the sun. Bohr's Nobel Prize-winning model was reconsidered over the next two decades but remains an important conceptualization of atomic behavior. In particular, remember that we now know that electrons are *not* restricted to specific pathways, but tend to be localized in certain regions of space.

Applications of the Bohr Model

The Bohr model of the hydrogen atom (and other one-electron systems, such as He^+ and Li^{2+}) is useful for explaining the atomic emission and absorption spectra of atoms.

MNEMONIC

As electrons go from a lower energy level to a higher energy level, they get **AHED**:

- **A**bsorb light
- **H**igher potential
- **E**xcited
- **D**istant (from the nucleus)

Atomic Emission Spectra

At room temperature, the majority of atoms in a sample are in the ground state. However, electrons can be excited to higher energy levels by heat or other energy forms to yield excited states. Because the lifetime of an excited state is brief, the electrons will return rapidly to the ground state, resulting in the emission of discrete amounts of energy in the form of photons, as shown in Figure 1.8.

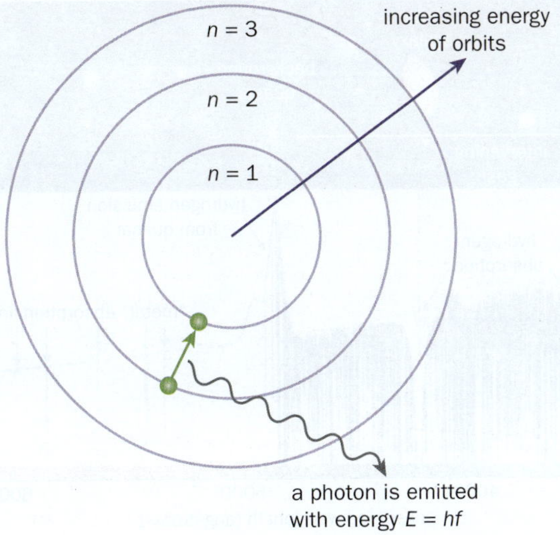

Figure 1.8 Atomic Emission of a Photon as a Result of a Ground State Transition

The electromagnetic energy of these photons can be determined using the following equation:

$$E = \frac{hc}{\lambda}$$

Equation 1.4

where h is Planck's constant, c is the speed of light in a vacuum $\left(3.00 \times 10^{8} \ \frac{\text{m}}{\text{s}}\right)$, and λ is the wavelength of the radiation. Note that Equation 1.4 is just a combination of two other equations: $E = hf$ and $c = f\lambda$.

The electrons in an atom can be excited to different energy levels. When these electrons return to their ground states, each will emit a photon with a wavelength characteristic of the specific energy transition it undergoes. As described above, these energy transitions do not form a continuum, but rather are quantized to certain values. Thus, the spectrum is composed of light at specified frequencies. It is sometimes called a **line spectrum**, where each line on the emission spectrum corresponds to a specific electron transition. Because each element can have its electrons excited to a different set of distinct energy levels, each possesses a unique **atomic emission spectrum**, which can be used as a fingerprint for the element. Figure 1.9 depicts the emission spectrum for oxygen, along with its absorption spectrum (discussed below).

REAL WORLD

Emissions from electrons dropping from an excited state to a ground state give rise to fluorescence. What we see is the color of the emitted light.

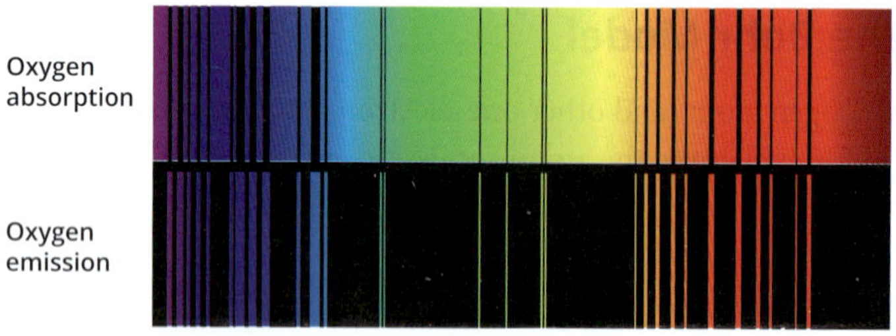

Figure 1.9 Absorption and Emission Spectra for Oxygen Gas

One particular application of atomic emission spectroscopy is in the analysis of stars and planets: while a physical sample may be impossible to procure, the light from a star can be resolved into its component wavelengths, which are then matched to the known line spectra of the elements as shown in Figure 1.10.

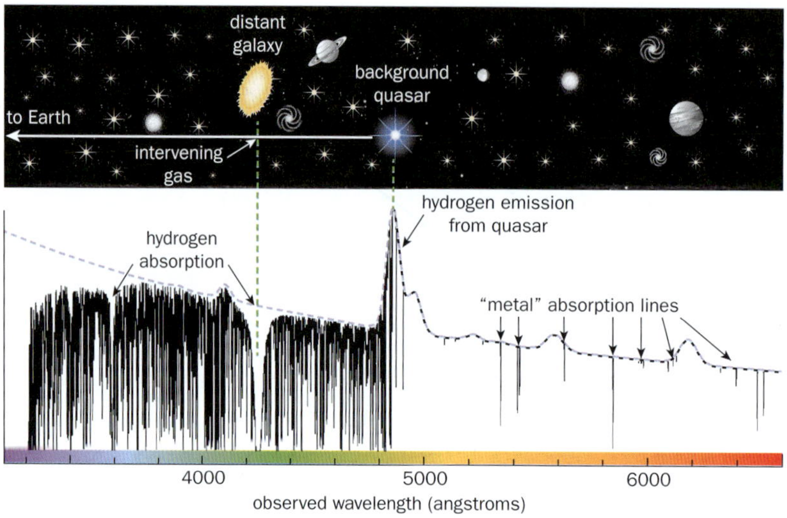

Figure 1.10 Line Spectrum with Transition Wavelengths for Various Celestial Bodies

The Bohr model of the hydrogen atom explained the atomic emission spectrum of hydrogen, which is the simplest emission spectrum among all the elements. The group of hydrogen emission lines corresponding to transitions from energy levels $n \geq 2$ to $n = 1$ is known as the **Lyman series**. The group corresponding to transitions from energy levels $n \geq 3$ to $n = 2$ is known as the **Balmer series** and includes four wavelengths in the visible region. The Lyman series includes larger energy transitions than the Balmer series; it therefore has shorter photon wavelengths in the UV region of the electromagnetic spectrum. The **Paschen series** corresponds to transitions from $n \geq 4$ to $n = 3$. These energy transition series can be seen in Figure 1.11.

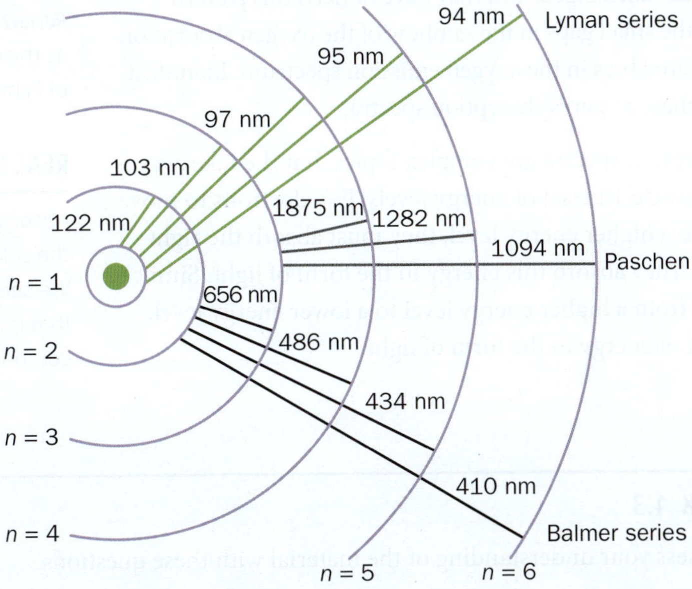

Figure 1.11 Wavelengths of Electron Orbital Transitions
Energy is inversely proportional to wavelength: $E = hf = \frac{hc}{\lambda}$.

The energy associated with a change in the principal quantum number from a higher initial value n_i to a lower final value n_f is equal to the energy of the photon predicted by Planck's quantum theory. Combining Bohr's and Planck's calculations, we can derive:

$$E = \frac{hc}{\lambda} = R_H\left[\frac{1}{n_i^2} - \frac{1}{n_f^2}\right]$$

Equation 1.5

This complex-appearing equation essentially says: *The energy of the emitted photon corresponds to the difference in energy between the higher-energy initial state and the lower-energy final state.*

KEY CONCEPT

It may seem strange to see an equation that has *initial* minus *final*, where most equations usually have final minus initial. But ultimately, this equation is designed to work just like you'd expect: If an atom emits a photon, the equation gives a negative value for energy, indicating a decrease. You can easily check this for yourself by using $n_i = 2$ and $n_f = 1$.

Atomic Absorption Spectra

When an electron is excited to a higher energy level, it must absorb exactly the right amount of energy to make that transition. This means that exciting the electrons of a particular element results in energy absorption at specific wavelengths. Thus, in addition to a unique emission spectrum, every element possesses a characteristic **absorption spectrum**. Not surprisingly, the wavelengths of absorption correspond exactly to the wavelengths of emission because the difference in energy between levels remains unchanged. You may have noticed this pattern earlier in Figure 1.9, where the small gaps in the rainbow of the oxygen absorption spectrum correspond to colored bars in the oxygen emission spectrum. Identification of elements in the gas phase requires absorption spectra.

Atomic emission and absorption spectra are complex topics, but the takeaway is that each element has a characteristic set of energy levels. For electrons to move from a lower energy level to a higher energy level, they must absorb the right amount of energy to do so. They absorb this energy in the form of light. Similarly, when electrons move from a higher energy level to a lower energy level, they emit the same amount of energy in the form of light.

BRIDGE

ΔE is the same for absorption or emission between any two energy levels according to the conservation of energy, as discussed in Chapter 2 of *MCAT Physics and Math Review*. This is also the same as the energy of the photon of light absorbed or emitted.

REAL WORLD

Absorption is the basis for the color of compounds. We see the color of the light that is *not* absorbed by the compound.

MCAT CONCEPT CHECK 1.3

Before you move on, assess your understanding of the material with these questions.

Note: *For these questions, try to estimate the calculations without a calculator to mimic Test Day conditions. Double-check your answers with a calculator and refer to the answers for confirmation of your results.*

1. The valence electron in a lithium atom jumps from energy level $n = 2$ to $n = 4$. What is the energy of this transition in joules? In eV? (Note: $R_H = 2.18 \times 10^{-18} \frac{\text{J}}{\text{electron}} = 13.6 \frac{\text{eV}}{\text{electron}}$)

____

2. If an electron emits 3 eV of energy, what is the corresponding wavelength of the emitted photon? (Note: $1\ \text{eV} = 1.60 \times 10^{-19}\ \text{J}$, $h = 6.626 \times 10^{-34}\ \text{J} \cdot \text{s}$)

____

3. Calculate the energy of a photon of wavelength 662 nm. (Note: $h = 6.626 \times 10^{-34}\ \text{J} \cdot \text{s}$)

____

1.4 Quantum Mechanical Model of Atoms

LEARNING OBJECTIVES

After Chapter 1.4, you will be able to:

- Identify the four quantum numbers, the potential range of values for each, and their relationship to the electron they represent
- Compare the orbital diagram for a neutral atom, such as sulfur (S), to an ion such as S^{2-}
- Differentiate between paramagnetic and diamagnetic compounds
- Determine the number of valence electrons in a given atom

While Bohr's model marked a significant advancement in the understanding of the structure of atoms, his model ultimately proved inadequate to explain the structure and behavior of atoms containing more than one electron. The model's failure was a result of not taking into account the repulsion between multiple electrons surrounding the nucleus. Modern quantum mechanics has led to a more rigorous and generalizable study of the electronic structure of atoms. The most important difference between Bohr's model and the modern quantum mechanical model is that Bohr postulated that electrons follow a clearly defined circular pathway or orbit at a fixed distance from the nucleus, whereas modern quantum mechanics has shown that this is not the case. Rather, we now understand that electrons move rapidly and are localized within regions of space around the nucleus called **orbitals**. The confidence by which those in Bohr's time believed they could identify the location (or pathway) of the electron was now replaced by a more modest suggestion that the best we can do is describe the probability of finding an electron within a given region of space surrounding the nucleus. In the current quantum mechanical model, it is impossible to pinpoint exactly where an electron is at any given moment in time. This is expressed best by the **Heisenberg uncertainty principle**: *It is impossible to simultaneously determine, with perfect accuracy, the momentum and the position of an electron.* If we want to assess the position of an electron, the electron has to stop (thereby removing its momentum); if we want to assess its momentum, the electron has to be moving (thereby changing its position). This can be seen visually in Figure 1.12.

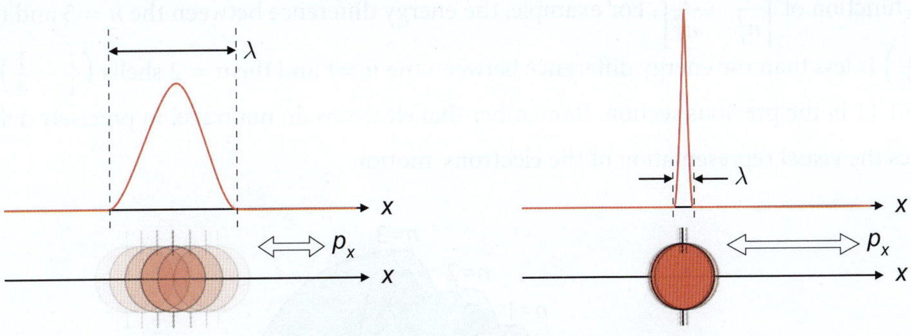

Figure 1.12 Heisenberg Uncertainty Principle
Known momentum and uncertain position (left); known position but uncertain momentum (right). λ = confidence interval of position; p_x = confidence interval of momentum.

Quantum Numbers

Modern atomic theory postulates that any electron in an atom can be completely described by four quantum numbers: n, l, m_l, and m_s. Furthermore, according to the **Pauli exclusion principle**, no two electrons in a given atom can possess the same set of four quantum numbers. The position and energy of an electron described by its quantum numbers are known as its *energy state*. The value of n limits the values of l, which in turn limit the values of m_l. In other words, for a given value of n, only particular values of l are permissible; given a value of l, only particular values of m_l are permissible. The values of the quantum numbers qualitatively give information about the size, shape, and orientation of the orbitals. As we examine the four quantum numbers more closely, pay attention especially to l and m_l because these two tend to give students the greatest difficulty.

MCAT EXPERTISE

Think of the quantum numbers as becoming more specific as one goes from n to l to m_l to m_s. This is like an address: one lives in a particular state (n), in a particular city (l), on a particular street (m_l), at a particular house number (m_s).

Principal Quantum Number (n)

The first quantum number is commonly known as the **principal quantum number** and is denoted by the letter ***n***. This is the quantum number used in Bohr's model that can theoretically take on any positive integer value. The larger the integer value of n, the higher the energy level and radius of the electron's **shell**, as seen in Figure 1.13 below. Within each shell, there is a capacity to hold a certain number of electrons, given by:

$$\text{Maximum number of electrons within a shell} = 2n^2$$

Equation 1.6

where n is the principal quantum number. The higher the principal quantum number, the more electrons can be held in the shell. Additionally, the higher the shell number, the further its position relative to the nucleus, thus increasing its energy. The difference in energy between two adjacent shells decreases as the distance from the nucleus increases because the energy difference is a function of $\left[\frac{1}{n_i^2} - \frac{1}{n_f^2}\right]$. For example, the energy difference between the $n = 3$ and the $n = 4$ shells $\left(\frac{1}{9} - \frac{1}{16}\right)$ is less than the energy difference between the $n = 1$ and the $n = 2$ shells $\left(\frac{1}{1} - \frac{1}{4}\right)$. This can be seen in Figure 1.11 in the previous section. Remember that electrons do not travel in precisely defined orbits; it just simplifies the visual representation of the electrons' motion.

BRIDGE

Remember, a larger integer value for the principal quantum number indicates a larger radius and higher energy. This is similar to gravitational potential energy, as discussed in Chapter 2 of *MCAT Physics Review*, where the higher or farther the object is above the Earth, the higher its potential energy will be.

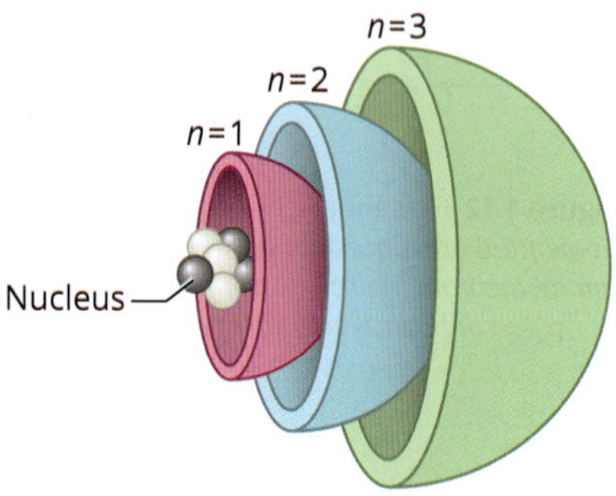

Figure 1.13 Electron Shells and Their Principal Quantum Numbers

Azimuthal Quantum Number (l)

The second quantum number is called the **azimuthal (angular momentum) quantum number** and is designated by the letter ***l***. The second quantum number refers to the shape and number of **subshells** within a given principal energy level (shell). The azimuthal quantum number is very important because it has important implications for chemical bonding and bond angles. The value of n limits the value of l in the following way: for any given value of n, the range of possible values for l is 0 to $(n - 1)$. For example, within the first principal energy level, $n = 1$, the only possible value for l is 0; within the second principal energy level, $n = 2$, the possible values for l are 0 and 1. A simpler way to remember this relationship is that the n-value also tells you the number of possible subshells. Therefore, there's only one subshell ($l = 0$) in the first principal energy level; there are two subshells ($l = 0$ and 1) within the second principal energy level; there are three subshells ($l = 0$, 1, and 2) within the third principal energy level, and so on.

KEY CONCEPT

For any principal quantum number n, there will be n possible values for l, ranging from 0 to $(n - 1)$.

s = 0
p = 1
d = 2
f = 3

Figure 1.14 Spectroscopic Notation Letter Designations

Spectroscopic notation refers to the shorthand representation of the principal and azimuthal quantum numbers. The principal quantum number remains a number, but the azimuthal quantum number is designated by a letter: the $l = 0$ subshell is called *s*; the $l = 1$ subshell is called *p*; the $l = 2$ subshell is called *d*; and the $l = 3$ subshell is called *f*, as summarized for easy reference in Figure 1.14. Thus, an electron in the shell $n = 4$ and subshell $l = 2$ is said to be in the 4*d* subshell. The spectroscopic notation for each subshell is demonstrated in Figure 1.15.

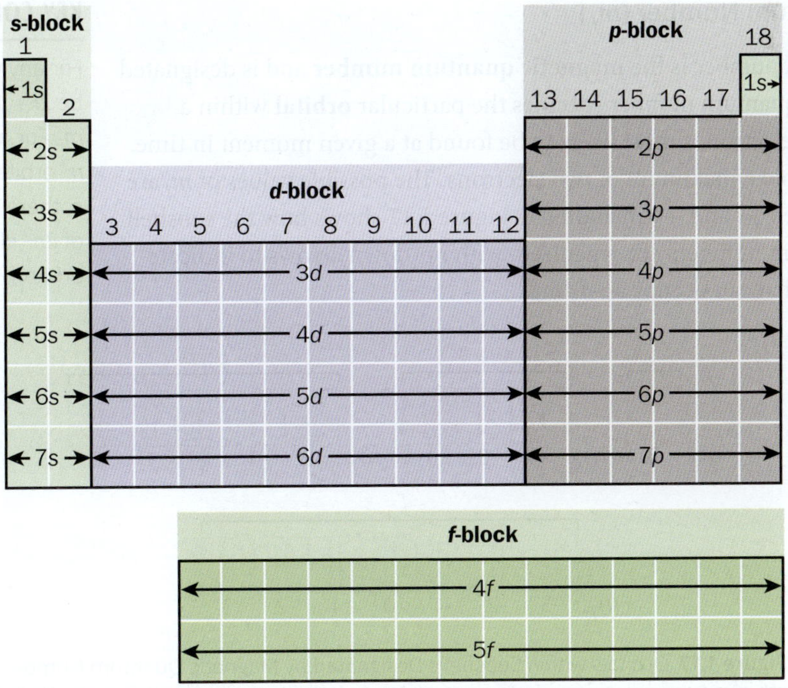

Figure 1.15 Spectroscopic Notation for Every Subshell on the Periodic Table

Within each subshell, there is a capacity to hold a certain number of electrons, given by:

$$\text{Maximum number of electrons within a subshell} = 4l + 2$$

Equation 1.7

where l is the azimuthal quantum number. The energies of the subshells increase with increasing l value; however, the energies of subshells from different principal energy levels may overlap. For example, the 4*s* subshell will have a lower energy than the 3*d* subshell.

Figure 1.16 provides an example of computer-generated probability maps of the first few electron clouds in a hydrogen atom. This provides a rough visual representation of the shapes of different subshells.

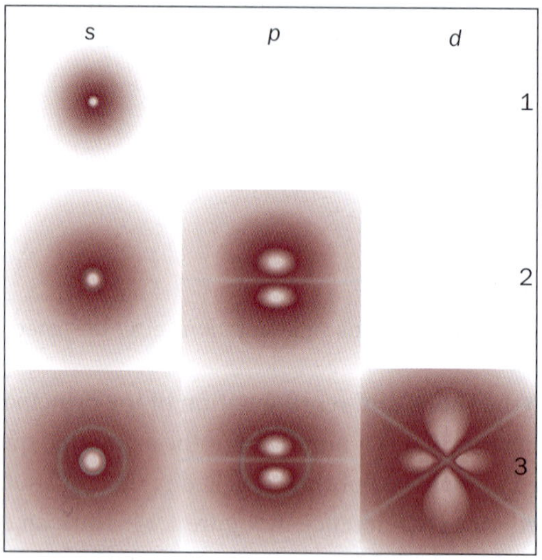

Figure 1.16 Electron Clouds of Various Subshells

Magnetic Quantum Number (m_l)

The third quantum number is the **magnetic quantum number** and is designated $\boldsymbol{m_l}$. The magnetic quantum number specifies the particular **orbital** within a subshell where an electron is most likely to be found at a given moment in time. Each orbital can hold a maximum of two electrons. The possible values of m_l are the integers between $-l$ and $+l$, including 0. Figure 1.17 shows how the subshell and orbital quantum numbers are organized, with up-down arrows to indicate the two electrons that can occupy an orbital.

KEY CONCEPT

For any value of l, there will be $2l + 1$ possible values for m_l. For any n, this produces n^2 orbitals. For any value of n, there will be a maximum of $2n^2$ electrons (two per orbital).

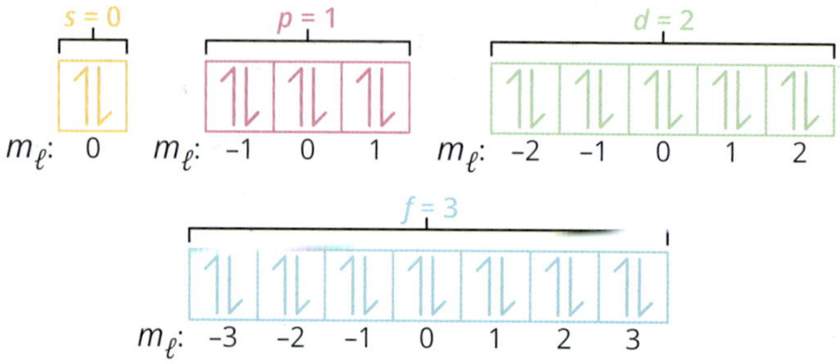

Figure 1.17 Orbitals within Subshells Designated by Magnetic Quantum Number
Each arrow represents one electron occupying an individual orbital within each subshell.

For example, the *s* subshell, with $l = 0$, limits the possible m_l values to 0, and because there is a single value of m_l, there is only one orbital in the *s* subshell. The *p* subshell, with $l = 1$, limits the possible m_l values to -1, 0, and $+1$, and because there are three values for m_l, there are three orbitals in the *p* subshell. The *d* subshell has five orbitals (-2 to $+2$), and the *f* subshell has seven orbitals (-3 to $+3$). In fact, the *p*-orbitals are often referred to as p_x, p_y, and p_z. The first five orbitals—1*s*, 2*s*, $2p_x$, $2p_y$, and $2p_z$—are demonstrated in Figure 1.18 Note the similarity to the images in Figure 1.16.

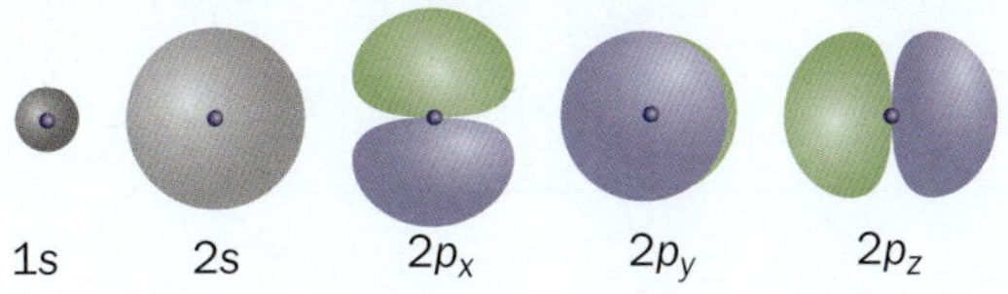

Figure 1.18 The First Five Atomic Orbitals

The three-dimensional orientation of the *s*, *p*, and *d* orbitals are shown in Figure 1.19. The shape of the orbitals, like the number of orbitals, is dependent on the subshell in which they are found. The orbitals in the *s* subshell are spherical, while the three orbitals in the *p* subshell are each dumbbell-shaped and align along the *x*-, *y*-, and *z*-axes. The five orbitals in the *d* subshell are mostly clover-shaped. The *f* subshell orbitals are much more complex, and the MCAT will not ask you about their appearance. The shapes of orbitals are defined in terms of a concept called probability density, the likelihood that an electron will be found in a particular region of space.

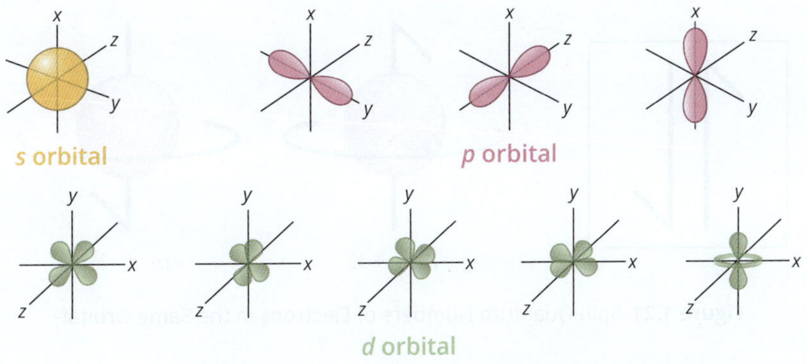

Figure 1.19 Shapes of the *s*, *p*, and *d* Orbitals

Take a look at the 2*p* block in the periodic table. As mentioned above, 2*p* contains three orbitals. If each orbital can contain two electrons, then six electrons can be added during the course of filling the 2*p*-orbitals. This is also seen in Figure 1.20, which shows the maximum number of electrons each subshell can hold. As atomic number increases, so too does the number of electrons (assuming the species is neutral). Therefore, it should be no surprise that the *p* block contains six groups of elements. The *s* block contains two elements in each row of the periodic table, the *d* block contains ten elements, and the *f* block contains fourteen elements.

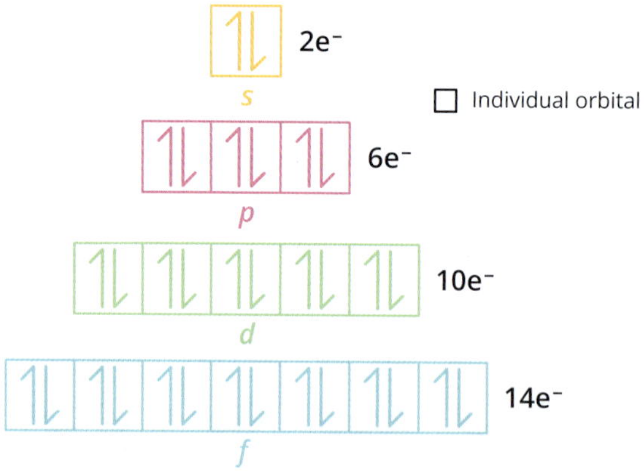

Figure 1.20 Electron Capacity in Orbital Levels

Spin Quantum Number (m_s)

The fourth quantum number is called the **spin quantum number** and is denoted by $\boldsymbol{m_s}$. In classical mechanics, an object spinning about its axis has an infinite number of possible values for its angular momentum. However, this does not apply to the electron, which has two spin orientations designated $+\frac{1}{2}$ and $-\frac{1}{2}$. Whenever two electrons are in the same orbital, they must have opposite spins (shown in Figure 1.21, this is typically represented with two oppositely oriented half-headed arrows). In this case, they are often referred to as being **paired**. Electrons in different orbitals with the same m_s values are said to have **parallel spins**.

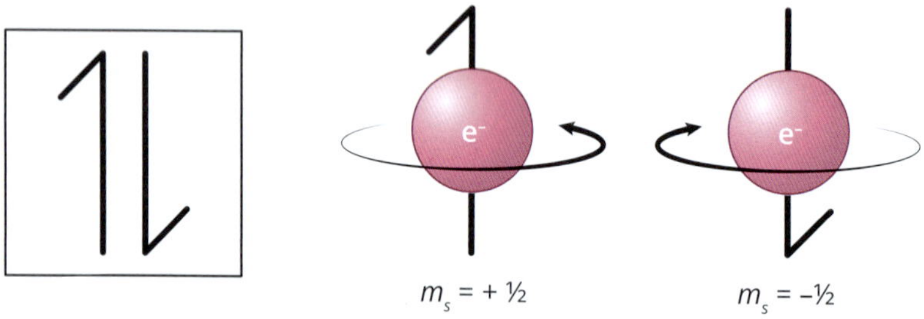

Figure 1.21 Spin Quantum Numbers of Electrons in the Same Orbital

Electron Configurations

For a given atom or ion, the pattern by which subshells are filled, as well as the number of electrons within each principal energy level and subshell, are designated by its **electron configuration**. Electron configurations use spectroscopic notation, wherein the first number denotes the principal energy level, the letter designates the subshell, and the superscript gives the number of electrons in that subshell. For example, $2p^4$ indicates that there are four electrons in the second (p) subshell of the second principal energy level. This also implies that the energy levels below $2p$ (that is, $1s$ and $2s$) have already been filled, as shown in Figure 1.22.

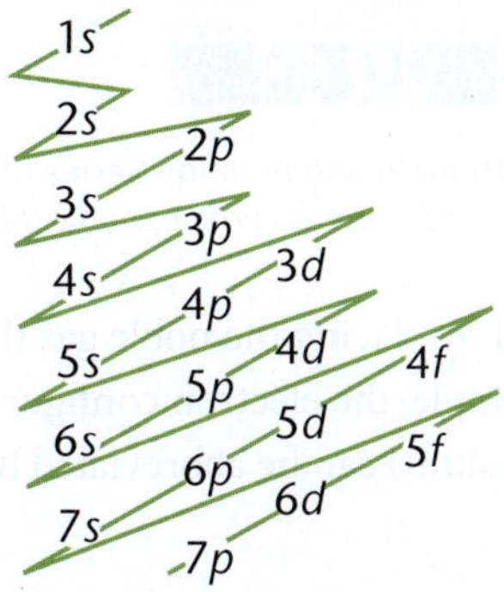

Figure 1.22 Electron Subshell Flow Diagram

MCAT EXPERTISE

Remember that the shorthand used to describe the electron configuration is derived directly from the quantum numbers.

To write out an atom's electron configuration, one needs to know the order in which subshells are filled. Electrons fill from lower- to higher-energy subshells, according to the **Aufbau principle** (also called the **building-up principle**), and each subshell will fill completely before electrons begin to enter the next one. The order need not be memorized because there are two very helpful ways of recalling this. The $\boldsymbol{n + l}$ **rule** can be used to rank subshells by increasing energy. This rule states that the lower the sum of the values of the first and second quantum numbers, $n + l$, the lower the energy of the subshell. This is a helpful rule to remember for Test Day. If two subshells possess the same $n + l$ value, the subshell with the lower n value has a lower energy and will fill with electrons first.

Example: Which will fill first, the 5*d* subshell or the 6*s* subshell?

Solution: For 5*d*, $n = 5$ and $l = 2$, so $n + l = 7$. For 6*s*, $n = 6$ and $l = 0$, so $n + l = 6$. Therefore, the 6*s* subshell has lower energy and will fill first.

An alternative way to approach electron configurations is through simply reading the periodic table. One must remember that the lowest *s* subshell is 1*s*, the lowest *p* subshell is 2*p*, the lowest *d* subshell is 3*d*, and the lowest *f* subshell is 4*f*. This can be seen in Figure 1.15. Then, we can simply read across the periodic table to get to the element of interest, filling subshells along the way. To do this, we must know the correct position of the lanthanide and actinide series (the *f* block), as shown in Figure 1.23. In most representations of the periodic table, the *f* block is pulled out and placed below the rest of the table. This is purely an effect of graphic design—placing the *f* block in its correct location results in a lot of excess white space on a page.

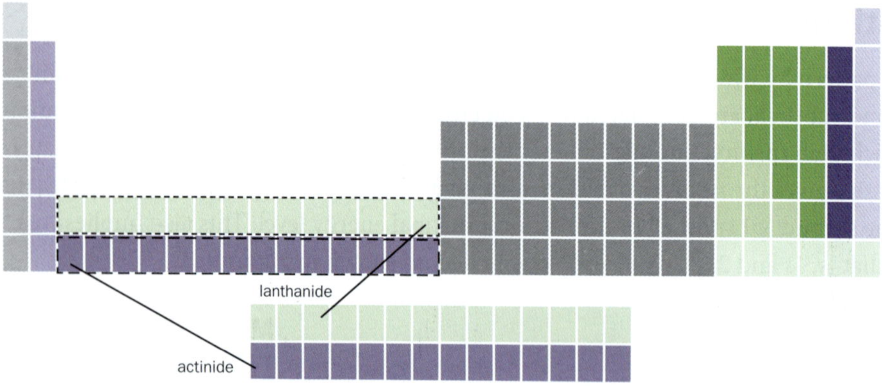

Figure 1.23 Periodic Table with Lanthanide and Actinide Series Inserted
The f *block fits between the* s *block and* d *block in the periodic table.*

MCAT EXPERTISE

Many general chemistry courses teach the flow diagram in Figure 1.22 as a method to determine the order of subshell filling in electron configurations. However, on Test Day, it can be both time-consuming and error-prone, resulting in incorrect electron configurations. Learning to read the periodic table, as described here, is the best method.

Electron configurations can be abbreviated by placing the noble gas that precedes the element of interest in brackets. For example, the electron configuration of any element in period four (starting with potassium) can be abbreviated by starting with [Ar].

Example: What is the electron configuration of osmium ($Z = 76$)?

Solution: The noble gas that comes just before osmium is xenon ($Z = 54$). Therefore, the electron configuration can begin with [Xe]. Continuing across the periodic table, we pass through the 6*s* subshell (cesium and barium), the 4*f* subshell (the lanthanide series; remember its position on the periodic table!), and into the 5*d* subshell. Osmium is the sixth element in the 5*d* subshell, so the configuration is [Xe] $6s^2 4f^{14} 5d^6$.

This method works for neutral atoms, but how does one write the electron configuration of an ion? Negatively charged ions (**anions**) have additional electrons that fill according to the same rules as above; for example, if fluorine's electron configuration is [He] $2s^2 2p^5$, then F^- is [He] $2s^2 2p^6$. Positively charged ions (**cations**) are a bit more complicated: start with the neutral atom, and remove electrons from the subshells with the highest value for *n* first. If multiple subshells are tied for the highest *n* value, then electrons are removed from the subshell with the highest *l* value among these.

Example: What is the electron configuration of Fe^{3+}?

Solution: The electron configuration of iron is [Ar] $4s^2 3d^6$. Electrons are removed from the 4*s* subshell before the 3*d* subshell because it has a higher principal quantum number. Therefore, Fe^{3+} has a configuration of [Ar] $3d^5$, not [Ar] $4s^2 3d^3$.

Hund's Rule

In subshells that contain more than one orbital, such as the 2*p* subshell with its three orbitals, the orbitals will fill according to **Hund's rule**, which states that, within a given subshell, orbitals are filled such that there are a maximum number of half-filled orbitals with parallel spins. As seen in Figure 1.24, the incorrect orbital diagram for oxygen has two paired electron in one orbital and an empty orbital. The correct placement will move one of the paired electrons into the empty orbital.

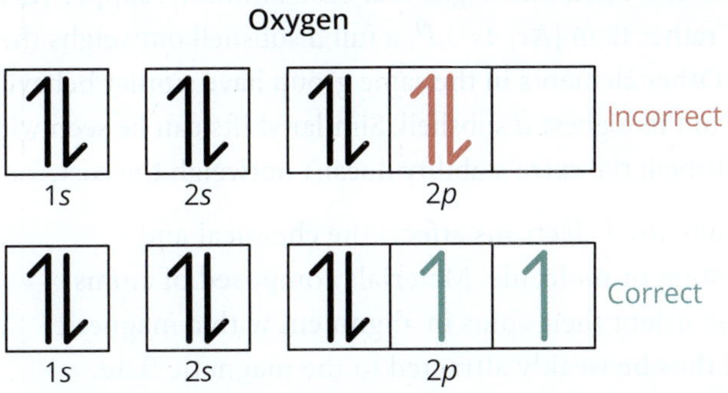

Figure 1.24 Hund's Rule as Applied to Oxygen

Like finding a seat on a crowded bus, electrons would prefer to have their own seat (orbital) before being forced to double up with another electron. Of course, the basis for this preference is electron repulsion: electrons in the same orbital tend to be closer to each other and thus repel each other more than electrons placed in different orbitals.

Example: According to Hund's rule, what are the orbital diagrams for nitrogen and iron?

Solution: Nitrogen has an atomic number of 7. Thus, its electron configuration is $1s^22s^22p^3$. According to Hund's rule, the two *s*-orbitals will fill completely, while the three *p*-orbitals will each contain one electron, all with parallel spins.

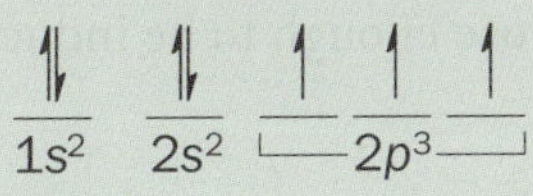

Iron has an atomic number of 26. As determined earlier, its electron configuration is [Ar] $4s^23d^6$. The electrons will fill all of the subshells except for the 3*d*, which will contain four orbitals with parallel (upward) spin and one orbital with electrons of both spin directions.

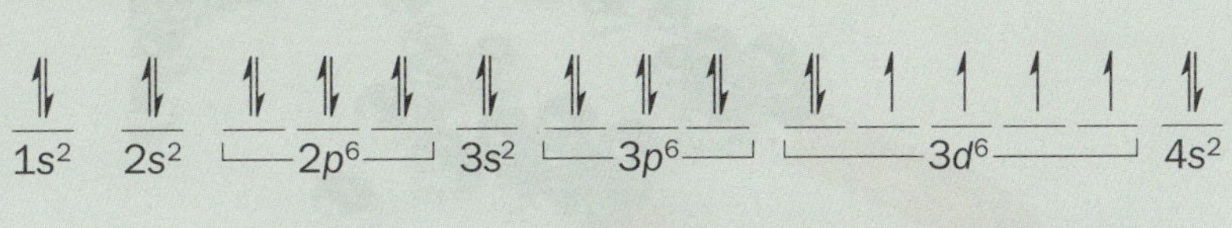

Subshells may be listed either in the order in which they fill (4*s* before 3*d*) or with subshells of the same principal quantum number grouped together, as shown here. Both methods are correct.

An important corollary from Hund's rule is that half-filled and fully filled orbitals have lower energies (higher stability) than other states. This creates two notable exceptions to electron configuration that are often tested on the MCAT: chromium (and other elements in its group) and copper (and other elements in its group). Chromium ($Z = 24$) should have the electron configuration [Ar] $4s^2 3d^4$ according to the rules established earlier. However, moving one electron from the 4*s* subshell to the 3*d* subshell allows the 3*d* subshell to be half-filled: [Ar] $4s^1 3d^5$ (remember that *s* subshells can hold two electrons and *d* subshells can hold ten). While moving the 4*s* electron up to the 3*d*-orbital is energetically unfavorable, the extra stability from making the 3*d* subshell half-filled outweighs that cost. Similarly, copper ($Z = 29$) has the electron configuration [Ar] $4s^1 3d^{10}$, rather than [Ar] $4s^2 3d^9$; a full *d* subshell outweighs the cost of moving an electron out of the 4*s* subshell. Other elements in the same group have similar behavior, moving one electron from the highest *s* subshell to the highest *d* subshell. Similar shifts can be seen with *f* subshells, but they are *never* observed for the *p* subshell; the extra stability doesn't outweigh the cost.

The presence of paired or unpaired electrons affects the chemical and magnetic properties of an atom or molecule. Materials composed of atoms with unpaired electrons will orient their spins in alignment with a magnetic field, and the material will thus be weakly attracted to the magnetic field. These materials are considered **paramagnetic**. Materials consisting of atoms that have only paired electrons will be slightly repelled by a magnetic field and are said to be **diamagnetic**. Figure 1.25 shows the electron distribution for paramagnetic and diamagnetic elements.

MNEMONIC

Remember that **para**magnetic means that a magnetic field will cause **para**llel spins in unpaired electrons and therefore cause an attraction.

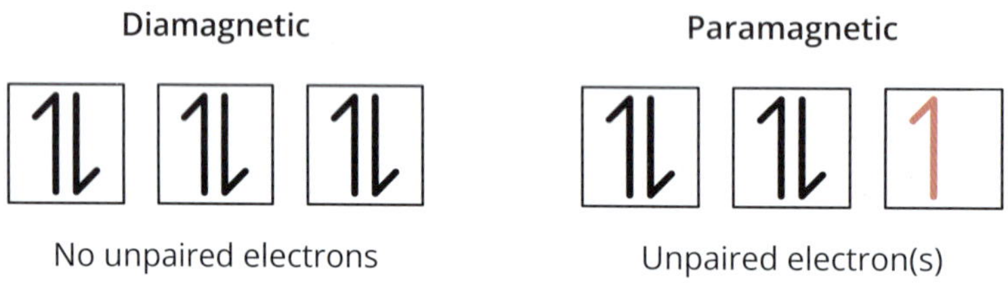

Figure 1.25 Electron Orbitals in Diamagnetic and Paramagnetic Atoms

An example of a paramagnetic material is shown in Figure 1.26, where a set of iron orbs is influenced by a magnet. The metallic spheres that are close enough to be induced by the magnet are attracted to the magnet and move toward it.

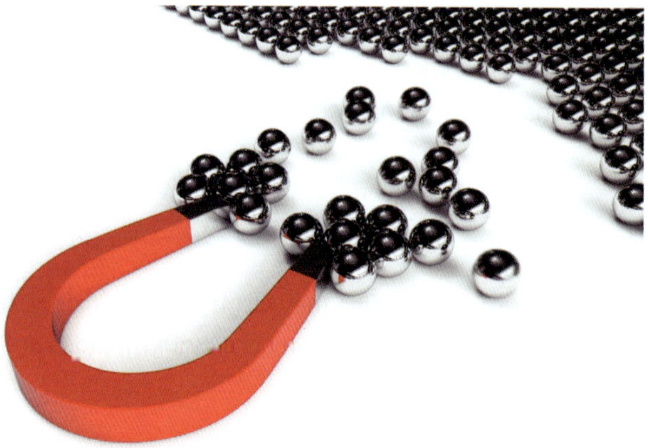

Figure 1.26 Attraction of Paramagnetic Iron Spheres to a Magnet

An example of a diamagnetic material is seen in Figure 1.27, where a piece of pyrolytic graphite is suspended in the air over strong neodymium magnets. All the electrons in this *allotrope* (configuration) of carbon are paired because of covalent bonding between layers of the material, and are thus opposed to being reoriented. Given sufficiently strong magnetic fields beneath an object, any diamagnetic substance can be made to levitate.

REAL WORLD

The concept behind "maglev" or magnetic levitation is no longer science fiction. Using powerful magnetic fields and strongly diamagnetic materials, some transportation systems have developed frictionless, high speed rail networks such as Japan's SCMaglev.

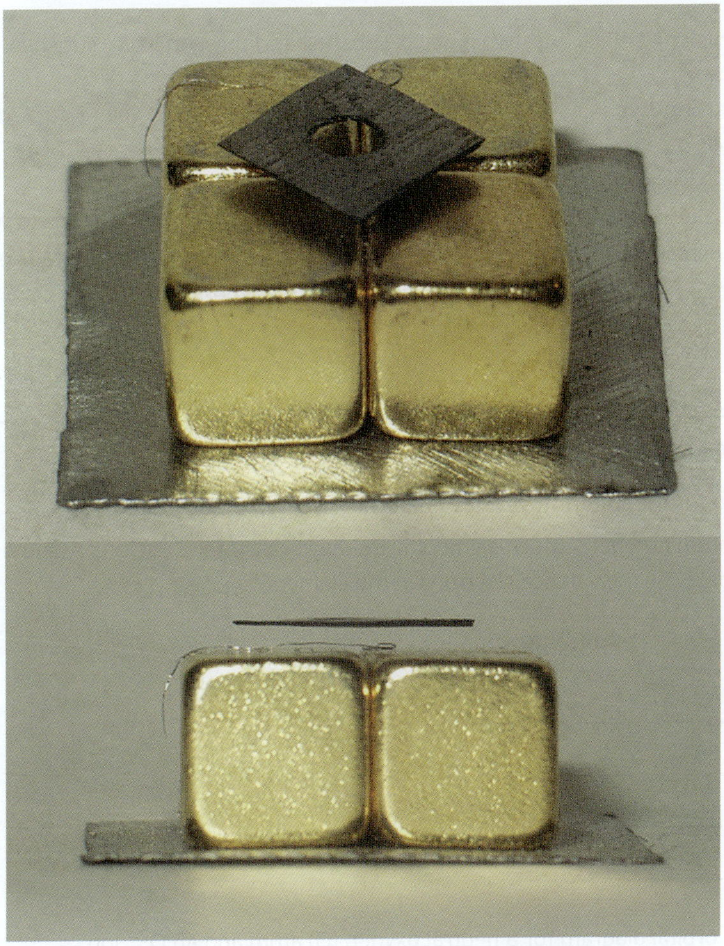

Figure 1.27 Diamagnetic Pyrolytic Graphite

Valence Electrons

The valence electrons of an atom are those electrons that are in its outermost energy shell, are most easily removed, and are available for bonding. In other words, the valence electrons are the "active" electrons of an atom and to a large extent dominate the chemical behavior of the atom. For elements in Groups IA and IIA (Groups 1 and 2), only the highest *s* subshell electrons are valence electrons. For elements in Groups IIIA through VIIIA (Groups 13 through 18), the highest *s* and *p* subshell electrons are valence electrons. For transition elements, the valence electrons are those in the highest *s* and *d* subshells, even though they have different principal quantum numbers. For the lanthanide and actinide series, the valence electrons are those in the highest *s* and *f* subshells, even though they have different principal quantum numbers. All elements in period three (starting with sodium) and below may accept electrons into their *d* subshell, which allows them to hold more than

MCAT EXPERTISE

The valence electron configuration of an atom helps us understand its properties and is ascertainable from the periodic table (the only "cheat sheet" available on the MCAT!). On Test Day, you will be able to access a periodic table by clicking on the button labeled "Periodic Table" on the bottom left of the screen. Use it as needed!

eight electrons in their valence shell. This allows them to violate the octet rule, as discussed in Chapter 3 of *MCAT General Chemistry Review*.

Example: Which electrons are the valence electrons of elemental vanadium, elemental selenium, and the sulfur atom in a sulfate ion?

Solution: Vanadium has five valence electrons: two in its 4*s* subshell and three in its 3*d* subshell.

Selenium has six valence electrons: two in its 4*s* subshell and four in its 4*p* subshell. Selenium's 3*d* electrons are not part of its valence shell.

Sulfur in a sulfate ion has 12 valence electrons: its original six plus six more from the oxygens to which it is bonded. Sulfur's 3*s* and 3*p* subshells can contain only eight of these 12 electrons; the other four electrons have entered the sulfur atom's 3*d* subshell, which is normally empty in elemental sulfur.

MCAT CONCEPT CHECK 1.4

Before you move on, assess your understanding of the material with these questions.

1. If given the following quantum numbers, which element(s) do they likely refer to? (Note: Assume that these quantum numbers describe the valence electrons in the element.)

n	*l*	Possible Elements
2	1	
3	0	
5	3	
4	2	

2. Write out and compare an orbital diagram for a neutral oxygen (O) atom and an O^{2-} ion.

---

3. Magnetic resonance angiography (MRA) is a technique that can resolve defects like stenotic (narrowed) arteries. A contrast agent like gadolinium or manganese injected into the blood stream interacts with the strong magnetic fields of the MRI device to produce such images. Based on their orbital configurations, are these contrast agents paramagnetic or diamagnetic?

---

4. Determine how many valence electrons come from each subshell in the following atoms:

Atom	*s*-electrons	*p*-electrons	*d*-electrons	*f*-electrons	Total Valence Electrons
P in PO_4^{3-}					
O in PO_4^{3-}					
Ir					
Cf					

Conclusion

Congratulations! You've made it through the first chapter! Now that we have covered topics related to the most fundamental unit of matter—the atom—you're set to advance your understanding of the physical world in more complex ways. This chapter described the characteristics and behavior of the three subatomic particles: the proton, neutron, and electron. In addition, it compared and contrasted two models of the atom. The Bohr model is adequate for describing the structure of one-electron systems, such as the hydrogen atom or the helium ion, but fails to adequately describe the structure of more complex atoms. The quantum mechanical model theorizes that electrons are found not in discrete orbits, but in "clouds of probability," or orbitals, by which we can predict the likelihood of finding electrons within given regions of space surrounding the nucleus. Both theories tell us that the energy levels available to electrons are not infinite but discrete and that the energy difference between levels is a precise amount called a quantum. The four quantum numbers completely describe the location and energy of any electron within a given atom. Finally, we learned two simple recall methods for the order in which electrons fill the shells and subshells of an atom and that the valence electrons are the reactive electrons in an atom. In the next chapter, we'll take a look at how the elements are organized on the periodic table and will then turn our attention to their bonding behavior—based on valence electrons—in Chapter 3 of *MCAT General Chemistry Review.*

GO ONLINE

You've reviewed the content, now test your knowledge and critical thinking skills by completing a test-like passage set in your online resources!

CONCEPT SUMMARY

Subatomic Particles

- **A proton** has a positive charge and mass around 1 amu; a **neutron** has no charge and mass around 1 amu; an **electron** has a negative charge and negligible mass.
- The **nucleus** contains the protons and neutrons, while the electrons move around the nucleus.
- The **atomic number** is the number of protons in a given element.
- The **mass number** is the sum of an element's protons and neutrons.

Atomic Mass vs. Atomic Weight

- **Atomic mass** is essentially equal to the mass number, the sum of an element's protons and neutrons.
  - **Isotopes** are atoms of a given element (same atomic number) that have different mass numbers. They differ in the number of neutrons.
  - Most isotopes are identified by the element followed by the mass number (such as carbon-12, carbon-13, and carbon-14).
  - The three isotopes of hydrogen go by different names: protium, deuterium, and tritium.
- **Atomic weight** is the weighted average of the naturally occurring isotopes of an element. The periodic table lists atomic weights, not atomic masses.

Rutherford, Planck, and Bohr

- Rutherford first postulated that the atom had a dense, positively charged nucleus that made up only a small fraction of the volume of the atom.
- In the **Bohr model of the atom**, a dense, positively charged nucleus is surrounded by electrons revolving around the nucleus in orbits with distinct energy levels.
- The energy difference between energy levels is called a **quantum**, first described by Planck.
  - Quantization means that there is not an infinite range of energy levels available to an electron; electrons can exist only at certain energy levels. The energy of an electron increases the farther it is from the nucleus.
  - The **atomic absorption spectrum** of an element is unique; for an electron to jump from a lower energy level to a higher one, it must absorb an amount of energy precisely equal to the energy difference between the two levels.
  - When electrons return from the excited state to the ground state, they emit an amount of energy that is exactly equal to the energy difference between the two levels; every element has a characteristic **atomic emission spectrum**, and sometimes the electromagnetic energy emitted corresponds to a frequency in the visible light range.

Quantum Mechanical Model of Atoms

- The **quantum mechanical model** posits that electrons do not travel in defined orbits but rather are localized in orbitals; an **orbital** is a region of space around the nucleus defined by the probability of finding an electron in that region of space.
- The **Heisenberg uncertainty principle** states that it is impossible to know both an electron's position and its momentum *exactly* at the same time.
- There are four **quantum numbers**; these numbers completely describe any electron in an atom.
  - The **principal quantum number, *n***, describes the average energy of a **shell**.
  - The **azimuthal quantum number, *l***, describes the **subshells** within a given principal energy level (*s*, *p*, *d*, and *f*).
  - The **magnetic quantum number, m_l**, specifies the particular **orbital** within a subshell where an electron is likely to be found at a given moment in time.
  - The **spin quantum number, m_s**, indicates the spin orientation $\left(\pm\frac{1}{2}\right)$ of an electron in an orbital.
- The **electron configuration** uses **spectroscopic notation** (combining the *n* and *l* values as a number and letter, respectively) to designate the location of electrons.
  - For example, $1s^2 2s^2 2p^6 3s^2$ is the electron configuration for magnesium: a neutral magnesium atom has 12 electrons—two in the *s* subshell of the first energy level, two in the *s* subshell of the second energy level, six in the *p* subshell of the second energy level, and two in the *s* subshell of the third energy level; the two electrons in the 3*s* subshell are the valence electrons for the magnesium atom.
- Electrons fill the principal energy levels and subshells according to increasing energy, which can be determined by the **$n + l$ rule**.
- Electrons fill orbitals according to **Hund's rule**, which states that subshells with multiple orbitals (*p*, *d*, and *f*) fill electrons so that every orbital in a subshell gets one electron before any of them gets a second.
  - **Paramagnetic** materials have unpaired electrons that align with magnetic fields, attracting the material to a magnet.
  - **Diamagnetic** materials have all paired electrons, which cannot easily be realigned; they are repelled by magnets.
- **Valence electrons** are those electrons in the outermost shell available for interaction (bonding) with other atoms.
  - For the representative elements (those in Groups 1, 2, and 13–18), the valence electrons are found in *s*- and/or *p*-orbitals.
  - For the transition elements, the valence electrons are found in *s*- and either *d*- or *f*-orbitals.
  - Many atoms interact with other atoms to form bonds that complete an octet in the valence shell.

ANSWERS TO CONCEPT CHECKS

1.1

1. Charge is determined by the number of electrons present. Atomic number is determined by the number of protons. Isotope is determined by the number of neutrons (while protons make up part of the mass number, it is the number of neutrons that explains the variability between isotopes).
2. ^{18}O: 8 p^+, 10 n^0, 8 e^-. ^{18}F: 9 p^+, 9 n^0, 9 e^-.

1.2

1. Atomic mass is (just slightly less than) the sum of the masses of protons and neutrons in a given atom of an element. Atoms of the same element with different mass numbers are isotopes of each other. The atomic weight is the weighted average of the naturally occurring isotopes of an element.
2. This ratio is an equivalent concept. It is therefore acceptable, as long as units can be cancelled in dimensional analysis.
3.

Isotope	Protons	Neutrons	Electrons
^{19}O	8	11	8
^{16}O	8	8	8
^{17}O	8	9	8
^{19}F	9	10	9
^{16}F	9	7	9
^{238}U	92	146	92
^{240}U	92	148	92

1.3

1. $E = R_H\left[\frac{1}{n_i^2} - \frac{1}{n_f^2}\right] = 2.18 \times 10^{-18}\left[\frac{1}{2^2} - \frac{1}{4^2}\right] \approx 2 \times 10^{-18}\left[\frac{3}{16}\right]$

$\approx 3.75 \times 10^{-19}\ \text{J} \approx 4 \times 10^{-19}\ \text{J}$ (actual value is 4.09×10^{-19} J).

$E = R_H\left[\frac{1}{n_i^2} - \frac{1}{n_f^2}\right] = 13.6\left[\frac{1}{2^2} - \frac{1}{4^2}\right] \approx (14)\left[\frac{3}{16}\right]$

$= \left(\frac{14 \times 3}{16}\right) = \left(\frac{7}{8} \times 3\right) = \left(\frac{21}{8}\right) \approx 2.5$ (actual value is 2.55 eV).

2. $3 \text{ eV}\left(1.60 \times 10^{-19}\frac{\text{J}}{\text{eV}}\right) = 4.8 \times 10^{-19}\text{J}$

$$E = \frac{hc}{\lambda} \rightarrow \lambda = \frac{hc}{E} = \frac{(6.626 \times 10^{-34}\text{J}\cdot\text{s})\left(3.00 \times 10^{8}\ \frac{\text{m}}{\text{s}}\right)}{(4.8 \times 10^{-19}\ \text{J})}$$

$$\approx \frac{(6.6 \times 3)(10^{-34} \times 10^{8})}{4.8 \times 10^{-19}} = \frac{6.6 \times 10^{-26}}{1.6 \times 10^{-19}} \approx \frac{6.4 \times 10^{-26}}{1.6 \times 10^{-19}} = \frac{64}{16} \times 10^{-26+19}$$

$$= 4 \times 10^{-7}\ \text{m} = 400\ \text{nm (actual value} = 4.14 \times 10^{-7} = 414\ \text{nm)}$$

3. $$E = \frac{hc}{\lambda} = \frac{(6.626 \times 10^{-34}\text{J}\cdot\text{s})\left(3.00 \times 10^{8}\ \frac{\text{m}}{\text{s}}\right)}{(6.62 \times 10^{-7}\ \text{m})}$$

$$= \frac{(6.626 \times 3.00)(10^{-34} \times 10^{8})}{6.62 \times 10^{-7}} = \frac{3.00 \times 10^{-26}}{10^{-7}} = 3.00 \times 10^{-26+7}$$

$$= 3.00 \times 10^{-19}\text{J}$$

1.4

1.

n	l	Possible Elements
2	1	2*p*: B, C, N, O, F, Ne
3	0	3*s*: Na, Mg
5	3	5*f*: Actinide series
4	2	4*d*: Y, Zr, Nb, Mo, Tc, Ru, Rh, Pd, Ag, Cd

2. Both O and O^{2-} have fully filled 1*s*- and 2*s*-orbitals. O has four electrons in the 2*p* subshell; two are paired, and the other two each have their own orbital. O^{2-} has six electrons in the 2*p* subshell, all of which are paired in the three *p*-orbitals.

3. Both these molecules have unfilled valence electron shells with relatively few paired electrons; therefore, they are paramagnetic.

4.

Atom	*s*-electrons	*p*-electrons	*d*-electrons	*f*-electrons	Total Valence Electrons
P in PO_4^{3-}	2	6	2	0	10
O in PO_4^{3-}	2	6	0	0	8
Ir	2	0	7	0	9
Cf	2	0	0	10	12

SCIENCE MASTERY ASSESSMENT EXPLANATIONS

1. **A**

Remember that when electrons are removed from an element, forming a cation, they will be removed from the subshell with the highest *n* value first. Zn^0 has 30 electrons, so it would have an electron configuration of $1s^22s^22p^63s^23p^64s^23d^{10}$. The 4*s* subshell has the highest principal quantum number, so it is emptied first, forming $1s^22s^22p^63s^23p^64s^03d^{10}$. **(B)** implies that electrons are pulled out of the *d* subshell, **(C)** presents the configuration of the uncharged zinc atom, and **(D)** shows the configuration that would exist if four electrons were removed.

2. **B**

The azimuthal quantum number *l* cannot be higher than $n - 1$, ruling out **(A)**. The m_l number, which describes the chemical's magnetic properties, can only be an integer value between $-l$ and l. It cannot be equal to ±1 if $l = 0$; this would imply that the *s* subshell has three orbitals (-1, 0, and 1) when we know it can only have one. This rules out **(C)** and **(D)**.

3. **C**

For any value of *n*, there will be a maximum of $2n^2$ electrons; that is, two per orbital. This can also be determined from the periodic table. There are only two elements (H and He) that have valence electrons in the $n = 1$ shell. Eight elements (Li to Ne) have valence electrons in the $n = 2$ shell. This is the only equation that matches this pattern.

4. **B**

This formula describes the number of electrons in terms of the azimuthal quantum number *l*, which ranges from 0 to $n - 1$, with *n* being the principal quantum number. A table of the maximum number of electrons per subshell is provided here:

Subshell	Azimuthal Quantum Number (*l*)	Number of Electrons
s	0	2
p	1	6
d	2	10
f	3	14

5. **D**

The only answer choice without unpaired electrons in its ground state is helium. Recall from the chapter that a diamagnetic substance is identified by the lack of unpaired electrons in its shell. A substance without unpaired electrons, like helium, cannot be magnetized by an external magnetic field and is actually slightly repelled. Elements that come at the end of a block (Group IIA, the group containing Zn, and the noble gases, most notably) have only paired electrons.

6. **D**

The problem requires the MCAT favorite equation $E = \frac{hc}{\lambda}$, where $h = 6.626 \times 10^{-34}\ \text{J} \cdot \text{s}$ (Planck's constant), $c = 3.00 \times 10^{8}\ \frac{\text{m}}{\text{s}}$ is the speed of light, and λ is the wavelength of the light. This question asks for the energy of one mole of photons, so we must multiply by Avogadro's number, $N_A = 6.02 \times 10^{23}\ \text{mol}^{-1}$.

The setup is: $E = \frac{hc}{\lambda} \times N_A$

$$= \frac{(6.626 \times 10^{-34}\ \text{J} \cdot \text{s})(3.00 \times 10^{8}\ \frac{\text{m}}{\text{s}})}{(500 \times 10^{-9}\ \text{m})} \times (6.02 \times 10^{23}\ \text{mol}^{-1})$$

$$= \frac{(6.626 \times 3 \times 6.02)(10^{-34} \times 10^{8} \times 10^{23})}{500 \times 10^{-9}}$$

$$\approx \frac{(7 \times 3 \times 6)(10^{-3})}{500 \times 10^{-9}}$$

$$= \frac{(21 \times 6)(10^{-3})}{500 \times 10^{-9}} \approx \frac{125}{500} \times 10^{-3+9} = \frac{1}{4} \times 10^{6}$$

$$= 2.5 \times 10^{5}\ \text{J}$$

As we rounded during calculation, we must find the answer choice that most closely matches this value. **(D)** is the closest match.

7. **B**

Because the electron is moving into the $n = 1$ shell, the only subshell available is the 1s subshell, which eliminates **(C)** and **(D)**. There will be some energy change, however, as the electron must lose energy to return to the minimum-energy ground state. That will require emitting radiation in the form of a photon.

8. **A**

Recall that the superscript refers to the mass number of an atom, which is equal to the number of protons plus the number of neutrons present in an element. Sometimes a text will list the atomic number, Z, as a subscript under the mass number, A. According to the periodic table, carbon contains six protons; therefore, its atomic number is 6. Isotopes all have the same number of protons, but differ in the number of neutrons. Almost all atoms with $Z > 1$ have at least one neutron. Carbon is most likely to have a mass number of 12, for six protons and six neutrons, as in **(B)**. **(C)** and **(D)** are possible isotopes that would have more neutrons than ^{12}C. The ^{6}C isotope is unlikely. It would mean that there are 6 protons and 0 neutrons. As shown in Figure 1.5, this would be a highly unstable isotope.

9. **C**

The limitations placed by the Heisenberg uncertainty principle are caused by limitations inherent in the measuring process: if a particle is moving, it has momentum, but trying to measure that momentum necessarily creates uncertainty in the position. Even if we had an exact definition of the meter, as in **(A)**, or perfect measuring devices, as in **(B)**, we still wouldn't be able to measure position *and* momentum simultaneously *and* exactly.

10. **B**

For the electron to *gain* energy, it must absorb energy from photons to jump up to a higher energy level. There is a bigger jump between $n = 2$ and $n = 6$ than there is between $n = 3$ and $n = 4$.

11. **A**

The MCAT covers the topics in this chapter qualitatively more often than quantitatively. It is critical to be able to distinguish the fundamental principles that determine electron organization, which are usually known by the names of the scientists who discovered or postulated them. The Heisenberg uncertainty principle, **(B)**, refers to the inability to know the momentum and position of a single electron simultaneously. The Bohr model, **(C)**, was an early attempt to describe the behavior of the single electron in a hydrogen atom. The Rutherford model, **(D)**, described a dense, positively charged nucleus. The element shown here, phosphorus, is often used to demonstrate Hund's rule because it contains a half-filled *p* subshell. Hund's rule explains that electrons fill empty orbitals first before doubling up electrons in the same orbital.

12. **A**

The quickest way to solve this problem is to use the periodic table and find out how many protons are in Cs atoms; there are 55. Neutral Cs atoms would also have 55 electrons. A stable Cs cation will have a single positive charge because it has one unpaired *s*-electron. This translates to one fewer electron than the number of protons or 54 electrons.

13. **B**

The easiest way to approach this problem is to set up a system of two algebraic equations, where H and D are the percentages of H (mass = 1 amu) and D (mass = 2 amu), respectively. Your setup should look like the following system:

$$\text{H} + \text{D} = 1 \text{ (percent H + percent D = 100\%)}$$

$$1\,\text{H} + 2\,\text{D} = 1.008 \text{ (atomic weight calculation)}$$

Rearranging the first equation and substituting into the second yields $(1 - \text{D}) + 2\text{D} = 1.008$, or $\text{D} = 0.008$. 0.008 is 0.8%, so there is 0.8% D.

14. **A**

The terms in the answer choices refer to the magnetic spin of the two electrons. The quantum number m_s represents this property as a measure of an electron's intrinsic spin. These electrons' spins are parallel, in that their spins are aligned in the same direction ($m_s = +\frac{1}{2}$ for both species).

15. **B**

When dealing with ions, you cannot directly approach electronic configurations based on the number of electrons they currently hold. First examine the neutral atom's configuration, and then determine which electrons are removed.

Neutral Atom's Configuration	Ion's Configuration
Cr^0: [Ar] $4s^1 3d^5$	—
Mn^0: [Ar] $4s^2 3d^5$	Mn^+: [Ar] $4s^1 3d^5$
Fe^0: [Ar] $4s^2 3d^6$	Fe^{2+}: [Ar] $4s^0 3d^6$

Due to the stability of half-filled *d*-orbitals, neutral chromium assumes the electron configuration of [Ar] $4s^1 3d^5$. Mn must lose one electron from its initial configuration to become the Mn^+ cation. That electron would come from the 4*s* subshell according to the rule that the first electron removed comes from the highest-energy shell. Fe must lose two electrons to become Fe^{2+}. They'll both be lost from the same orbital; the only way Fe^{2+} could hold the configuration in the question stem would be if one *d*-electron and one *s*-electron were lost together.

GO ONLINE

Consult your online resources for additional practice.

EQUATIONS TO REMEMBER

(1.1) **Planck relation (frequency):** $E = hf$

(1.2) **Angular momentum of an electron (Bohr model):** $L = \frac{nh}{2\pi}$

(1.3) **Energy of an electron (Bohr model):** $E = -\frac{R_H}{n^2}$

(1.4) **Planck relation (wavelength):** $E = \frac{hc}{\lambda}$

(1.5) **Energy of electron transition (Bohr model):** $E = R_H \left[\frac{1}{n_i^2} - \frac{1}{n_f^2}\right]$

(1.6) **Maximum number of electrons within a shell:** $2n^2$

(1.7) **Maximum number of electrons within a subshell:** $4l + 2$

SHARED CONCEPTS

General Chemistry Chapter 2
The Periodic Table

General Chemistry Chapter 3
Bonding and Chemical Interactions

Organic Chemistry Chapter 3
Bonding

Physics and Math Chapter 2
Work and Energy

Physics and Math Chapter 8
Light and Optics

Physics and Math Chapter 9
Atomic and Nuclear Phenomena

CHAPTER 2

THE PERIODIC TABLE

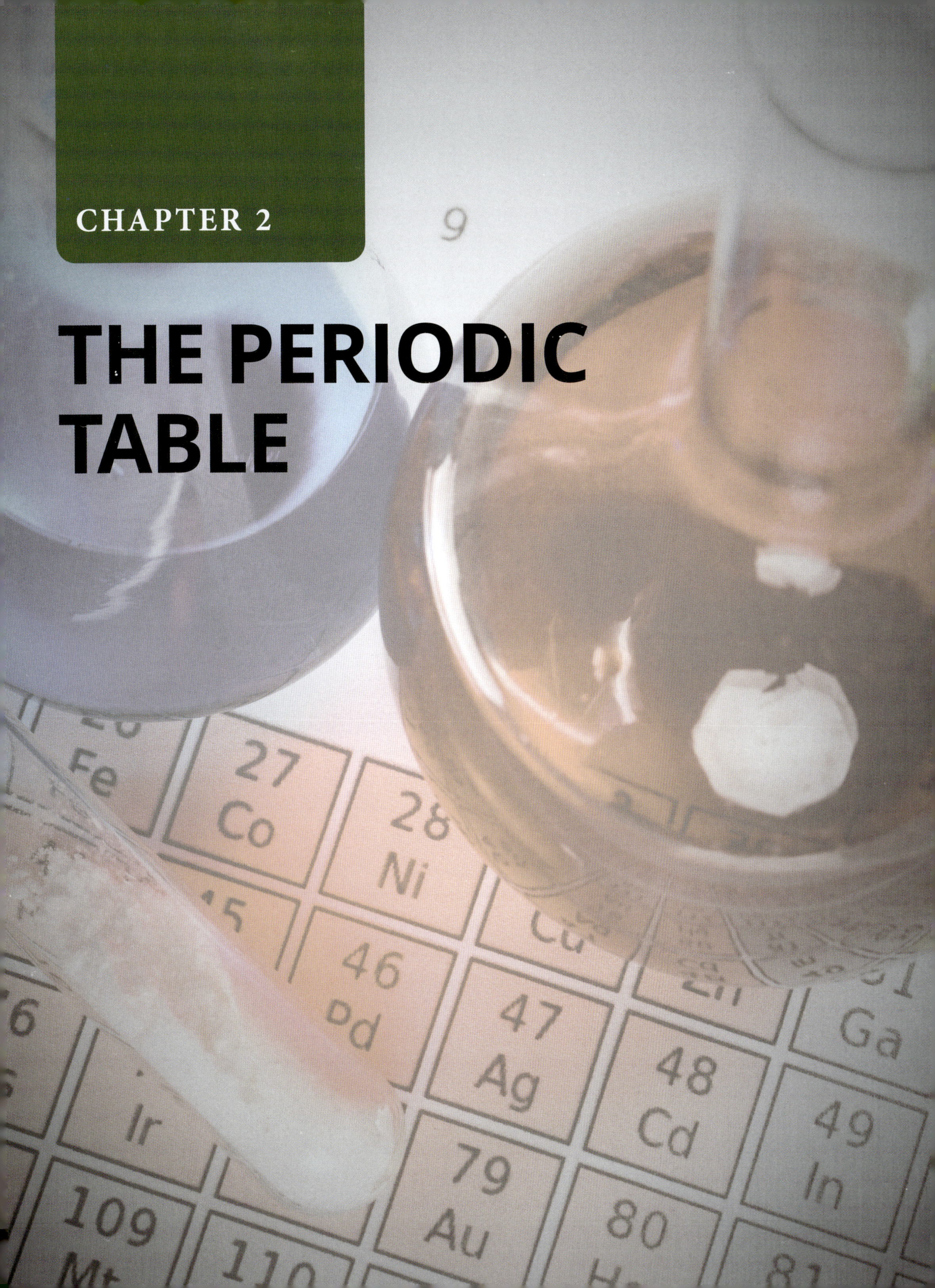

SCIENCE MASTERY ASSESSMENT

Every pre-med knows this feeling: there is so much content I have to know for the MCAT! How do I know what to do first or what's important?

While the high-yield badges throughout this book will help you identify the most important topics, this Science Mastery Assessment is another tool in your MCAT prep arsenal. This quiz (which can also be taken in your online resources) and the guidance below will help ensure that you are spending the appropriate amount of time on this chapter based on your personal strengths and weaknesses. Don't worry though—skipping something now does not mean you'll never study it. Later on in your prep, as you complete full-length tests, you'll uncover specific pieces of content that you need to review and can come back to these chapters as appropriate.

How to Use This Assessment

If you answer 0–7 questions correctly:

Spend about 1 hour to read this chapter in full and take limited notes throughout. Follow up by reviewing **all** quiz questions to ensure that you now understand how to solve each one.

If you answer 8–11 questions correctly:

Spend 20–40 minutes reviewing the quiz questions. Beginning with the questions you missed, read and take notes on the corresponding subchapters. For questions you answered correctly, ensure your thinking matches that of the explanation and you understand why each choice was correct or incorrect.

If you answer 12–15 questions correctly:

Spend less than 20 minutes reviewing all questions from the quiz. If you missed any, then include a quick read-through of the corresponding subchapters, or even just the relevant content within a subchapter, as part of your question review. For questions you answered correctly, ensure your thinking matches that of the explanation and review the Concept Summary at the end of the chapter.

1. Lithium and sodium have similar chemical properties. For example, both can form ionic bonds with chloride. Which of the following best explains this similarity?
   - A. Both lithium and sodium ions are positively charged.
   - B. Lithium and sodium are in the same group of the periodic table.
   - C. Lithium and sodium are in the same period of the periodic table.
   - D. Both lithium and sodium have low atomic weights.

2. Carbon and silicon are the basis of biological life and synthetic computing, respectively. While these elements share many chemical properties, which of the following best describes a difference between the two elements?
   - A. Carbon has a smaller atomic radius than silicon.
   - B. Silicon has a smaller atomic radius than carbon.
   - C. Carbon has fewer valence electrons than silicon.
   - D. Silicon has fewer valence electrons than carbon.

3. Which of the following elements has the highest electronegativity?
   - A. Mg
   - B. Cl
   - C. Zn
   - D. I

4. Ionization energy contributes to an atom's chemical reactivity. Which of the following shows an accurate ranking of ionization energies from lowest to highest?
   - A. First ionization energy of Be < second ionization energy of Be < first ionization energy of Li
   - B. First ionization energy of Be < first ionization energy of Li < second ionization energy of Be
   - C. First ionization energy of Li < first ionization energy of Be < second ionization energy of Be
   - D. First ionization energy of Li < second ionization energy of Be < first ionization energy of Be

5. Antimony is used in some antiparasitic medications—specifically those targeting *Leishmania donovani*. What type of element is antimony?
   - A. Metal
   - B. Metalloid
   - C. Halogen
   - D. Nonmetal

6. The properties of atoms can be predicted, to some extent, by their location within the periodic table. Which property or properties increase in the direction of the arrows shown?

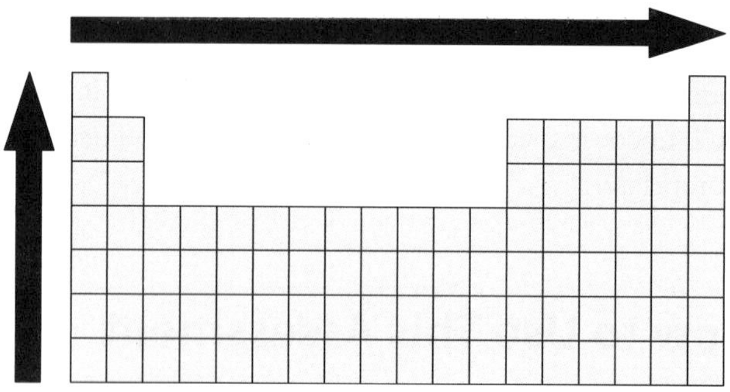

   - I. Electronegativity
   - II. Atomic radius
   - III. First ionization energy

   - A. I only
   - B. I and II only
   - C. I and III only
   - D. II and III only

7. Metals are often used for making wires that conduct electricity. Which of the following properties of metals explains why?
   - A. Metals are malleable.
   - B. Metals have low electronegativities.
   - C. Metals have valence electrons that can move freely.
   - D. Metals have high melting points.

8. Which of the following is an important property of the group of elements shaded in the periodic table below?

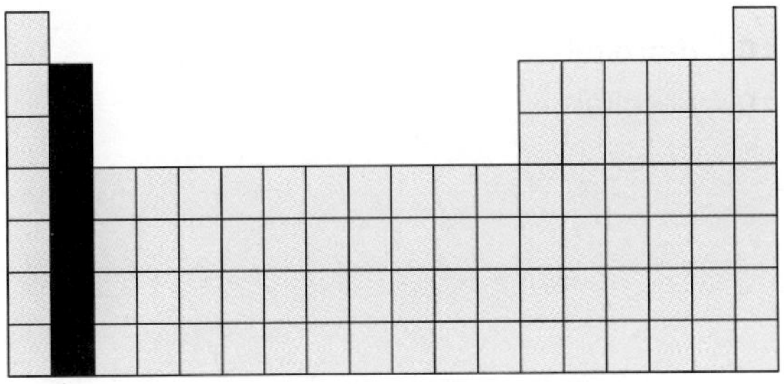

A. These elements are the best electrical conductors in the periodic table.
B. These elements form divalent cations.
C. The second ionization energy for these elements is lower than the first ionization energy.
D. The atomic radii of these elements decrease as one moves down the column.

9. When dissolved in water, which of the following ions is most likely to form a complex ion with H_2O?
A. Na^+
B. Fe^{2+}
C. Cl^-
D. S^{2-}

10. How many valence electrons are present in elements in the third period?
A. 2
B. 3
C. The number decreases as the atomic number increases.
D. The number increases as the atomic number increases.

11. Arsenic mediates some of its toxic effects via the inhibition of acetyl-CoA formation and the inhibition of the enzyme succinic dehydrogenase to decrease ATP production. In addition to its metabolic effects, arsenic can also replace phosphorus in many reactions. Which of the following best explains the similarity between these two elements?
A. Similar atomic numbers
B. Similar number of electrons
C. Similar valence configuration
D. Similar atomic radius

12. Of the four atoms depicted here, which has the highest electron affinity?
A.
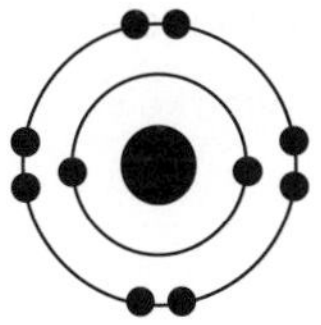
B.
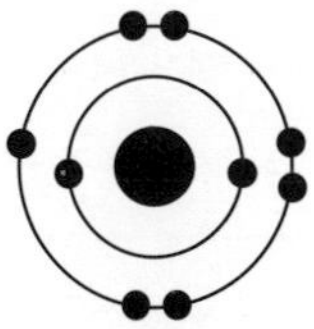
C.
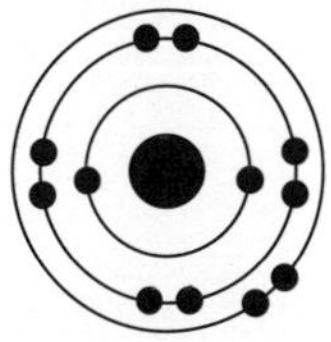
D.
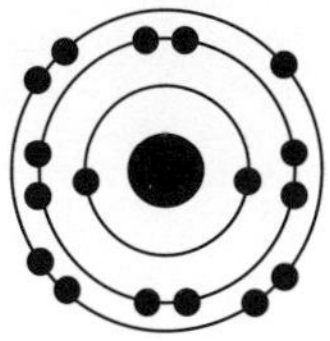

13. Which of the following atoms or ions has the largest effective nuclear charge?
   A. Cl
   B. Cl^-
   C. K
   D. K^+

14. Why do halogens often form ionic bonds with alkaline earth metals?
   A. The alkaline earth metals have much higher electron affinities than the halogens.
   B. By sharing electrons equally, the alkaline earth metals and halogens both form full octets.
   C. Within the same row, the halogens have smaller atomic radii than the alkaline earth metals.
   D. The halogens have much higher electron affinities than the alkaline earth metals.

15. What is the highest-energy orbital of elements with valence electrons in the $n = 3$ shell?
   A. *s*-orbital
   B. *p*-orbital
   C. *d*-orbital
   D. *f*-orbital

Answer Key follows on next page.

Answer Key

1. **B** (See section 2.4)
2. **A** (See section 2.2)
3. **B** (See section 2.2)
4. **C** (See section 2.3)
5. **B** (See section 2.2)
6. **C** (See section 2.3)
7. **C** (See section 2.3)
8. **B** (See section 2.3)
9. **B** (See section 2.3)
10. **D** (See section 2.1)
11. **C** (See section 2.1)
12. **D** (See section 2.3)
13. **D** (See section 2.3)
14. **D** (See section 2.4)
15. **C** (See section 2.1)

The relevant section of the chapter to review for each question is given in parentheses after the correct answer. Detailed explanations can be found at the end of the chapter.

CHAPTER 2

THE PERIODIC TABLE

In This Chapter

CHAPTER PROFILE

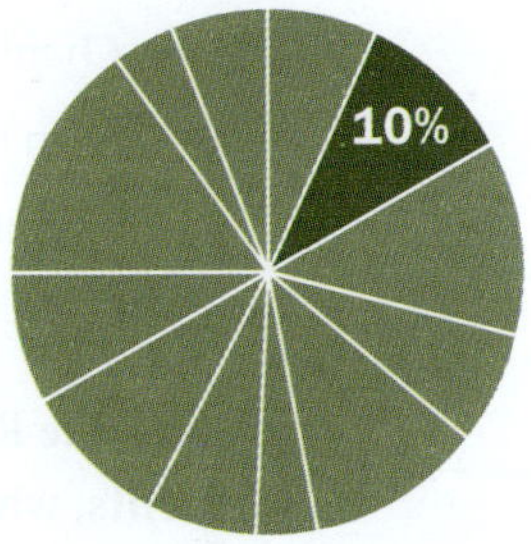

The content in this chapter should be relevant to about 10% of all questions about general chemistry on the MCAT.

This chapter covers material from the following AAMC content category:

4E: Atoms, nuclear decay, electronic structure, and atomic chemical behavior

Introduction

The pharmacological history of lithium is an interesting window into the scientific and medical communities' attempts to take advantage of the chemical and physical properties of an element for human benefit. By the mid-1800s, the medical community was showing great interest in theories that linked uric acid to a myriad of maladies. When it was discovered that solutions of lithium carbonate dissolved uric acid, therapeutic preparations containing lithium carbonate salt became popular. Even nonmedical companies tried to profit from lithium's reputation as a cure-all by adding it to their soft drinks.

Eventually, fascination with theories of uric acid wore off, and lithium's time in the spotlight seemed to be coming to an end. Then, in the 1940s, doctors began to recommend salt-restricted diets for cardiac patients. Lithium chloride was made commercially available as a sodium chloride (table salt) substitute. Unfortunately, lithium is quite toxic at fairly low concentrations, and when medical literature in the late 1940s reported several incidents of severe poisonings and multiple deaths—some associated with only minor lithium overdosing—U.S. companies voluntarily withdrew all lithium salts from the market. Right around this time, John Cade, a psychiatrist from Australia, proposed the use of lithium salts for the treatment of mania. Cade's clinical trials were quite successful. In fact, his use of lithium salts to control mania was the first instance of successful medical treatment of a mental illness, and lithium carbonate became commonly prescribed in Europe for manic behavior. Not until 1970 did the U.S. Food and Drug Administration finally approve the use of lithium carbonate for manic symptoms.

Lithium (Li) is the element with the atomic number 3. It is a very soft alkali metal, and under standard conditions, it is the least dense solid element (specific gravity = 0.53). Lithium is so reactive that it does not naturally occur on earth in its elemental form and is found only in various salt compounds.

Why would medical scientists pay attention to this particular element? What would make doctors believe that lithium chloride would be a good substitute for sodium chloride for patients on salt-restricted diets? The answers lie in the periodic table.

2.1 The Periodic Table

LEARNING OBJECTIVES

After Chapter 2.1, you will be able to:

- Explain how the modern periodic table is organized
- Differentiate between representative and nonrepresentative elements

In 1869, the Russian chemist Dmitri Mendeleev published the first version of his **Periodic Table of the Elements**, which showed that ordering the known elements according to atomic weight revealed a pattern of periodically recurring physical and chemical properties. Since then, the periodic table has been revised, using the work of English physicist Henry Moseley, to organize the elements based on increasing atomic number (the number of protons in an element) rather than atomic weight. Using this revised table, many properties of elements that had not yet been discovered could be predicted. The periodic table creates a visual representation of the **periodic law**, which states: *the chemical and physical properties of the elements are dependent, in a periodic way, upon their atomic numbers.*

The modern periodic table arranges the elements into **periods** (rows) and **groups** or **families** (columns), based on atomic number, as seen in Figure 2.1. There are seven periods representing the principal quantum numbers $n = 1$ through $n = 7$ for the *s*- and *p*-block elements. Each period is filled sequentially, and each element in a given period has one more proton and one more electron than the element to its left (in their neutral states). Groups contain elements that have the same electronic configuration in their **valence shell** and share similar chemical properties.

The electrons in the valence shell, known as the **valence electrons**, are the farthest from the nucleus and have the greatest amount of potential energy. Their higher potential energy and the fact that they are held less tightly by the nucleus allows them to become involved in chemical bonds with the valence electrons of other atoms; thus, the valence shell electrons largely determine the chemical reactivity and properties of the element.

BRIDGE

Recall from Chapter 1 of *MCAT General Chemistry Review* that periods (rows) graphically represent the principal quantum number, and groups (columns) help to determine the valence electron configuration.

MCAT EXPERTISE

Relating valence electrons to reactivity is important. Elements with similar valence electron configurations generally behave in similar ways, as long as they are the same type (metal, nonmetal, or metalloid).

Period ↓ / Group →	IA	IIA	IIIB	IVB	VB	VIB	VIIB	VIIIB	VIIIB	VIIIB	IB	IIB	IIIA	IVA	VA	VIA	VIIA	VIIIA
1	1 **H** 1.0																	2 **He** 4.0
2	3 **Li** 6.9	4 **Be** 9.0											5 **B** 10.8	6 **C** 12.0	7 **N** 14.0	8 **O** 16.0	9 **F** 19.0	10 **Ne** 20.2
3	11 **Na** 23.0	12 **Mg** 24.3											13 **Al** 27.0	14 **Si** 28.1	15 **P** 31.0	16 **S** 32.1	17 **Cl** 35.5	18 **Ar** 39.9
4	19 **K** 39.1	20 **Ca** 40.1	21 **Sc** 45.0	22 **Ti** 47.9	23 **V** 50.9	24 **Cr** 52.0	25 **Mn** 54.9	26 **Fe** 55.8	27 **Co** 58.9	28 **Ni** 58.7	29 **Cu** 63.5	30 **Zn** 65.4	31 **Ga** 69.7	32 **Ge** 72.6	33 **As** 74.9	34 **Se** 79.0	35 **Br** 79.9	36 **Kr** 83.8
5	37 **Rb** 85.5	38 **Sr** 87.6	39 **Y** 88.9	40 **Zr** 91.2	41 **Nb** 92.9	42 **Mo** 95.9	43 **Tc** (98)	44 **Ru** 101.1	45 **Rh** 102.9	46 **Pd** 106.4	47 **Ag** 107.9	48 **Cd** 112.4	49 **In** 114.8	50 **Sn** 118.7	51 **Sb** 121.8	52 **Te** 127.6	53 **I** 126.9	54 **Xe** 131.3
6	55 **Cs** 132.9	56 **Ba** 137.3	57 **La*** 138.9	72 **Hf** 178.5	73 **Ta** 180.9	74 **W** 183.9	75 **Re** 186.2	76 **Os** 190.2	77 **Ir** 192.2	78 **Pt** 195.1	79 **Au** 197.0	80 **Hg** 200.6	81 **Tl** 204.4	82 **Pb** 207.2	83 **Bi** 209.0	84 **Po** (209)	85 **At** (210)	86 **Rn** (222)
7	87 **Fr** (223)	88 **Ra** (226)	89 **Ac†** (227)	104 **Rf** (267)	105 **Db** (268)	106 **Sg** (271)	107 **Bh** (270)	108 **Hs** (269)	109 **Mt** (278)	110 **Ds** (281)	111 **Rg** (282)	112 **Cn** (285)	113 **Nh** (286)	114 **Fl** (289)	115 **Mc** (289)	116 **Lv** (293)	117 **Ts** (294)	118 **Og** (294)

*	58 **Ce** 140.1	59 **Pr** 140.9	60 **Nd** 144.2	61 **Pm** (145)	62 **Sm** 150.4	63 **Eu** 152.0	64 **Gd** 157.3	65 **Tb** 158.9	66 **Dy** 162.5	67 **Ho** 164.9	68 **Er** 167.3	69 **Tm** 168.9	70 **Yb** 173.0	71 **Lu** 173.0
†	90 **Th** 232.0	91 **Pa** (231)	92 **U** 238.0	93 **Np** (237)	94 **Pu** (244)	95 **Am** (243)	96 **Cm** (247)	97 **Bk** (247)	98 **Cf** (251)	99 **Es** (252)	100 **Fm** (257)	101 **Md** (258)	102 **No** (259)	103 **Lr** (266)

Figure 2.1 The Periodic Table of Elements

The Roman numeral above each group represents the number of valence electrons elements in that group have in their neutral state. The Roman numeral is combined with the letter A or B to separate the elements into two larger classes. The **A elements** are known as the **representative elements** and include groups IA through VIIIA. The elements in these groups have their valence electrons in the orbitals of either *s* or *p* subshells. The **B elements** are known as the **nonrepresentative elements** and include both the **transition elements**, which have valence electrons in the *s* and *d* subshells, and the **lanthanide** and **actinide series**, which have valence electrons in the *s* and *f* subshells. For the representative elements, the Roman numeral and the letter designation determine the electron configuration. For example, an element in Group VA has five valence electrons with the configuration s^2p^3. As described in Chapter 1 of *MCAT General Chemistry Review*, the nonrepresentative elements may have unexpected electron configurations, such as chromium ($4s^13d^5$) and copper ($4s^13d^{10}$). In the modern IUPAC identification system, the groups are numbered 1 to 18 and are not subdivided into Group A and Group B elements.

MCAT CONCEPT CHECK 2.1

Before you move on, assess your understanding of the material with these questions.

1. Mendeleev's table was arranged by atomic weight, but the modern periodic table is arranged by:

____

2. Which of the following are representative elements (A), and which are nonrepresentative (B)?

Element	A or B	Element	A or B	Element	A or B	Element	A or B
Ag		Al		K		P	
Pb		Li		Pu		U	
Cu		Cf		Zn		B	
N		Np		O		He	

2.2 Types of Elements

LEARNING OBJECTIVES

After Chapter 2.2, you will be able to:

- Classify elements as metal, nonmetal, or metalloid
- Predict the traits of an element given its location on a periodic table:

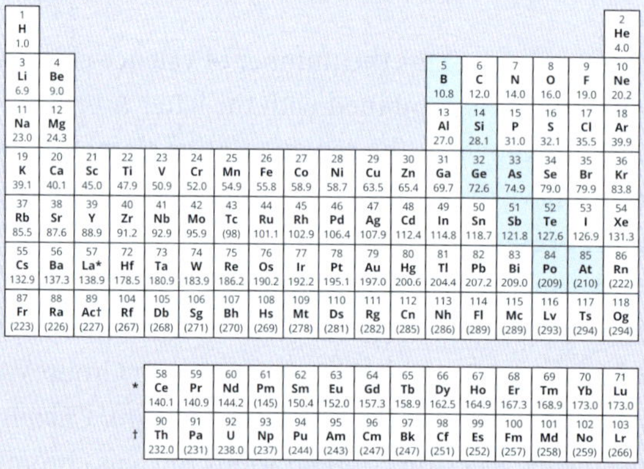

When we consider the trends of chemical reactivity and physical properties together, we can begin to identify groups of elements with similar characteristics. These larger collections are divided into three categories: metals, nonmetals, and metalloids (also called semimetals).

Metals

Metals are found on the left side and in the middle of the periodic table, as seen in Figure 2.2. They include the active metals, the transition metals, and the lanthanide and actinide series of elements. Metals are **lustrous** (shiny) solids, except for mercury, which is a liquid under standard conditions. They generally have high melting points and densities, but there are exceptions, such as lithium, which has a density about half that of water. Metals have the ability to be deformed without breaking; the ability of metal to be hammered into shapes is called **malleability**, and its ability to be pulled or drawn into wires is called **ductility**. At the atomic level, a metal is defined by a low effective nuclear charge, low electronegativity (high **electropositivity**), large atomic radius, small ionic radius, low ionization energy, and low electron affinity. All of these characteristics are manifestations of the ability of metals to easily give up electrons.

Metal properties

- Malleable
- Ductile
- Conductors

1 **H** 1.0																	2 **He** 4.0
3 **Li** 6.9	4 **Be** 9.0											5 **B** 10.8	6 **C** 12.0	7 **N** 14.0	8 **O** 16.0	9 **F** 19.0	10 **Ne** 20.2
11 **Na** 23.0	12 **Mg** 24.3											13 **Al** 27.0	14 **Si** 28.1	15 **P** 31.0	16 **S** 32.1	17 **Cl** 35.5	18 **Ar** 39.9
19 **K** 39.1	20 **Ca** 40.1	21 **Sc** 45.0	22 **Ti** 47.9	23 **V** 50.9	24 **Cr** 52.0	25 **Mn** 54.9	26 **Fe** 55.8	27 **Co** 58.9	28 **Ni** 58.7	29 **Cu** 63.5	30 **Zn** 65.4	31 **Ga** 69.7	32 **Ge** 72.6	33 **As** 74.9	34 **Se** 79.0	35 **Br** 79.9	36 **Kr** 83.8
37 **Rb** 85.5	38 **Sr** 87.6	39 **Y** 88.9	40 **Zr** 91.2	41 **Nb** 92.9	42 **Mo** 95.9	43 **Tc** (98)	44 **Ru** 101.1	45 **Rh** 102.9	46 **Pd** 106.4	47 **Ag** 107.9	48 **Cd** 112.4	49 **In** 114.8	50 **Sn** 118.7	51 **Sb** 121.8	52 **Te** 127.6	53 **I** 126.9	54 **Xe** 131.3
55 **Cs** 132.9	56 **Ba** 137.3	57 **La*** 138.9	72 **Hf** 178.5	73 **Ta** 180.9	74 **W** 183.9	75 **Re** 186.2	76 **Os** 190.2	77 **Ir** 192.2	78 **Pt** 195.1	79 **Au** 197.0	80 **Hg** 200.6	81 **Tl** 204.4	82 **Pb** 207.2	83 **Bi** 209.0	84 **Po** (209)	85 **At** (210)	86 **Rn** (222)
87 **Fr** (223)	88 **Ra** (226)	89 **Act** (227)	104 **Rf** (267)	105 **Db** (268)	106 **Sg** (271)	107 **Bh** (270)	108 **Hs** (269)	109 **Mt** (278)	110 **Ds** (281)	111 **Rg** (282)	112 **Cn** (285)	113 **Nh** (286)	114 **Fl** (289)	115 **Mc** (289)	116 **Lv** (293)	117 **Ts** (294)	118 **Og** (294)

*	58 **Ce** 140.1	59 **Pr** 140.9	60 **Nd** 144.2	61 **Pm** (145)	62 **Sm** 150.4	63 **Eu** 152.0	64 **Gd** 157.3	65 **Tb** 158.9	66 **Dy** 162.5	67 **Ho** 164.9	68 **Er** 167.3	69 **Tm** 168.9	70 **Yb** 173.0	71 **Lu** 173.0
†	90 **Th** 232.0	91 **Pa** (231)	92 **U** 238.0	93 **Np** (237)	94 **Pu** (244)	95 **Am** (243)	96 **Cm** (247)	97 **Bk** (247)	98 **Cf** (251)	99 **Es** (252)	100 **Fm** (257)	101 **Md** (258)	102 **No** (259)	103 **Lr** (266)

Figure 2.2 Metals of the Periodic Table

Many of the transition metals (Group B elements) have two or more **oxidation states** (charges when forming bonds with other atoms). Because the valence electrons of all metals are only loosely held to their atoms, they are free to move, which makes metals good **conductors** of heat and electricity. The valence electrons of the active metals are found in the *s* subshell; those of the transition metals are found in the *s* and *d* subshells; and those of the lanthanide and actinide series elements are in the *s* and *f* subshells. Some transition metals—copper, nickel, silver, gold, palladium, and platinum—are relatively nonreactive, a property that makes them ideal for the production of coins and jewelry.

KEY CONCEPT

Alkali and alkaline earth metals are both metallic in nature because they easily lose electrons from the *s* subshell of their valence shells.

An example of a metal is shown in Figure 2.3 with a copper wire. The wire exhibits luster, malleability, and ductility. It is used as a wire because it also exhibits good heat and electrical conductivity.

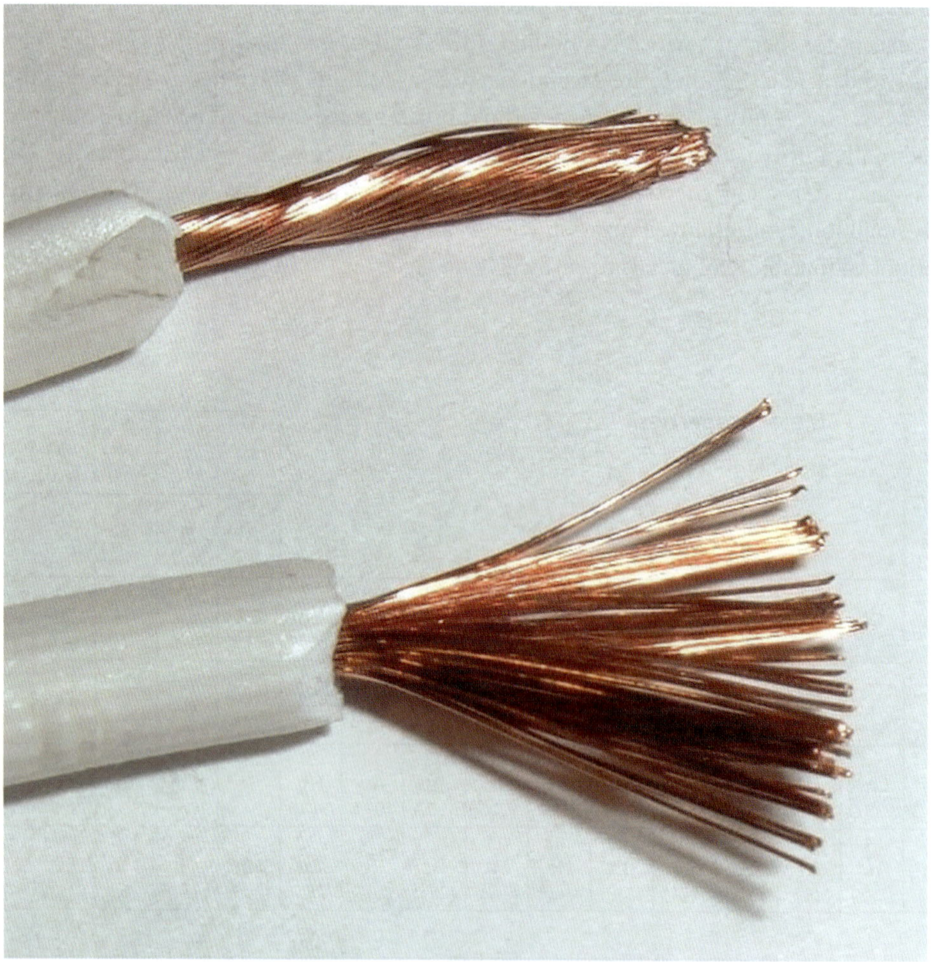

Figure 2.3 Copper (Cu) Metal Wire

Nonmetals

Nonmetals are found predominantly on the upper right side of the periodic table, as shown in Figure 2.4. Nonmetals are generally brittle in the solid state and show little or no metallic luster. They have high ionization energies, electron affinities, and electronegativities, as well as small atomic radii and large ionic radii. They are usually poor conductors of heat and electricity. All of these characteristics are manifestations of the *inability* of nonmetals to easily give up electrons. Nonmetals are less unified in their chemical and physical properties than the metals.

Nonmetal properties

- Brittle
- Poor conductors

1 **H** 1.0																	2 **He** 4.0
3 **Li** 6.9	4 **Be** 9.0											5 **B** 10.8	6 **C** 12.0	7 **N** 14.0	8 **O** 16.0	9 **F** 19.0	10 **Ne** 20.2
11 **Na** 23.0	12 **Mg** 24.3											13 **Al** 27.0	14 **Si** 28.1	15 **P** 31.0	16 **S** 32.1	17 **Cl** 35.5	18 **Ar** 39.9
19 **K** 39.1	20 **Ca** 40.1	21 **Sc** 45.0	22 **Ti** 47.9	23 **V** 50.9	24 **Cr** 52.0	25 **Mn** 54.9	26 **Fe** 55.8	27 **Co** 58.9	28 **Ni** 58.7	29 **Cu** 63.5	30 **Zn** 65.4	31 **Ga** 69.7	32 **Ge** 72.6	33 **As** 74.9	34 **Se** 79.0	35 **Br** 79.9	36 **Kr** 83.8
37 **Rb** 85.5	38 **Sr** 87.6	39 **Y** 88.9	40 **Zr** 91.2	41 **Nb** 92.9	42 **Mo** 95.9	43 **Tc** (98)	44 **Ru** 101.1	45 **Rh** 102.9	46 **Pd** 106.4	47 **Ag** 107.9	48 **Cd** 112.4	49 **In** 114.8	50 **Sn** 118.7	51 **Sb** 121.8	52 **Te** 127.6	53 **I** 126.9	54 **Xe** 131.3
55 **Cs** 132.9	56 **Ba** 137.3	57 **La*** 138.9	72 **Hf** 178.5	73 **Ta** 180.9	74 **W** 183.9	75 **Re** 186.2	76 **Os** 190.2	77 **Ir** 192.2	78 **Pt** 195.1	79 **Au** 197.0	80 **Hg** 200.6	81 **Tl** 204.4	82 **Pb** 207.2	83 **Bi** 209.0	84 **Po** (209)	85 **At** (210)	86 **Rn** (222)
87 **Fr** (223)	88 **Ra** (226)	89 **Ac†** (227)	104 **Rf** (267)	105 **Db** (268)	106 **Sg** (271)	107 **Bh** (270)	108 **Hs** (269)	109 **Mt** (278)	110 **Ds** (281)	111 **Rg** (282)	112 **Cn** (285)	113 **Nh** (286)	114 **Fl** (289)	115 **Mc** (289)	116 **Lv** (293)	117 **Ts** (294)	118 **Og** (294)

*	58 **Ce** 140.1	59 **Pr** 140.9	60 **Nd** 144.2	61 **Pm** (145)	62 **Sm** 150.4	63 **Eu** 152.0	64 **Gd** 157.3	65 **Tb** 158.9	66 **Dy** 162.5	67 **Ho** 164.9	68 **Er** 167.3	69 **Tm** 168.9	70 **Yb** 173.0	71 **Lu** 173.0
†	90 **Th** 232.0	91 **Pa** (231)	92 **U** 238.0	93 **Np** (237)	94 **Pu** (244)	95 **Am** (243)	96 **Cm** (247)	97 **Bk** (247)	98 **Cf** (251)	99 **Es** (252)	100 **Fm** (257)	101 **Md** (258)	102 **No** (259)	103 **Lr** (266)

Figure 2.4 Nonmetals of the Periodic Table

Carbon, shown in Figure 2.5, is a stereotypical nonmetal that retains a solid structure but is brittle, nonlustrous, and generally a poor conductor of heat and electricity.

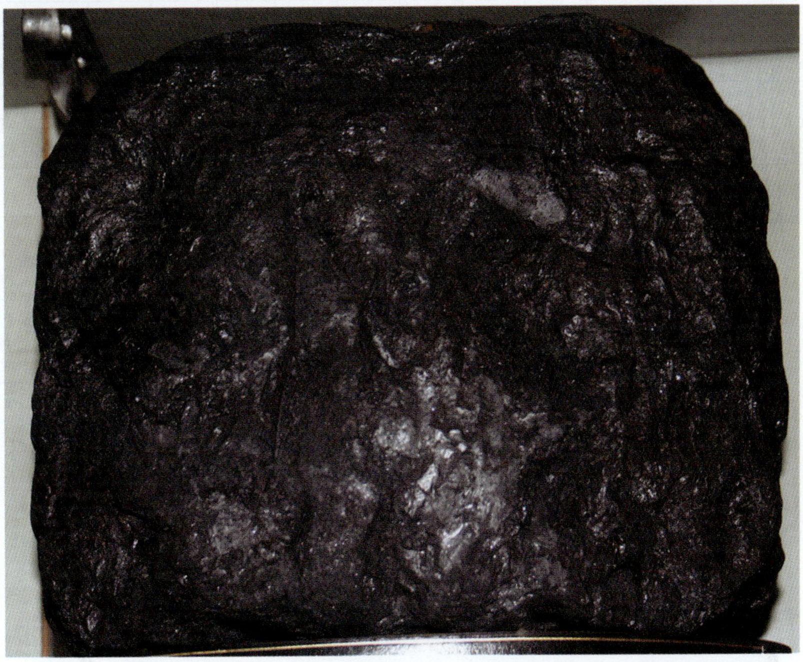

Figure 2.5 Charcoal, Composed of the Nonmetal Carbon (C)

Metalloids

Separating the metals and nonmetals are a stair-step group of elements called the **metalloids**, as seen in Figure 2.6. The metalloids are also called **semimetals** because they share some characteristics with both metals and nonmetals. The electronegativities and ionization energies of the metalloids lie between those of metals and nonmetals. Their physical properties—densities, melting points, and boiling points—vary widely and can be combinations of metallic and nonmetallic characteristics. For example, silicon (Si) has a metallic luster but is brittle and a poor conductor. The reactivities of the metalloids are dependent on the elements with which they are reacting. Boron (B), for example, behaves like a nonmetal when reacting with sodium (Na) and like a metal when reacting with fluorine (F). The elements classified as metalloids form a "staircase" on the periodic table and include boron, silicon, germanium (Ge), arsenic (As), antimony (Sb), tellurium (Te), polonium (Po), and astatine (At). While there is debate over polonium and astatine's status as metalloids, most sources label them as such.

REAL WORLD

Metalloids share some properties with metals and others with nonmetals. For instance, metalloids make good semiconductors due to their partial conductivity of electricity.

1 **H** 1.0																	2 **He** 4.0
3 **Li** 6.9	4 **Be** 9.0											5 **B** 10.8	6 **C** 12.0	7 **N** 14.0	8 **O** 16.0	9 **F** 19.0	10 **Ne** 20.2
11 **Na** 23.0	12 **Mg** 24.3											13 **Al** 27.0	14 **Si** 28.1	15 **P** 31.0	16 **S** 32.1	17 **Cl** 35.5	18 **Ar** 39.9
19 **K** 39.1	20 **Ca** 40.1	21 **Sc** 45.0	22 **Ti** 47.9	23 **V** 50.9	24 **Cr** 52.0	25 **Mn** 54.9	26 **Fe** 55.8	27 **Co** 58.9	28 **Ni** 58.7	29 **Cu** 63.5	30 **Zn** 65.4	31 **Ga** 69.7	32 **Ge** 72.6	33 **As** 74.9	34 **Se** 79.0	35 **Br** 79.9	36 **Kr** 83.8
37 **Rb** 85.5	38 **Sr** 87.6	39 **Y** 88.9	40 **Zr** 91.2	41 **Nb** 92.9	42 **Mo** 95.9	43 **Tc** (98)	44 **Ru** 101.1	45 **Rh** 102.9	46 **Pd** 106.4	47 **Ag** 107.9	48 **Cd** 112.4	49 **In** 114.8	50 **Sn** 118.7	51 **Sb** 121.8	52 **Te** 127.6	53 **I** 126.9	54 **Xe** 131.3
55 **Cs** 132.9	56 **Ba** 137.3	57 **La*** 138.9	72 **Hf** 178.5	73 **Ta** 180.9	74 **W** 183.9	75 **Re** 186.2	76 **Os** 190.2	77 **Ir** 192.2	78 **Pt** 195.1	79 **Au** 197.0	80 **Hg** 200.6	81 **Tl** 204.4	82 **Pb** 207.2	83 **Bi** 209.0	84 **Po** (209)	85 **At** (210)	86 **Rn** (222)
87 **Fr** (223)	88 **Ra** (226)	89 **Ac†** (227)	104 **Rf** (267)	105 **Db** (268)	106 **Sg** (271)	107 **Bh** (270)	108 **Hs** (269)	109 **Mt** (278)	110 **Ds** (281)	111 **Rg** (282)	112 **Cn** (285)	113 **Nh** (286)	114 **Fl** (289)	115 **Mc** (289)	116 **Lv** (293)	117 **Ts** (294)	118 **Og** (294)

*	58 **Ce** 140.1	59 **Pr** 140.9	60 **Nd** 144.2	61 **Pm** (145)	62 **Sm** 150.4	63 **Eu** 152.0	64 **Gd** 157.3	65 **Tb** 158.9	66 **Dy** 162.5	67 **Ho** 164.9	68 **Er** 167.3	69 **Tm** 168.9	70 **Yb** 173.0	71 **Lu** 173.0
†	90 **Th** 232.0	91 **Pa** (231)	92 **U** 238.0	93 **Np** (237)	94 **Pu** (244)	95 **Am** (243)	96 **Cm** (247)	97 **Bk** (247)	98 **Cf** (251)	99 **Es** (252)	100 **Fm** (257)	101 **Md** (258)	102 **No** (259)	103 **Lr** (266)

Figure 2.6 Metalloids of the Periodic Table

MCAT CONCEPT CHECK 2.2

Before you move on, assess your understanding of the material with these questions.

1. Based on their location in the periodic table, identify a few elements that likely possess the following properties:
   - Luster:

   ___

   - Poor conductivity of heat and electricity:

   ___

   - Good conductivity but brittle:

   ___

2. Classify the following elements as metals (M), nonmetals (NM), or metalloids (MO):

Element	Class	Element	Class	Element	Class	Element	Class
Ag		Al		K		P	
Pb		Li		Pu		U	
Cu		As		Zn		B	
Si		Np		O		He	

2.3 Periodic Properties of the Elements High Yield

LEARNING OBJECTIVES

After Chapter 2.3, you will be able to:

- Compare the atomic radius of neutral atoms to their ions
- Rank elements by ionization energy, electron affinity, electronegativity, or atomic radius:

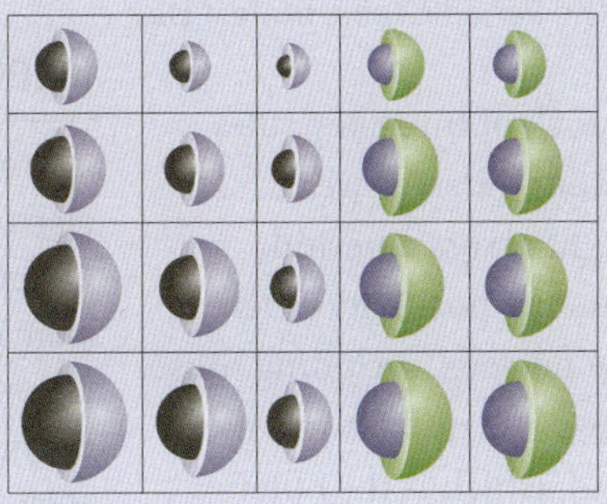

The MCAT does *not* expect you to have memorized the entire periodic table. On Test Day, the MCAT interface includes a Periodic Table button (shortcut: Alt + T) that brings up a full-screen table like the one appearing in Figure 2.7. Fortunately, the periodic table is a guide unto itself, a self-referencing localization system for all of the elements. Remember, the modern table is organized in such a way to represent visually the periodicity of chemical and physical properties of the elements. The periodic table, then, can provide you with a tremendous amount of information that otherwise would have to be memorized. Note, though, that while you do not need to memorize the periodic table for the MCAT, you *do* need to understand the trends within the periodic table that help predict the chemical and physical behaviors of the elements.

MCAT EXPERTISE

Don't try to memorize the periodic table. You will have access to it on Test Day through the test interface. *Do* understand its configuration and trends so that you can use it efficiently to get a higher score!

1 **H** 1.0																	2 **He** 4.0
3 **Li** 6.9	4 **Be** 9.0											5 **B** 10.8	6 **C** 12.0	7 **N** 14.0	8 **O** 16.0	9 **F** 19.0	10 **Ne** 20.2
11 **Na** 23.0	12 **Mg** 24.3											13 **Al** 27.0	14 **Si** 28.1	15 **P** 31.0	16 **S** 32.1	17 **Cl** 35.5	18 **Ar** 39.9
19 **K** 39.1	20 **Ca** 40.1	21 **Sc** 45.0	22 **Ti** 47.9	23 **V** 50.9	24 **Cr** 52.0	25 **Mn** 54.9	26 **Fe** 55.8	27 **Co** 58.9	28 **Ni** 58.7	29 **Cu** 63.5	30 **Zn** 65.4	31 **Ga** 69.7	32 **Ge** 72.6	33 **As** 74.9	34 **Se** 79.0	35 **Br** 79.9	36 **Kr** 83.8
37 **Rb** 85.5	38 **Sr** 87.6	39 **Y** 88.9	40 **Zr** 91.2	41 **Nb** 92.9	42 **Mo** 95.9	43 **Tc** (98)	44 **Ru** 101.1	45 **Rh** 102.9	46 **Pd** 106.4	47 **Ag** 107.9	48 **Cd** 112.4	49 **In** 114.8	50 **Sn** 118.7	51 **Sb** 121.8	52 **Te** 127.6	53 **I** 126.9	54 **Xe** 131.3
55 **Cs** 132.9	56 **Ba** 137.3	57 **La*** 138.9	72 **Hf** 178.5	73 **Ta** 180.9	74 **W** 183.9	75 **Re** 186.2	76 **Os** 190.2	77 **Ir** 192.2	78 **Pt** 195.1	79 **Au** 197.0	80 **Hg** 200.6	81 **Tl** 204.4	82 **Pb** 207.2	83 **Bi** 209.0	84 **Po** (209)	85 **At** (210)	86 **Rn** (222)
87 **Fr** (223)	88 **Ra** (226)	89 **Ac†** (227)	104 **Rf** (267)	105 **Db** (268)	106 **Sg** (271)	107 **Bh** (270)	108 **Hs** (269)	109 **Mt** (278)	110 **Ds** (281)	111 **Rg** (282)	112 **Cn** (285)	113 **Nh** (286)	114 **Fl** (289)	115 **Mc** (289)	116 **Lv** (293)	117 **Ts** (294)	118 **Og** (294)

58 **Ce** 140.1	59 **Pr** 140.9	60 **Nd** 144.2	61 **Pm** (145)	62 **Sm** 150.4	63 **Eu** 152.0	64 **Gd** 157.3	65 **Tb** 158.9	66 **Dy** 162.5	67 **Ho** 164.9	68 **Er** 167.3	69 **Tm** 168.9	70 **Yb** 173.0	71 **Lu** 173.0
90 **Th** 232.0	91 **Pa** (231)	92 **U** 238.0	93 **Np** (237)	94 **Pu** (244)	95 **Am** (243)	96 **Cm** (247)	97 **Bk** (247)	98 **Cf** (251)	99 **Es** (252)	100 **Fm** (257)	101 **Md** (258)	102 **No** (259)	103 **Lr** (266)

Figure 2.7 The Periodic Table on Test Day

Before exploring the periodic trends, let's take stock of three key rules that control how valence electrons work in an atom. First, as we've already mentioned, as one moves from left to right across a period, electrons and protons are added one at a time. As the positivity of the nucleus increases, the electrons surrounding the nucleus, including those in the valence shell, experience a stronger electrostatic pull toward the center of the atom. This causes the electron cloud, which is the outer boundary defined by the valence shell electrons, to move closer and bind more tightly to the nucleus. This pull is somewhat mitigated by nonvalence electrons that reside closer to the nucleus. The electrostatic

BRIDGE

Z_{eff} relies on the principles of electrostatic forces defined in Chapter 5 of *MCAT Physics and Math Review.* The values q_1 and q_2 can represent the net charge of the nucleus and valence electron shell, respectively. The larger each charge gets (going to the right in the periodic table), the higher the value of Z_{eff}.

attraction between the valence shell electrons and the nucleus is known as the **effective nuclear charge** (**Z_{eff}**), a measure of the net positive charge experienced by the outermost electrons. For elements in the same period, Z_{eff} increases from left to right. The parts of an atom responsible for Z_{eff} are illustrated in Figure 2.8.

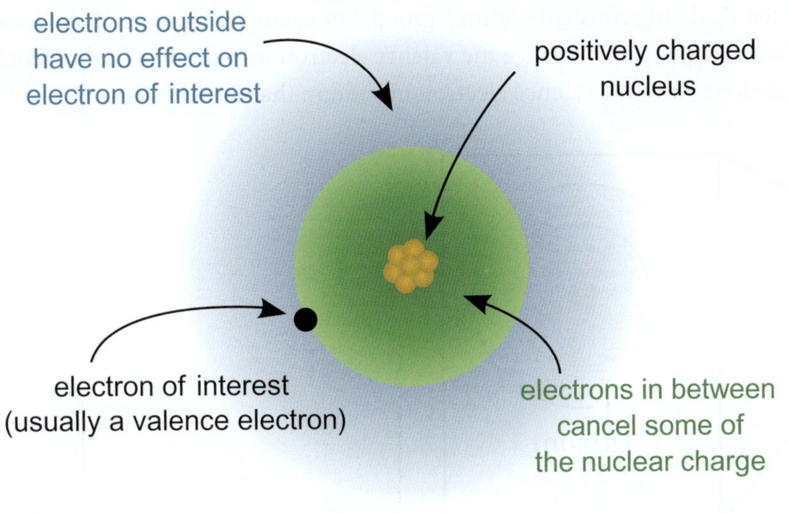

Figure 2.8 Factors that Determine Effective Nuclear Charge (Z_{eff})

A simple approximation for the effective nuclear charge is given by the equation $Z_{eff} = Z - S$, where Z is the atomic number (number of protons) and S is the number of core (nonvalence) electrons. As such, Z_{eff} is calculated by subtracting the nonvalence electrons from the total number of protons in an atom. A larger positive value indicates a stronger electrostatic attraction. For elements in the same period, Z_{eff} increases from left to right. An example of this is seen in Figure 2.9, which compares the effective nuclear charge of lithium to fluorine. Lithium, with three protons and two nonvalence electrons, has a Z_{eff} of $+1$. In comparison, fluorine, with nine protons and two nonvalence electrons, has a Z_{eff} of $+7$. The Z_{eff} approximates the pull the nucleus has for the electrons, so the higher the Z_{eff}, the more electrons are held closer to the nucleus, resulting in a smaller atomic radius for fluorine compared to lithium. For elements in the same period, Z_{eff} increases from left to right.

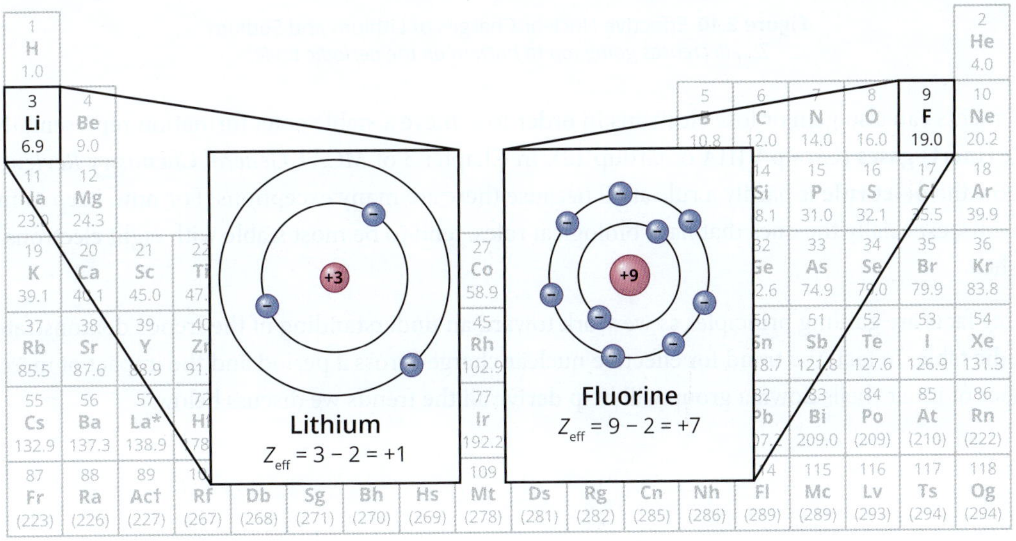

Figure 2.9 Effective Nuclear Charges of Lithium and Fluorine
Z_{eff} increases from left to right across the periodic table.

Second, as one moves down the elements of a given group, the **principal quantum number**—the number of filled energy levels or shells—increases by one each time. This results in a larger physical distance between the valence electrons and the nucleus, as well as an increased shielding created by the inner shell electrons that cancels out the increased positivity of the nucleus. Both factors contribute to the valence electrons being held less tightly despite the Z_{eff} being constant within a group. For example, Figure 2.10 demonstrates that lithium and sodium both have a Z_{eff} of +1, but since the valence electron in sodium is farther from the nucleus than in lithium, it is easier to remove the valence electron in sodium than in lithium.

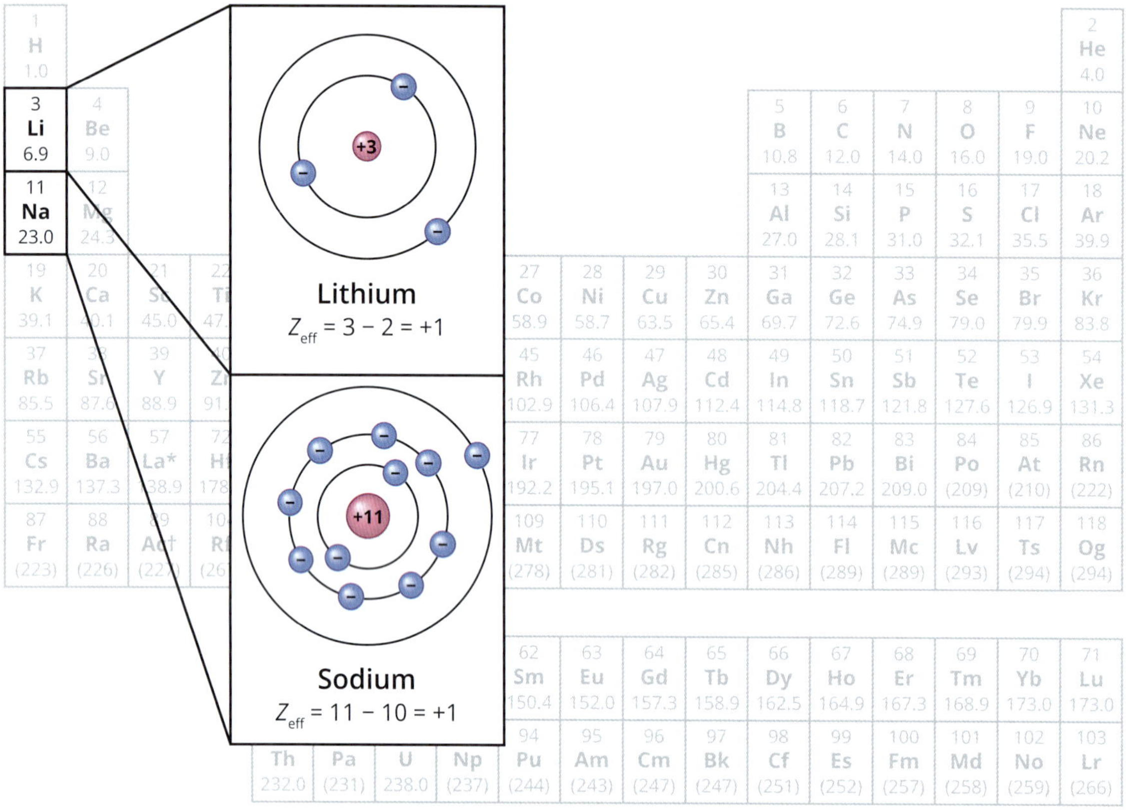

Figure 2.10 Effective Nuclear Charges of Lithium and Sodium
Z_{eff} decreases going top to bottom on the periodic table.

Third, elements can also gain or lose electrons in order to achieve a stable octet formation representative of the **noble (inert) gases** (Group VIIIA or Group 18). In Chapter 3 of *MCAT General Chemistry Review*, we will discuss how the **octet rule** is hardly a rule at all because there are many exceptions. For now, keep in mind that elements, especially the ones that have biological roles, tend to be most stable with eight electrons in their valence shell.

These three facts are guiding principles as we work toward an understanding of the trends demonstrated in the periodic table. In fact, the trend for effective nuclear charge across a period and the impact of increasing the number of inner shells down a group will help derive all the trends we discuss below.

Atomic and Ionic Radii

Think of an atom as a cloud of electrons surrounding a dense core of protons and neutrons. The **atomic radius** of an element is thus equal to one-half of the distance between the centers of two atoms of an element that are briefly in contact with each other. The distance between two centers of circles in contact is akin to a diameter, making this radius calculation simple. The atomic radius cannot be measured by examining a single atom because the electrons are constantly moving around, making it impossible to mark the outer boundary of the electron cloud.

KEY CONCEPT

Atomic radius refers to the size of a neutral element, while an ionic radius is dependent on *how* the element ionizes based on its element type and group number.

As we move across a period from left to right, protons and electrons are added one at a time to the atoms. Because the electrons are being added only to the outermost shell and the number of inner-shell electrons remains constant, the increasing positive charge of the nucleus pulls the outer electrons more closely inward and holds them more tightly. The Z_{eff} increases left to right across a period, and as a result, atomic radius decreases from left to right across a period.

MCAT EXPERTISE

Atomic radius is essentially opposite that of all other periodic trends. While others increase going up and to the right, atomic radius increases going down and to the left.

As we move down a group, the increasing principal quantum number implies that the valence electrons will be found farther away from the nucleus because the number of inner shells is increasing, separating the valence shell from the nucleus. Although the Z_{eff} remains essentially constant, the atomic radius increases down a group. Within each group, the largest atom will be at the bottom, and within each period, the largest atom will be in Group IA (Group 1). For reference, the largest atomic radius in the periodic table belongs to cesium (Cs, 260 pm), and the smallest belongs to helium (He, 25 pm). Francium is typically not considered because it is exceptionally rare in nature. Figure 2.11 displays a graph of atomic radius vs. atomic number, with Group IA elements possessing the largest atomic radius in each row.

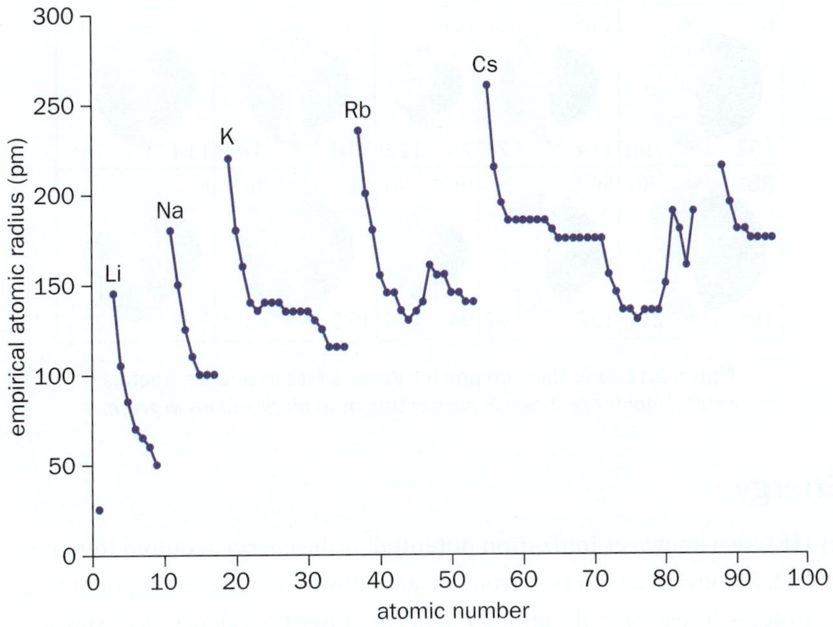

Figure 2.11 Atomic Radius (in pm) vs. Atomic Number

Unlike atomic radii, **ionic radii** will require some critical thinking and periodic table geography to determine. In order to understand ionic radii, we must make two generalizations. One is that metals lose electrons and become positive, while nonmetals gain electrons and become negative. The other is that metalloids can go in either direction, but tend to follow the trend based on which side of the metalloid line they fall on. Thus, silicon (Si) behaves more like a nonmetal, while germanium (Ge) tends to act more like a metal. On the MCAT, these generalizations can also be inferred from information found in passages and questions, such as oxidation states in compounds.

For nonmetals close to the metalloid line, their group number dictates that they require more electrons than other nonmetals to achieve the electronic configuration seen in Group VIIIA (Group 18). These nonmetals gain electrons while their nuclei maintain the same charge. Therefore, these nonmetals close to the metalloid line possess a larger ionic radius than their counterparts closer to Group VIIIA.

For metals, the trend is similar but opposite. Metals closer to the metalloid line have more electrons to lose to achieve the electronic configuration seen in Group VIIIA. Because of this, the ionic radius of metals near the metalloid line is dramatically smaller than that of other metals. Metals closer to Group IA have fewer electrons to lose and therefore experience a less drastic reduction in radius during ionization. These changes are illustrated in Figure 2.12. Note that tellurium (Te) behaves as a nonmetal and boron (B) behaves as a metal; under varying conditions, these metalloids can have opposite behavior.

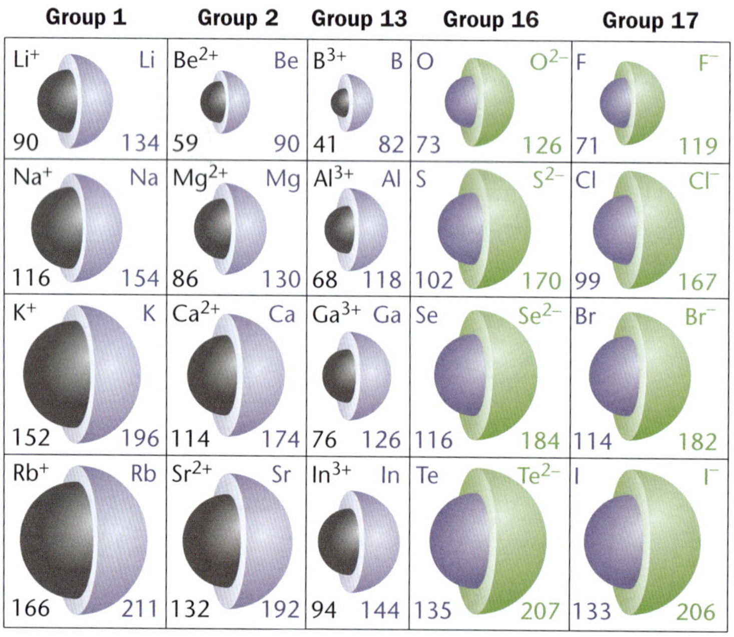

Figure 2.12 Ionic Radii (in pm) for Various Metals and Nonmetals
Neutral atoms are shown in purple; cations in black; anions in green.

Ionization Energy

Ionization energy (IE), also known as **ionization potential**, is the energy required to remove an electron from a gaseous species. Removing an electron from an atom always requires an input of heat, which makes it an **endothermic process**. The greater the atom's Z_{eff} or the closer the valence electrons are to the nucleus, the more tightly bound they are. This makes it more difficult to remove one or more electrons, increasing the ionization energy. Thus, ionization energy increases from left to right across a period and from bottom to top in a group. The subsequent removal of a second or third electron requires increasing amounts of energy because the removal of more than one electron means that the electrons are being removed from an increasingly cationic (positive) species. The energy necessary to remove the first electron is called the **first ionization energy**; the energy necessary to remove the second electron from the univalent cation (X^+) to form the divalent cation (X^{2+}) is called the **second ionization energy**, and so on. For example:

$$Mg\,(g) \rightarrow Mg^+(g) + e^- \qquad \text{first ionization energy} = 738\ \frac{kJ}{mol}$$

$$Mg^+(g) \rightarrow Mg^{2+}(g) + e^- \qquad \text{second ionization energy} = 1450\ \frac{kJ}{mol}$$

Elements in Groups IA and IIA (Groups 1 and 2), such as lithium and beryllium, have such low ionization energies that they are called the **active metals**. The active metals do not exist naturally in their neutral forms; they are always found in ionic compounds, minerals, or ores. The loss of one electron from the alkali metals (Group IA) or the loss of two electrons from the alkaline earth metals (Group IIA) results in the formation of a stable, filled valence shell. In contrast, the Group VIIA (Group 17) elements—the halogens—do not typically give up their electrons. In fact, in their ionic form, they are generally anions. The first ionization energies of the elements are shown in Figure 2.13.

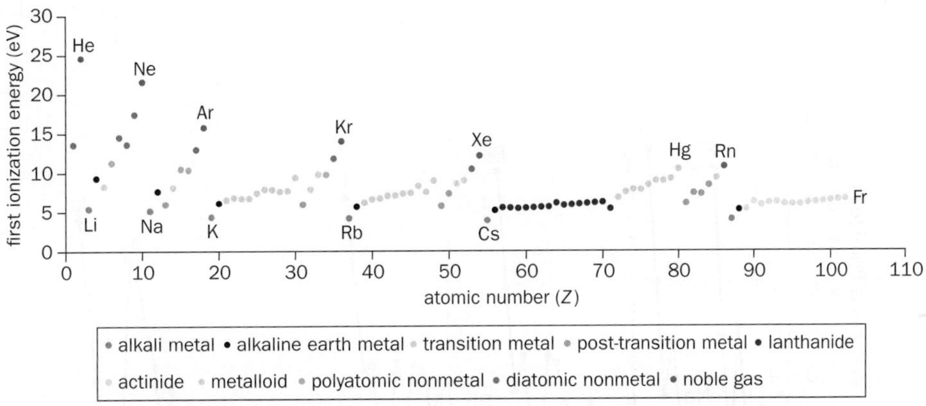

Figure 2.13 First Ionization Energies (in eV) of the Elements

The values for second ionization energies are disproportionally larger for Group IA monovalent cations (like Na^+) but generally not that much larger for Group IIA or subsequent monovalent cations (like Mg^+). This is because removing one electron from a Group IA metal results in a noble gas-like electron configuration.

Group VIIIA (Group 18) elements, or noble or inert gases, are the least likely to give up electrons. They already have a stable electron configuration and are unwilling to disrupt that stability by giving up an electron. Therefore, noble gases are among the elements with the highest ionization energies.

MCAT EXPERTISE

First ionization energy (IE) will always be smaller than second IE, which will always be smaller than third IE. However, the degree to which the IE increases provides clues about the identity of the atom. If losing a certain number of electrons gives an element a noble gas-like electron configuration, then removing a subsequent electron will cost much more energy. For example:

$$Mg^{2+}\,(g) \rightarrow Mg^{3+}\,(g) + e^-$$

$$\text{third ionization energy} = 7730\ \frac{kJ}{mol}$$

Electron Affinity

Halogens are the most "greedy" group of elements on the periodic table when it comes to electrons. By acquiring one additional electron, a halogen is able to complete its octet and achieve a noble gas configuration. This **exothermic** process expels energy in the form of heat. **Electron affinity** refers to the energy dissipated by a gaseous species when it gains an electron. Note the electron affinity is essentially the opposite concept from ionization energy. Because this is an exothermic process, ΔH_{rxn} has a negative sign; however, the electron affinity is reported as a positive number. This is because electron affinity refers to the energy dissipated: if $200\ \frac{kJ}{mol}$ of energy is released, $\Delta H_{rxn} = -200\ \frac{kJ}{mol}$, and the electron affinity is $200\ \frac{kJ}{mol}$. The stronger the electrostatic pull (the higher the Z_{eff}) between the nucleus and the valence shell electrons, the greater the energy release will be when the atom gains the electron. Thus, electron affinity increases across a period from left to right. Because the valence shell is farther away from the nucleus as the principal quantum number increases, electron affinity decreases in a group from top to bottom. Groups IA and IIA (Groups 1 and 2) have very low electron affinities, preferring to give up electrons to achieve the octet configuration of the noble gas in the previous period. Conversely, Group VIIA (Group 17) elements have very high electron affinities because they need to gain only one electron to achieve the octet configuration of the noble gases (Group VIIIA or Group 18) in the same period. Although the noble gases would be predicted to have the highest electron affinities according to the trend, they actually have electron affinities on the order of zero because they already possess a stable octet and cannot readily accept an electron. Most metals also have low electron affinity values, as can be seen in Figure 2.14.

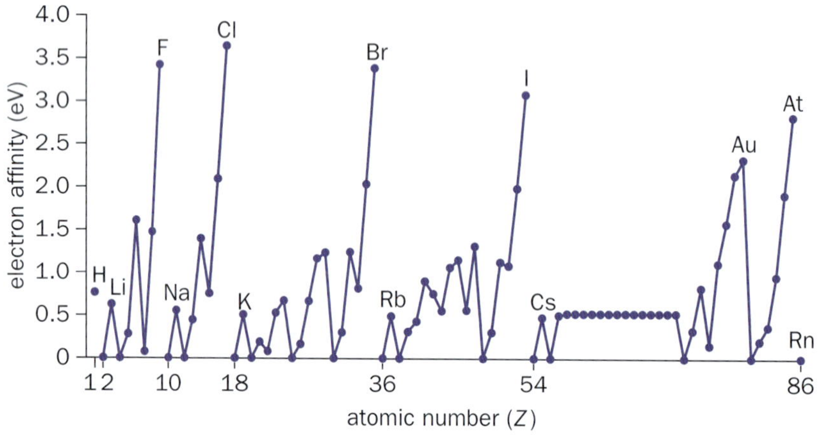

Figure 2.14 Electron Affinities (in eV) of the Elements

Electronegativity

Electronegativity is a measure of the attractive force that an atom will exert on an electron in a chemical bond. The greater the electronegativity of an atom, the more it attracts electrons within a bond. Figure 2.15 demonstrates this by showing the distribution of electrons in a bond between two carbon atoms vs. two atoms with a large difference in electronegativity, carbon and fluorine. More of the electrons in the latter bond are closer to the fluorine atom compared to the carbon atom, resulting in a polar bond with an uneven distribution of electrons. Electronegativity values are related to ionization energies: the lower the ionization energy, the lower the electronegativity; the higher the ionization energy, the higher the electronegativity. The first three noble gases are exceptions: despite their high ionization energies, these elements have negligible electronegativity because they do not often form bonds.

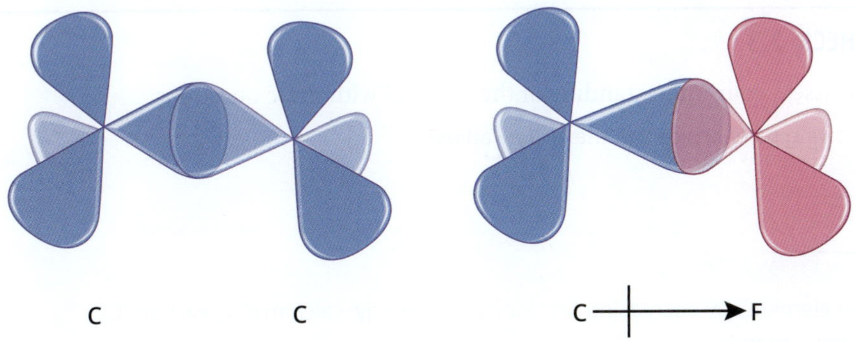

Figure 2.15 Electronegativity Influences Electron Distribution in a Covalent Bond

The electronegativity value is a relative measure, and there are different scales used to express it. The most common scale is the **Pauling electronegativity scale**, which ranges from 0.7 for cesium, the least electronegative (most electropositive) element, to 4.0 for fluorine, the most electronegative element. Electronegativity increases across a period from left to right and decreases in a group from top to bottom. Figure 2.16 shows the electronegativity values of the elements.

H 2.1																	He
Li 1.0	Be 1.5											B 2.0	C 2.5	N 3.0	O 3.5	F 4.0	Ne
Na 0.9	Mg 1.2											Al 1.5	Si 1.8	P 2.1	S 2.5	Cl 3.0	Ar
K 0.8	Ca 1.0	Sc 1.3	Ti 1.5	V 1.6	Cr 1.6	Mn 1.5	Fe 1.8	Co 1.9	Ni 1.8	Cu 1.9	Zn 1.6	Ga 1.6	Ge 1.8	As 2.0	Se 2.4	Br 2.8	Kr
Rb 0.8	Sr 1.0	Y 1.2	Zr 1.4	Nb 1.6	Mo 1.8	Tc 1.9	Ru 2.2	Rh 2.2	Pd 2.2	Ag 1.9	Cd 1.7	In 1.7	Sn 1.8	Sb 1.9	Te 2.1	I 2.5	Xe
Cs 0.7	Ba 0.9	La	Hf 1.3	Ta 1.5	W 1.7	Re 1.9	Os 2.2	Ir 2.2	Pt 2.2	Au 2.4	Hg 1.9	Tl 1.8	Pb 1.9	Bi 1.9	Po 2.0	At 2.2	Rn
Fr 0.7	Ra 0.9	Ac	Rf	Db	Sg	Bh	Hs	Mt	Ds	Rg	Cn	Nh	Fl	Mc	Lv	Ts	Og

Figure 2.16 Pauling Electronegativity Values of the Elements

The periodic trends are summarized together in Figure 2.17.

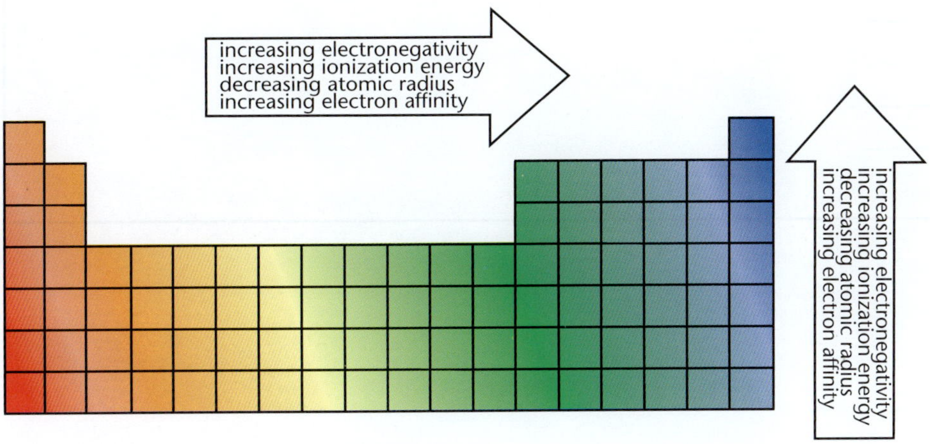

Figure 2.17 Periodic Trends

KEY CONCEPT

- Cs = largest, least electronegative
- F = smallest, most electronegative

KEY CONCEPT

Periodic Trends

Left → Right

- Atomic radius ↓
- Ionization energy ↑
- Electron affinity ↑
- Electronegativity ↑

Top → Bottom

- Atomic radius ↑
- Ionization energy ↓
- Electron affinity ↓
- Electronegativity ↓

Note: Atomic radius is always opposite the other trends. Ionic radius is variable.

MCAT CONCEPT CHECK 2.3

Before you move on, assess your understanding of the material with these questions.

1. In each of the following pairs, which has the larger radius?
   - F or F^- ______________
   - K or K^+______________

2. Rank the following elements by decreasing first ionization energy: calcium (Ca), carbon (C), germanium (Ge), potassium (K)
   1. ______________
   2. ______________
   3. ______________
   4. ______________

3. Rank the following elements by increasing electron affinity: barium (Ba), copper (Cu), sulfur (S), yttrium (Y)
   1. ______________
   2. ______________
   3. ______________
   4. ______________

4. Rank the following elements by decreasing electronegativity: antimony (Sb), neon (Ne), oxygen (O), thallium (Tl)
   1. ______________
   2. ______________
   3. ______________
   4. ______________

5. Rank the following elements by increasing atomic radius: niobium (Nb), praseodymium (Pr), tantalum (Ta), xenon (Xe)
   1. ______________
   2. ______________
   3. ______________
   4. ______________

2.4 The Chemistry of Groups

LEARNING OBJECTIVES

After Chapter 2.4, you will be able to:

- Identify the groups on the periodic table by the properties they exhibit
- Connect periodic table groups 1, 2, 16, 17, 18, and 3–12 to their common names

What follows is a discussion of the major groups you are likely to encounter on the MCAT. While it is rare to be tested on every group, it is important to understand the overarching trends we have already discussed and how they relate across different groups.

Alkali Metals (IA)

The **alkali metals** (Group IA or Group 1) possess most of the classic physical properties of metals, except that their densities are lower than those of other metals (as described for lithium earlier in this chapter). The alkali metals have only one loosely bound electron in their outermost shells. Their Z_{eff} values are very low, giving them the largest atomic radii of all the elements in their respective periods. This low Z_{eff} value also explains the other trends: low ionization energies, low electron affinities, and low electronegativities. Alkali metals easily lose one electron to form univalent cations, and they react readily with nonmetals—especially the halogens—as in NaCl. Figure 2.18 illustrates the reaction of an alkali metal with water, a stereotypically violent reaction.

REAL WORLD

Due to their high reactivity with water and air, most alkali metals are stored in mineral oil.

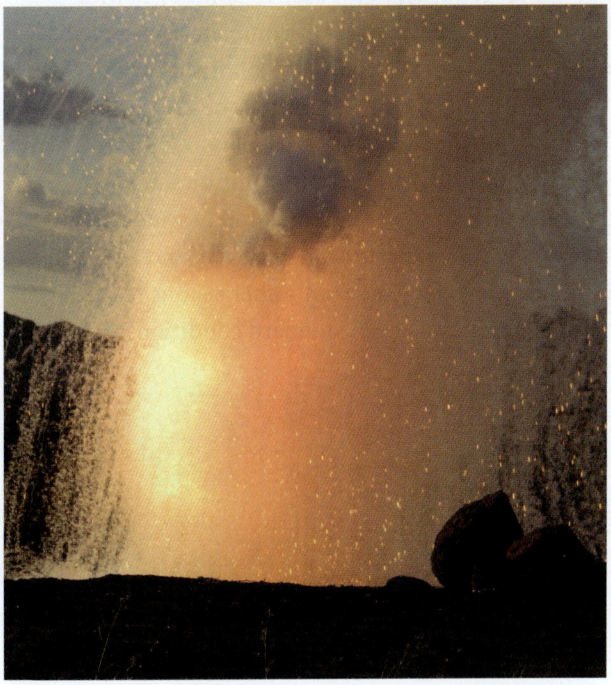

Figure 2.18 Reaction of Sodium with Water
Group IA metals react violently with water, forming strong bases.

Alkaline Earth Metals (IIA)

The **alkaline earth metals** (Group IIA or Group 2) also possess many properties characteristic of metals. They share most of the characteristics of the alkali metals, except that they have slightly higher effective nuclear charges and thus slightly smaller atomic radii. They have two electrons in their valence shell, both of which are easily removed to form divalent cations. Together, the alkali and alkaline earth metals are called the active metals because they are so reactive that they are not naturally found in their elemental (neutral) state.

Chalcogens (VIA)

The **chalcogens** (Group VIA or Group 16) are an eclectic group of nonmetals and metalloids. While not as reactive as the halogens, they are crucial for normal biological functions. They each have six electrons in their valence electron shell and, due to their proximity to the metalloids, generally have small atomic radii and large ionic radii. Oxygen is the most important element in this group for many reasons; it is one of the primary constituents of water, carbohydrates, and other biological molecules. Sulfur is also an important component of certain amino acids and vitamins. Selenium also is an important nutrient for microorganisms and has a role in protection from oxidative stress. The remainder of this group is primarily metallic and generally toxic to living organisms. It is important to note that, at high concentrations, many of these elements—no matter how biologically useful—can be toxic or damaging.

BRIDGE

Many of the molecules discussed in metabolism, covered in Chapters 9 through 12 of *MCAT Biochemistry Review,* utilize lighter nontoxic elements from the chalcogen group (oxygen and sulfur). Many of the heavier chalcogens are toxic metals.

Halogens (VIIA)

The **halogens** (Group VIIA or Group 17) are highly reactive nonmetals with seven valence electrons. These elements are desperate to complete their octets by gaining one additional electron. The physical properties of this group are variable. At standard conditions, the halogens range from gaseous (F_2 and Cl_2) to liquid (Br_2) to solid (I_2) forms. Their chemical reactivity is more uniform, and, due to their very high electronegativities and electron affinities, they are especially reactive toward the alkali and alkaline earth metals. Fluorine (F) has the highest electronegativity of all the elements. The halogens are so reactive that they are not naturally found in their elemental state but rather as ions (called **halides**) or diatomic molecules. Diatomic iodine at standard conditions can be seen in Figure 2.19.

MCAT EXPERTISE

Halogens are frequently tested on the MCAT. Remember that they only need one more electron to have a noble gas-like electron configuration (full valence shell).

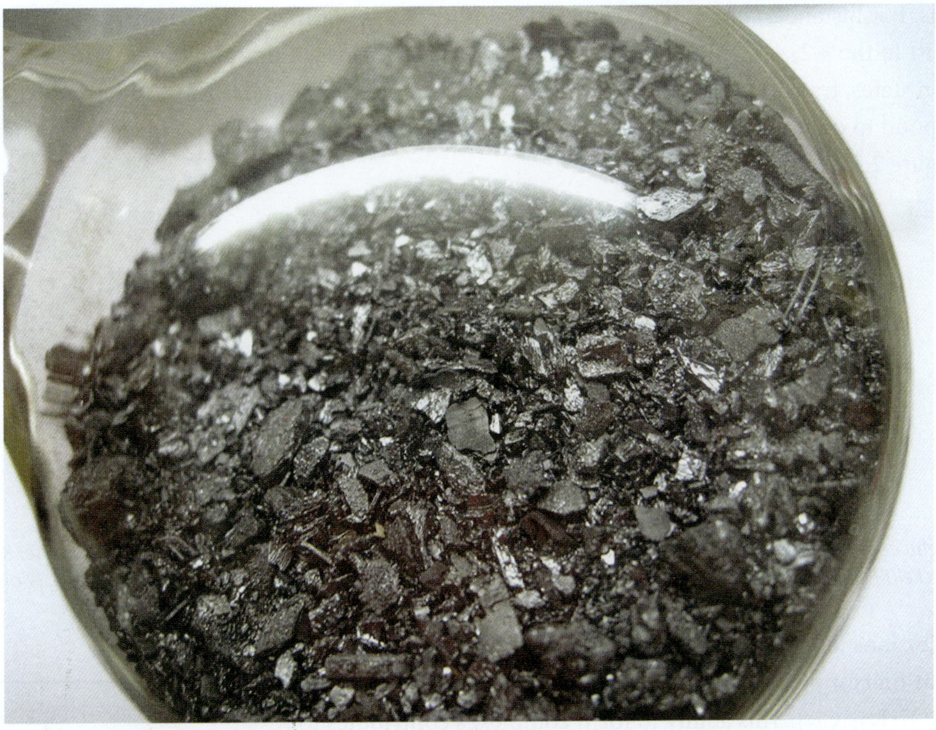

Figure 2.19 Iodine in Standard State (Diatomic Iodine)

Noble Gases (VIIIA)

The **noble gases** (Group VIIIA or Group 18) are also known as **inert gases** because they have minimal chemical reactivity due to their filled valence shells. They have high ionization energies, little or no tendency to gain or lose electrons, and (for He, Ne, and Ar, at least), no measurable electronegativities. The noble gases have extremely low boiling points and exist as gases at room temperature. Noble gases have found a commercial niche as lighting sources, as seen in Figure 2.20, due to their lack of reactivity.

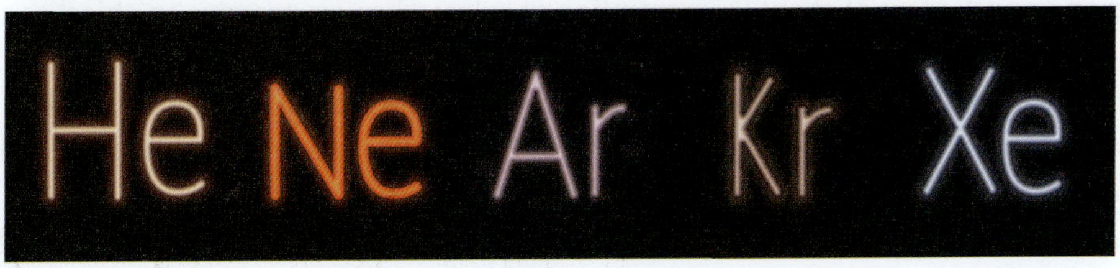

Figure 2.20 Noble Gases Used in "Neon" Signs

Transition Metals (B)

The **transition elements** (Groups IB to VIIIB or Groups 3 to 12) are considered to be metals and as such have low electron affinities, low ionization energies, and low electronegativities. These metals are very hard and have high melting and boiling points. They tend to be quite malleable and are good conductors due to the loosely held electrons that progressively fill the *d*-orbitals in their valence shells. One of the unique properties of the transition metals is that many of them can have different possible charged forms or **oxidation states** because they are capable of losing different numbers of electrons from the *s*- and *d*-orbitals in their valence shells. For instance, copper (Cu) can exist in either the +1 or the +2 oxidation state, and manganese (Mn) can exist in the +2, +3, +4, +6, or +7 oxidation state. Because of this ability to attain different positive oxidation states, transition metals form many different ionic compounds. These different oxidation states often correspond to different colors; solutions with transition metal-containing complexes are often vibrant, as shown in Figure 2.21.

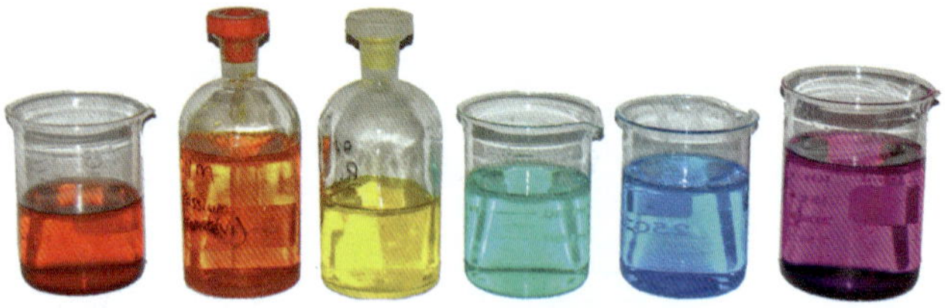

Figure 2.21 Solutions of Transition Metal-Containing Compounds
From left to right: cobalt(II) nitrate, $Co(NO_3)_2$ (red); potassium dichromate, $K_2Cr_2O_7$ (orange); potassium chromate, K_2CrO_4 (yellow); nickel(II) chloride, $NiCl_2$ (green); copper(II) sulfate, $CuSO_4$ (blue); potassium permanganate, $KMnO_4$ (violet)

These complex ions tend to associate in solution either with molecules of water (**hydration complexes**, such as $CuSO_4 \cdot 5\ H_2O$) or with nonmetals (such as $[Co(NH_3)_6]Cl_3$). This ability to form complexes contributes to the variable solubility of certain transition metal-containing compounds. For example, AgCl is insoluble in water but quite soluble in aqueous ammonia due to the formation of the complex ion $[Ag(NH_3)_2]^+$. The formation of complexes causes the *d*-orbitals to split into two energy sublevels. This enables many of the complexes to absorb certain frequencies of light—those containing the precise amount of energy required to raise electrons from the lower- to the higher-energy *d*-orbitals. The frequencies not absorbed (known as the subtraction frequencies) give the complexes their characteristic colors.

BRIDGE

Many transition metals act as cofactors for enzymes, including vanadium, chromium, manganese, iron, cobalt, nickel, copper, and zinc. Cofactors and coenzymes are discussed in Chapter 2 of *MCAT Biochemistry Review*.

This brings up an important point about the perception of color: when we perceive an object as a particular color, it is because that color is *not* absorbed—but rather reflected—by the object. If an object absorbs a given color of light and reflects all others, our brain mixes these **subtraction frequencies** and we perceive the **complementary color** of the frequency that was absorbed. This is best illustrated with an example. *Carotene* is a photosynthetic pigment that strongly absorbs blue light but reflects other colors. Thus, our brains interpret the color of carotene as the result of white light *minus* blue light, which is yellow light. The complementary colors are shown in Figure 2.22. It should also be noted that the manner in which colors mix in this scheme is distinctly different from mixing, say, paint colors. The differences between these two schemes, termed additive and subtractive color mixing, respectively, are outside the scope of the MCAT.

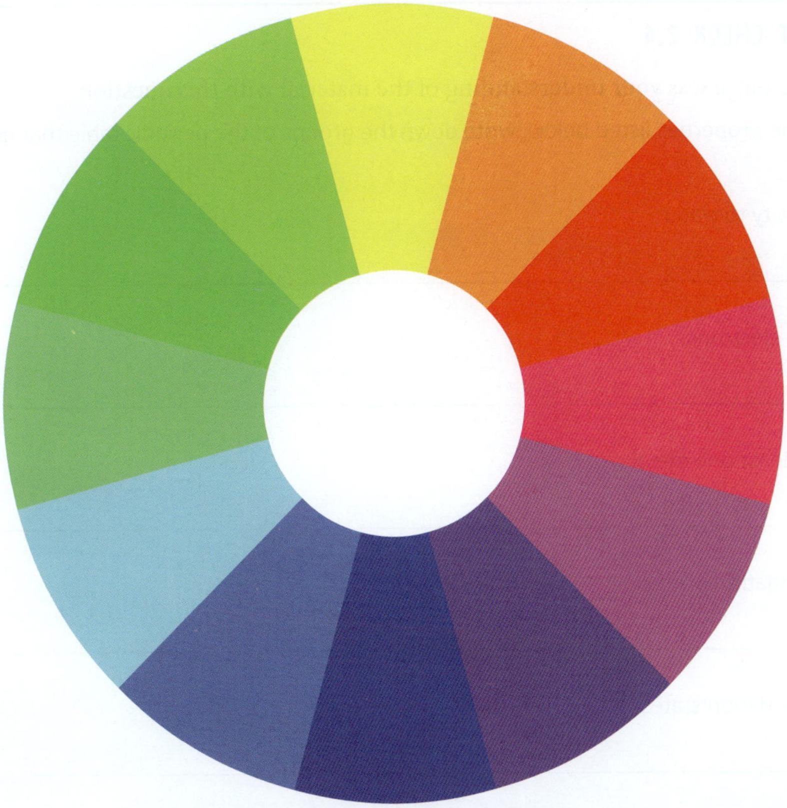

Figure 2.22 Red–Green–Blue (Additive) Color Wheel
Each color is directly across the circle from its complementary color; commonly referenced complementary pairs include red/cyan, green/magenta, and blue/yellow.

MCAT CONCEPT CHECK 2.4

Before you move on, assess your understanding of the material with this question.

1. For each of the properties listed below, write down the groups of the periodic table that exhibit those properties.
   - High reactivity to water:

   ____

   - Six valence electrons:

   ____

   - Contain at least one metal:

   ____

   - Multiple oxidation states:

   ____

   - Negative oxidation states:

   ____

   - Possess a full octet in the neutral state:

   ____

Conclusion

Now that we have completed our review of the Periodic Table of the Elements, commit to understanding (not just memorizing) the trends of physical and chemical properties of the elements. They will help you quickly answer many questions on the MCAT. As you progress through the chapters of this book, a foundational understanding of the elements will help you develop a richer, more nuanced understanding of their general and particular behaviors. Topics in general chemistry that may have given you trouble in the past will be understandable from the perspective of the behaviors and characteristics that you have reviewed here.

More broadly, you will see a diverse array of elements from the groups we have discussed here that are critical or detrimental to biological function. In addition, you may begin to see why the human body utilizes certain elements for specific purposes, taking advantage of the periodic trends discussed here.

GO ONLINE

You've reviewed the content, now test your knowledge and critical thinking skills by completing a test-like passage set in your online resources!

CONCEPT SUMMARY

The Periodic Table

- The **Periodic Table of the Elements** organizes the elements according to their atomic numbers and reveals a pattern of similar chemical and physical properties among elements.
  - Rows are called **periods** and are based on the same principal energy level, *n*.
  - Columns are called **groups**. Elements in the same group have the same valence shell electron configuration.

Types of Elements

- The elements on the periodic table belong to one of three types.
  - **Metals** are shiny (**lustrous**), conduct electricity well, and are **malleable** and **ductile**. Metals are found on left side and middle of the periodic table.
  - **Nonmetals** are dull, poor conductors of electricity, and are brittle. Nonmetals are found on right side of the periodic table.
  - **Metalloids** possess characteristics of both metals and nonmetals and are found in a stair-step pattern starting with boron (B).

Periodic Properties of the Elements

- **Effective nuclear charge** (Z_{eff}) is the net positive charge experienced by electrons in the valence shell and forms the foundation for all periodic trends.
  - Z_{eff} increases from left to right across a period, with little change in value from top to bottom in a group.
  - Valence electrons become increasingly separated from the nucleus as the principal energy level, *n*, increases from top to bottom in a group.
- **Atomic radius** decreases from left to right across a period and increases from top to bottom in a group.
- **Ionic radius** is the size of a charged species. The largest nonmetallic ionic radii and the smallest metallic ionic radii exist at the metalloid boundary.
  - Cations are generally smaller than their corresponding neutral atom.
  - Anions are generally larger than their corresponding neutral atom.
- **Ionization energy** is the amount of energy necessary to remove an electron from the valence shell of a gaseous species; it increases from left to right across a period and decreases from top to bottom in a group.
- **Electron affinity** is the amount of energy released when a gaseous species gains an electron in its valence shell; it increases from left to right across a period and decreases from top to bottom in a group.
- **Electronegativity** is a measure of the attractive force of the nucleus for electrons within a bond; it increases from left to right across a period and decreases from top to bottom in a group.

The Chemistry of Groups

- **Alkali metals** typically take on an oxidation state of +1 and prefer to lose an electron to achieve a noble gas-like configuration; they and the alkaline earth metals are the most reactive of all metals.
- **Alkaline earth metals** take on an oxidation state of +2 and can lose two electrons to achieve noble gas-like configurations.
- **Chalcogens** take on oxidation states of −2 or +6 (depending on whether they are nonmetals or metals, respectively) in order to achieve noble gas configuration. They are very biologically important.
- **Halogens** typically take on an oxidation state of −1 and prefer to gain an electron to achieve noble gas-like configurations; these nonmetals have the highest electronegativities.
- **Noble gases** have a fully filled valence shell in their standard state and prefer not to give up or take on additional electrons; they have very high ionization energies and (for He, Ne, and Ar), virtually nonexistent electronegativities and electron affinities.
- **Transition metals** are unique because they take on multiple oxidation states, which explains their ability to form colorful complexes with nonmetals in solution and their utility in certain biological systems.

ANSWERS TO CONCEPT CHECKS

2.1

1. The modern periodic table is arranged in order by atomic number.
2.

Element	A or B	Element	A or B	Element	A or B	Element	A or B
Ag	B	**Al**	A	**K**	A	**P**	A
Pb	A	**Li**	A	**Pu**	B	**U**	B
Cu	B	**Cf**	B	**Zn**	B	**B**	A
N	A	**Np**	B	**O**	A	**He**	A

2.2

1. Metals have luster. Nonmetals have poor conductivity. Metalloids exhibit brittleness but good conductivity. Any answers within each of these categories are acceptable.
2.

Element	Class	Element	Class	Element	Class	Element	Class
Ag	M	**Al**	M	**K**	M	**P**	NM
Pb	M	**Li**	M	**Pu**	M	**U**	M
Cu	M	**As**	MO	**Zn**	M	**B**	MO
Si	MO	**Np**	M	**O**	NM	**He**	NM

2.3

1. $F^- > F$; $K > K^+$. The ionic radii of anions are larger than the associated atomic radii, while the ionic radii of cations are smaller.
2. Ionization energy: carbon > germanium > calcium > potassium
3. Electron affinity: barium < yttrium < copper < sulfur
4. Electronegativity: oxygen > antimony > thallium > neon
5. Atomic radius: xenon < niobium < tantalum < praseodymium

2.4

1. - High reactivity to water: Groups 1 and 2
   - Six valence electrons: Groups 6 and 16
   - Contain at least one metal: Groups 1 through 15
   - Multiple oxidation states: All groups; most notably Groups 3 through 12 (transition metals)
   - Negative oxidation states: Almost all groups; most notably Groups 14 through 17 (nonmetals)
   - Possess a full octet in the neutral state: Group 18

SCIENCE MASTERY ASSESSMENT EXPLANATIONS

1. **B**

The periodic table is organized into periods (rows) and groups (columns). Groups (columns) are particularly significant because they represent sets of elements with the same valence electron configuration, which in turn will dictate many of the chemical properties of those elements. Although **(A)** is true, the fact that both ions are positively charged does not explain the similarity in chemical properties; most metals produce positively charged ions. **(C)** is not true because lithium and sodium are in the same group, not period. Finally, although lithium and sodium do have relatively low atomic weights, so do several other elements that do not share the same properties, eliminating **(D)**.

2. **A**

As one moves from top to bottom in a group (column), extra electron shells accumulate, despite the fact that the valence configurations remain identical. These extra electron shells provide shielding between the positive nucleus and the outermost electrons, decreasing the electrostatic attraction and increasing the atomic radius. Because carbon and silicon are in the same group, and silicon is farther down in the group, silicon will have a larger atomic radius because of its extra electron shell.

3. **B**

This question requires knowledge of the trends of electronegativity within the Periodic Table. Electronegativity increases as one moves from left to right for the same reasons that effective nuclear charge increases. Electronegativity decreases as one moves down the Periodic Table because there are more electron shells separating the nucleus from the outermost electrons. In this question, chlorine is the furthest toward the top-right corner of the Periodic Table, making **(B)** the correct answer.

4. **C**

Ionization energy increases from left to right, so the first ionization energy of lithium is lower than that of beryllium. Second ionization energy is always larger than first ionization energy, so beryllium's second ionization energy should be the highest value. This is because removing an additional electron from Be^+ requires one to overcome a significantly larger electrostatic force.

5. **B**

Antimony (Sb) is on the right side of the periodic table, but not far right enough to be a nonmetal, **(D)**. It certainly does not lie far enough to the right to fall in Group VIIA (Group 17), which would classify it as a halogen, **(C)**. While sources have rarely classified antimony as a metal, **(A)**, it is usually classified as a metalloid, **(B)**.

6. **C**

Electronegativity describes how strong an attraction an element will have for electrons in a bond. A nucleus with a larger effective nuclear charge will have a higher electronegativity; Z_{eff} increases toward the right side of a period. A stronger nuclear pull will also lead to increased first ionization energy, as the forces make it more difficult to remove an electron. The vertical arrow can be explained by the size of the atoms. As size decreases, the positive charge becomes more effective at attracting electrons in a chemical bond (higher electronegativity), and the energy required to remove an electron (ionization energy) increases.

7. **C**

All four descriptions of metals are true, but the most significant property that contributes to the ability of metals to conduct electricity is the fact that they have valence electrons that can move freely. Malleability, **(A)**, is the ability to shape a material with a hammer, which does not play a role in conducting electricity. The low electronegativity and high melting points of metals, **(B)** and **(D)**, also do not play a major role in the conduction of electricity.

8. **B**

This block represents the alkaline earth metals, which form divalent cations, or ions with a +2 charge. All of the elements in Group IIA have two electrons in their outermost *s* subshell. Because loss of these two electrons would leave a full octet as the outermost shell, becoming a divalent cation is a stable configuration for all of the alkaline earth metals. Although some of these elements might be great conductors, they are not as effective as the alkali metals, eliminating **(A)**. **(C)** is also incorrect because, although forming a divalent cation is a stable configuration for the alkaline earth metals, the second ionization energy is still always higher than the first. Finally, **(D)** is incorrect because atomic radii increase when moving down a group of elements because the number of electron shells increases.

9. **B**

Iron is a transition metal. Transition metals can often form more than one ion. Iron, for example, can be Fe^{2+} or Fe^{3+}. The transition metals, in these various oxidation states, can often form hydration complexes with water. Part of the significance of these complexes is that, when a transition metal can form a complex, its solubility within the related solvent will increase. The other ions given might dissolve readily in water, but because none of them are transition metals, they will not likely form complexes.

10. **D**

This question is simple if one recalls that periods refer to the rows in the periodic table, while groups or families refer to the columns. Within the same period, an additional valence electron is added with each step toward the right side of the table.

11. **C**

Phosphorous and arsenic are both found in group 5A, indicating that they have a similar number of valence electrons. Since the valence electron configuration is one of the main determinants of bonding, elements with similar valence states react similarly, supporting **(C)**.

12. **D**

The correct answer to this question may be surprising because this question illustrates an important exception to a trend. Electron affinity generally increases as one moves up and to the right on the periodic table. Based on this trend alone, one might expect that the atom fluorine, depicted in **(B)**, would be correct. However, the correct answer is chlorine, **(D)**, even despite the fact that chlorine is below fluorine on the periodic table. The diagrams in the answer choices help make sense of this apparent exception: Fluorine and chlorine have the same valence electron configuration and have a similar amount of effective nuclear charge. However, when an electron is added to fluorine's valence shell, that negative charge is added to the second energy shell, which is quite small in physical size, meaning that the new electron is crowded into a small energy shell with seven other electrons. As a result, energy is still released when an electron is added to fluorine, but not as much energy as might be predicted by the general trend alone. By contrast, when an additional electron is added to a chlorine atom, that new electron adds to the third energy shell, so there is less repulsion among the valence electrons, leading to a slightly greater electron affinity for chlorine. Thus, chlorine, **(D)**, has the highest electron affinity and is the right answer.

13. **D**

The effective nuclear charge refers to the strength with which the protons in the nucleus can pull on electrons. This phenomenon helps to explain electron affinity, electronegativity, and ionization energy. The effective nuclear charge can be calculated by subtracting the number of non-valence electrons from the number of protons. In **(A)** and **(B)**, chlorine has 17 protons and 10 non-valence electrons, giving it a Z_{eff} of 7. Next, elemental potassium, **(C)**, has the lowest effective nuclear charge because it contains additional inner shells that shield its valence electron from the nucleus. With 19 protons and 18 non-valence electrons, it has a Z_{eff} of 1. **(D)**, ionic potassium, has a higher effective nuclear charge than any of the other options. It has the same electron configuration as Cl^- (10 non-valence electrons) but contains two extra protons in its nucleus, and thus has a Z_{eff} of 9.

14. **D**

Ionic bonds are formed through unequal sharing of electrons. These bonds typically occur because the electron affinities of the two bonded atoms differ greatly. For example, the halogens have high electron affinities because adding a single electron to their valence shells would create full valence shells. In contrast, the alkaline earth metals have very low electron affinities and are more likely to be electron donors because the loss of two electrons would leave them with full valence shells. **(A)** states the opposite and is incorrect because the halogens have high electron affinity and the alkaline earth metals have low electron affinity. **(B)** is incorrect because equal sharing of electrons is a classic description of covalent bonding, not ionic. **(C)** is a true statement, but is not relevant to why ionic bonds form.

15. **C**

When $n = 3$, $l = 0$, 1, or 2. The highest value for l in this case is 2, which corresponds to the d subshell. Although the 3d block appears to be part of the fourth period, it still has the principal quantum number $n = 3$. In general, the subshells within an energy shell increase in energy as follows: $s < p < d < f$ (although there is no 3f subshell).

GO ONLINE

Consult your online resources for additional practice.

SHARED CONCEPTS

General Chemistry Chapter 1
Atomic Structure

General Chemistry Chapter 3
Bonding and Chemical Interactions

General Chemistry Chapter 4
Compounds and Stoichiometry

Organic Chemistry Chapter 3
Bonding

Physics and Math Chapter 5
Electrostatics and Magnetism

Physics and Math Chapter 9
Atomic and Nuclear Phenomena

CHAPTER 3

BONDING AND CHEMICAL INTERACTIONS

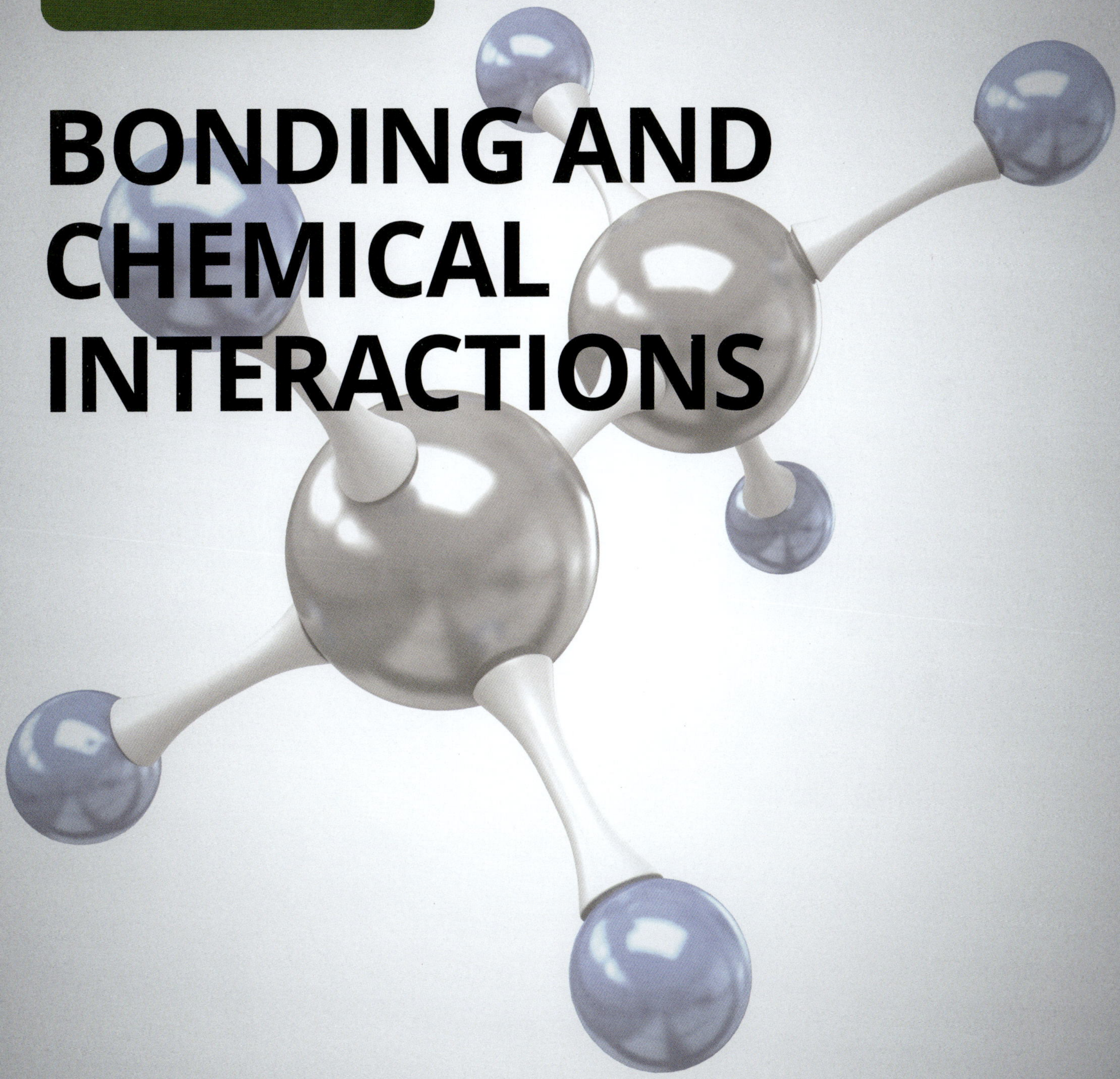

SCIENCE MASTERY ASSESSMENT

Every pre-med knows this feeling: there is so much content I have to know for the MCAT! How do I know what to do first or what's important?

While the high-yield badges throughout this book will help you identify the most important topics, this Science Mastery Assessment is another tool in your MCAT prep arsenal. This quiz (which can also be taken in your online resources) and the guidance below will help ensure that you are spending the appropriate amount of time on this chapter based on your personal strengths and weaknesses. Don't worry though—skipping something now does not mean you'll never study it. Later on in your prep, as you complete full-length tests, you'll uncover specific pieces of content that you need to review and can come back to these chapters as appropriate.

How to Use This Assessment

If you answer 0–7 questions correctly:

Spend about 1 hour to read this chapter in full and take limited notes throughout. Follow up by reviewing **all** quiz questions to ensure that you now understand how to solve each one.

If you answer 8–11 questions correctly:

Spend 20–40 minutes reviewing the quiz questions. Beginning with the questions you missed, read and take notes on the corresponding subchapters. For questions you answered correctly, ensure your thinking matches that of the explanation and you understand why each choice was correct or incorrect.

If you answer 12–15 questions correctly:

Spend less than 20 minutes reviewing all questions from the quiz. If you missed any, then include a quick read-through of the corresponding subchapters, or even just the relevant content within a subchapter, as part of your question review. For questions you answered correctly, ensure your thinking matches that of the explanation and review the Concept Summary at the end of the chapter.

1. What is the character of the bonds in carbon dioxide?
   - **A.** Ionic
   - **B.** Polar covalent
   - **C.** Nonpolar covalent
   - **D.** Coordinate covalent

2. Which of the following molecules contains the oxygen atoms with the most negative average formal charge?
   - **A.** H_2O
   - **B.** CO_3^{2-}
   - **C.** O_3
   - **D.** CH_2O

3. Which of the following elements does NOT break the octet rule?
   - **A.** Be
   - **B.** S
   - **C.** Na
   - **D.** P

4. Which of the following correctly ranks the compounds below by ascending boiling point?
   - **I.** Acetone
   - **II.** KCl
   - **III.** Kr
   - **IV.** Isopropyl alcohol

   - **A.** I < II < IV < III
   - **B.** III < IV < I < II
   - **C.** II < IV < I < III
   - **D.** III < I < IV < II

5. Both CO_3^{2-} and ClF_3 have three atoms bonded to a central atom. What is the best explanation for why CO_3^{2-} has trigonal planar electronic geometry, while ClF_3 has trigonal bipyramidal electronic geometry?
   - **A.** CO_3^{2-} has multiple resonance structures, while ClF_3 does not.
   - **B.** CO_3^{2-} has a charge of −2, while ClF_3 has no charge.
   - **C.** ClF_3 has lone pairs on its central atom, while CO_3^{2-} has none.
   - **D.** CO_3^{2-} has lone pairs on its central atom, while ClF_3 has none.

6. Which of the following elements, when paired together, would form ionic bonds?
   - **I.** Mg
   - **II.** Cl
   - **III.** O
   - **IV.** H

   - **A.** II and IV
   - **B.** I and II
   - **C.** II and III
   - **D.** III and IV

7. Despite the fact that both C_2H_2 and HCN contain triple bonds, the lengths of these triple bonds are not equal. Which of the following is the best explanation for this finding?
   - **A.** In C_2H_2, the bond is shorter because it is between atoms of the same element.
   - **B.** The two molecules have different resonance structures.
   - **C.** Carbon is more electronegative than hydrogen.
   - **D.** Nitrogen is more electronegative than carbon.

8. Which of the following is the best explanation of the phenomenon of hydrogen bonding?
   A. Hydrogen has a strong affinity for holding onto valence electrons.
   B. Hydrogen can only hold two valence electrons.
   C. Electronegative atoms disproportionately carry shared electron pairs when bonded to hydrogen.
   D. Hydrogen bonds have ionic character.

9. Which of the following best describes the number and character of the bonds in an ammonium cation?
   A. Three polar covalent bonds
   B. Four polar covalent bonds, of which none are coordinate covalent bonds
   C. Four polar covalent bonds, of which one is a coordinate covalent bond
   D. Four polar covalent bonds, of which two are coordinate covalent bonds

10. Although the octet rule dictates much of molecular structure, some atoms can violate the octet rule by being surrounded by more than eight electrons. Which of the following is the best explanation for why some atoms can exceed the octet?
   A. Atoms that exceed the octet already have eight electrons in their outermost electron shell.
   B. Atoms that exceed the octet only do so when bonding with transition metals.
   C. Atoms that exceed the octet can do so because they have *d*-orbitals in which extra electrons can reside.
   D. Some atoms can exceed the octet because they are highly electronegative.

11. Which of the following types of intermolecular forces provides the most accurate explanation for why noble gases can liquefy?
   A. Hydrogen bonding
   B. Ion–dipole interactions
   C. Dispersion forces
   D. Dipole–dipole interactions

12. In the structure shown, which atom(s) have the most positive charge?

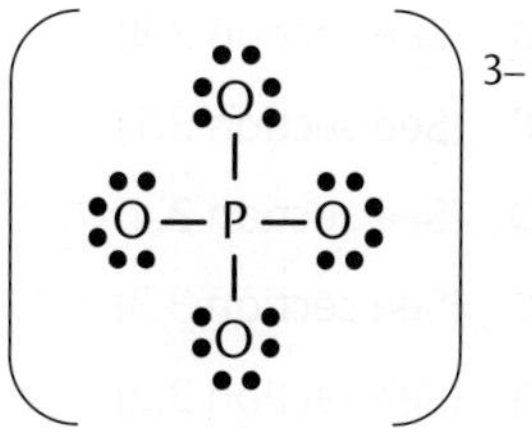

   A. The phosphorus atom has the most positive charge.
   B. All atoms share the charge equally.
   C. The four oxygen atoms share the highest charge.
   D. The oxygen atom at the peak of the trigonal pyramidal geometry has the most positive charge.

13. Which of the following is the best name for the new bond formed in the reaction shown?

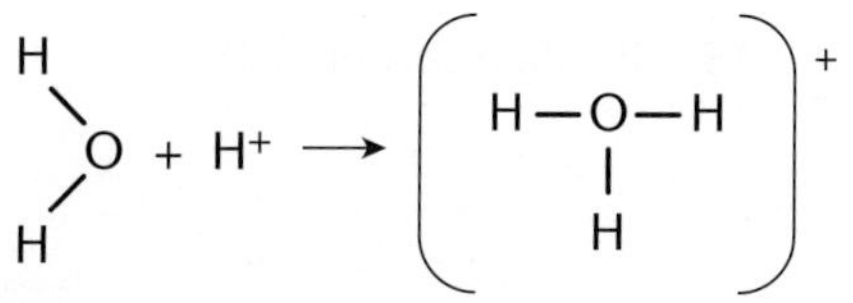

   A. Nonpolar covalent bond
   B. Ionic bond
   C. Coordinate covalent bond
   D. Hydrogen bond

14. Both BF_3 and NH_3 have three atoms bonded to the central atom. Which of the following is the best explanation for why the geometry of these two molecules is different?
   A. BF_3 has three bonded atoms and no lone pairs, which makes its geometry trigonal pyramidal.
   B. NH_3 is nonpolar, while BF_3 is polar.
   C. NH_3 has three bonded atoms and one lone pair, which makes its geometry trigonal pyramidal.
   D. BF_3 is nonpolar, while NH_3 is polar.

15. Which of the following compounds has the highest melting point?
   A. Sucrose
   B. NaCl
   C. Glycerol
   D. H_2O

Answer Key

1. **B** (See section 3.3)
2. **B** (See section 3.3)
3. **C** (See section 3.1)
4. **D** (See section 3.4)
5. **C** (See section 3.3)
6. **B** (See section 3.2)
7. **D** (See section 3.3)
8. **C** (See section 3.4)
9. **C** (See section 3.3)
10. **C** (See section 3.1)
11. **C** (See section 3.4)
12. **A** (See section 3.3)
13. **C** (See section 3.3)
14. **C** (See section 3.3)
15. **B** (See section 3.2)

The relevant section of the chapter to review for each question is given in parentheses after the correct answer. Detailed explanations can be found at the end of the chapter.

CHAPTER 3

BONDING AND CHEMICAL INTERACTIONS

In This Chapter

CHAPTER PROFILE

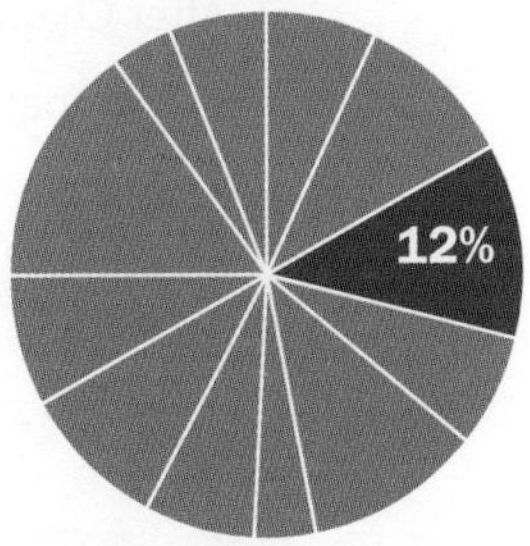

The content in this chapter should be relevant to about 12% of all questions about general chemistry on the MCAT.

This chapter covers material from the following AAMC content categories:

4C: Electrochemistry and electrical circuits and their elements

5B: Nature of molecules and intermolecular interactions

Introduction

The Maillard reaction is one of the most important chemical processes that occurs while cooking. The reaction mechanism itself is one with which you are closely familiar from your studies of organic chemistry: a nucleophilic reaction between the amino terminus of the peptide chain of a protein and the carbonyl functionality of a sugar to form an *N*-substituted glycosylamine. This compound undergoes a complex series of rearrangements and other reactions to produce a set of compounds that gives cooked food its pleasing color and delectable flavor. This reaction is especially important for browning meat.

When the surface of the meat comes into contact with the hot surface of a pan or grill, the proteins and sugars on the meat's exterior begin interacting via the Maillard reaction. The pan must be sufficiently hot to bring the exterior of the meat to a temperature of 155°C (310°F), the optimal temperature for the reaction to occur. So how does a grill master achieve the impossible: generating very high heat for the exterior but not over-cooking the interior? The answer lies, in part, in drying the meat. When meat that has a lot of water on its exterior surface hits the hot pan, the first process that takes place is the boiling of the water. Boiling is a phase change from liquid to gas and occurs at a constant temperature; water's boiling point is 100°C (212°F). Because this temperature is considerably lower than that necessary for the Maillard reaction, no browning will occur and the flavor compounds will not form. The lesson here is: if you want a tasty steak, always dry the surface of your meat!

Of course, the real lesson is the topic of discussion for this chapter: bonding and chemical interactions. We will not address complex chemical bonding, such as that which takes place in the Maillard reaction, in this chapter. Rather, this chapter will address the basics of chemical bonding and interactions. Here, we will investigate the nature and behavior of covalent and ionic bonds. We will also review a system—Lewis structures—by which bonding electrons are accounted for, and we will address the main principles of valence shell electron pair repulsion (VSEPR) theory. Finally, we will recount the various modes of interaction between molecules: intermolecular forces.

3.1 Bonding

LEARNING OBJECTIVES

After Chapter 3.1, you will be able to:

- Compare and contrast ionic and covalent compounds
- Identify elements that do not obey the octet rule
- Apply periodic trends to determine whether a covalent bond is polar or nonpolar:

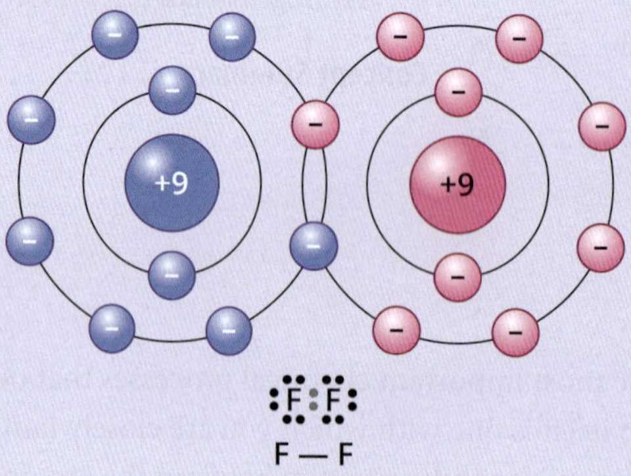

The atoms of most elements, except for a few noble gases, can combine to form **molecules**. The atoms within these molecules are held together by strong attractive forces called **chemical bonds**, which are formed via the interaction of the valence electrons of the combining atoms. The chemical and physical properties of the resulting compound are usually very different from those of the constituent elements. For example, elemental sodium, an alkali metal, is so reactive that it can actually produce fire when reacting with water because the reaction is highly exothermic. Diatomic chlorine gas is so toxic that it was used for chemical warfare during World War I. However, when sodium and chlorine react, the biologically important compound NaCl (table salt) is produced.

The Octet Rule

How do atoms join together to form compounds? In the example above, how do the sodium and the chlorine atoms form sodium chloride? For many molecules, the constituent atoms bond according to the **octet rule**, which states that an atom tends to bond with other atoms so that it has eight electrons in its outermost shell, thereby forming a stable electron configuration similar to that of the noble gases. An example of an octet configuration is shown for the noble gas argon (Ar) in Figure 3.1.

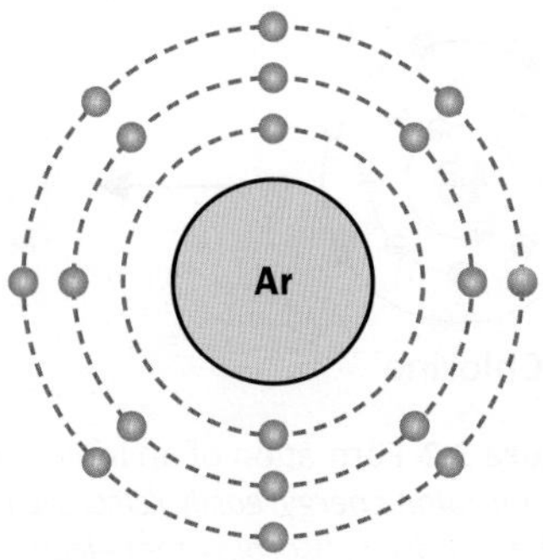

Figure 3.1 Electron Configuration of Argon
As a noble gas, argon has a complete octet in its valence shell.

However, this is more of a "rule of thumb," because there are more elements that can be exceptions to the rule than those that follow the rule. These "exceptional" elements include hydrogen, which can only have two valence electrons (achieving the configuration of helium); lithium and beryllium, which bond to attain two and four valence electrons, respectively; boron, which bonds to attain six valence electrons; and all elements in period 3 and greater, which can expand the valence shell to include more than eight electrons by incorporating *d*-orbitals. For example, in certain compounds, chlorine can form seven covalent bonds, thereby holding 14 electrons in its valence shell.

KEY CONCEPT

The octet rule is the desire of all atoms to achieve noble gas configuration. However, keep in mind that there are many exceptions to this rule.

A simple way to remember all the exceptions is as follows:

- **Incomplete octet:** These elements are stable with fewer than 8 electrons in their valence shell and include hydrogen (stable with 2 electrons), helium (2), lithium (2), beryllium (4), and boron (6).
- **Expanded octet:** Any element in period 3 and greater can hold more than 8 electrons, including phosphorus (10), sulfur (12), chlorine (14), and many others.
- **Odd numbers of electrons:** Any molecule with an odd number of valence electrons cannot distribute those electrons to give eight to each atom; for example, nitric oxide (NO) has eleven valence electrons.

Another way to remember the exceptions is to remember the common elements that almost always abide by the octet rule: carbon, nitrogen, oxygen, fluorine, sodium, and magnesium. Note that nonmetals gain electrons and metals lose electrons to achieve their respective complete octets.

Types of Bonds

We classify chemical bonds into two distinct types: ionic and covalent.

In **ionic bonding**, one or more electrons from an atom with a low ionization energy, typically a metal, are transferred to an atom with a high electron affinity, typically a nonmetal. An illustration of such a process is shown for our initial example, sodium chloride, in Figure 3.2.

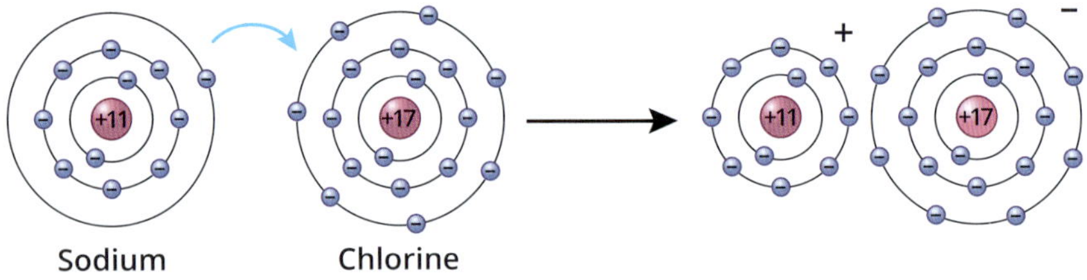

Figure 3.2 Formation of an Ionic Bond
Sodium (Na) has a low ionization energy, easily releasing an electron; chlorine (Cl) has a high electron affinity, easily absorbing that electron into its valence shell. In this example, both atoms achieve an octet formation.

The resulting electrostatic attraction between opposite charges is what holds the ions together. This is the nature of the bond in sodium chloride, where the positively charged sodium cation is electrostatically attracted to the negatively charged chloride anion. It is important to note that this type of electrostatic attraction creates lattice structures consisting of repeating rows of cations and anions, rather than individual molecular bonds, as shown in Figure 3.3.

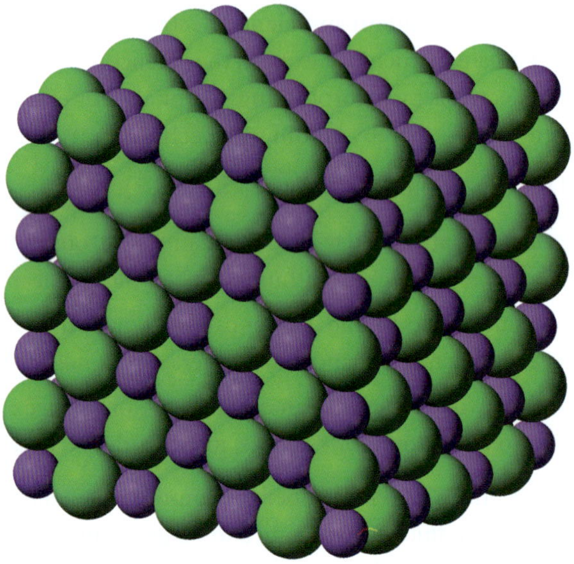

Figure 3.3 Crystal Lattice Structure of Sodium Chloride
Sodium = purple; chloride = green

In **covalent bonding**, an electron pair is shared between two atoms, typically nonmetals, that have relatively similar values of electronegativity. The degree to which the pair of electrons is shared equally or unequally between the two atoms determines the degree of polarity in the covalent bond. For example, if the electron pair is shared equally, the covalent bond is nonpolar; and if the pair is shared unequally, the bond is polar. If both of the shared electrons are contributed by only one of the two atoms, the bond is called **coordinate covalent**.

An example of nonpolar covalent bonding is shown for diatomic fluorine in Figure 3.4. Each atom has seven electrons in its valence shell, and by sharing one of these electrons from each atom, they can each form an octet. Unlike ionic crystal lattices, covalent compounds consist of individually bonded molecules.

BRIDGE

Electronegativity, discussed in Chapter 2 of *MCAT General Chemistry Review*, is a property that addresses how an individual atom acts within a bond and will help us understand the formation of molecules from atoms with different electronegativities.

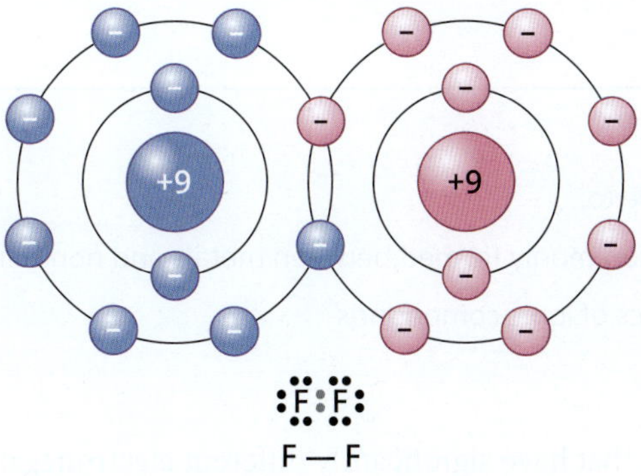

Figure 3.4 Formation of a Covalent Bond
Fluorine (F) has seven valence electrons; by sharing one electron from each atom, both fluorine atoms achieve an octet formation.

MCAT CONCEPT CHECK 3.1

Before you move on, assess your understanding of the material with these questions.

1. Describe the atomic differences between ionic and covalent compounds:
   - Ionic:

   ____

   - Covalent:

   ____

2. List three elements that do not follow the octet rule and explain why:

Element	Why It Violates the Octet Rule

3. Which periodic trend determines whether a covalent bond is polar or nonpolar?

____

3.2 Ionic Bonds

LEARNING OBJECTIVES

After Chapter 3.2, you will be able to:

- Explain why ionic bonds are commonly formed between metals and nonmetals
- Recall the major characteristics of ionic compounds

Ionic bonds form between atoms that have significantly different electronegativities. The atom that loses the electrons becomes a **cation**, and the atom that gains electrons becomes an **anion**. The ionic bond is the result of an electrostatic force of attraction between the opposite charges of these ions. Electrons are not shared in an ionic bond. For this electron transfer to occur, the difference in electronegativity must be greater than 1.7 on the Pauling scale.

MNEMONIC

Me**T**als lose electrons to become ca**T**ions = posi**T**ive (+) ions

Nonmetals gain electrons to become a**N**ions = **N**egative (–) ions

The MCAT won't expect you to memorize the Pauling scale, but recognize that ionic bonds are generally formed between a metal and a nonmetal. Figure 3.5 uses color coding to represent the Pauling scale on the periodic table. Elements with a low value are blue and are found on the left, whereas the highly electronegative elements are colored pink on the far right. For example, alkali and alkaline earth metals of Groups IA and IIA (Groups 1 and 2, respectively) readily form ionic bonds with the halogens of Group VIIA (Group 17). The atoms of the active metals loosely hold onto their electrons, whereas the halogens are more likely to gain an electron to complete their valence shell. The differences in bonding behavior for these classes of elements, and their differences in electronegativity values (ΔEN), explain the formation of ionic compounds such as cesium chloride ($\Delta EN = 2.3$), potassium iodide ($\Delta EN = 1.7$), and sodium fluoride ($\Delta EN = 3.1$).

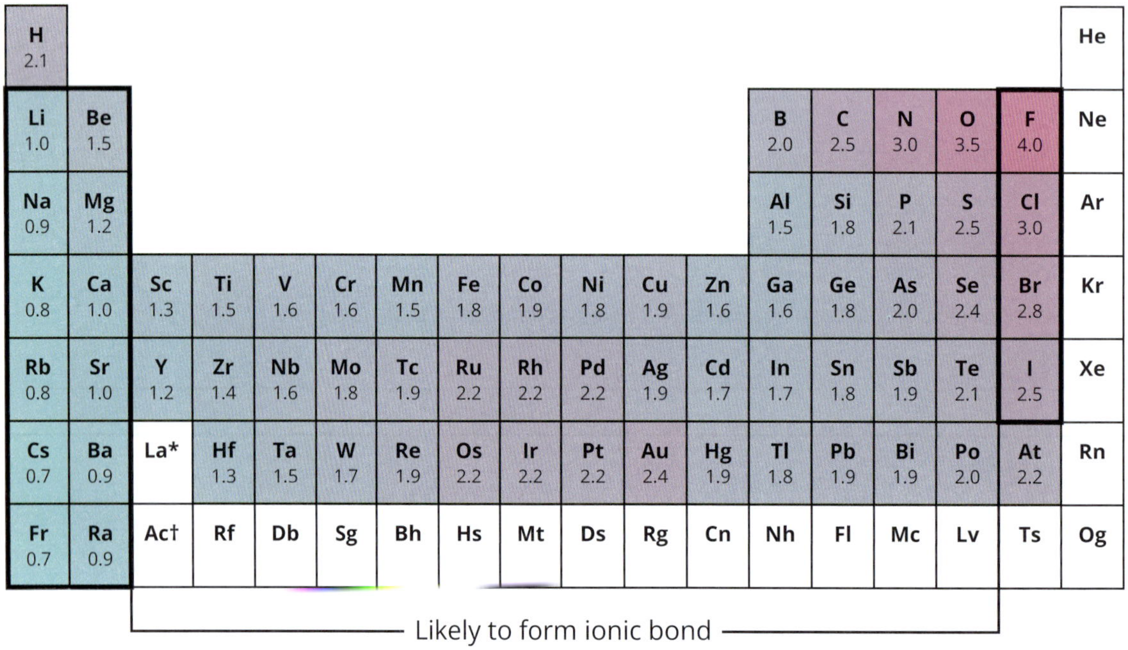

Figure 3.5 Pauling Scale Periodic Table
Due to their large difference in electronegativity, metals in Groups IA and IIA are likely to form ionic bonds with halogens in Group VIIA, highlighted in the table.

Ionic compounds have characteristic physical properties that you should recognize for Test Day. Because of the strength of the electrostatic force between the ionic constituents of the compound, ionic compounds have very high melting and boiling points. For example, the melting point of sodium chloride is 801°C. Many ionic compounds dissolve readily in water and other polar solvents and, in the molten or aqueous state, are good conductors of electricity. In the solid state, the ionic constituents of the compound form a **crystalline lattice** consisting of repeating positive and negative ions, as shown earlier in Figure 3.3. With this arrangement, the attractive forces between oppositely charged ions are maximized, and the repulsive forces between ions of like charge are minimized.

MCAT CONCEPT CHECK 3.2

Before you move on, assess your understanding of the material with these questions.

1. Why do ionic bonds tend to form between metals and nonmetals?

____

____

2. Describe five characteristics of ionic compounds.

- ______________________________
- ______________________________
- ______________________________
- ______________________________
- ______________________________

3.3 Covalent Bonds

High Yield

LEARNING OBJECTIVES

After Chapter 3.3, you will be able to:

- Explain the relationship between bond strength, bond length, and bond energy
- Identify the values of ΔEN for which polar covalent, nonpolar covalent, and ionic bonds will form
- Predict the molecular geometry of a molecule given its formula
- Draw Lewis dot structures for simple molecules, including resonance structures, such as:

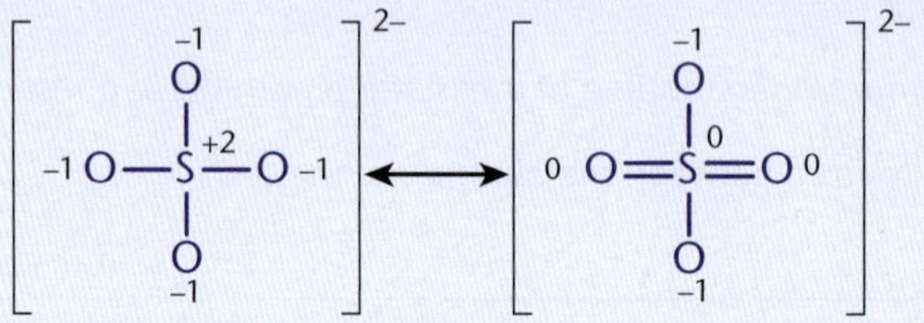

When two or more atoms with similar electronegativities interact, the energy required to form ions through the complete transfer of one or more electrons is greater than the energy that would be released upon the formation of an ionic bond. That is, when two atoms of similar tendency to attract electrons form a compound, it is energetically unfavorable to create ions. Rather than transferring electrons to form octets, the atoms share electrons. The bonding force between the atoms is not ionic; instead, there is an attraction that each electron in the shared pair has for the two positive nuclei of the bonded atoms.

Covalent compounds contain discrete molecular units with relatively weak intermolecular interactions. As a result, compounds like carbon dioxide (CO_2) tend to have lower melting and boiling points. In addition, because they do not break down into constituent ions, they are poor conductors of electricity in the liquid state or in aqueous solutions.

MCAT EXPERTISE

Think of bonds as a tug-of-war between two atoms. When the difference in electronegativity is great (more than 1.7), then the "stronger" atom wins all of the electrons and becomes the anion. When the electronegativity values are relatively similar, then we have a stalemate, or a covalent bond with mostly equal sharing of electrons.

Properties of Covalent Compounds

The formation of one covalent bond may not be sufficient to fill the valence shell for a given atom. Thus, many atoms can form bonds with more than one other atom, and most atoms can form multiple bonds with other atoms. Two atoms sharing one, two, or three pairs of electrons are said to be joined by a **single**, **double**, or **triple covalent bond**, respectively. The number of shared electron pairs between two atoms is called the **bond order**; hence, a single bond has a bond order of one, a double bond has a bond order of two, and a triple bond has a bond order of three. There are three important characteristics of a covalent bond to explain: bond length, bond energy, and polarity.

Bond Length

Bond length is the average distance between the two nuclei of atoms in a bond. Atoms with larger atomic radii will naturally have a longer bond length than atoms of a smaller size, as seen in Figure 3.6. A carbon-carbon bond is longer than a carbon-hydrogen bond since the hydrogen has a smaller atomic radius. Additionally, as the number of shared electron pairs increases, the two atoms are pulled closer together, resulting in a decrease in bond length. Thus, for a given pair of atoms, a triple bond is shorter than a double bond, which is shorter than a single bond.

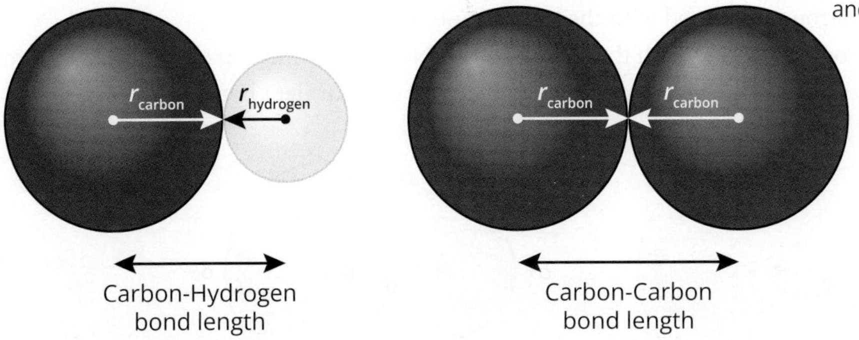

Figure 3.6 Bond Length Varies Based on Atomic Radius

KEY CONCEPT

You will see this inverse relationship between bond length and strength in both organic and general chemistry.

	Bond Length	Bond Strength
C–C	longest	weakest
C=C	medium	medium
C≡C	shortest	strongest

Know this relationship on Test Day and you'll earn quick points!

Bond Energy

Bond energy is the energy required to break a bond by separating its components into their isolated, gaseous atomic states. The greater the number of pairs of electrons shared between the atomic nuclei, the more energy is required to break the bonds holding the atoms together. Thus, triple bonds have the greatest bond energy, and single bonds have the lowest bond energy. We will discuss bond energy and calculations involving bond enthalpy in Chapter 7 of *MCAT General Chemistry Review*. By convention, the greater the bond energy is, the stronger the bond.

Polarity

Polarity is the unequal distribution of electron density in a molecule or a bond, resulting from a difference in electronegativity between two atoms. When these atoms come together in covalent bonds, they must negotiate the degree to which the electron pairs will be shared. The atom with the higher electronegativity gets the larger share of the electron density.

Nonpolar Covalent Bonds

When two atoms have similar or identical electronegativities (usually a difference in electronegativity, ΔEN, of less than 0.5 using the Pauling scale), they share electrons almost equally, forming a **nonpolar covalent bond**. The electron density is distributed evenly and there is no separation of charge. An important nonpolar covalent bond for the MCAT is the one that exists between carbon and hydrogen. Note that only atoms of the same element have exactly the same electronegativity, and therefore only diatomic molecules contain bonds with a purely equal distribution of electrons. The seven common diatomic molecules are H_2, N_2, O_2, F_2, Cl_2, Br_2, and I_2. Figure 3.7 shows the electron distribution in the bond between two fluorine atoms. The yellow spheres represent the valence electrons associated with the left fluorine, and the orange spheres are valence electrons associated with the right fluorine. Notice how the two electrons, one from each fluorine, are shared equally between the two atoms to form the nonpolar covalent bond.

MNEMONIC

Here's a quick way to remember the naturally occurring diatomic elements on the periodic table: they form the number **7** on the periodic table (except for H), there are **7** of them, and most of them are in Group **VIIA**: H_2, N_2, O_2, F_2, Cl_2, Br_2, I_2.

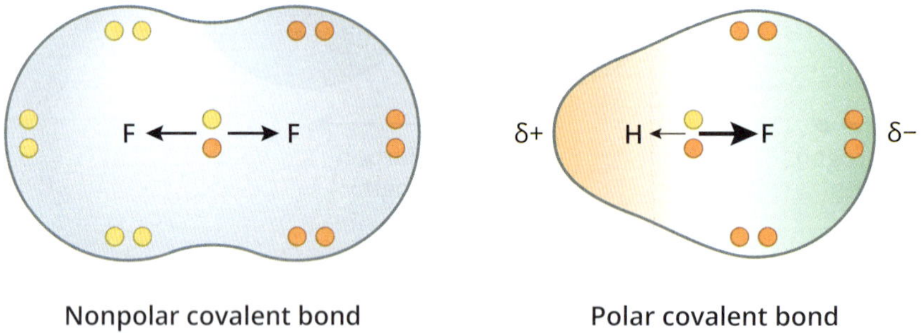

Figure 3.7 Nonpolar vs. Polar Covalent Bonds
Dipole moment of a polar covalent bond, HF, compared to a nonpolar covalent bond, F_2

Polar Covalent Bonds and Dipole Moments

A **polar covalent bond** forms when there's a moderate difference in electronegativity between two atoms (typically ΔEN between 0.5 and 1.7). The more electronegative atom attracts the shared electrons more strongly, gaining a **partial negative charge** (δ^-), while the less electronegative element acquires a **partial positive charge** (δ^+). This separation of charge creates a **dipole moment (p)**, a vector quantity that represents the polarity of the bond or molecule. The dipole moment vector points from the positive to the negative charge and is calculated by:

$$\mathbf{p} = q\mathbf{d}$$

Equation 3.1

where **p** is the dipole moment, q is the magnitude of the charge, and **d** is the distance between the charges. The unit for the dipole moment is the **Debye** (coulomb–meter).

MCAT EXPERTISE

The range of electronegativities for nonpolar bonds is roughly 0 to 0.5. Polar bonds are found from 0.5 to 1.7, and ionic bonds are at 1.7 and above. Some chemistry courses allude to a grey area from 1.7 to 2.0. For the MCAT, if a molecule in this range has a metal and nonmetal, then it is effectively ionic; otherwise, it is polar covalent.

An example of a polar covalent bond with a dipole moment is shown in Figure 3.7. The single electron associated with the hydrogen in yellow is shared in the covalent bond with fluorine, but since the fluorine is more electronegative, the covalent bond in HF is polar due to the large ΔEN, with the partial negative charge on the fluorine and the partial positive charge on the hydrogen.

BRIDGE

The chemistry that creates coordinate covalent bonds appears in many forms. These reactions can be called nucleophile–electrophile reactions, described in Chapter 4 of *MCAT Organic Chemistry Review*; Lewis acid–base reactions, described in Chapter 10 of *MCAT General Chemistry Review*, or complexation reactions, described in Chapter 9 of *MCAT General Chemistry Review.*

Coordinate Covalent Bonds

In a **coordinate covalent bond**, both of the shared electrons originated on the same atom. Generally, this means that a lone pair of one atom attacked another atom with an unhybridized *p*-orbital to form a bond, as shown in Figure 3.8. Once such a bond forms, however, it is indistinguishable from any other covalent bond. The distinction is only helpful for keeping track of the valence electrons and formal charges. Coordinate covalent bonds are typically found in Lewis acid–base reactions, described in Chapter 10 of *MCAT General Chemistry Review*. A Lewis acid is any compound that will accept a lone pair of electrons, while a Lewis base is any compound that will donate a pair of electrons to form a covalent bond.

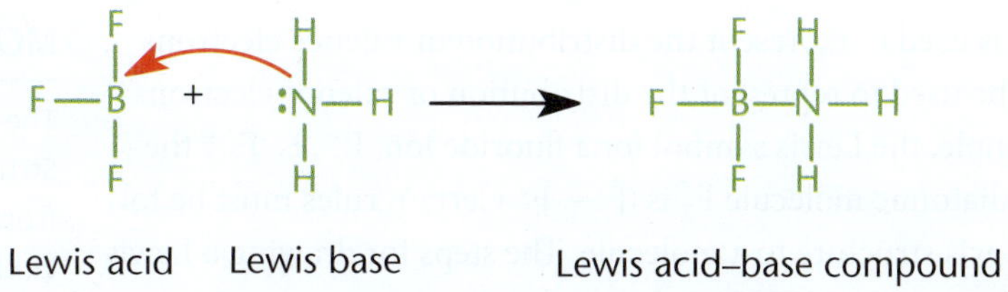

Figure 3.8 Coordinate Covalent Bond

Here, NH_3 donates a pair of electrons to form a coordinate covalent bond; thus, it acts as a Lewis base. At the same time, BF_3 accepts this pair of electrons to form the coordinate covalent bond; thus, it acts as a Lewis acid.

Covalent Bond Notation

The electrons involved in a covalent bond are in the valence shell and are **bonding electrons**, while those electrons in the valence shell that are not involved in covalent bonds are **nonbonding electrons**. The unshared electron pairs are also known as lone pairs because they are associated only with one atomic nucleus. Because atoms can bond with other atoms in many different combinations, the **Lewis structure** system of notation was developed to keep track of the bonded and nonbonded electron pairs.

Think of Lewis structures as a bookkeeping method for electrons. The number of valence electrons attributed to a particular atom in the Lewis structure of a molecule is not necessarily the same as the number of valence electrons in the neutral atom. This difference accounts for the **formal charge** of an atom in a Lewis structure. Often, more than one Lewis structure can be drawn for a molecule. If the possible Lewis structures differ in their bond connectivity or arrangement, then the Lewis structures represent different possible compounds. However, if the Lewis structures show the same bond connectivity and differ only in the arrangement of the electron pairs, then these structures represent different resonance forms of a single compound. Note that Lewis structures do not represent the actual or even theoretical geometry of a real compound. Their usefulness lies in showing the different possible ways in which atoms may be combined to form different compounds or resonance forms of a single compound.

When more than one arrangement can be made, one can assess the likelihood of each arrangement by checking the formal charges on the atoms in each arrangement. The arrangement that minimizes the number and magnitude of formal charges is usually the most stable arrangement of the compound.

Lewis Structures

A Lewis structure, or **Lewis dot diagram**, is the chemical symbol of an element surrounded by dots, each representing one of the *s* or *p* valence electrons of the atom. The Lewis symbols of the elements in the second period of the periodic table are shown in Table 3.1.

·Li	Lithium	·N̈· (with one dot below)	Nitrogen
·Be·	Beryllium	·Ö:	Oxygen
·Ḃ·	Boron	·F̤̈:	Fluorine
·Ċ· (with one dot below)	Carbon	:N̤̈e:	Neon

Table 3.1 Lewis Symbols for Period 2 Elements

KEY CONCEPT

In drawing Lewis dot structures, remember that some atoms can expand their octets by utilizing the *d*-orbitals in their outer shell. This will only take place with atoms in period 3 or greater.

Just as a Lewis symbol is used to represent the distribution of valence electrons in an atom, it can also be used to represent the distribution of valence electrons in a molecule. For example, the Lewis symbol for a fluoride ion, F^-, is :F̤̈:$^-$ the Lewis structure of the diatomic molecule F_2 is :F̤̈ – F̤̈:. Certain rules must be followed in assigning a Lewis structure to a molecule. The steps for drawing a Lewis structure are outlined here, using HCN as an example.

MCAT EXPERTISE

The number of dots in Lewis Structure notation comes from group numbers. Lithium is in Group IA and therefore has one electron (dot). Carbon is in Group IVA and has four dots.

- Draw out the backbone of the compound—that is, the arrangement of atoms. In general, the least electronegative atom is the central atom. Hydrogen (always) and the halogens F, Cl, Br, and I (usually) occupy a terminal position.

  In HCN, H must occupy an end position. Of the remaining two atoms, C is the least electronegative and, therefore, occupies the central position. Therefore, the skeletal structure is as follows:

  H—C—N

- Count all the valence electrons of the atoms. The number of valence electrons of the molecule is the sum of the valence electrons of all atoms present:

  H has 1 valence electron
  C has 4 valence electrons
  N has 5 valence electrons; therefore,
  HCN has a total of 10 valence electrons.

- Draw single bonds between the central atom and the atoms surrounding it. Each single bond corresponds to a pair of electrons:

$$H:C:N$$

- Complete the octets of all atoms bonded to the central atom, using the remaining valence electrons left to be assigned. Recall that H is an exception to the octet rule because it can only have two valence electrons. In this example, H already has two valence electrons from its bond with C.

$$H{:}C{:}\ddot{\underset{..}{N}}{:}$$

- Place any extra electrons on the central atom. If the central atom has less than an octet, try to write double or triple bonds between the central and surrounding atoms using the lone pairs on the surrounding atoms.

The HCN structure above does not satisfy the octet rule for C because C only has four valence electrons. Therefore, two lone electron pairs from the N atom must be moved to form two more bonds with C, creating a triple bond between C and N. To make it easier to visualize, bonding electron pairs are represented as lines. You should be familiar with both dot and line notation for bonds.

$$H-C\equiv N:$$

Now, the octet rule is satisfied for all three atoms; C and N have eight valence electrons, and H has two valence electrons.

Formal Charge

To determine if a Lewis structure is representative of the actual arrangement of atoms in a compound, one must calculate the formal charge of each atom. In doing so, assume a perfectly equal sharing of all bonded electron pairs, regardless of actual differences in electronegativity. In other words, assume that each electron pair is split evenly between the two nuclei in the bond. The difference between the number of electrons assigned to an atom in a Lewis structure and the number of electrons normally found in that atom's valence shell is the **formal charge**. A simple equation you can use to calculate formal charge is:

$$\text{formal charge} = V - N_{\text{nonbonding}} - \frac{1}{2} N_{\text{bonding}}$$

Equation 3.2

where V is the normal number of electrons in the atom's valence shell, $N_{\text{nonbonding}}$ is the number of nonbonding electrons, and N_{bonding} is the number of bonding electrons (double the number of bonds because each bond has two electrons). The charge of an ion or compound is equal to the sum of the formal charges of the individual atoms comprising the ion or compound.

MNEMONIC

A less formal way to calculate formal charge is with the formula:

Formal charge = valence electrons − dots − sticks

Where a "dot" refers to a lone electron and a "stick" refers to a bond.

Example: Calculate the formal charge on the central N atom of $[NH_4]^+$.

Solution: The Lewis structure of $[NH_4]^+$ is:

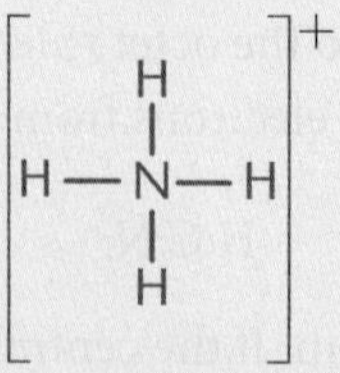

Nitrogen is in Group VA; thus, it has five valence electrons. In $[NH_4]^+$, N has four bonds (eight bonding electrons and zero nonbonding electrons).

Thus, $V = 5$; $N_{bonding} = 8$; $N_{nonbonding} = 0$

$$\text{Formal charge} = 5 - 0 - \frac{1}{2}(8) = +1$$

Thus, the formal charge on the N atom in $[NH_4]^+$ is $+1$.

One can also use logic to determine formal charge. As drawn, N has four bonds. Assuming equal sharing of the electrons in the bonds, this means N has four valence electrons. In its normal state, N has five valence electrons. Thus, nitrogen has one fewer electron than its normal state, and has a $+1$ charge.

Let us offer a brief note of explanation on the difference between formal charge and oxidation number: formal charge underestimates the effect of electronegativity differences, whereas oxidation numbers overestimate the effect of electronegativity differences, assuming that the more electronegative atom has a 100 percent share of the bonding electron pair. For example, in a molecule of CO_2 (carbon dioxide), the formal charge on each of the atoms is 0, but the oxidation number of each of the oxygen atoms is -2 and of the carbon is $+4$. In reality, the distribution of electron density between the carbon and oxygen atoms lies somewhere between the extremes predicted by the formal charges and the oxidation states.

Resonance

As suggested earlier, it may be possible to draw two or more Lewis structures that demonstrate the same arrangement of atoms but that differ in the specific placement of the electrons. These are called **resonance structures** and are represented with a double-headed arrow between them. The actual electronic distribution in the compound is a hybrid, or composite, of all of the possible resonance structures. For example, SO_2 has three resonance structures, as shown in Figure 3.9.

BRIDGE

Resonance is an important topic in both general and organic chemistry. It allows for greater stability, delocalizing electrons and charges over what is known as a π (pi) system. Resonance in organic molecules is discussed in Chapter 3 of *MCAT Organic Chemistry Review.*

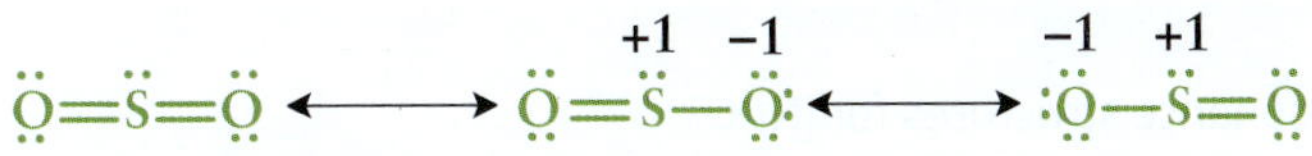

Figure 3.9 Resonance Structures for SO_2
The double-headed arrows indicate that these molecules are involved in a resonance hybrid.

The nature of the bonds within the actual compound is a hybrid of these three structures. If one were to evaluate the spectral data, it would indicate that the two S—O bonds are identical and equivalent. This phenomenon is known as resonance, and the actual structure of the compound is called the **resonance hybrid**. Another example of a resonance hybrid can be seen in Figure 3.10, a carbonate ion, CO_3^{2-}. The average charge on each oxygen is shown in the resonance hybrid structure, resulting in a negative charge that is slightly less than 1 for each oxygen. Adding up the charges on all oxygens results in an overall charge of −2.

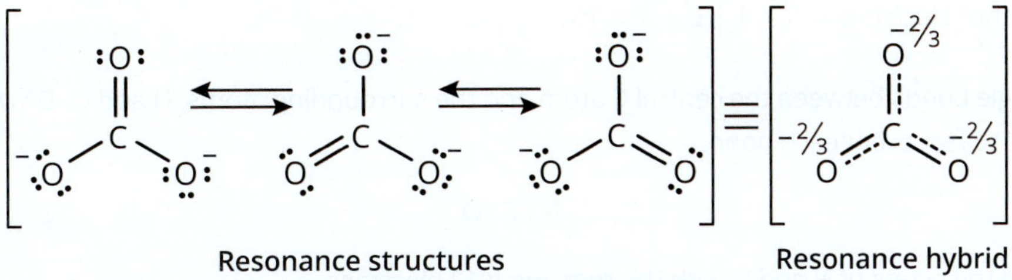

Figure 3.10 Resonance Structures and Hybrid for the Carbonate Ion

The first resonance structure in Figure 3.9 is significantly more stable than the other two structures. Consequently, it is the major contributor to the resonance hybrid. In general, the more stable the structure, the more it contributes to the character of the resonance hybrid. In Figure 3.9, the minor contributors contain formal charges, indicating decreased stability. In contrast, for the carbonate ion in Figure 3.10, all resonance structures have the same formal charge, so each contributes equally to the resonance hybrid. One can use formal charge to assess the stability of resonance structures according to the following guidelines:

- A Lewis structure with small or no formal charges is preferred over a Lewis structure with large formal charges.
- A Lewis structure with less separation between opposite charges is preferred over a Lewis structure with a large separation of opposite charges.
- A Lewis structure in which negative formal charges are placed on more electronegative atoms is more stable than one in which the negative formal charges are placed on less electronegative atoms.

Example: Write the resonance structures for $[NCO]^-$.

Solution:

1. C is the least electronegative of the three given atoms. Therefore, the C atom occupies the central position in the skeletal structure of $[NCO]^-$:

$$N - C - O$$

2. N has 5 valence electrons;
C has 4 valence electrons;
O has 6 valence electrons;
and the species has one negative charge.
Total valence electrons $= 5 + 4 + 6 + 1 = 16$

3. Draw single bonds between the central C atom and the surrounding atoms, N and O. Draw a pair of electrons to represent each bond.

$$N : C : O$$

4. Complete the octets of N and O with the remaining 12 electrons.

$$:\ddot{\underset{..}{N}} : C : \ddot{\underset{..}{O}}:$$

5. The C octet is incomplete. There are three ways in which double and triple bonds can be formed to complete the C octet: two lone pairs from the O atom can be used to form a triple bond between the C and O atoms:

$$:\overset{-2}{\ddot{\underset{..}{N}}} - \overset{0}{C} \equiv \overset{+1}{\ddot{O}}$$

Or one lone electron pair can be taken from both O and N to form two double bonds, one between N and C, the other between O and C:

$$:\overset{-1}{\ddot{N}} = \overset{0}{C} = \overset{0}{\ddot{O}}:$$

Or two lone electron pairs can be taken from the N atom to form a triple bond between the C and N atoms:

$$:\overset{0}{N} \equiv \overset{0}{C} - \overset{-1}{\ddot{\underset{..}{O}}}:$$

All three are resonance structures of $[NCO]^-$

6. Assign formal charges to each atom of each resonance structure.

The most stable structure is this:

$$:\overset{0}{N} \equiv \overset{0}{C} - \overset{-1}{\ddot{\underset{..}{O}}}:$$

because the charges are minimized, and the negative formal charge is on the most electronegative atom, O.

Exceptions to the Octet Rule

As stated previously, the octet rule has many exceptions. In addition to hydrogen, helium, lithium, beryllium, and boron, which are exceptions because they cannot or do not usually reach the octet, all elements in or beyond the third period may be exceptions because they can take on more than eight electrons in their valence shells. These electrons can be placed into orbitals of the *d* subshell, and as a result, atoms of these elements can form more than four bonds. On Test Day, don't automatically discount a Lewis structure with a central atom that has more than four bonds—the testmakers may be testing your ability to recognize that many atoms can expand their valence shells beyond the octet.

MCAT EXPERTISE

Don't be surprised if you can draw more than two resonance structures for a molecule or ion. Becoming proficient at drawing and, more importantly, recognizing resonance structures will save you time on Test Day.

Consider the sulfate ion, SO_4^{2-}. In the Lewis structure for the sulfate ion, giving the sulfur 12 valence electrons permits three of the five atoms to be assigned a formal charge of zero. The sulfate ion can be drawn in at least six resonance forms, many of which have two double bonds attached to a different combination of oxygen atoms. Figure 3.11 shows two of the possible forms.

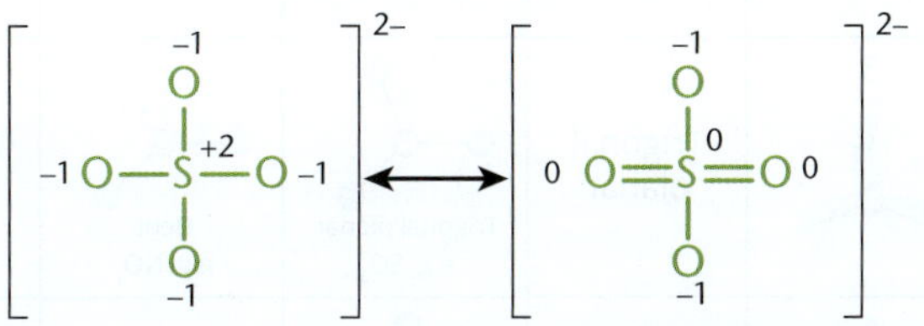

Figure 3.11 Two Different Resonance Forms of the Sulfate Ion

Geometry and Polarity

Because Lewis dot structures do not suggest or reflect the actual geometric arrangement of atoms in a compound, we need another system to provide this information. One such system is known as the **valence shell electron pair repulsion** (**VSEPR**) **theory**.

Valence Shell Electron Pair Repulsion (VSEPR) Theory

VSEPR theory uses Lewis dot structures to predict the molecular geometry of covalently bonded molecules. It states that the three-dimensional arrangement of atoms surrounding a central atom is determined by the repulsions between bonding and nonbonding electron pairs in the valence shell of the central atom. These electron pairs arrange themselves as far apart as possible, thereby minimizing repulsive forces. The following steps are used to predict the geometrical structure of a molecule using the VSEPR theory:

- Draw the Lewis dot structure of the molecule.
- Count the total number of bonding and nonbonding electron pairs in the valence shell of the central atom.

- Arrange the electron pairs around the central atom so that they are as far apart as possible. For example, the compound AX_2 has the Lewis structure X : A : X. The A atom has two bonding electron pairs in its valence shell. To position these electron pairs as far apart as possible, their geometric structure should be linear:

$$X - A - X$$

Electronic geometry describes the spatial arrangement of all electrons, bonded and lone pairs. **Molecular geometry** describes only the arrangement of atoms themselves. A summary of electronic and molecular geometries as predicted by VSEPR theory is shown in Table 3.2.

MCAT EXPERTISE

According to the AAMC's official content lists, you need to be prepared to draw and identify structural formulas for molecules involving H, C, N, O, F, S, P, Si, and Cl. Rather than memorizing these elements, however, just be familiar with the process of creating a Lewis diagram for any element and predicting its three-dimensional shape from VSEPR theory.

Number of electron dense areas	Electron pair geometry	Molecular geometry			
		No lone pairs	1 lone pair	2 lone pairs	3 lone pairs
2	Linear	Linear e.g. CO_2			
3	Trigonal planar	Trigonal planar e.g. SO_3	Bent e.g. NO_2^-	Linear e.g. O_2	
4	Tetrahedral	Tetrahedral e.g. CH_4	Trigonal bipyramidal e.g. NH_3	Bent e.g. H_2O	Linear e.g. HCl
5	Trigonal bipyramidal	Trigonal bipyramidal e.g. PCl_5	Seesaw e.g. SF_4	T-shaped e.g. ClF_3	Linear e.g. I_3^-
6	Octahedral	Octahedral e.g. SF_6	Square pyramidal e.g. ClF_5	Square planar e.g. ICl_4^-	

Lone pair · Ligand · Central atom

Table 3.2 VSEPR Theory
This table lists the most common electronic and molecular configurations of molecules.

Example: Predict the molecular geometry of NH_3.

Solution:

1. The Lewis structure of NH_3 is:

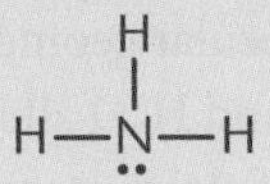

2. The central atom, N, has three bonding electron pairs and one nonbonding electron pair, for a total of four electron pairs.

3. The four electron pairs will be farthest apart when they occupy the corners of a tetrahedron. Because one of the four electron pairs is a lone pair, the observed molecular geometry is trigonal pyramidal, shown below.

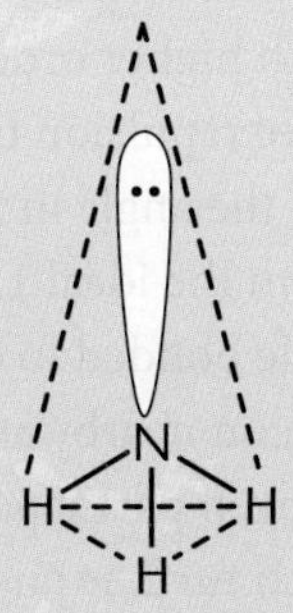

In describing the shape of a molecule, only the arrangement of atoms (not electrons) is considered. Even though the electron pairs are arranged tetrahedrally, the shape of NH_3 is pyramidal. It is not trigonal planar because the lone pair repels the three bonding electron pairs, causing them to move as far apart as possible.

KEY CONCEPT

The shapes from Table 3.2 refer to *electronic geometry,* which is different from *molecular geometry.* In the worked example, notice that the ammonia molecule has a tetrahedral *electronic* structure, but is considered to have a *molecular* structure that is trigonal pyramidal.

Example: Predict the geometry of CO_2.

Solution: The Lewis structure of CO_2 is $\ddot{\underset{..}{O}}::C::\ddot{\underset{..}{O}}$

The double bond behaves just like a single bond for the purposes of predicting molecular shape. This compound has two groups of electrons around the carbon. According to the VSEPR theory, the two sets of electrons will orient themselves 180° apart, on opposite sides of the carbon atom, minimizing electron repulsion. Therefore, the molecular structure of CO_2 is linear: $\ddot{\underset{..}{O}}=C=\ddot{\underset{..}{O}}$

One subtlety that the MCAT loves to test is the difference between electronic geometry and molecular geometry. **Electronic geometry** describes the spatial arrangement of all pairs of electrons around the central atom, including both the bonding and the lone pairs. In contrast, the **molecular geometry** describes the spatial arrangement of only the bonding pairs of electrons. The **coordination number**, which is the number of atoms that surround and are bonded to a central atom, is the relevant factor when determining molecular geometry. For example, consider that CH_4 (methane), NH_3 (ammonia), and H_2O all have the same electronic geometry: in each compound, four pairs of electrons surround the central atom. This is tetrahedral electronic geometry. However, because each molecule has a different coordination number, they have different molecular geometries. In molecular geometry, methane has tetrahedral geometry, ammonia has trigonal pyramidal geometry, and water is identified as angular or bent.

MCAT EXPERTISE

CH_4, NH_3, and H_2O all have a tetrahedral electronic geometry, but differ in their molecular shapes:

CH_4 is tetrahedral, NH_3 is pyramidal, and H_2O is bent or angular.

The distinction is important, and the MCAT will primarily focus on molecular geometry. However, there is one important implication of electronic geometry: the determination of the **ideal bond angle**. Trigonal planar electronic geometry, for example, is associated with an ideal bond angle of 120°, as seen in Figure 3.12 with BH_3. However, nonbonding electron pairs, along with higher order bonds like double bonds, contain greater electron density. This increased density exerts more repulsion than bonding pairs and single bonds because these electrons reside closer to the nucleus. Thus, the angle in molecules with lone pairs or double bonds in a trigonal planar arrangement would deviate from the ideal 120°. An example of this can be seen in Figure 3.12 with an amide, O=C–N. The carbon double bonded to oxygen has a greater electron density than that of a single bond, which creates greater repulsion on nearby atoms and bonds, resulting in deviation from ideal angles. Additionally, the lone pairs on the nitrogen participate in resonance to form a partial double bond between the nitrogen and carbonyl carbon, which further pushes the bonds away from the ideal.

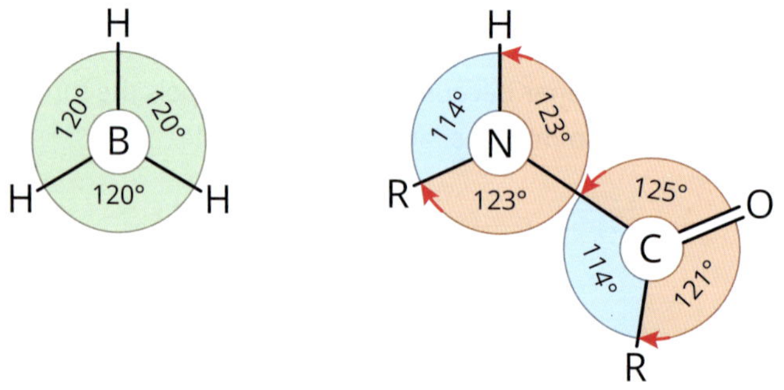

Figure 3.12 Bond Angles of BH_3 and the Amide Functional Group
BH_3 has ideal bond angles of 120°, whereas the bond angles in amide deviate away from the ideal.

Polarity of Molecules

When two atoms of different electronegativities bond covalently, sharing one or more pairs of electrons, the resulting bond is polar, with the more electronegative atom possessing the greater share of the electron density. However, the presence of bond dipoles does not necessarily result in a molecular dipole; that is, an overall separation of charge across the molecule. We must first consider the molecular geometry and the vector addition of the bond dipoles based upon that molecular geometry. A compound with nonpolar bonds is always nonpolar. However, a compound with polar bonds may be polar or nonpolar, depending upon the spatial orientation of the polar bonds in the molecule. If the compound has a molecular geometry such that the bond dipole moments cancel each other out (that is, if the vector sum is zero), then the result is a nonpolar compound. For example, CCl_4 (carbon tetrachloride) has four polar C–Cl bonds, but because the molecular geometry of carbon tetrachloride is tetrahedral, the four bond dipoles point to the vertices of the tetrahedron and, therefore, cancel each other out, resulting in a nonpolar compound, as shown in Figure 3.13.

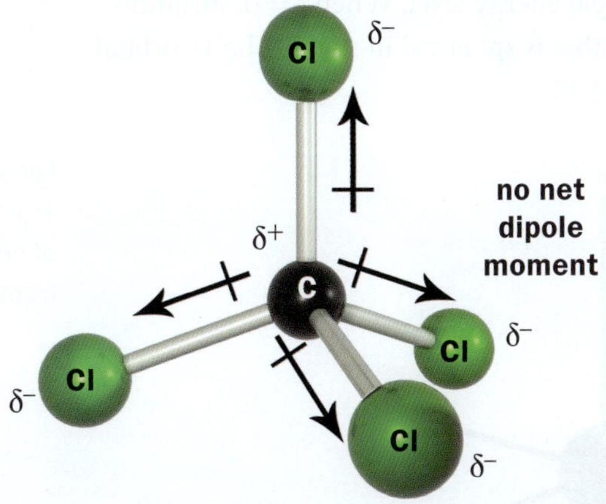

Figure 3.13 CCl_4 is a Nonpolar Compound with Four Polar Bonds

However, when the molecular geometry is arranged such that the bond dipoles do not cancel each other out, the molecule will have a net dipole moment and will therefore be polar. For instance, the O–H bonds in H_2O are polar, with each hydrogen atom assuming a partial positive charge and the oxygen assuming a partial negative charge. Recall that the molecular geometry of water is angular (bent). Therefore, the vector summation of the bond dipoles results in a molecular dipole moment from the partially positive hydrogen end to the partially negative oxygen end, as illustrated in Figure 3.14.

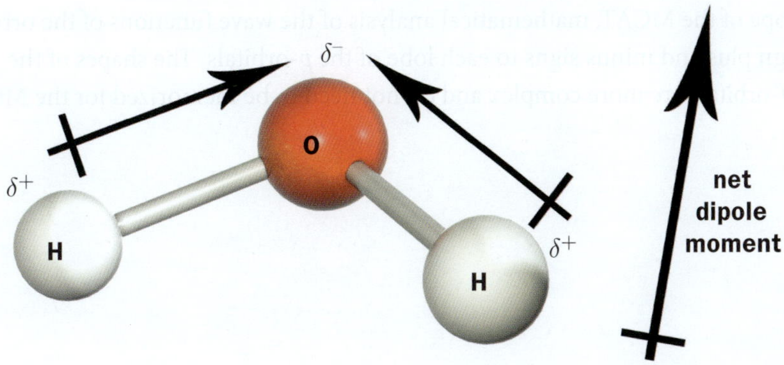

Figure 3.14 H_2O is a Polar Molecule with Two Polar Bonds

MCAT EXPERTISE

Be careful! If you spot a polar bond in a molecule, the molecule can be either polar or nonpolar. On the contrary, when you see only nonpolar bonds in a molecule, the structure *must* be nonpolar. When in doubt, draw out relevant structures on your scratch paper on Test Day.

Atomic and Molecular Orbitals

To finish the discussion of covalent bonds, we need to address the concept of atomic and molecular orbitals. Recall the model of the atom as a dense, positively charged nucleus surrounded by a cloud of electrons organized into orbitals (regions in space surrounding the nucleus within which there are certain probabilities of finding an electron). The four quantum numbers describe the energy and position of an electron in an atom. While the principal quantum number, n, indicates the average energy level of the shell, the azimuthal quantum number, l, describes the subshells within each principal energy level. When $l = 0$, this indicates the *s* subshell, which has one orbital that is spherical in shape. The 1*s*-orbital ($n = 1, l = 0, m_l = 0$) is plotted in Figure 3.15.

BRIDGE

Quantum Numbers (Chapter 1 of *MCAT General Chemistry Review*) revisited:

For any value of n, there are n values of l ($0 \rightarrow n - 1$).

- $l = 0 \rightarrow s$
- $l = 1 \rightarrow p$
- $l = 2 \rightarrow d$
- $l = 3 \rightarrow f$

For any value of l, there are $2l + 1$ values of ml (number of orbitals); values range from $-l$ to l.

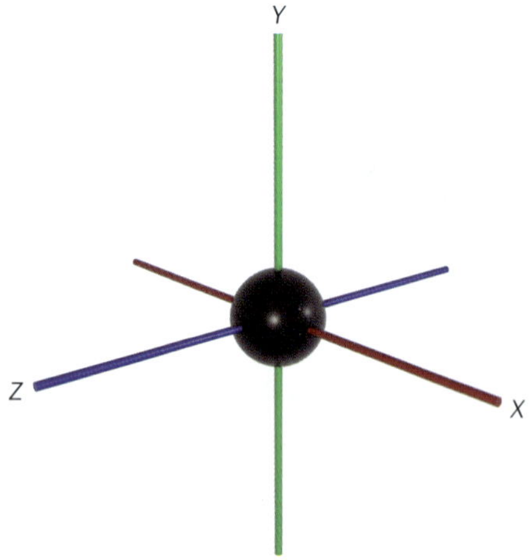

Figure 3.15 1*s*-Orbital

When $l = 1$, this indicates the *p* subshell, which has three orbitals shaped like barbells along the *x*-, *y*-, and *z*-axes at right angles to each other. The 2*p*-orbitals ($n = 2, l = 1, m_l = -1, 0,$ and $+1$) are plotted in Figure 3.16.

Although well beyond the scope of the MCAT, mathematical analysis of the wave functions of the orbitals is used to determine and assign plus and minus signs to each lobe of the *p*-orbitals. The shapes of the five *d*-orbitals and the seven *f*-orbitals are more complex and do not need to be memorized for the MCAT.

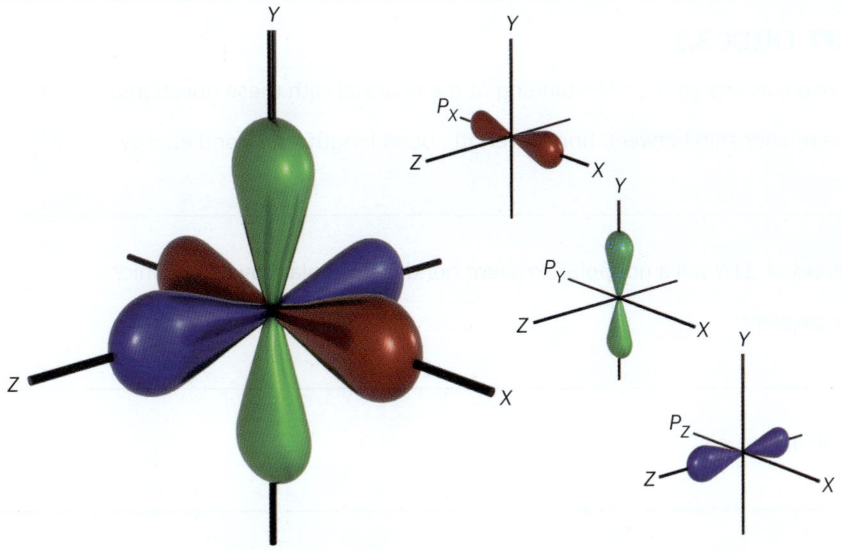

Figure 3.16 *p*-Orbitals on the *x*-, *y*-, and *z*-Axes

When two atoms bond to form a compound, the atomic orbitals interact to form a **molecular orbital** that describes the probability of finding the bonding electrons in a given space. Molecular orbitals are obtained by combining the wave functions of the atomic orbitals. Qualitatively, the overlap of two atomic orbitals describes this molecular orbital. If the signs of the two atomic orbitals are the same, a **bonding orbital** forms. If the signs are different, an **antibonding orbital** forms.

Two different patterns of overlap are observed in the formation of molecular bonds. When orbitals overlap head-to-head, the resulting bond is a **sigma (σ) bond**. σ bonds allow for free rotation about their axes because the electron density of the bonding orbital is a single linear accumulation between the atomic nuclei.

When the orbitals overlap in such a way that there are two parallel electron cloud densities, a **pi (π) bond** is formed. π bonds do not allow for free rotation because the electron densities of the orbitals are parallel and cannot be twisted in such a way that allows continuous overlapping of the clouds of electron densities. Sigma and pi bond orbitals can be seen in Figure 3.17. The presence of a σ bond alone corresponds to a single bond. A double bond is a σ bond plus a π bond. A triple bond is a σ bond plus two π bonds.

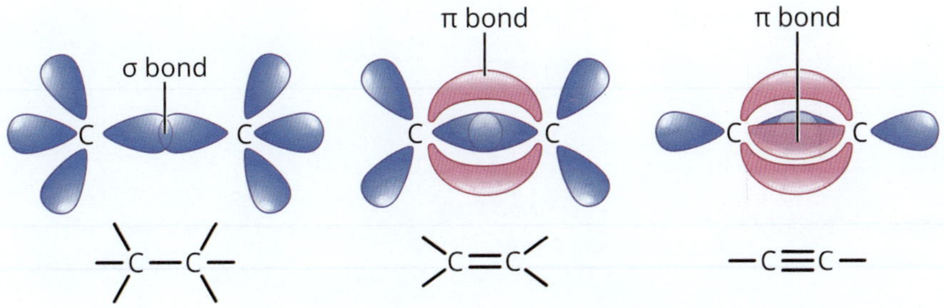

Figure 3.17 Sigma and Pi Bond Orientation

MCAT CONCEPT CHECK 3.3

Before you move on, assess your understanding of the material with these questions.

1. Describe the relationship between bond strength, bond length, and bond energy.

2. For what values of ΔEN will a nonpolar covalent bond form? Polar covalent? Ionic?
   - Nonpolar covalent:
   - Polar covalent:
   - Ionic:

3. Draw a Lewis dot structure for the carbonate ion (CO_3^{2-}) and its two other resonance structures.

4. Predict the molecular geometries of the following molecules:
   - PCl_5:
   - MgF_2:
   - AlF_3:
   - UBr_6:
   - SiH_4:

3.4 Intermolecular Forces

LEARNING OBJECTIVES

After Chapter 3.4, you will be able to:

- Order the intermolecular forces from strongest to weakest
- Describe what occurs during dipole-dipole, hydrogen bonding, and London dispersion force interactions
- Predict what intermolecular forces are possible for given interacting molecules:

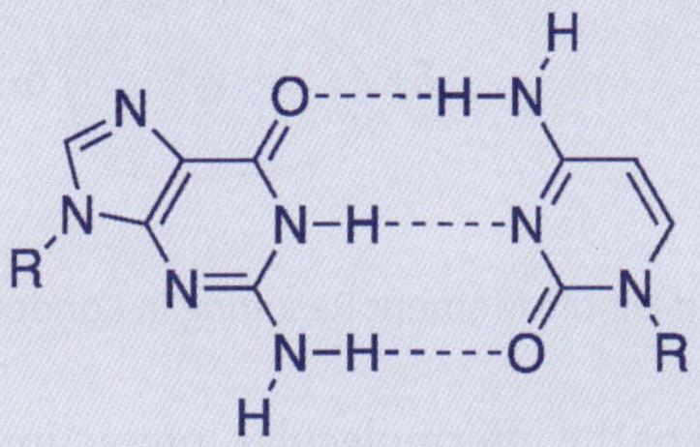

Atoms and compounds participate in weak electrostatic interactions. The strength of these **intermolecular forces** can impact certain physical properties, such as melting and boiling points. The weakest of the intermolecular interactions are the dispersion forces, also known as London forces. Next are the dipole–dipole interactions, which are of intermediate strength. Finally, we have the strongest type of interaction, the hydrogen bond, which is a misnomer because there is no actual sharing or transfer of electrons. We must keep in mind, however, that even hydrogen bonds, the strongest of these interactions, only have about 10 percent of the strength of a covalent bond. Therefore, these electrostatic interactions can be overcome with small or moderate amounts of energy.

BRIDGE

These intermolecular forces are the bonding forces that keep a substance together in its solid or liquid state and determine whether two substances are miscible or immiscible in solution. Solutions and solubility are discussed in Chapter 9 of *MCAT General Chemistry Review.*

London Dispersion Forces

The bonding electrons in nonpolar covalent bonds may appear to be shared equally between two atoms, but at any point in time, they will be located randomly throughout the orbital. In a given moment, the electron density may be unequally distributed between the two atoms. As shown in Figure 3.18, this results in a rapid polarization and counterpolarization of the electron cloud and the formation of short-lived dipole moments, creating temporary partially negative and positive charged ends to the atom. Subsequently, these dipoles interact with the electron clouds of neighboring compounds, inducing the formation of more dipoles. The momentarily negative end of one molecule will cause the closest region in any neighboring molecule to become temporarily positive itself. This causes the other end of the neighboring molecule to become temporarily negative, which in turn induces other molecules to become temporarily polarized, and the cycle begins again. The attractive or repulsive interactions of these short-lived and rapidly shifting dipoles are known as **London dispersion forces**, a type of van der Waals force.

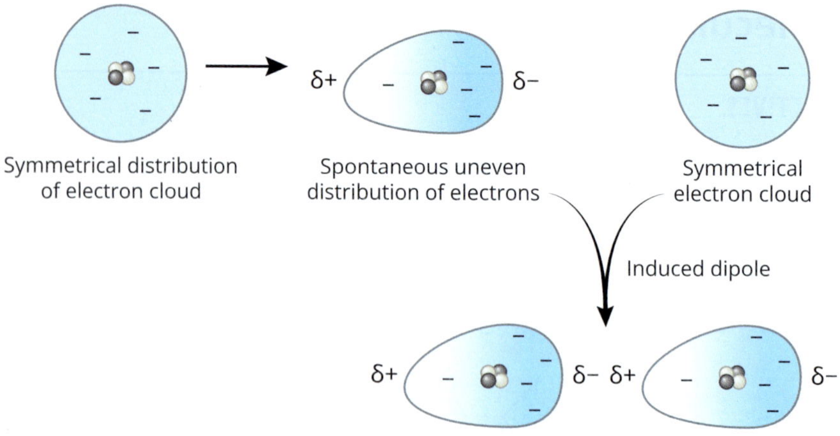

Figure 3.18 Induced Dipole Moment Resulting in London Dispersion Forces

Dispersion forces are the weakest of all of the intermolecular interactions because they are the result of induced dipoles that change and shift moment to moment. They do not extend over long distances and are, therefore, significant only when molecules are in close proximity. The strength of the London force also depends on the degree and ease by which the molecules can be polarized—that is, how easily the electrons can be shifted around. Large molecules are more easily polarizable than comparable smaller molecules and thus possess greater dispersion forces.

Despite their weak nature, don't underestimate the importance of dispersion forces. If it weren't for them, the noble gases would not liquefy at any temperature because no other intermolecular forces exist between the noble gas atoms. The low temperatures at which noble gases liquefy are indicative of the very small magnitude of the dispersion forces between the atoms.

REAL WORLD

While dispersion forces (a type of van der Waals force) are the weakest of the intermolecular attractions, when there are millions of these interactions there is an amazing power of adhesion. This is demonstrated by geckos' feet; the animal's ability to climb smooth, vertical, and even inverted surfaces is due to dispersion forces.

Dipole–Dipole Interactions

Polar molecules tend to orient themselves in such a way that the oppositely charged ends of the respective molecular dipoles are closest to each other: the positive region of one molecule is close to the negative region of another molecule. This arrangement is energetically favorable because an attractive electrostatic force is formed between the two molecules. This attractive force is denoted by dashed lines in most molecular notations and indicates a temporary bonding interaction, as shown in Figure 3.19.

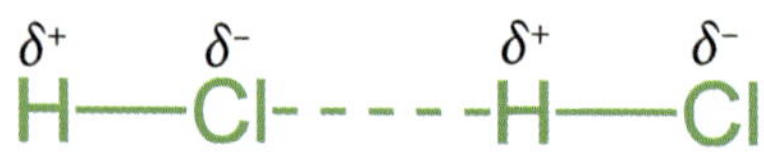

Figure 3.19 Dipole–Dipole Interactions in HCl

Dipole–dipole interactions are present in the solid and liquid phases but become negligible in the gas phase because of the significantly increased distance between gas particles. Polar species tend to have higher melting and boiling points than nonpolar species of comparable molecular weight due to these interactions. Realize that London forces and dipole–dipole interactions are different not in kind but in duration. Both are electrostatic forces between opposite partial charges; the difference is only in the transience or permanence of the molecular dipole.

BRIDGE

In organic chemistry, carbonyl groups possess distinct dipoles that facilitate nucleophilic attacks. This is the focus of almost all of the reactions in Chapters 6 to 9 of *MCAT Organic Chemistry Review*.

Hydrogen Bonds

Hydrogen bonds are a favorite topic on the MCAT. A hydrogen bond is a specific, unusually strong form of dipole–dipole interaction that may be intra- or intermolecular. Hydrogen bonds are not actually bonds—there is no sharing or transferring of electrons between two atoms. When hydrogen is bonded to one of three highly electronegative atoms—nitrogen, oxygen, or fluorine—the hydrogen atom carries only a small amount of the electron density in the covalent bond.

MNEMONIC

Hydrogen bonds: Pick up the **FON** (phone):

Hydrogen bonds exist in molecules containing a hydrogen bonded to **F**luorine, **O**xygen, or **N**itrogen.

The hydrogen atom essentially acts as a naked proton. The positively charged hydrogen atom interacts with the partial negative charge of fluorine, oxygen, or nitrogen on nearby molecules. Substances that display hydrogen bonding tend to have unusually high boiling points compared to compounds of similar molecular weights that do not exhibit hydrogen bonding. The difference derives from the energy required to break the hydrogen bonds. Hydrogen bonding, shown in Figure 3.20, is particularly important in the behavior of water, alcohols, amines, and carboxylic acids.

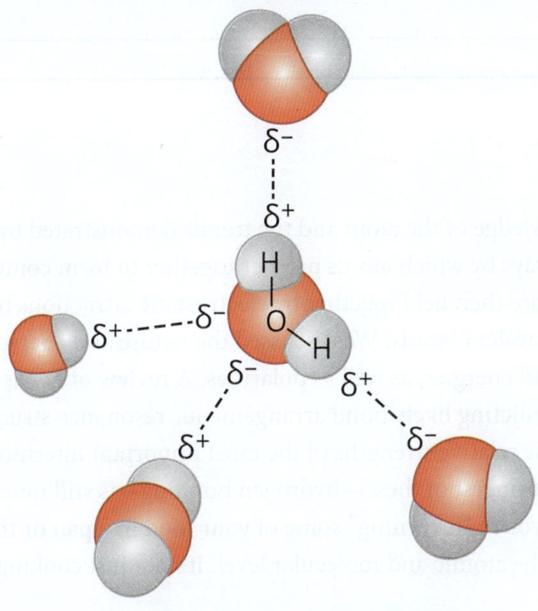

Figure 3.20 Hydrogen Bonding in Water

Many biochemical molecules, such as nucleotides, have different regions that are stabilized by hydrogen bonding, as shown in Figure 3.21. It is not an overstatement to say that, were it not for water's ability to form hydrogen bonds and exist in the liquid state at room temperature, we would not exist (at least not in the form we recognize as "human").

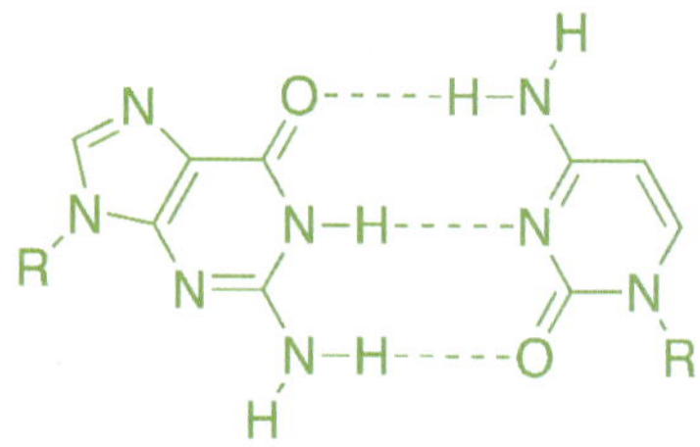

Figure 3.21 Hydrogen Bonding between Guanine and Cytosine

MCAT CONCEPT CHECK 3.4

Before you move on, assess your understanding of the material with these questions.

1. Rank the major intermolecular forces from strongest to weakest:

    1. ______________________
    2. ______________________
    3. ______________________

2. Describe what occurs during dipole–dipole interactions.

    ____

3. In order to exhibit hydrogen bonding, what must be true of a given molecule?

    ____

Conclusion

This chapter built on our knowledge of the atom and the trends demonstrated by the elements in the periodic table to explain the different ways by which atoms partner together to form compounds, either by exchanging electrons to form ions, which are then held together by electrostatic attractions between opposite charges; or by sharing electrons to form covalent bonds. We discussed the nature and characteristics of covalent bonds, noting their relative lengths and energies, as well as polarities. A review of Lewis dot structures and VSEPR theory will prepare you for predicting likely bond arrangements, resonance structures, and molecular geometries. Finally, we compared the relative strengths of the most important intermolecular electrostatic interactions, noting that even the strongest of these—hydrogen bonding—is still much weaker than an actual covalent bond. The next time you're "browning" some of your food in a pan or the oven, take a moment to consider what's happening at the atomic and molecular level. It's not just cooking; it's science!

GO ONLINE

You've reviewed the content, now test your knowledge and critical thinking skills by completing a test-like passage set in your online resources!

CONCEPT SUMMARY

Bonding

- Chemical bonds can be ionic or covalent.
- Elements will form bonds to attain a noble gas-like electron configuration.
- The **octet rule** states that elements will be most stable with eight valence electrons. However, there are many exceptions to this rule:
  - Elements with an incomplete octet are stable with fewer than eight electrons and include H, He, Li, Be, and B.
  - Elements with an expanded octet are stable with more than eight electrons and include all elements in period 3 or greater.
  - Compounds with an odd number of electrons cannot have eight electrons on each element.

Ionic Bonds

- An **ionic bond** is formed via the transfer of one or more electrons from an element with a relatively low ionization energy to an element with a relatively high electron affinity.
  - Ionic bonds occur between elements with large differences in electronegativity ($\Delta EN > 1.7$), usually between metals and nonmetals.
  - A positively charged ion is called a **cation**. A negatively charged ion is called an **anion**.
  - The resulting electrostatic attraction between the ions causes them to remain in close proximity, forming the bond.
  - Ionic compounds form **crystalline lattices**—large, organized arrays of ions.
- Ionic compounds have unique physical and chemical properties.
  - Ionic compounds tend to dissociate in water and other polar solvents.
  - Ionic solids tend to have high melting points.

Covalent Bonds

- A **covalent bond** is formed via the sharing of electrons between two elements of similar electronegativities.
- **Bond order** refers to whether a covalent bond is a single bond, double bond, or triple bond. As bond order increases, **bond strength** increases, **bond energy** increases, and **bond length** decreases.

- Covalent bonds can be categorized as nonpolar or polar based on the nature of the elements involved.
  - **Nonpolar bonds** result in molecules in which both atoms have exactly the same electronegativity; some bonds are considered nonpolar when there is a very small difference in electronegativity between the atoms ($\Delta EN < 0.5$), even though they are technically slightly polar.
  - **Polar bonds** form when there is a significant difference in electronegativities ($\Delta EN = 0.5$ to 1.7), but not enough to transfer electrons and form an ionic bond. In a polar bond, the more electronegative element takes on a partial negative charge, and the less electronegative element takes on a partial positive charge.
- **Coordinate covalent bonds** result when a single atom provides both bonding electrons while the other atom does not contribute any; coordinate covalent bonds are most often found in Lewis acid–base chemistry.
- **Lewis dot symbols** are a chemical representation of an atom's valence electrons.
- Drawing a complete Lewis dot structure requires a balance of valence, bonding, and nonbonding electrons in a molecule or ion.
- **Formal charges** exist when an atom is surrounded by more or fewer valence electrons than it has in its neutral state (assuming equal sharing of electrons in a bond).
- For any molecule with a π (pi) system of electrons, **resonance structures** exist; these represent all of the possible configurations of electrons—stable and unstable—that contribute to the overall structure.
- The **valence shell electron pair repulsion (VSEPR) theory** predicts the three-dimensional molecular geometry of covalently bonded molecules. In this theory, electrons—whether bonding or nonbonding—arrange themselves to be as far apart as possible from each other in three-dimensional space, leading to characteristic geometries.
  - Nonbonding electrons exert more repulsion than bonding electrons because they reside closer to the nucleus.
  - **Electronic geometry** refers to the position of all electrons in a molecule, whether bonding or nonbonding. **Molecular geometry** refers to the position of only the bonding pairs of electrons in a molecule.
- The **polarity of molecules** is dependent on the dipole moment of each bond and the sum of the dipole moments in a molecular structure.
  - All polar molecules contain polar bonds.
  - Nonpolar molecules may contain nonpolar bonds, or polar bonds with dipole moments that cancel each other.
- σ and π bonds describe the patterns of overlap observed when molecular bonds are formed.
  - **Sigma (σ) bonds** are the result of head-to-head overlap.
  - **Pi (π) bonds** are the result of the overlap of two parallel electron cloud densities.

Intermolecular Forces

- **Intermolecular forces** are electrostatic attractions between molecules. They are significantly weaker than covalent bonds (which are weaker than ionic bonds).
  - **London dispersion forces** are the weakest interactions, but are present in all atoms and molecules. As the size of the atom or structure increases, so does the corresponding London dispersion force.
  - **Dipole–dipole interactions**, which occur between the oppositely charged ends of polar molecules, are stronger than London forces; these interactions are evident in the solid and liquid phases but negligible in the gas phase due to the distance between particles.
  - **Hydrogen bonds** are a specialized subset of dipole–dipole interactions involved in intra- and intermolecular attraction; hydrogen bonding occurs when hydrogen is bonded to one of three very electronegative atoms—fluorine, oxygen, or nitrogen.

ANSWERS TO CONCEPT CHECKS

3.1

1. Ionic bonds form between ions and involve gain or loss of electrons. Covalent bonds occur when electrons are shared between atoms.
2. Any three examples that form incomplete octets (H, He, Li, Be, B) or expanded octets (Period 3 and greater) are acceptable.
3. The polarity in a covalent bond is determined by differences in electronegativity between the two atoms involved.

3.2

1. Metals lose electrons because they have low ionization energies, while nonmetals gain electrons because they have high electron affinities. These processes are complementary, leading to the formation of an ionic bond.
2. Some characteristics of ionic compounds include high melting and boiling points due to electrostatic attractions, solubility of ions in water due to interactions with polar solvents, good conductors of heat and electricity, crystal lattice arrangement to minimize repulsive forces, and large electronegativity differences between ions, among other possible answers.

3.3

1. Bond strength is defined by the electrostatic attraction between nuclei and electrons; multiple bonds (higher bond order) increases strength. Bond length is a consequence of these attractions. The stronger the bond, the shorter it is. Bond energy is the minimum amount of energy needed to break a bond. The stronger the bond, the higher the bond energy.
2. Nonpolar covalent bonds form with $\Delta EN = 0$ to 0.5. Polar covalent bonds form with $\Delta EN = 0.5$ to 1.7. Ionic bonds form with $\Delta EN = 1.7$ or higher.
3. 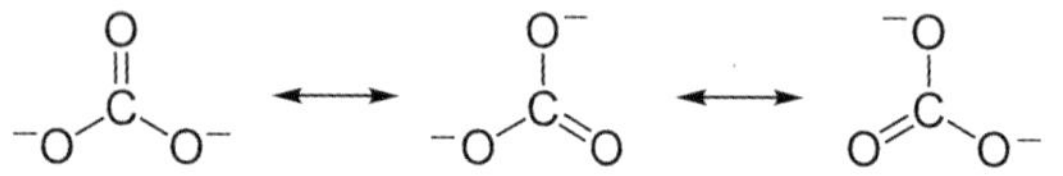
4. PCl_5: trigonal bipyramidal, MgF_2: linear, AlF_3: trigonal planar, UBr_6: octahedral, SiH_4: tetrahedral

3.4

1. Hydrogen bonding > dipole–dipole interactions > dispersion (London) forces
2. A dipole consists of a segment of a molecule with partial positive and partial negative regions. The positive end of one molecule is attracted to the negative end of another molecule, and vice-versa.
3. To experience hydrogen bonding, a molecule must contain a hydrogen bonded to a very electronegative atom (nitrogen, oxygen, or fluorine).

SCIENCE MASTERY ASSESSMENT EXPLANATIONS

1. **B**

Carbon dioxide, CO_2, has a double bond between carbon and each of its oxygen atoms. In polar covalent bonds, the difference in electronegativity between the bonded atoms is great enough to cause electrons to move disproportionately toward the more electronegative atom; hence the bonds are polar. But the electronegativity difference is not great enough to completely transfer electrons to the more electronegative atom; hence the bonds are covalent. Because oxygen has somewhat greater electronegativity compared to carbon, the bonds of carbon dioxide are polar covalent.

2. **B**

To answer this question, one must understand the contribution of resonance structures to average formal charge. In **(B)**, there are three possible resonance structures. Each of the three oxygen atoms carries a formal charge of -1 in two out of the three structures. This averages to approximately $-\frac{2}{3}$ charge on each oxygen atom, which is more negative than in the other answer choices. Both water and formaldehyde, **(A)** and **(D)**, have no formal charge on the oxygen. Ozone, **(C)**, has a $-\frac{1}{2}$ on two of the three oxygens and a $+1$ charge on the central oxygen.

3. **C**

This question is asking for an element that reliably follows the octet rule. There are only a few elements that do not break the octet rule, including carbon, nitrogen, oxygen, fluorine, sodium, and magnesium. Thus, **(C)** is correct. To eliminate **(A)**, **(B)**, and **(D)**, observe that the remaining elements can have other valences; Be is stable with a valence of four electrons, while both S and P can expand their octets.

4. **D**

The key to answering this question is to understand the types of intermolecular forces that exist in each of these molecules because larger intermolecular forces correspond to higher boiling points. Kr is a noble gas with a full octet, so the only intermolecular forces present are London dispersion forces, the weakest type of intermolecular forces. Acetone and isopropyl alcohol are both polar, so both have dipole–dipole interactions, which are stronger than dispersion forces. However, isopropyl alcohol can also form hydrogen bonds, increasing its boiling point. Finally, the strongest interactions are ionic bonds, which exist in potassium chloride.

5. **C**

The central carbon in carbonate has no lone pairs. It has three resonance structures, each of which involves a double bond between carbon and one of the three oxygens. Having made four bonds, carbon has no further orbitals for bonding or to carry lone pairs. This makes carbonate's geometry trigonal planar. Alternatively, ClF_3 also has three bonds; however, chloride still maintains two extra lone pairs. These lone pairs each inhabit one orbital, meaning that the central chloride must organize five items about itself: three bonds to fluorides and two lone pairs. The best configuration for maximizing the distance between all of these groups is trigonal bipyramidal. **(A)** and **(B)** are true statements but do not account for the difference in geometry.

6. **B**

Ionic bonds are formed between elements with large differences in electronegativity, i.e. between metals and nonmetals. Mg is a metal, whereas Cl, O, and H are all nonmetals. Since **(B)** contains a metal and nonmetal, it is correct. **(A)**, **(C)**, and **(D)** all describe covalent bonds. While HCl does ionize in aqueous solution, it exists as a polar covalent compound in the gaseous state.

7. **D**

Bond lengths decrease as the bond order increases, and they also decrease with larger differences in electronegativity. In this case, because both C_2H_2 and HCN have triple bonds, we cannot compare the bond lengths based on bond order. We must then rely on other periodic trends. The bond length decreases when moving to the right along the periodic table's rows because more electronegative atoms have shorter atomic radii. The nitrogen in HCN is likely to hold its electrons closer, or in a shorter radius, than the carbons in C_2H_2.

8. **C**

Electronegative atoms bonded to hydrogen disproportionately pull covalently bonded electrons toward themselves, which leaves hydrogen with a partial positive character. That partial positive charge is attracted to nearby negative or partial negative charges, such as those on other electronegative atoms.

9. **C**

First recall that ammonium is NH_4^+, while ammonia is NH_3. Ammonium is formed by the association of NH_3, an uncharged molecule with a lone pair on the nitrogen, with a positively charged hydrogen cation. In other words, NH_3 is a Lewis base, while H^+ is a Lewis acid. This type of bonding between a Lewis acid and base is a coordinate covalent bond.

10. **C**

All atoms in the third period or greater have *d*-orbitals, which can hold an additional 10 electrons. The typical "octet" electrons reside in *s*- and *p*-orbitals, but elements in period 3 or higher can place electrons into these *d*-orbitals.

11. **C**

All of the listed types of forces describe interactions between different types of molecules. However, noble gases are entirely uncharged and do not have polar covalent bonds, ionic bonds, or dipole moments. Therefore, the only intermolecular forces experienced by noble gases are London dispersion forces. Although these interactions are small in magnitude, they are necessary for condensation into a liquid.

12. **A**

In this Lewis diagram, the phosphate molecule has an overall formal charge of -3. The four oxygen atoms would each be assigned a formal charge of -1. Given the overall charge of -3 and the -1 charge on each oxygen, the phosphorus must have a formal charge of $+1$.

13. **C**

The reaction in this question shows a water molecule, which has two lone pairs of electrons on the central oxygen, combining with a free hydrogen cation. The resulting molecule, H_3O^+ has formed a new bond between H^+ and H_2O. This bond is created via the sharing of one of oxygen's lone pairs with the free H^+ ion. This represents the donation of a shared pair of electrons from a Lewis base (H_2O) to a Lewis acid (H^+, electron acceptor). This type of bond is called a coordinate covalent bond.

14. **C**

NH_3 has three hydrogen atoms bonded to the central nitrogen, which also has a lone pair. These four groups—three atoms, one lone pair—lead NH_3 to assume tetrahedral electronic geometry yet trigonal pyramidal molecular geometry. The nitrogen in ammonia is sp^3-hybridized. By hybridizing all three *p*-orbitals and the one *s*-orbital, four groups are arranged about the central atom, maximizing the distances between the groups to minimize the energy of the molecule with a tetrahedral configuration. In contrast, BF_3 has three atoms and no lone pairs, resulting in sp^2-hybridization. Its shape is called trigonal planar.

15. **B**

When a compound melts, the interactions between molecules must be broken to a sufficient extent to enable movement. In NaCl, these interactions are ionic. On the other hand, solids made of molecules of sucrose, glycerol, or water are held together by hydrogen bonds. Due to the greater electrostatic attraction between the full charges of ionic bonds, the ionic bonds of NaCl are significantly stronger than hydrogen bonds of other molecules. Thus, NaCl has the highest melting point, consistent with **(B)**.

GO ONLINE

Consult your online resources for additional practice.

EQUATIONS TO REMEMBER

(3.1) **Dipole moment:** $\mathbf{p} = q\mathbf{d}$

(3.2) **Formal charge:** $V - N_{\text{nonbonding}} - \frac{1}{2}N_{\text{bonding}}$

SHARED CONCEPTS

General Chemistry Chapter 1
Atomic Structure

General Chemistry Chapter 2
The Periodic Table

General Chemistry Chapter 4
Compounds and Stoichiometry

Organic Chemistry Chapter 3
Bonding

Organic Chemistry Chapter 4
Analyzing Organic Reactions

Physics and Math Chapter 5
Electrostatics and Magnetism

CHAPTER 4

COMPOUNDS AND STOICHIOMETRY

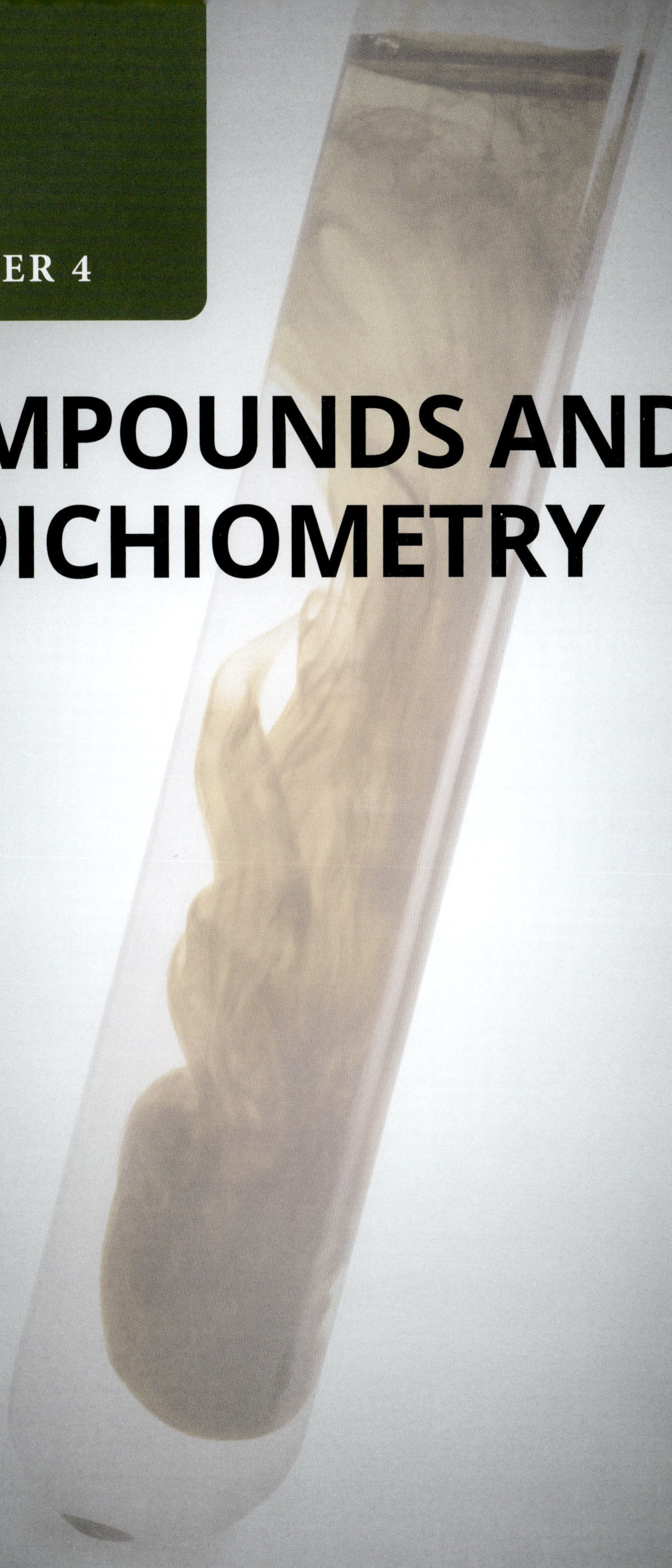

SCIENCE MASTERY ASSESSMENT

Every pre-med knows this feeling: there is so much content I have to know for the MCAT! How do I know what to do first or what's important?

While the high-yield badges throughout this book will help you identify the most important topics, this Science Mastery Assessment is another tool in your MCAT prep arsenal. This quiz (which can also be taken in your online resources) and the guidance below will help ensure that you are spending the appropriate amount of time on this chapter based on your personal strengths and weaknesses. Don't worry though—skipping something now does not mean you'll never study it. Later on in your prep, as you complete full-length tests, you'll uncover specific pieces of content that you need to review and can come back to these chapters as appropriate.

How to Use This Assessment

If you answer 0–7 questions correctly:

Spend about 1 hour to read this chapter in full and take limited notes throughout. Follow up by reviewing **all** quiz questions to ensure that you now understand how to solve each one.

If you answer 8–11 questions correctly:

Spend 20–40 minutes reviewing the quiz questions. Beginning with the questions you missed, read and take notes on the corresponding subchapters. For questions you answered correctly, ensure your thinking matches that of the explanation and you understand why each choice was correct or incorrect.

If you answer 12–15 questions correctly:

Spend less than 20 minutes reviewing all questions from the quiz. If you missed any, then include a quick read-through of the corresponding subchapters, or even just the relevant content within a subchapter, as part of your question review. For questions you answered correctly, ensure your thinking matches that of the explanation and review the Concept Summary at the end of the chapter.

CHAPTER 4

COMPOUNDS AND STOICHIOMETRY

1. Which of the following best describes ionic compounds?

A. Ionic compounds are formed from molecules containing two or more atoms.

B. Ionic compounds are formed of charged particles and are measured by molecular weight.

C. Ionic compounds are formed of charged particles that share electrons equally.

D. Ionic compounds are three-dimensional arrays of charged particles.

2. Which of the following compounds has a formula weight between 74 and 75 grams per mole?

A. KCl

B. $C_4H_{10}O$

C. $MgCl_2$

D. BF_3

3. Which of the following is the gram equivalent weight of H_2SO_4 with respect to protons?

A. 49.1 g

B. 98.1 g

C. 147.1 g

D. 196.2 g

4. Which of the following molecules CANNOT be expressed by the empirical formula CH?

A. Benzene

B. Ethyne

C. 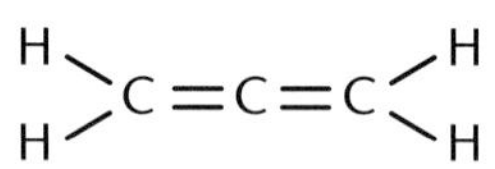

D. 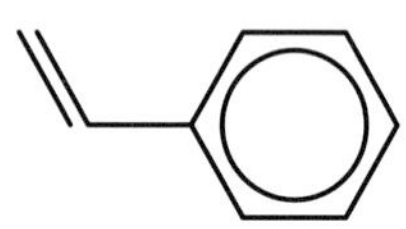

5. In which of the following compounds is the percent composition of carbon by mass closest to 62 percent?

A. Acetone

B. Ethanol

C. Propane

D. Methanol

6. What is the most specific characterization of the reaction shown?

$$Ca(OH)_2\ (aq) + H_2SO_4\ (aq) \rightarrow CaSO_4\ (aq) + H_2O\ (l)$$

A. Single-displacement

B. Neutralization

C. Double-displacement

D. Oxidation–reduction

7. In the reaction shown, if 39.05 g of Na_2S are reacted with 85.5 g of $AgNO_3$, how much of the excess reagent will be left over once the reaction has gone to completion?

$$Na_2S + 2\ AgNO_3 \rightarrow Ag_2S + 2\ NaNO_3$$

A. 19.5 g Na_2S

B. 26.0 g Na_2S

C. 41.4 g $AgNO_3$

D. 74.3 g $AgNO_3$

8. Using a given mass of $KClO_3$, how would one calculate the mass of oxygen produced in the following reaction, assuming it goes to completion?

$$2\ KClO_3 \rightarrow 2\ KCl + 3\ O_2$$

A. $$\frac{\substack{(\text{grams } KClO_3 \text{ consumed})(3 \text{ moles } O_2) \\ (\text{molar mass } O_2)}}{(\text{molar mass } KClO_3)(2 \text{ moles } KClO_3)}$$

B. $$\frac{(\text{grams } KClO_3 \text{ consumed})(\text{molar mass } O_2)}{(\text{molar mass } KClO_3)(2 \text{ moles } KClO_3)}$$

C. $$\frac{(\text{molar mass } KClO_3)(2 \text{ moles } KClO_3)}{(\text{grams } KClO_3 \text{ consumed})(\text{molar mass } O_2)}$$

D. $$\frac{(\text{grams } KClO_3 \text{ consumed})(3 \text{ moles } O_2)}{\substack{(\text{molar mass } KClO_3)(2 \text{ moles } KClO_3) \\ (\text{molar mass } O_2)}}$$

9. Aluminum metal can be used to remove tarnish from silver when the two solid metals are placed in water, according to the following reaction:

$$3\ AgO + 2\ Al \rightarrow 3\ Ag + Al_2O_3$$

This reaction is a:

I. double-displacement reaction.
II. single-displacement reaction.
III. oxidation–reduction reaction.
IV. combination reaction.

A. II only
B. IV only
C. I and III only
D. II and III only

10. Which of the following types of reactions generally have the same number of reactants and products?

I. Double-displacement reactions
II. Single-displacement reactions
III. Combination reactions

A. I only
B. II only
C. I and II only
D. II and III only

11. Diethyl zinc is a very unstable compound. When exposed to air, it reacts with oxygen to produce zinc oxide, carbon dioxide, and water. The unbalanced reaction is shown below.

$$Zn(C_2H_5)_2 + O_2 \rightarrow ZnO + CO_2 + H_2O$$

What is the coefficient for carbon dioxide in the balanced reaction?

A. 4
B. 5
C. 6
D. 7

12. In the process of photosynthesis, carbon dioxide and water combine with energy to form glucose and oxygen, according to the following equation:

$$CO_2 + H_2O \xrightarrow{hv} C_6H_{12}O_6 + O_2$$

What is the theoretical yield of glucose if 30 grams of water are reacted with excess carbon dioxide and energy, according to the equation above?

A. 30.0 g
B. 50.0 g
C. 300.1 g
D. 1801 g

13. In the following reaction:

$$Au_2S_3\ (s) + H_2\ (g) \rightarrow Au\ (s) + H_2S\ (g)$$

If 2 moles of Au_2S_3 (*s*) is reacted with 5 moles of hydrogen gas, what is the limiting reagent?

A. Au_2S_3 (*s*)
B. H_2 (*g*)
C. Au (*s*)
D. H_2S (*g*)

14. Which of the following would make the strongest electrolytic solution?

A. A nonpolar covalent compound with significant solubility.
B. An ionic compound composed of one cation with +3 charge and three anions with −1 charge.
C. A polar covalent compound with a small dissociation constant.
D. An ionic compound composed of two cations with +1 charge and one anion with −2 charge.

15. Carbon disulfide and nitrous oxide, when ignited, react exothermically to produce elemental sulfur, nitrogen, and carbon dioxide. Since this reaction produces a "woof" sound, it is sometimes referred to as the Barking Dog reaction. Which of the following represents the balanced chemical reaction?

A. $8\ N_2O + 4\ CS_2 \rightarrow S_8 + 4\ CO_2 + 8\ N_2$
B. $6\ N_2O + 4\ CS_2 \rightarrow S_8 + 4\ CO_2 + 6\ N_2$
C. $8\ N_2O + 2\ CS_2 \rightarrow S_8 + 2\ CO_2 + 8\ N_2$
D. $7\ N_2O + 5\ CS_2 \rightarrow S_8 + 4\ CO_2 + 7\ N_2$

Answer Key

1. **D** (See section 4.6)
2. **A** (See section 4.1)
3. **A** (See section 4.1)
4. **C** (See section 4.2)
5. **A** (See section 4.2)
6. **B** (See section 4.3)
7. **A** (See section 4.5)
8. **A** (See section 4.5)
9. **D** (See section 4.3)
10. **C** (See section 4.3)
11. **A** (See section 4.4)
12. **B** (See section 4.5)
13. **B** (See section 4.5)
14. **B** (See section 4.6)
15. **A** (See section 4.4)

The relevant section of the chapter to review for each question is given in parentheses after the correct answer. Detailed explanations can be found at the end of the chapter.

CHAPTER 4

COMPOUNDS AND STOICHIOMETRY

In This Chapter

CHAPTER PROFILE

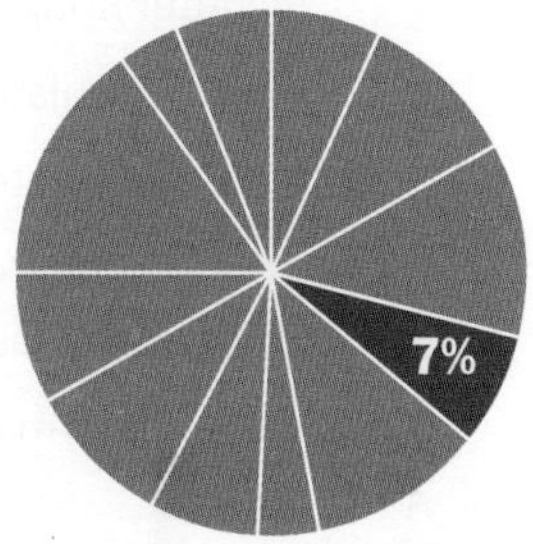

The content in this chapter should be relevant to about 7% of all questions about general chemistry on the MCAT.

This chapter covers material from the following AAMC content categories:

4C: Electrochemistry and electrical circuits and their elements

4E: Atoms, nuclear decay, electronic structure, and atomic chemical behavior

5A: Unique nature of water and its solutions

Introduction

Oh—what is that smell? It smells like rancid almonds. Then you notice a few green bugs whose backs give the impression of a shield. *Stink bugs!* A stink bug "stinks" because it produces a highly concentrated solution of volatile compounds that we perceive as malodorous, noxious, and irritating. Interestingly enough, the primary compounds in the stink bug's stink bomb are hydrogen cyanide—a highly toxic compound that inhibits *cytochrome c oxidase*, thereby blocking aerobic respiration—and benzaldehyde. Like many other aromatic compounds, benzaldehyde vaporizes at room temperature and reaches the olfactory system as gas particles. Benzaldehyde is also the key ingredient in artificial almond extract. At low concentrations, it produces a pleasant aroma of toasted almonds. However, at high concentrations, its odor is that of rotten almonds, and it is a noxious irritant to the skin, eyes, and respiratory tract.

Benzaldehyde is a compound composed of seven carbon atoms, six hydrogen atoms, and one oxygen atom. One mole of benzaldehyde has a mass of approximately 106 grams. It can react with other atoms or compounds to form new **compounds**—pure substances composed of two or more elements in a fixed proportion. Compounds can be broken down by chemical means to produce their constituent elements or other compounds. They are characterized by describing their physical and chemical properties.

This chapter focuses on compounds and their reactions. It reviews the various ways in which compounds are represented, using empirical and molecular formulas and percent composition. There is a brief overview of the major classes of chemical reactions, which we will examine more closely in subsequent chapters, and finally, there is a recap of the steps involved in balancing chemical equations with a particular focus on identifying limiting reagents and calculating reaction yields.

4.1 Molecules and Moles

LEARNING OBJECTIVES

After Chapter 4.1, you will be able to:

- Calculate the molar mass of a given substance, such as AgCN
- Calculate the number of moles of a molecule given its mass in grams
- Compare the number of molecules in two different compounds given their gram weights and molecular formulas
- Determine the normality of a solution

A **molecule** is a combination of two or more atoms held together by covalent bonds. Molecules are the smallest units of compounds that display their identifying properties. Molecules can be composed of two or more atoms of the same element (such as N_2 and O_2) or may be composed of atoms of different elements, as in CO_2 (carbon dioxide), $SOCl_2$ (thionyl chloride), and C_6H_5CHO (benzaldehyde). Because reactions usually involve a very large number of molecules—far too many to count individually—we usually measure amounts of compounds in terms of moles or grams, using molar mass to interconvert between these units.

Ionic compounds do not form true molecules because of the way in which the oppositely charged ions arrange themselves in the solid state. As solids, they can be considered as nearly infinite three-dimensional arrays of the charged particles that comprise the compound. As described in Chapter 3 of *MCAT General Chemistry Review*, solid NaCl is a coordinated lattice in which each of the Na^+ ions is surrounded by Cl^- ions and each of the Cl^- ions is surrounded by Na^+ ions. This makes it rather difficult to clearly define a sodium chloride molecule, and the term **formula unit**, representing the empirical formula of the compound, is used instead. Because no molecule actually exists, molecular weight becomes meaningless, and the term **formula weight** is used instead.

BRIDGE

Ionic compounds form from combinations of elements with large electronegativity differences, such as sodium and chlorine. Molecular compounds form from elements of similar electronegativity, such as carbon with oxygen. The difference between ionic and covalent bonds is discussed in Chapter 3 of *MCAT General Chemistry Review.*

Molecular Weight

Remember that the term **atomic weight** is a misnomer because it is actually a weighted average of the masses of the naturally occurring isotopes of an element, not their weights. The same applies here to our discussion of **molecular weight**. Molecular weight, then, is simply the sum of the atomic weights of all the atoms in a molecule, and its units are atomic mass units (amu) per molecule. Similarly, the **formula weight** of an ionic compound is found by adding up the atomic weights of the constituent ions according to its empirical formula, and its units are also amu per molecule.

Example: What is the molecular weight of $SOCl_2$?

Solution: To find the molecular weight of $SOCl_2$, add together the atomic weights of each of the atoms.

1 S: 1×32.1 amu	=	32.1 amu
1 O: 1×16.0 amu	=	16.0 amu
2 Cl: 2×35.5 amu	=	71.0 amu
Total molecular weight	=	119.1 amu per molecule

Mole

A **mole** is a quantity of any substance (atoms, molecules, dollar bills, kittens—anything) equal to the number of particles that are found in 12 grams of carbon-12 $\left({}^{12}_{6}\text{C}\right)$. This number of particles is defined as **Avogadro's number** (N_A), $6.022 \times 10^{23}\ \text{mol}^{-1}$. One mole of a compound has a mass in grams equal to the molecular or formula weight of the compound in amu. For example, one molecule of H_2CO_3 (carbonic acid) has a mass of 62 amu; one mole of the compound has a mass of 62 grams. The mass of one mole of a compound is called its **molar mass** and is usually expressed in $\frac{\text{g}}{\text{mol}}$. The term *molecular weight* is sometimes used incorrectly to imply molar mass; remember, molecular weight is measured in $\frac{\text{amu}}{\text{molecule}}$, not $\frac{\text{g}}{\text{mol}}$.

KEY CONCEPT

Remember that Avogadro's number (and the mole) are just units of convenience, like the dozen is a convenient unit for eggs.

The formula for determining the number of moles of a sample substance is:

$$\text{Moles} = \frac{\text{Mass of sample (g)}}{\text{Molar mass}\left(\frac{\text{g}}{\text{mol}}\right)}$$

Equation 4.1

This equation is often used in stoichiometry and titration problems.

Example: How many moles are in 9.53 g of $MgCl_2$?

Solution: First, find the molar mass of $MgCl_2$.

$$\left(1 \times 24.3\ \frac{\text{g}}{\text{mol}}\right) + \left(2 \times 35.5\ \frac{\text{g}}{\text{mol}}\right) = 95.3\ \frac{\text{g}}{\text{mol}}$$

Now, solve for the number of moles.

$$\frac{9.53\ \text{g}}{95.3\ \frac{\text{g}}{\text{mol}}} = 0.10\ \text{mol MgCl}_2$$

Equivalent Weight

Equivalent weight and the related concept of **equivalents** are a source of confusion for many students. Part of the problem may be the context in which equivalents and equivalent weights are usually discussed: acid–base reactions, oxidation–reduction reactions, and precipitation reactions, all three of which can be sources of confusion and anxiety on their own. Therefore, let's start with a more basic discussion of equivalents.

Often, certain elements or compounds can act more potently than others in performing certain reactions. For example, one mole of HCl has the ability to donate one mole of hydrogen ions (H^+) in solution, but one mole of H_2SO_4 has the ability to donate two moles of hydrogen ions, and one mole of H_3PO_4 has the ability to donate three moles of hydrogen ions. To gather one mole of hydrogen ions for a particular acid–base reaction, we could use one mole of HCl, a half-mole of H_2SO_4, or one-third of a mole of H_3PO_4. Or, consider the difference between Na and Mg: one mole of sodium has the ability to donate one mole of electrons, while one mole of magnesium has the ability to donate two moles of electrons. This provides context for the concept of **equivalents**: How many moles of the *thing we are interested in* (protons, hydroxide ions, electrons, or ions) will one mole of a given compound produce? Sodium will donate one mole of electrons (one equivalent), but magnesium will donate two moles of electrons (two equivalents).

BRIDGE

The idea of *equivalents* is related to the concept of normality, which is explained in the discussion of acids and bases in Chapter 10 of *MCAT General Chemistry Review*.

So far, this discussion has been focused on the mole-to-mole relationship between, say, an acid compound and the hydrogen ions it donates. However, sometimes we need to work in units of mass rather than moles. Just as one mole of HCl will donate one mole of hydrogen ions, a certain mass of HCl (about 36.5 g) will also donate one equivalent of hydrogen ions. This amount of a compound, measured in grams, that produces one equivalent of the particle of interest is called the **gram equivalent weight** and can be calculated from:

$$\text{Gram equivalent weight} = \frac{\text{Molar mass}}{n}$$

Equation 4.2

where n is the number of particles of interest produced or consumed per molecule of the compound in the reaction. For example, one would need 31 grams of H_2CO_3 $\left(\text{molar mass} = 62\ \frac{\text{g}}{\text{mol}}\right)$ to produce one equivalent of hydrogen ions because each molecule of H_2CO_3 can donate two hydrogen ions ($n = 2$). Simply put, the equivalent weight of a compound is the mass that provides one mole of the particle of interest.

MCAT EXPERTISE

Whenever confronting a stoichiometry problem, always look for normality by identifying an equivalent unit (protons, hydroxide ions, electrons, ions) and then multiplying it by the number of moles or molar concentration to find the normal concentration.

If the amount of a compound in a reaction is known and we need to determine how many equivalents are present, use the equation:

$$\text{Equivalents} = \frac{\text{Mass of compound (g)}}{\text{Gram equivalent weight (g)}}$$

Equation 4.3

Finally, we can now introduce the measurement of normality. **Normality** (**N**) is a measure of concentration, given in the units $\frac{\text{equivalents}}{\text{L}}$. On the MCAT, it is most commonly used for hydrogen ion concentration. Thus, a 1 N solution of acid contains a concentration of hydrogen ions equal to 1 mole per liter; a 2 N solution of acid contains a concentration of hydrogen ions equal to 2 moles per liter. The actual concentration of the acidic compound may be the same or different from the normality because different compounds are able to donate different numbers of hydrogen ions. In a 1 N HCl solution, the molarity of HCl is 1 M because HCl is a monoprotic acid; in a 1 N H_2CO_3 solution, the molarity of H_2CO_3 is 0.5 M because H_2CO_3 is a diprotic acid. Note that normality calculations always assume that a reaction will proceed to completion; while carbonic acid does not fully dissociate in solution, it can be reacted with enough base for each molecule to give up both of its protons. The conversion from normality to molarity of a given solute is:

$$\text{Molarity} = \frac{\text{Normality}}{n}$$

Equation 4.4

where n is the number of protons, hydroxide ions, electrons, or ions produced or consumed by the solute.

Figure 4.1 shows the titration curves of HCl and H_2CO_3 using NaOH to titrate. The x-axis indicates that equivalents of base needed to neutralize the protons from the acid. Since HCl is monoprotic, it only requires one equivalent of NaOH to fully neutralize the acid. All of the HCl and NaOH has been converted into NaCl and H_2O at the equivalence point, resulting in a solution with a pH of 7. H_2CO_3 is diprotic, and requires two equivalents of NaOH to fully neutralize the acid. The first equivalence point results in all of the H_2CO_3 and NaOH converted to $NaHCO_3$, which is mildly acidic due to the presence of the hydrogen, resulting in a slightly acidic pH of 6.4 solution. At the second equivalence point, all of the $NaHCO_3$ has reacted with NaOH, resulting in Na_2CO_3. As CO_3^{2-} is mildly basic, the solution at the second equivalence point is basic with a pH of 10.3.

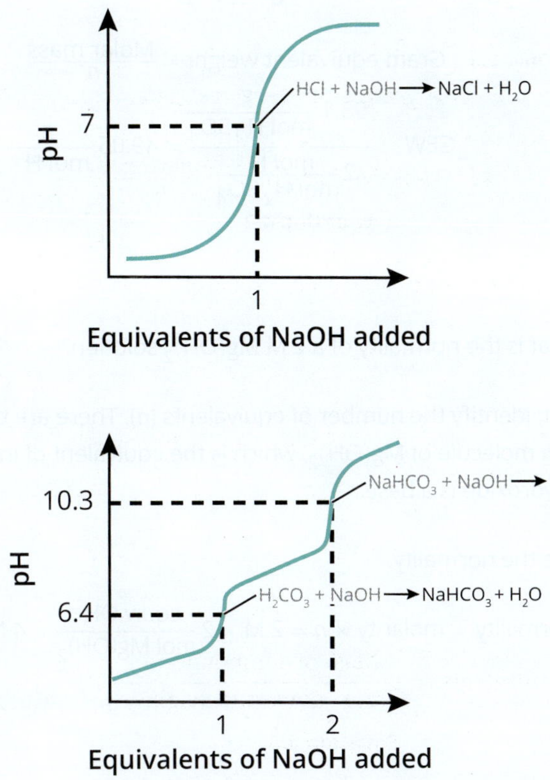

Figure 4.1 Monoprotic vs. Diprotic Acid Titrations
Hydrochloric acid is monoprotic and only one equivalent of base is needed to neutralize it. Carbonic acid is diprotic, so two equivalents of base are required to neutralize both protons of the acid.

There is a real benefit to working with equivalents and normality because it allows a direct comparison of the quantities of the entity we are most interested in. In an acid–base reaction, we care about the hydrogen or hydroxide ions; where the ions come from is not really the primary concern. It is convenient to be able to say that one equivalent of acid (hydrogen ions) will neutralize one equivalent of base (hydroxide ions), but the same could not necessarily be said if we were dealing with moles of acidic compounds and moles of basic compounds. For example, one mole of HCl will not completely neutralize one mole of $Ca(OH)_2$ because one mole of HCl will donate one equivalent of acid, but $Ca(OH)_2$ will donate two equivalents of base.

Example: What is the gram equivalent weight (GEW) of sulfuric acid?

Solution: First, find the molar mass of H_2SO_4.

$$\left(2 \times 1.0\frac{\text{g}}{\text{mol H}}\right) + \left(1 \times 32.1\frac{\text{g}}{\text{mol S}}\right) + \left(4 \times 16.0\frac{\text{g}}{\text{mol O}}\right) = 98.1\frac{\text{g}}{\text{mol H}_2\text{SO}_4}$$

Next, identify the equivalents: protons (H^+), because these are transferred in acid–base reactions. The number of protons in sulfuric acid (n) is 2.

Now, calculate the gram equivalent weight.

$$\text{Gram equivalent weight} = \frac{\text{Molar mass}}{n}$$

$$\text{GEW} = \frac{98.1\ \frac{\text{g}}{\text{mol H}_2\text{SO}_4}}{2\frac{\text{mol H}^+}{\text{mol H}_2\text{SO}_4}} = 49.05\ \frac{\text{g}}{\text{mol H}^+}$$

KEY CONCEPT

In acid–base chemistry, the gram equivalent weight represents the mass of acid that yields one mole of protons, or the mass of base that yields one mole of hydroxide ions.

Example: What is the normality of a 2 M $Mg(OH)_2$ solution?

Solution: First, identify the number of equivalents (n). There are two hydroxide ions (OH^-) for each molecule of $Mg(OH)_2$, which is the equivalent of interest because magnesium hydroxide is a base.

Then, calculate the normality.

$$\text{Normality} = \text{molarity} \times n = 2\text{ M} \times 2\frac{\text{equiv OH}^-}{\text{mol Mg(OH)}_2} = 4\text{ N Mg(OH)}_2$$

MCAT CONCEPT CHECK 4.1

Before you move on, assess your understanding of the material with these questions.

1. Calculate the molar masses of the following substances:
   - $NaBr$:
   - $SrCl_2$:
   - $C_6H_{12}O_6$:
2. Calculate the number of moles in 100 g of each of the following substances:
   - $NaBr$:
   - $SrCl_2$:
   - $C_6H_{12}O_6$:
3. How do the number of molecules in 18 g of H_2O compare to the number of formula units in 58.5 g of NaCl?
4. Determine the normality of the following solutions: (Note: The species of interest is H^+.)
   - 0.25 M H_3PO_4:
   - 95 g PO_4^{3-} in 100 mL solution:

4.2 Representation of Compounds

LEARNING OBJECTIVES

After Chapter 4.2, you will be able to:

- Recall the similarities and differences between molecular and empirical formulas
- Calculate the percent composition by mass of a compound, such as $C_6H_{12}O_6$
- Determine the empirical formula of a compound given its percent composition by mass

There are different ways of representing compounds and their constituent atoms. We've already reviewed a couple of these systems in Chapter 3 of *MCAT General Chemistry Review*: Lewis dot structures and VSEPR theory. In organic chemistry, it is common to encounter skeletal representations of compounds, called **structural formulas**, that show the various bonds between the constituent atoms of a compound. Inorganic (general) chemistry typically represents compounds by showing the constituent atoms without representing the actual bond connectivity or atomic arrangement. For example, the formula $C_6H_{12}O_6$ (glucose) tells us that this particular compound consists of six atoms of carbon, twelve atoms of hydrogen, and six atoms of oxygen, but there is no indication of how the different atoms are arranged or how many bonds exist between each of the atoms.

BRIDGE

Many of these representations are discussed in more detail in Chapter 2 of *MCAT Organic Chemistry Review*. Understanding the theory behind such representations will help convert between different projections and representations with ease.

Law of Constant Composition

The **law of constant composition** states that any pure sample of a given compound will contain the same elements in an identical mass ratio. For example, every sample of water will contain two hydrogen atoms for every one oxygen atom, or—in terms of mass—for every one gram of hydrogen, there will be eight grams of oxygen.

REAL WORLD

Even biologically important molecules, such as water and amino acids on Earth are, by composition, the same anywhere else in the universe, even though densities and other physical properties may differ.

Empirical and Molecular Formulas

There are two ways to express the formula of a compound. The **empirical formula** gives the simplest whole-number ratio of the elements in the compound. The **molecular formula** gives the exact number of atoms of each element in the compound and is a multiple of the empirical formula. For example, the empirical formula for benzene is CH, while the molecular formula is C_6H_6. For some compounds, the empirical and molecular formulas are identical, as is the case for H_2O. As previously discussed, ionic compounds, such as NaCl or $CaCO_3$, will only have empirical formulas.

BRIDGE

An empirical formula of CH_2O is indicative of a monosaccharide. Common monosaccharides include glucose, fructose, and galactose. The structures of these monosaccharides—and of carbohydrates in general—are discussed in Chapter 4 of *MCAT Biochemistry Review*.

Percent Composition

The **percent composition** of an element (by mass) is the percent of a specific compound that is made up of a given element. To determine the percent composition of an element in a compound, the following formula is used:

$$\text{Percent composition} = \frac{\text{Mass of element in formula}}{\text{Molar mass}} \times 100\%$$

Equation 4.5

MCAT EXPERTISE

Percent composition is a common way for stoichiometry to be tested on the MCAT. Practice these problems to build up speed and efficiency for Test Day.

One can calculate the percent composition of an element by using either the empirical or the molecular formula. It is also possible to determine the molecular formula given both the percent compositions and molar mass of a compound. The following examples demonstrate such calculations.

Example: What is the percent composition of chromium in $K_2Cr_2O_7$?

Solution: The molar mass of $K_2Cr_2O_7$ is:

$$\left(2 \times 39.1 \frac{g}{mol}\right) + \left(2 \times 52.0 \frac{g}{mol}\right) + \left(7 \times 16.0 \frac{g}{mol}\right)$$

$$\approx (2 \times 40) + (2 \times 50) + (7 \times 16)$$

$$= 292 \frac{g}{mol} \left(\text{actual value} = 294.2 \frac{g}{mol}\right)$$

Calculate the percent composition of Cr:

$$\text{Percent composition} = \frac{2 \times 52.0 \frac{g}{mol}}{294.2 \frac{g}{mol}} \times 100\%$$

$$\approx \frac{2 \times 50}{300} \times 100\% = \frac{100}{300} \times 100\%$$

$$= 33\% \text{ (actual value} = 35.4\%)$$

Example: What are the empirical and molecular formulas of a carbohydrate that contains 40.9% carbon, 4.58% hydrogen, and 54.52% oxygen and has a molar mass of $264 \frac{g}{mol}$?

Method One: First, determine the number of moles of each element in the compound by assuming a 100-gram sample; this converts the percentage of each element present directly into grams of that element. Then convert grams to moles:

$$\text{moles C} = \frac{40.9 \text{ g}}{12 \frac{g}{mol}} \approx 3.4 \text{ mol}$$

$$\text{moles H} = \frac{4.58 \text{ g}}{1 \frac{g}{mol}} \approx 4.6 \text{ mol}$$

$$\text{moles O} = \frac{54.52 \text{ g}}{16 \frac{g}{mol}} \approx 3.4 \text{ mol}$$

Next, find the simplest whole number ratio of the elements by dividing the number of moles for each compound by the smallest number out of all obtained in the previous step.

$$\text{C: } \frac{3.4}{3.4} = 1.00;\ \text{H: } \frac{4.6}{3.4} \approx 1.33;\ \text{O: } \frac{3.4}{3.4} = 1.00$$

Finally, the empirical formula is obtained by converting the numbers obtained into whole numbers by multiplying them by an integer value.

$$\text{Empirical formula} = C_1H_{1.33}O_1 \times 3 = C_3H_4O_3$$

To determine the molecular formula, divide the molar mass (264 g/mol, given in the question stem) by the empirical formula weight. The resulting value gives the number of empirical formula units in the molecular formula.

The formula weight of the empirical formula $C_3H_4O_3$ is:

$$\left(3 \times 12.0\ \frac{\text{g}}{\text{mol C}}\right) + \left(4 \times 1.0\ \frac{\text{g}}{\text{mol H}}\right) + \left(3 \times 16.0\ \frac{\text{g}}{\text{mol O}}\right) = 88\ \frac{\text{g}}{\text{mol total}}$$

$$\text{ratio of } \frac{\text{molecular formula}}{\text{empirical formula}} = \frac{264\ \frac{\text{g}}{\text{mol}}}{88\ \frac{\text{g}}{\text{mol}}} = 3$$

Finally, find the molecular formula by multiplying by this ratio:

$C_3H_4O_3 \times 3 = C_9H_{12}O_9$. The molecular formula is $C_9H_{12}O_9$.

Method Two: When the molar mass is given, it is generally easier to find the molecular formula first. This is accomplished by multiplying the molar mass by the given percentages to find the mass of each element present in one mole of compound, then dividing by the respective atomic weights to find the mole ratio of the elements:

$$\text{moles C} = \frac{(0.409)(264\ \text{g})}{12\ \frac{\text{g}}{\text{mol}}} \approx \frac{(0.4)(270)}{12} \approx \frac{270}{30} = 9\ \text{mol}$$

$$\text{moles H} = \frac{(0.0458)(264\ \text{g})}{1\ \frac{\text{g}}{\text{mol}}} \approx \frac{(0.05)(270)}{1} \approx 13\ \text{mol}$$

$$\text{moles O} = \frac{(0.5452)(264\ \text{g})}{16\ \frac{\text{g}}{\text{mol}}} \approx \frac{(0.5)(270)}{16} \approx \frac{270}{30} = 9\ \text{mol}$$

At first glance, this gives a molecular formula of $C_9H_{13}O_9$. However, familiarity with carbohydrates indicates that a molecular formula of $C_9H_{12}O_9$ fits the ratio CH_2O, and takes rounding error into account. The empirical formula can now be found by reducing the subscript ratio to the simplest integer values ($C_3H_4O_3$).

MCAT EXPERTISE

When there are two methods for approaching a problem, be well-versed in both. Knowing multiple ways to solve a problem will help you tackle questions efficiently.

KEY CONCEPT

The molecular formula is either the same as the empirical formula or a multiple of it. To calculate the molecular formula, you need to know the mole ratio (this will give you the empirical formula) and the molar mass (molar mass divided by empirical formula weight will give the multiplier for the empirical formula-to-molecular formula conversion).

MCAT CONCEPT CHECK 4.2

Before you move on, assess your understanding of the material with these questions.

1. What are some similarities and differences between molecular and empirical formulas?
   - Similarities:

   - Differences:

   ---

2. Find the percent composition (by mass) of sodium, carbon, and oxygen in sodium carbonate (Na_2CO_3):
   - Sodium:

   - Carbon:

   - Oxygen:

   ---

3. Experimental data from the combustion of an unknown compound indicates that it is 28.5% iron, 24.0% sulfur, and 49.7% oxygen by mass. What is its empirical formula?

4.3 Types of Chemical Reactions

LEARNING OBJECTIVES

After Chapter 4.3, you will be able to:

- Describe the series of events in a single displacement, double displacement, neutralization, or combustion reaction
- Classify a reaction and predict its products given the reactants:

$$CH_4 + 2O_2 \rightarrow$$

This section reviews the major classes of chemical reactions. We will begin with a classification of major types of reactions seen on the MCAT and then discuss methods to recognize their products. It is important to understand the conventions of reaction mechanisms. In the following section, we will discuss how to properly balance chemical equations.

BRIDGE

Many of the reactions we will discuss here have analogs in *MCAT Organic Chemistry Review* and *MCAT Biochemistry Review*. Be sure to understand the relationships between the products and reactants because it will help simplify more advanced reactions.

Combination Reactions

A **combination reaction** has two or more reactants forming one product. The formation of water by burning hydrogen gas in air is an example of a combination reaction. This reaction is highlighted in Figure 4.2.

$$2\ H_2\ (g) + O_2\ (g) \rightarrow 2\ H_2O\ (g)$$

KEY CONCEPT

Combination reactions have more reactants than products: **A + B → C**

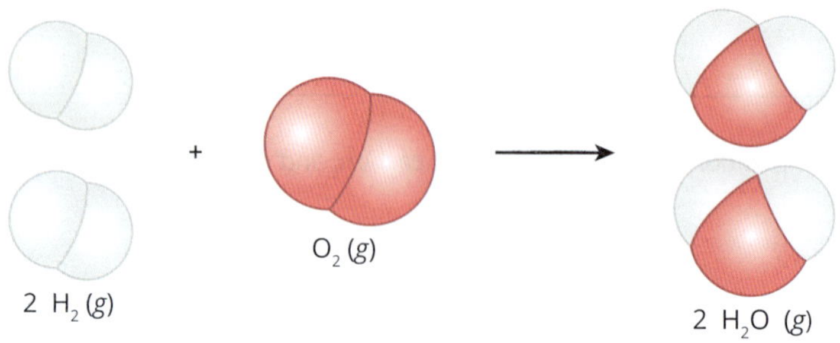

Figure 4.2 Formation of Water from Hydrogen and Oxygen

Decomposition Reactions

A **decomposition** reaction is the opposite of a combination reaction: a single reactant breaks down into two or more products, usually as a result of heating, high-frequency radiation, or electrolysis. An example of decomposition is the electrolysis of molten sodium chloride (NaCl) into molten sodium metal and chloride gas, as seen in Figure 4.3.

KEY CONCEPT

Decomposition reactions generally have more products than reactants. **A → B + C**

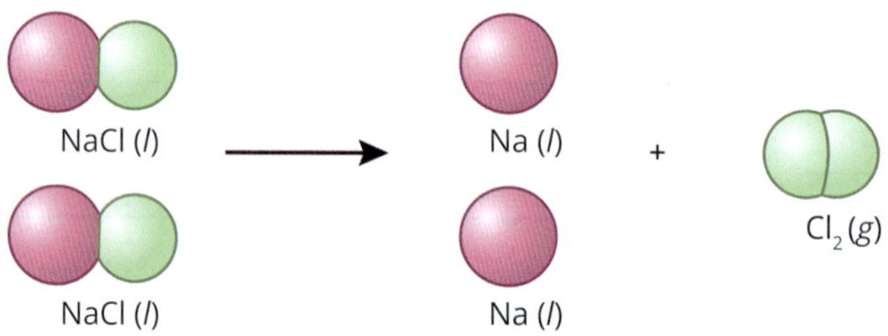

Figure 4.3 Decomposition of Molten Sodium Chloride

An example of a reaction that utilizes high-frequency light is the decomposition of silver chloride crystals, shown in Figure 4.4, in the presence of sunlight. The ultraviolet component of sunlight has sufficient energy to catalyze certain chemical reactions. For silver chloride, exposure to sunlight results in a decomposition reaction that yields a rust-colored product that consists of separated silver and chlorine.

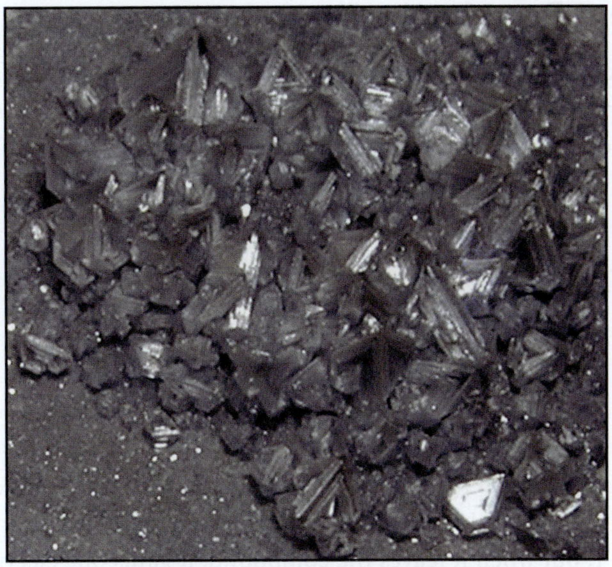

Figure 4.4 Silver Chloride (AgCl) Crystals
Silver chloride will decompose to a rust-colored product upon exposure to sunlight.

Combustion Reactions

A **combustion reaction** is a special type of reaction that involves a fuel—usually a hydrocarbon—and an oxidant (normally oxygen). In its most common form, these reactants form the two products of carbon dioxide and water. For example, the balanced equation expressing the combustion of methane is shown in Figure 4.5.

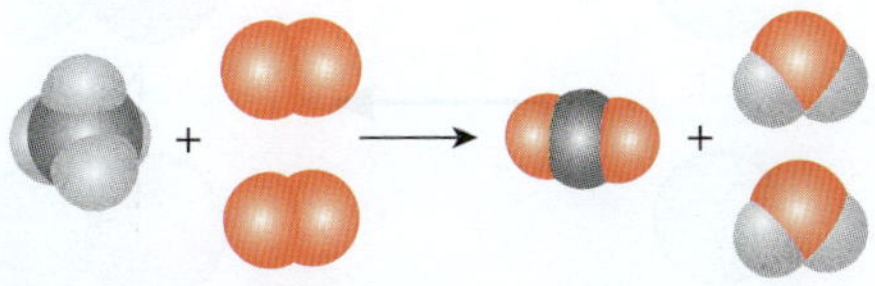

$$CH_4 + 2O_2 \longrightarrow CO_2 + 2H_2O$$

Figure 4.5 Combustion of Methane

KEY CONCEPT

Combustion involves oxidation (using O_2 or similar) of a fuel (typically a hydrocarbon).

MCAT EXPERTISE

Combustion reactions are usually conducted with hydrocarbon fuels, but they can also use elements such as sulfur or other compounds such as sugars. The products can differ, but carbon dioxide and water are almost always present. Therefore, it is important to recognize the reactants and products of this reaction type because you may see it in various contexts.

Single-Displacement Reactions

A **single-displacement reaction** occurs when an atom or ion in a compound is replaced by an atom or ion of another element. For example, solid copper metal will displace silver ions in a clear solution of silver nitrate to form a copper nitrate solution and solid silver metal, as seen in Figure 4.6.

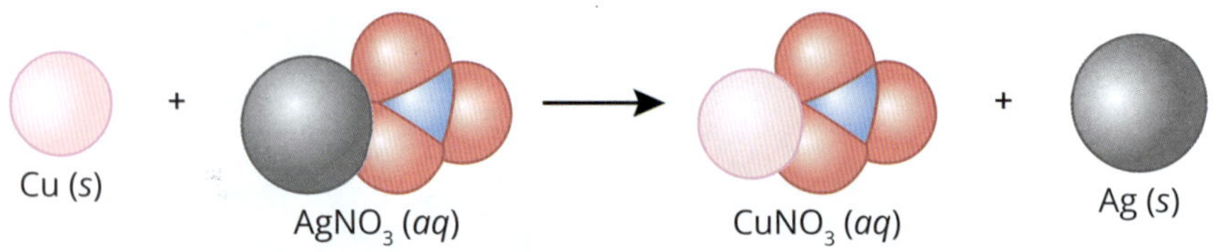

Figure 4.6 Single Displacement of Silver Nitrate with Copper

Single-displacement reactions are often further classified as oxidation–reduction reactions, which will be discussed in greater detail in Chapter 11 of *MCAT General Chemistry Review*. For example, Ag in $AgNO_3$ has an oxidation state of $+1$, but when it leaves the compound, it gains one electron (the Ag^+ is reduced to Ag). On the other hand, copper loses an electron (oxidation) when it joins the nitrate ion.

Double-Displacement Reactions

In **double-displacement reactions**, also called **metathesis reactions**, elements from two different compounds swap places with each other to form two new compounds. This type of reaction occurs when one of the products is removed from the solution as a precipitate or gas or when two of the original species combine to form a weak electrolyte that remains undissociated in solution. For example, when solutions of sodium sulfide and hydrochloric acid are combined, hydrogen sulfide gas evolves from the resulting solution of sodium chloride, as seen in Figure 4.7.

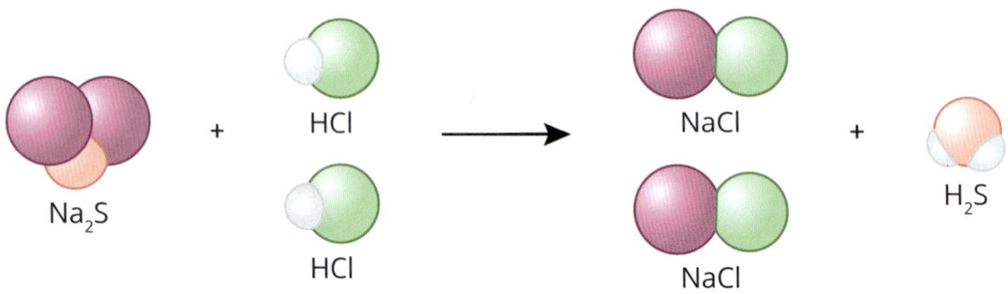

Figure 4.7 Double Displacement of Sodium Sulfide and Hydrochloric Acid

A series of double-displacement reactions is depicted in Figure 4.8. Shown are illustrations of test tubes in which $Zn(NO_3)_2$ is dissolved in solutions to precipitate solid zinc salts. From left to right, the solutions are $(NH_4)_2S$, NaOH, and Na_2CO_3.

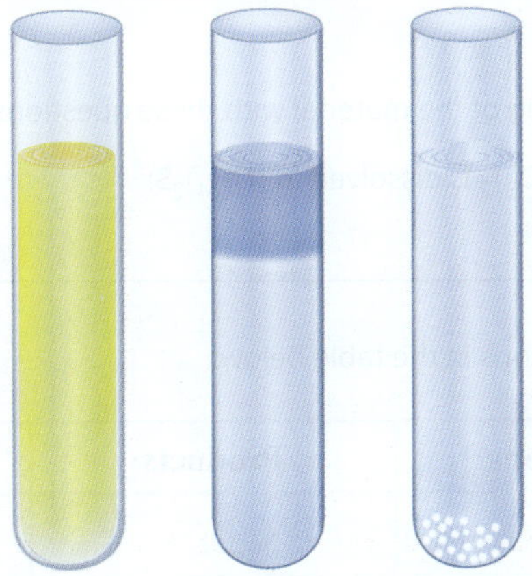

Figure 4.8 Illustration of Double-Displacement Reactions Forming Zinc Salts
Left: $(NH_4)_2S$ solution, producing ZnS (s). Middle: NaOH solution, producing $Zn(OH)_2$ (s). Right: Na_2CO_3 solution, producing $ZnCO_3$ (s).

Neutralization Reactions

Neutralization reactions are a specific type of double-displacement reaction in which an acid reacts with a base to produce a salt (and, usually, water). For example, hydrochloric acid and sodium hydroxide will react to form sodium chloride and water, as seen in Figure 4.9.

BRIDGE

Acids and bases combine in neutralization reactions to produce salts (and, usually, water). Acid–base chemistry is discussed in Chapter 10 of *MCAT General Chemistry Review*.

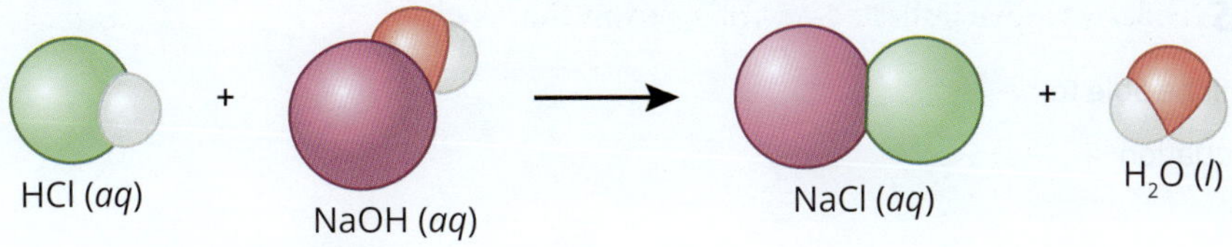

Figure 4.9 Neutralization of Hydrochloric Acid and Sodium Hydroxide

Reactions between acids and bases are not always visible. The addition of an indicator or use of indicator strips, as shown in Figure 4.10, can determine when the reaction has occurred.

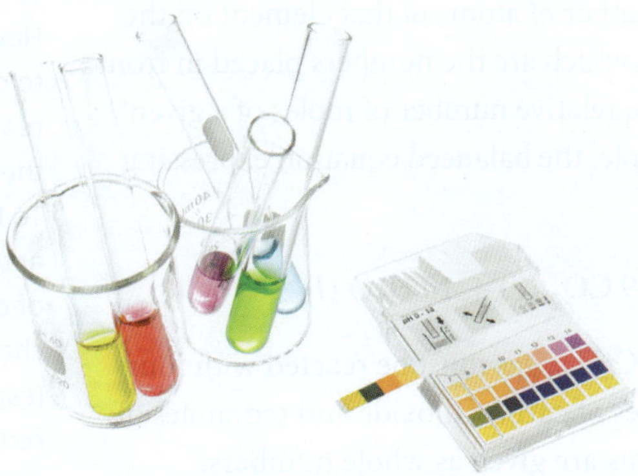

Figure 4.10 Indicator Strip Tested in Solutions of Varying pH
After an indicator strip is placed in a solution, the indicator strip (right) can be read using the indicator key.

MCAT CONCEPT CHECK 4.3

Before you move on, assess your understanding of the material with these questions.

1. Describe in words what occurs when $Zn(NO_3)_2$ is dissolved in $(NH_4)_2S$:

____

2. Complete and classify the most likely reactions in the table below:

Reactants	Conditions	Products	Reaction Type
$2\ H_2 + O_2$	$\rightarrow$		
$Al(OH)_3 + H_3PO_4$	$\rightarrow$		
$2\ H_2O$	$\xrightarrow{\text{electricity}}$		
$NaNO_3 + CuOH$	$\rightarrow$		
$Zn + AgCl$	$\rightarrow$		

4.4 Balancing Chemical Equations

High Yield

LEARNING OBJECTIVES

After Chapter 4.4, you will be able to:

- Balance a chemical equation

Because chemical equations express how much and what types of reactants must be used to obtain a given quantity of product, it is of utmost importance that the reaction be balanced so as to reflect the **laws of conservation of mass** and **charge**. The mass of the reactants consumed must equal the mass of products generated. More specifically, one must ensure that the number of atoms of each element on the reactant side equals the number of atoms of that element on the product side. **Stoichiometric coefficients**, which are the numbers placed in front of each compound, are used to indicate the relative number of moles of a given species involved in the reaction. For example, the balanced equation expressing the combustion of nonane is:

$$C_9H_{20}\ (g) + 14\ O_2\ (g) \rightarrow 9\ CO_2\ (g) + 10\ H_2O\ (l)$$

The coefficients indicate that one mole of C_9H_{20} gas must be reacted with fourteen moles of O_2 gas to produce nine moles of carbon dioxide and ten moles of water. In general, stoichiometric coefficients are given as whole numbers.

MCAT EXPERTISE

It is unlikely that you will come across a question that explicitly asks you to balance an equation. However, you will need to recognize unbalanced reactions and quickly add the necessary coefficients. To balance a reaction, look at the number of atoms of each element and the charge on both sides (especially for oxidation–reduction reactions).

The steps taken to balance a chemical reaction are necessary to ensure that calculations regarding the reaction are performed correctly. Let's review the steps involved in balancing a chemical equation, using an example.

Example: Balance the following reaction:

$$C_4H_{10}\ (l) + O_2\ (g) \rightarrow CO_2\ (g) + H_2O\ (l)$$

Method One: First, balance the carbons (4 on reactant side) in the products. Carbons are a good choice to start with because they appear only once on both sides of the reaction:

$$C_4H_{10}\ (l) + O_2\ (g) \rightarrow \mathbf{4}\ CO_2\ (g) + H_2O\ (l)$$

Then, balance the hydrogens (10 on reactant side) in the products. Again, hydrogens appear only once on each side, making them a good choice to work on next:

$$C_4H_{10}\ (l) + O_2\ (g) \rightarrow 4\ CO_2\ (g) + \mathbf{5}\ H_2O\ (l)$$

Next, balance the oxygens (now 13 on product side) in the reactants. Note that oxygens appear in multiple reactants and products, making them the most complex atom to balance and therefore the best to leave until the end:

$$C_4H_{10}\ (l) + \frac{13}{2}\ O_2\ (g) \rightarrow 4\ CO_2\ (g) + 5\ H_2O\ (l)$$

Next, produce a whole number ratio. In this case, double each coefficient.

$$2\ C_4H_{10}\ (l) + 13\ O_2\ (g) \rightarrow 8\ CO_2\ (g) + 10\ H_2O\ (l)$$

Finally, check that all of the elements and the total charges are balanced correctly. If there is a difference in total charge between the reactants and products, then the charge will also have to be balanced. (Instructions for balancing charge in oxidation–reduction reactions are found in Chapter 11 of *MCAT General Chemistry Review*.)

Method Two: First, if in doubt, take a guess. Assume there are 4 of the first reactant and balance the carbons appropriately.

$$\mathbf{4}\ C_4H_{10}\ (l) + O_2\ (g) \rightarrow \mathbf{16}\ CO_2\ (g) + H_2O\ (l)$$

Second, balance the hydrogens (40 on reactant side) in the products.

$$4\ C_4H_{10}\ (l) + O_2\ (g) \rightarrow 16\ CO_2\ (g) + \mathbf{20}\ H_2O\ (l)$$

Third, balance the oxygens (now 52 on product side) in the reactants.

$$4\ C_4H_{10}\ (l) + \mathbf{26}\ O_2\ (g) \rightarrow 16\ CO_2\ (g) + 20\ H_2O\ (l)$$

Fourth, produce the simplest whole number ratio through the greatest common factor. In this case, divide each side by 2.

$$2\ C_4H_{10}\ (l) + 13\ O_2\ (g) \rightarrow 8\ CO_2\ (g) + 10\ H_2O\ (l)$$

KEY CONCEPT

When balancing equations, focus on the least represented elements first and work your way to the most represented element of the reaction (usually oxygen or hydrogen). If you're stuck, take a guess at the coefficient of the first reactant and balance the remainder appropriately.

Finally, check that all of the elements and the total charges are balanced correctly. Notice that both methods produce a multiple of our final answer. These ratios are both correct, but in terms of the stoichiometry one performs on the MCAT, the simpler the numbers are, the easier calculations will become.

MCAT CONCEPT CHECK 4.4

Before you move on, assess your understanding of the material with this question.

1. Balance the following reactions:
   - __ Fe + __ Cl_2 → __ $FeCl_3$
   - __ Zn + __ HCl → __ $ZnCl_2$ + __ H_2
   - __ C_5H_{12} + __ O_2 → __ CO_2 + __ H_2O
   - __ $Pb(NO_3)_2$ + __ $AlCl_3$ → __ $PbCl_2$ + __ $Al(NO_3)_3$

4.5 Applications of Stoichiometry

LEARNING OBJECTIVES

After Chapter 4.5, you will be able to:

- Calculate the grams of product produced given the quantities of reactant
- Identify the limiting reagent within a reaction
- Calculate the mass of excess reagent in a reaction with a limiting reagent
- Calculate the percent yield of a reaction

KEY CONCEPT

Stoichiometry, an application of dimensional analysis, is often simplified to a series of three fractions. These fractions demonstrate an underlying three-step process:

- Convert from the given units to moles
- Use the mole ratio
- Convert from moles to the desired units

Perhaps the most useful information to glean from a balanced reaction is the mole ratio of reactants consumed-to-products generated. One can also generate the mole ratio of one reactant to another or one product to another. All of these ratios can be generated using the stoichiometric coefficients. In the formation of water ($2\ H_2 + O_2 \rightarrow 2\ H_2O$), for example, one can determine that, for every one mole of hydrogen gas consumed, one mole of water can be produced; for every one mole of oxygen gas consumed, two moles of water can be produced. Furthermore, mole-to-mole, hydrogen gas is being consumed at a rate twice that of oxygen gas.

Stoichiometry problems usually involve at least a few unit conversions, so take care when working through these types of problems to ensure that units cancel out appropriately to lead to the desired units of the answer choices. Pay close attention to the following problem, which demonstrates a clear and easy-to-follow method for keeping track of the numbers, calculations, and unit conversions.

Example: How many grams of calcium chloride are needed to prepare 71.7 g of silver chloride according to the following equation?

$$CaCl_2\,(aq) + 2\,AgNO_3\,(aq) \rightarrow Ca(NO_3)_2\,(aq) + 2\,AgCl\,(s)$$

Solution: Noting first that the equation is balanced, 1 mole of $CaCl_2$ is reacted with 2 moles of $AgNO_3$ to yield 2 moles of AgCl. The molar mass of $CaCl_2$ is 111.1 g, and the molar mass of AgCl is 143.4 g. The given quantity is 71.7 g AgCl.

$$71.7\text{ g AgCl} \times \left[\frac{1\text{ mol AgCl}}{143.4\text{ g AgCl}}\right]\left[\frac{1\text{ mol CaCl}_2}{2\text{ mol AgCl}}\right]\left[\frac{111.1\text{ g CaCl}_2}{1\text{ mol CaCl}_2}\right]$$

$$\approx \frac{72}{144} \times \frac{1}{2} \times \frac{110}{1} = \frac{1}{2} \times \frac{1}{2} \times \frac{110}{1} = \frac{110}{4}$$

$$= 27.5\text{ g CaCl}_2 \text{ (actual value} = 27.775\text{ g)}$$

Thus, about 27.8 g $CaCl_2$ are needed to produce 71.7 g AgCl.

MCAT EXPERTISE

Common conversions used in stoichiometry include:

- 1 mole of any ideal gas at STP = 22.4 L
- 1 mole of any substance = 6.022×10^{23} particles (Avogadro's number)
- 1 mole of any substance = its molar mass in grams (from the periodic table)

Limiting Reagent

Rarely are reactants added in the exact stoichiometric proportions shown in the balanced equation of a reaction. As a result, in most reactions, one reactant will be used up or consumed first. This reactant is known as the **limiting reagent** (or reactant) because it limits the amount of product that can be formed in the reaction. The reactants that remain after all the limiting reagent is used up are called **excess reagents** (or reactants).

MCAT EXPERTISE

When the quantities of two reactants are given on the MCAT, expect to have to figure out which is the limiting reagent.

Figure 4.11 shows a reaction vessel that has significant amounts of reactants A and B, which react in equal amounts to produce product C. On the left, before the reaction, there is more reactant A than B. After the reaction is over, there is more product C but there is reactant A left over. Thus, reactant A is considered in excess, and reactant B is considered limiting.

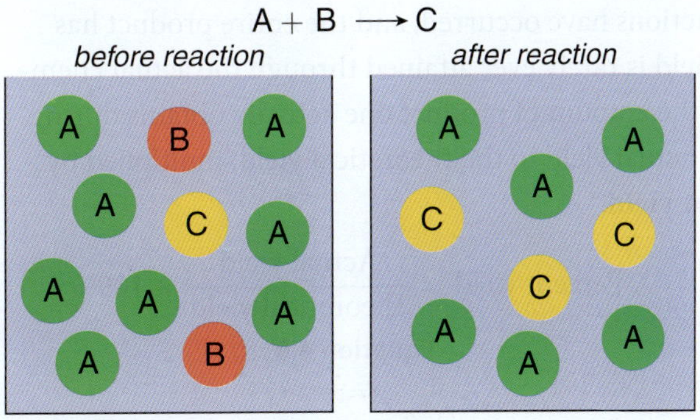

Figure 4.11 Reaction with a Limiting Reagent
A is considered an excess reagent; B is the limiting reagent.

For problems involving the determination of the limiting reagent, keep in mind two principles:

1. All comparisons of reactants must be done in units of moles. Gram-to-gram comparisons will be useless and may even be misleading.
2. It is not the absolute mole quantities of the reactants that determine which reactant is the limiting reagent. Rather, the rate at which the reactants are consumed (the stoichiometric ratios of the reactants), combined with the absolute mole quantities determines which reactant is the limiting reagent.

Example: If 27.9 g of Fe react with 24.1 g of S to produce FeS, what would be the limiting reagent? How many grams of excess reagent would be present in the vessel at the end of the reaction?

The balanced equation is $Fe + S \rightarrow FeS$.

Solution: First, determine the number of moles for each reactant.

$$27.9\text{ g Fe} \times \frac{1\text{ mol Fe}}{55.8\text{ g Fe}} \approx 28 \times \frac{1}{56} = 0.5\text{ mol Fe}$$
$$24.1\text{ g S} \times \frac{1\text{ mol S}}{32.1\text{ g S}} \approx 24 \times \frac{1}{32} = 0.75\text{ mol S}$$

Because 1 mole of Fe is needed to react with 1 mole of S and there are 0.5 moles Fe for the given 0.75 moles S, the limiting reagent is Fe. Thus, 0.5 moles of Fe will react with 0.5 moles of S, leaving an excess of 0.25 moles of S in the vessel. The mass of the excess reagent will be:

$$0.25\text{ mol} \times \frac{32.1\text{ g S}}{1\text{ mol S}} \approx 8\text{ g S}$$

Yield

The **yield** of a reaction can refer to either the amount of product predicted (theoretical yield) or actually obtained (raw or actual yield) when a reaction is carried out. **Theoretical yield** is the maximum amount of product that can be generated as predicted from the balanced equation, assuming that all of the limiting reactant is consumed, no side reactions have occurred, and the entire product has been collected. Theoretical yield is rarely ever attained through the actual chemical reaction. **Actual yield** is the amount of product one actually obtains during the reaction. The ratio of the actual yield to the theoretical yield, multiplied by 100 percent, gives the **percent yield**:

$$\text{Percent yield} = \frac{\text{Actual yield}}{\text{Theoretical yield}} \times 100\%$$

Equation 4.6

MCAT EXPERTISE

An experimentally based passage that involves a chemical reaction may include a pseudo-discrete question that involves finding the percent yield.

Example: What is the percent yield for a reaction in which 28 g of Cu is produced by reacting 32.7 g of Zn in excess $CuSO_4$ solution?

Solution: The balanced equation is as follows:

$$Zn\ (s) + CuSO_4\ (aq) \rightarrow Cu\ (s) + ZnSO_4\ (aq)$$

Calculate the theoretical yield for Cu.

$$32.7 \text{ g Zn} \times \left[\frac{1 \text{ mol Zn}}{65.4 \text{ g Zn}}\right]\left[\frac{1 \text{ mol Cu}}{1 \text{ mol Zn}}\right]\left[\frac{63.5 \text{ g Cu}}{1 \text{ mol Cu}}\right]$$

$$\approx 33 \times \frac{1}{66} \times \frac{1}{1} \times \frac{64}{1} = \frac{1}{2} \times \frac{64}{1} = 32 \text{ (actual value} = 31.8 \text{ g Cu)}$$

This 31.8 g represents the theoretical yield. Finally, determine the percent yield.

$$\frac{28 \text{ g}}{31.8 \text{ g}} \times 100\% \approx \frac{28}{32} \times 100\% = \frac{7}{8} \times 100\% = 87.5\%$$

MCAT CONCEPT CHECK 4.5

Before you move on, assess your understanding of the material with these questions.

Questions 1–3 refer to the following unbalanced equation:

$$Na\ (s) + O_2\ (g) \rightarrow Na_2O\ (s)$$

1. Balance the chemical equation:

   $$\_\_\ Na\ (s) + \_\_\ O_2\ (g) \rightarrow \_\_\ Na_2O\ (s)$$

2. If 46 g Na and 32 g O_2 are provided, find the maximum number of moles of sodium oxide produced.

   ____

3. Identify the limiting reagent, and find the mass of the excess reagent left over once the reaction has run to completion.

   ____

4. $Be(OH)_2$ is produced when water reacts with BeO. Starting with 2.5 kg BeO in excess water, and producing 1.1 kg $Be(OH)_2$, what is the percent yield of this reaction?

   ____

4.6 Ions

LEARNING OBJECTIVES

After Chapter 4.6, you will be able to:

- Determine whether a molecule will act as an electrolyte in solution
- Recall the common polyatomic ions, including their names and charges

Ionic compounds are of particular interest to chemists because certain important types of chemical reactions—acid–base and oxidation–reduction reactions, for instance—commonly take place in ionic solutions. For stoichiometry problems, the goal with ions is to identify oxidation states. This will allow us to determine electron equivalents, balance equations, and deduce chemical formulas from nomenclature.

BRIDGE

The magnitude of the electrostatic force in an ionic bond follows the same conventions described for Coulomb's law in Chapter 5 of *MCAT Physics and Math Review*. The distance between nuclei in ionic bonds is inversely proportional to the force. Therefore, ionic compounds with long bond distances are much more weakly held together.

Cations and Anions

In Chapter 3 of *MCAT General Chemistry Review*, we discussed how ionic compounds are made up of positively charged **cations**, usually metals, and negatively charged **anions**, usually nonmetals. This rule does not always hold true for elements like hydrogen, which can act like an anion or cation but is still classified as a nonmetal, as shown in Figure 4.12 Ionic compounds are held together by **ionic bonds**, which rely on the force of electrostatic attraction between oppositely charged particles.

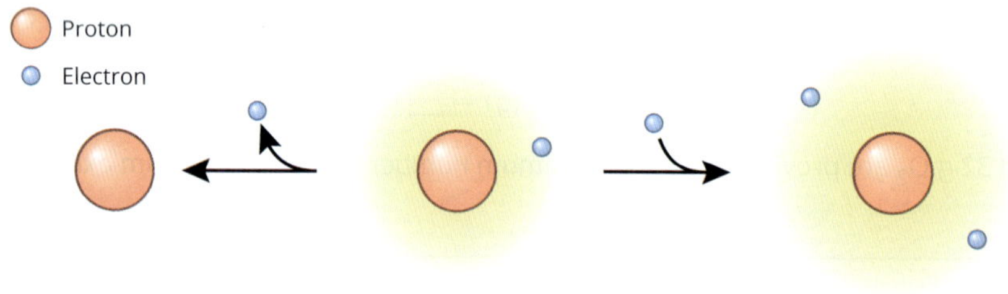

No. of protons	1	1	1
No. of electrons	0	1	2
Charge	+1	0	−1
Notation	H^+	H	H^-
Classification	cation	neutral (not an ion)	anion

Figure 4.12 Oxidation States of Hydrogen

The nomenclature of ionic compounds is based on the names of the component ions:

1. For elements (usually metals) that can form more than one positive ion, the charge is indicated by a Roman numeral in parentheses following the name of the element

Fe^{2+}	Iron(II)	Cu^+	Copper(I)
Fe^{3+}	Iron(III)	Cu^{2+}	Copper(II)

2. An older, less commonly used method is to add the endings –***ous*** or –***ic*** to the root of the Latin name of the element to represent the ions with lesser and greater charge, respectively.

Fe^{2+}	Ferrous	Cu^{+}	Cuprous
Fe^{3+}	Ferric	Cu^{2+}	Cupric

3. Monatomic anions are named by dropping the ending of the name of the element and adding –***ide***.

H^{-}	Hydride	S^{2-}	Sulfide
F^{-}	Fluoride	N^{3-}	Nitride
O^{2-}	Oxide	P^{3-}	Phosphide

4. Many polyatomic anions contain oxygen and are therefore called **oxyanions**. When an element forms two oxyanions, the name of the one with less oxygen ends in –***ite***, and the one with more oxygen ends in –***ate***.

NO_2^-	Nitrite	SO_3^{2-}	Sulfite
NO_3^-	Nitrate	SO_4^{2-}	Sulfate

5. In extended series of oxyanions, prefixes are also used. ***Hypo***– and hyper, written as ***per***–, are used to indicate less oxygen and more oxygen, respectively.

ClO^-	Hypochlorite
ClO_2^-	Chlorite
ClO_3^-	Chlorate
ClO_4^-	Perchlorate

6. Polyatomic anions often gain one or more H^+ ions to form anions of lower charge. The resulting ions are named by adding the word **hydrogen** or **dihydrogen** to the front of the anion's name. An older method uses the prefix ***bi***– to indicate the addition of a single hydrogen ion.

HCO_3^-	Hydrogen carbonate or bicarbonate
HSO_4^-	Hydrogen sulfate or bisulfate
$H_2PO_4^-$	Dihydrogen phosphate

MCAT EXPERTISE

It is unlikely that *–ous* or *–ic* endings will be required for most problem-solving. Passages tend to provide reaction schemes that allow you to deduce any unfamiliar compound's formulas. However, it is still important to understand the nomenclature for discrete questions.

MNEMONIC

The "**lite**st" anions have the fewest oxygens; the heaviest anions **ate** the most oxygens.

7. Other common polyatomic ions that may be useful to know are in Table 4.1. Note that Table 4.1 is not an exhaustive list of polyatomic ions.

Charge	Formula	Name
+1	NH_4^+	Ammonium
−1	$C_2H_3O_2^-$	Acetate
	CN^-	Cyanide
	MnO_4^-	Permanganate
	SCN^-	Thiocyanate
−2	CrO_4^{2-}	Chromate
	$Cr_2O_7^{2-}$	Dichromate
−3	BO_3^{3-}	Borate

Table 4.1 Other Common Polyatomic Ions

Ion Charges

Ionic species, by definition, have charge. Cations have positive charge, and anions have negative charge. Some elements are only found naturally in their charged forms, while others may exist naturally in the charged or uncharged state. Some elements can even have several different charges or **oxidation states**, depending on the other atoms in a compound, as can be seen in Figure 4.13.

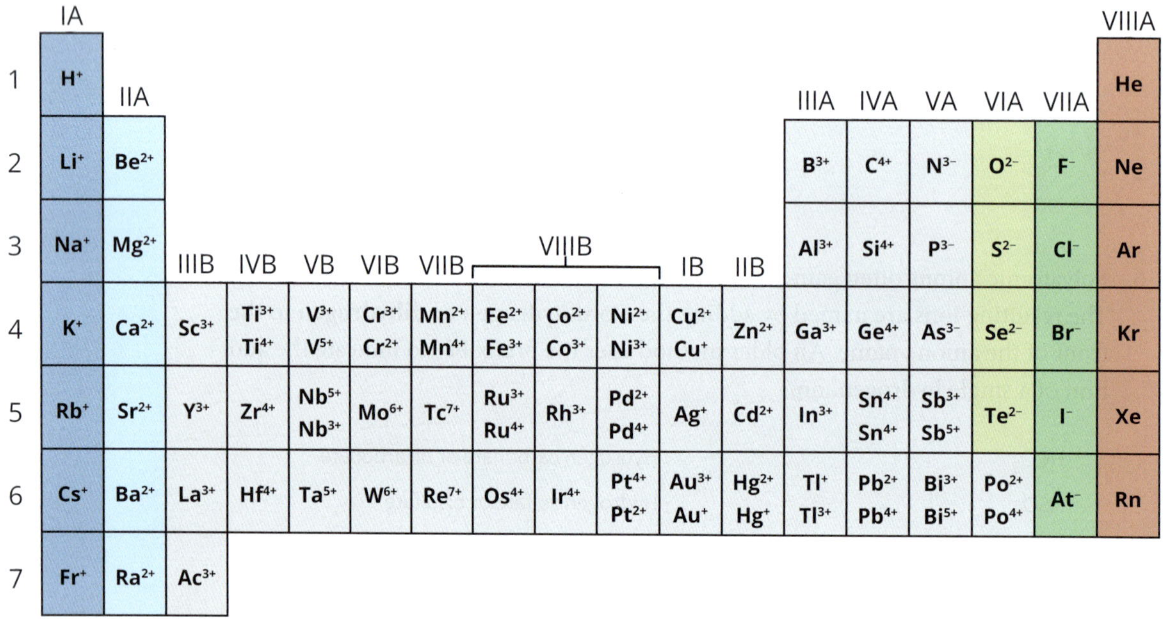

Figure 4.13 Common Oxidation States of Atoms

Some of the charged atoms or molecules that are on the MCAT include the active metals—the alkali metals (Group IA or Group 1), shown in dark blue, have a charge of +1. The alkaline earth metals (Group IIA or Group 2) have charges of +2 and are highlighted in light blue.

Nonmetals, which are found on the right side of the periodic table, generally form anions. The oxygen group (Group VIA or Group 16) in yellow typically has a −2 charge. All the halogens (Group VIIA or Group 17), shown in green, form monatomic anions with a charge of −1 because they already have 7 electrons and aim to fill an octet. The noble gases (Group VIIIA or Group 18) in red are highly stable and unreactive due to having a full shell of valence electrons, and do not typically ionize.

In summary, all elements in a given group tend to form monatomic ions with the same charge (for example, all Group IA elements have a charge of +1 in their ionic state). Note that there are anionic species that contain metallic elements (for example, MnO_4^- [permanganate] and CrO_4^{2-} [chromate]); even so, the metals have positive oxidation states. Also note that in the oxyanions of the halogens, such as ClO^- and ClO_2^-, the halogen is assigned a positive oxidation state.

For nonrepresentative elements like many of the transition metals, such as copper, iron, and chromium, there are numerous positively charged states. These states need not be memorized. Qualitatively, the color of a solution can be indicative of the oxidation state of a given element in the solution. The same element in different oxidation states can undergo different electron transitions and therefore absorb different frequencies of light. In Figure 4.14, this phenomenon is shown for various plutonium salts with different oxidation states for plutonium indicated in Roman numerals.

BRIDGE

Remember that alkali metals are not typically found in nature in their uncharged state because they are highly reactive with moisture. Instead, they are found as cations in salts (like NaCl).

BRIDGE

Oxyanions of transition metals like the MnO_4^- and CrO_4^{2-} ions have an inordinately high oxidation number on the metal. As such, they tend to gain electrons in order to reduce this oxidation number and thus make good oxidizing agents. Good oxidizing and reducing agents are discussed in Chapter 4 of *MCAT Organic Chemistry Review*.

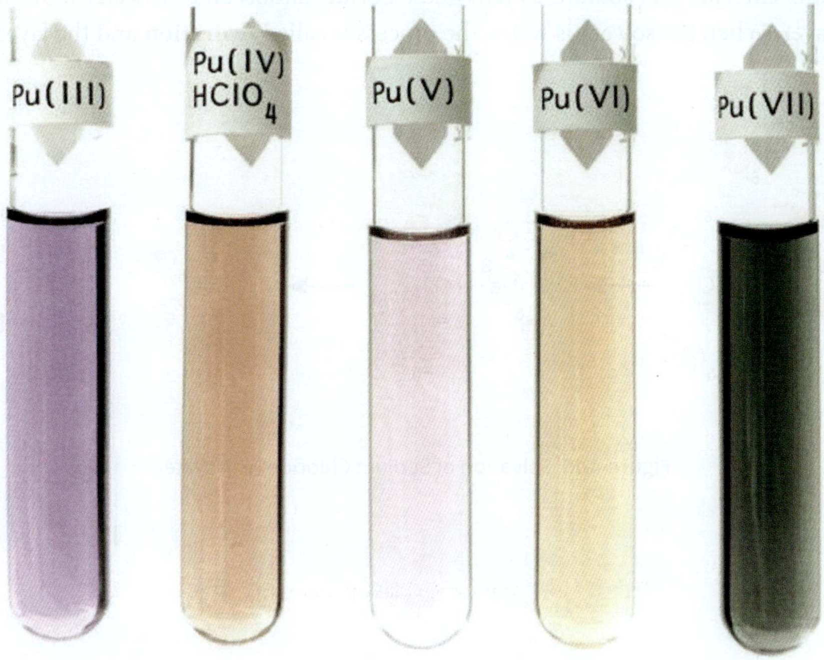

Figure 4.14 Solutions with Various Plutonium Oxidation States

The trends of **ionicity**, as we've described here, are helpful but are complicated by the fact that many elements have intermediate electronegativity and are consequently less likely to form ionic compounds, and by the left-to-right transition from metallic to nonmetallic character on the periodic table.

Electrolytes

In spite of the fact that ionic compounds are composed of ions, solid ionic compounds tend to be poor conductors of electricity because the charged particles are rigidly set in place by the lattice arrangement of the crystalline solid. In aqueous solutions, however, the lattice arrangement is disrupted by the ion–dipole interactions between the ionic components and the water molecules. The cations and anions are now free to move, and as a result, the solution of ions is able to conduct electricity.

Solutes that enable solutions to carry currents are called **electrolytes**. The electrical conductivity of aqueous solutions is governed by the presence and concentration of ions in the solution. Subsequently, the number of electron equivalents being transferred in such a system, such as in electrochemical cells, varies. Pure water, which has no ions other than the very few hydrogen ions and hydroxide ions that result from water's low-level autodissociation, is a very poor conductor.

MCAT EXPERTISE

Ionic compounds make good electrolytes because they dissolve most readily. Nonpolar covalent compounds are the weakest because they do not form current-carrying ions.

The tendency of an ionic solute to dissolve, or **solvate**, into its constituent ions in water may be high or low. A solute is considered a strong electrolyte if it dissociates completely into its constituent ions. Examples of strong electrolytes include certain ionic compounds, such as NaCl and KI, and molecular compounds with highly polar covalent bonds that dissociate into ions when dissolved, such as HCl in water. An example of solvation of such compounds is shown in Figure 4.15. When solid sodium chloride is introduced into a polar solvent like water, the water molecules orient in such a way that the oxygen atoms, which have a partial negative charge, surround the sodium atom and the hydrogen atoms, with a slightly positive charge, surround the chloride atom. This facilitates the separation of sodium chloride into sodium cations and chloride anions, and the water molecules organize into a **solvation layer**. When the solvent is water, the process is called **hydration** and the layer is known as a **hydration shell**.

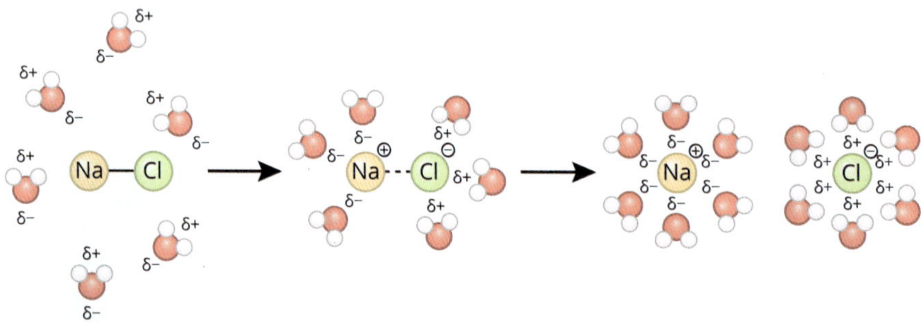

Figure 4.15 Solvation of Sodium Chloride with Water

A weak electrolyte, on the other hand, ionizes or hydrolyzes incompletely in aqueous solution, and only some of the solute is dissolved into its ionic constituents. Examples include Hg_2I_2 ($K_{sp} = 4.5 \times 10^{-29}$), acetic acid and other weak acids, and ammonia and other weak bases. Many compounds do not ionize at all in water, retaining their molecular structure in solution, which may also limit their solubility. These compounds are called nonelectrolytes and include many nonpolar gases and organic compounds, such as O_2 (*g*), CO_2 (*g*), and glucose.

BRIDGE

Because electrolytes ionize in solution, they will produce a larger effect on colligative properties, described in Chapter 9 of *MCAT General Chemistry Review*, than one would expect from the given concentration.

MCAT CONCEPT CHECK 4.6

Before you move on, assess your understanding of the material with these questions.

1. Label the following solutions as electrolytes or nonelectrolytes: (Note: Assume these compounds are all in aqueous solution.)

• HCl	Electrolyte	Nonelectrolyte
• Sucrose	Electrolyte	Nonelectrolyte
• $MgBr_2$	Electrolyte	Nonelectrolyte
• CH_4	Electrolyte	Nonelectrolyte

2. Identify the following ions as cations or anions, and then provide the formula or chemical symbol:

Ion	Cation or Anion	Formula
Phosphate		
Hypochlorite		
Ammonium		
Phosphide		
Bicarbonate		
Nitrite		
Chromium(II)		

Conclusion

We began our consideration of compounds with benzaldehyde. As a compound, it is made from constituent atoms of different elements in a set ratio defined by its empirical or molecular formula. Each molecule of a compound has a defined mass that is measured as its molecular weight. The mass of one mole of any compound is determined from its molar mass in the units of grams per mole. We reviewed the basic classifications of reactions commonly tested on the MCAT: combination, decomposition, combustion, single-displacement, double-displacement, and neutralization reactions. Furthermore, we are now confident in our understanding of the steps necessary to balance any chemical reaction; we are ready to tackle more stoichiometric problems in preparation for Test Day.

Before moving to the next chapters discussing chemical kinetics and thermodynamics, let us offer our congratulations to you. By completing these first four chapters, you have been introduced to the fundamental concepts of chemistry—everything from the structure of the atom and trends of the elements to bonding and the formation of compounds. The understanding you have gained so far will be the foundation for your comprehension of even the most difficult general chemistry concepts tested on the MCAT. Keep moving forward with your review of general chemistry; don't get stuck in the details. Those details will be learned best through the application of the basic principles to MCAT practice passages and questions.

GO ONLINE

You've reviewed the content, now test your knowledge and critical thinking skills by completing a test-like passage set in your online resources!

CONCEPT SUMMARY

Molecules and Moles

- **Compounds** are substances composed of two or more elements in a fixed proportion.
- **Molecular weight** is the mass (in amu) of the constituent atoms in a compound as indicated by the molecular formula.
- **Molar mass** is the mass of one mole (**Avogadro's number** or 6.022×10^{23} particles) of a compound; usually measured in grams per mole.
- **Gram equivalent weight** is a measure of the mass of a substance that can donate one equivalent of the species of interest.
- **Normality** is the ratio of equivalents per liter; it is related to **molarity** by multiplying the molarity by the number of equivalents present per mole of compound.
- **Equivalents** are moles of the species of interest; equivalents are most often seen in acid–base chemistry (hydrogen ions or hydroxide ions) and oxidation–reduction reactions (moles of electrons or other ions).

Representation of Compounds

- The **law of constant composition** states that any pure sample of a compound will contain the same elements in the same mass ratio.
- The **empirical formula** is the smallest whole-number ratio of the elements in a compound.
- The **molecular formula** is either the same as or a multiple of the empirical formula; it gives the exact number of atoms of each element in a compound.
- To calculate **percent composition** by mass, determine the mass of the individual element and divide by the molar mass of the compound.

Types of Chemical Reactions

- **Combination reactions** occur when two or more reactants combine to form one product.
- **Decomposition reactions** occur when one reactant is chemically broken down into two or more products.
- **Combustion reactions** occur when a fuel and an oxidant (typically oxygen) react, forming the products water and carbon dioxide (if the fuel is a hydrocarbon).
- **Displacement reactions** occur when one or more atoms or ions of one compound are replaced with one or more atoms or ions of another compound.
  - **Single-displacement reactions** occur when an ion of one compound is replaced with another element.
  - **Double-displacement reactions** occur when elements from two different compounds trade places with each other to form two new compounds.
- **Neutralization reactions** are those in which an acid reacts with a base to form a salt (and, usually, water).

Balancing Chemical Equations

- Chemical equations must be balanced to perform stoichiometric calculations.
- **Balanced equations** are determined using the following steps in order:
  - Balancing the least common atoms
  - Balancing the more common atoms (usually hydrogen and oxygen)
  - Balancing charge, if necessary

Applications of Stoichiometry

- Balanced equations can be used to determine the **limiting reagent**, which is the reactant that will be consumed first in a chemical reaction.
- The other reactants present are termed **excess reagents**.
- **Theoretical yield** is the amount of product generated if all of the limiting reactant is consumed with no side reactions.
- **Actual yield** is typically lower than theoretical yield.
- **Percent yield** is calculated by dividing actual yield by theoretical yield and converting to a percentage.

Ions

- Like organic chemistry, ions in general chemistry have a system of nomenclature:
  - Roman numerals are used for nonrepresentative elements to denote ionic charge.
  - –***ous*** endings can also be used to indicate lesser charge, while –***ic*** endings indicate greater charge.
  - All monatomic anions end in –***ide***.
  - Oxyanions are given a suffix indicating how oxidized the central atom is. Those that contain a lesser amount of oxygen are given the suffix –***ite***, and those with a greater amount are given the suffix –***ate***.
  - Oxyanion series with more than two members are given an additional level of nomenclature. The species with the fewest oxygens is given the prefix ***hypo***–, and the species with the most oxygens is given the prefix ***per***–.
  - Polyatomic ions containing hydrogen denote the number of hydrogens using ***hydrogen*** or ***bi***– to denote one, or ***dihydrogen*** to denote two.
- **Ionic charges** are predictable by group number and type of element (metal or nonmetal) for representative elements, but are generally unpredictable for nonrepresentative elements.
  - Metals form positively charged cations based on group number.
  - Nonmetals form negatively charged anions based on the number of electrons needed to achieve an octet.
- **Electrolytes** contain equivalents of ions from molecules that dissociate in solution. The strength of an electrolyte depends on its degree of dissociation or **solvation**.

ANSWERS TO CONCEPT CHECKS

4.1

1. NaBr: $23 + 79.9 \approx 23 + 80 = 103\ \frac{\text{g}}{\text{mol}}$

   $SrCl_2$: $87.6 + (2 \times 35.5) = 87.6 + 71 = 158.6\ \frac{\text{g}}{\text{mol}}$

   $C_6H_{12}O_6$: $(6 \times 12) + (12 \times 1) + (6 \times 16) = 180\ \frac{\text{g}}{\text{mol}}$

2. NaBr: $\dfrac{100\ \text{g}}{103\ \frac{\text{g}}{\text{mol}}} = 0.97$ moles

   Note that the denominator is greater than the numerator by approximately 3 percent, and the actual value is less than 1 by approximately 3 percent. This approximation can be used to quickly estimate answers that are close to one.

   $SrCl_2$: $\dfrac{100\ \text{g}}{158.6\ \frac{\text{g}}{\text{mol}}} \approx \dfrac{100}{160} = \dfrac{10}{16} = \dfrac{5}{8} = 0.625$ moles

   Note that the answer is a fraction based on eighths. As these are commonly used on the MCAT, knowing the values for 1/8 through 7/8 can be useful for many problems.

   $C_6H_{12}O_6$: $\dfrac{100\ \text{g}}{180\ \frac{\text{g}}{\text{mol}}} = \dfrac{10}{18} = \dfrac{5}{9} = 0.555$ moles

   Note that the final fraction is in ninths. Dividing by nine follows a standard pattern that is useful to know for the MCAT: $1/9 = 0.111$, $2/9 = 0.222$, $3/9 = 0.333$, etc.

3. Both values equal one mole of the given substance. The number of entities in a mole is always the same (Avogadro's number, $6.022 \times 10^{23}\ \text{mol}^{-1}$).

4. Normality is calculated as $N = M \times \dfrac{\text{equivalents}}{\text{mole}}$.

   For H_3PO_4: $0.25\ \text{M}\ H_3PO_4 \times \dfrac{3\ \text{equiv}\ H^+}{\text{mol}\ H_3PO_4} = 0.75\ \text{N}\ H_3PO_4$.

   For PO_4^{3-} the grams must first be converted to moles, then to normality. PO_4^{3-} has a molecular mass of 95, giving

   $$\frac{95\ \text{g}}{100\ \text{mL}} = \frac{950\ \text{g}}{1\ \text{L}} = \frac{10\ \text{mol}}{1\ \text{L}} = 10\ \text{M}\ PO_4^{3-}$$

   $$10\ \text{M}\ PO_4^{3-} \times \frac{3\ \text{equiv}\ H^+}{\text{mol}\ PO_4^{3-}} = 30\ \text{N}\ PO_4^{3-}.$$

4.2

1. Both molecular and empirical formulas contain the same elements in the same ratios. They differ in that molecular formulas give the actual number of atoms of each element in the compound; empirical formulas give only the ratio and therefore may or may not give the actual number of atoms.
2. The molar mass of sodium carbonate is given by $(2 \times 23) + (1 \times 12) + (3 \times 16) = 106\ \frac{\text{g}}{\text{mol}}$. The percent compositions are:

$$\text{Na: } \frac{2 \times \left(23\ \frac{\text{g}}{\text{mol}}\right)}{106\ \frac{\text{g}}{\text{mol}}} \times 100\% \approx \frac{46}{100} \times 100\% = 46\%\ (\text{actual value} = 43.4\%)$$

$$\text{O: } \frac{3 \times \left(16\ \frac{\text{g}}{\text{mol}}\right)}{106\ \frac{\text{g}}{\text{mol}}} \times 100\% \approx \frac{48}{100} \times 100\% = 48\%\ (\text{actual value} = 45.3\%)$$

$$\text{C: } \frac{1 \times \left(12\ \frac{\text{g}}{\text{mol}}\right)}{106\ \frac{\text{g}}{\text{mol}}} \times 100\% \approx \frac{12}{100} \times 100\% = 12\%\ (\text{actual value} = 11.3\%)$$

Note that in all three cases, the estimation reduces the value of the denominator, thus making the calculated value larger than the actual value.

3. Start by assuming a 100 g sample, which represents 28.5 g Fe, 24.0 g S, and 49.7 g O. Next, divide each number of grams by the atomic weight to determine the number of moles:

$$\text{Fe: } \frac{28.5\ \text{g}}{55.8\ \frac{\text{g}}{\text{mol}}} \approx \frac{28}{56} = 0.5\ \text{moles}$$

$$\text{S: } \frac{24\ \text{g}}{32.1\ \frac{\text{g}}{\text{mol}}} \approx \frac{24}{32} = \frac{3}{4} = 0.75\ \text{moles}$$

$$\text{O: } \frac{49.7\ \text{g}}{16\ \frac{\text{g}}{\text{mol}}} \approx \frac{48}{16} = 3\ \text{moles}$$

Next, find the multiplier that gives all three compounds integer values of moles. Using sulfur, multiplying 0.75 moles $\times$ 4 = 3 moles. Using 4 as a multiplier for all three compounds gives the ratio 2 Fe : 3 S : 12 O. This gives an empirical formula of $Fe_2S_3O_{12}$.

4.3

1. Ammonium cations swap places with (or displace) zinc cations yielding ammonium nitrate and zinc(II) sulfide. Zinc(II) sulfide then precipitates out of solution as a solid salt.

2.

Reactants	Conditions	Products	Reaction Type
$2\ H_2 + O_2$	$\longrightarrow$	$2\ H_2O$	Combination
$Al(OH)_3 + H_3PO_4$	$\longrightarrow$	$3\ H_2O + AlPO_4$	Neutralization (a type of double-displacement)
$2\ H_2O$	$\xrightarrow{\text{electricity}}$	$2\ H_2 + O_2$	Decomposition
$NaNO_3 + CuOH$	$\longrightarrow$	$NaOH + CuNO_3$	Double-displacement (metathesis)
$Zn + AgCl$	$\longrightarrow$	$ZnCl + Ag$	Single-displacement

4.4

1.
- $2\ Fe + 3\ Cl_2 \rightarrow 2\ FeCl_3$
- $Zn + 2\ HCl \rightarrow ZnCl_2 + H_2$
- $C_5H_{12} + 8\ O_2 \rightarrow 5\ CO_2 + 6\ H_2O$
- $3\ Pb(NO_3)_2 + 2\ AlCl_3 \rightarrow 3\ PbCl_2 + 2\ Al(NO_3)_3$

4.5

1. $4\ Na\ (s) + O_2\ (g) \rightarrow 2\ Na_2O\ (s)$

2. $46\text{ g Na} \times \left[\frac{1\text{ mol Na}}{23\text{ g Na}}\right] = 2\text{ mol Na}; 32\text{ g }O_2 \times \left[\frac{1\text{ mol }O_2}{32\text{ g }O_2}\right] = 1\text{ mol }O_2$

   Because 4 sodium atoms are needed for every oxygen molecule, sodium will run out first. To determine the amount of Na_2O formed:

$$2\text{ mol Na} \times \left[\frac{2\text{ mol }Na_2O}{4\text{ mol Na}}\right] = 1\text{ mol }Na_2O$$

3. The limiting reagent is Na because 4 sodium atoms are needed for every oxygen molecule.

$$2\text{ mol Na} \times \left[\frac{1\text{ mol }O_2}{4\text{ mol Na}}\right] = 0.5\text{ mol }O_2$$

   will be used, so $1.0 - 0.5\text{ mol }O_2 = 0.5\text{ mol }O_2$ will remain. In grams, this is:

$$0.5\text{ mol }O_2 \times \left[\frac{32\text{ g }O_2}{1\text{ mol }O_2}\right] = 16\text{ g excess }O_2$$

4. Reaction: $BeO + H_2O \rightarrow Be(OH)_2$

Theoretical yield:

$$2500 \text{ g BeO} \times \left[\frac{1 \text{ mol BeO}}{25 \text{ g BeO}}\right]\left[\frac{1 \text{ mol Be(OH)}_2}{1 \text{ mol BeO}}\right]\left[\frac{43 \text{ g Be(OH)}_2}{1 \text{ mol Be(OH)}_2}\right] = 4300 \text{ g Be(OH)}_2$$

$$\text{Percent yield} = \frac{\text{Actual yield}}{\text{Theoretical yield}} \times 100\% = \frac{1100 \text{ g}}{4300 \text{ g}} \times 100\% \approx \frac{11}{44} \times 100\%$$

$$= 25\% \text{ yield (actual value} = 25.6\%)$$

4.6

1. Electrolytes: HCl, $MgBr_2$; Nonelectrolytes: sucrose, CH_4

2.

Ion	Cation or Anion	Formula
Phosphate	Anion	PO_4^{3-}
Hypochlorite	Anion	ClO^-
Ammonium	Cation	NH_4^+
Phosphide	Anion	P^{3-}
Bicarbonate	Anion	HCO_3^-
Nitrite	Anion	NO_2^-
Chromium(II)	Cation	Cr^{2+}

SCIENCE MASTERY ASSESSMENT EXPLANATIONS

1. **D**

Ionic compounds are composed of atoms held together by ionic bonds. Ionic bonds associate charged particles with large differences in electronegativity. Rather than forming molecules or being measured by molecular weight, as in **(A)** and **(B)**, ionic compounds form large arrays of ions in crystalline solids and are measured with formula weights. In ionic bonds, electrons are not really shared but rather are donated from the less electronegative atom to the more electronegative atom, eliminating **(C)**.

2. **A**

Of the compounds listed, both **(B)** and **(D)** are covalent compounds and thus are measured in molecular weights, not formula weights. The formula weight of $MgCl_2$ is much too high ($24.3 \text{ amu} + 2 \times 35.5 \text{ amu} = 95.3 \text{ amu}$ per formula unit), eliminating **(C)**. Only KCl fits the criteria ($39.1 \text{ amu} + 35.5 \text{ amu} = 74.6 \text{ amu}$).

3. **A**

First, it is helpful to know the molar mass of one mole of H_2SO_4, which is found by adding the atomic weights of the atoms that constitute the molecule:

$$\left(2 \times 1.0 \frac{\text{g}}{\text{mol H}}\right) + \left(1 \times 32.1 \frac{\text{g}}{\text{mol S}}\right) + \left(4 \times 16.0 \frac{\text{g}}{\text{mol O}}\right) = 98.1 \frac{\text{g}}{\text{mol H}_2\text{SO}_4}.$$

Gram equivalent weight is the mass (in grams) that would release one mole of protons. Because sulfuric acid has two hydrogens per molecule, the gram equivalent weight is 98.1 g divided by 2, or 49.1 g.

4. **C**

The definition of an empirical formula is a formula that represents a molecule with the simplest ratio, in whole numbers, of the elements comprising the compound. In this case, given the empirical formula CH, any molecule with carbon and hydrogen atoms in a 1:1 ratio would be accurately represented by this empirical formula. **(C)** has three carbon atoms and four hydrogen atoms. Both its molecular and empirical formulas would be C_3H_4 because this formula represents the smallest whole-number ratio of its constituent elements.

5. **A**

The percent composition by mass of any given element within a molecule is equal to the mass of that element in the molecule divided by the molar mass of the compound, times 100%. In this case, acetone, C_3H_6O, has

$$\frac{3 \times 12 \frac{\text{g}}{\text{mol C}}}{\left(3 \times 12 \frac{\text{g}}{\text{mol C}}\right) + \left(6 \times 1 \frac{\text{g}}{\text{mol H}}\right) + \left(16 \frac{\text{g}}{\text{mol O}}\right)} = \frac{36 \frac{\text{g}}{\text{mol}}}{58 \frac{\text{g}}{\text{mol}}} = \frac{18}{29} \approx \frac{2}{3} \approx 66.7\%.$$

This is an overestimation, and the actual value will be lower; it is closest to 62% out of the four choices available. **(B)**, ethanol, is $\frac{24 \frac{\text{g}}{\text{mol C}}}{46 \frac{\text{g}}{\text{mol total}}} \approx 50\%$. This is an underestimation, and the actual value will be higher but nowhere near 62%. **(C)**, propane, is C_3H_8, and calculates to be $\frac{36 \frac{\text{g}}{\text{mol c}}}{44 \frac{\text{g}}{\text{mol total}}} \approx \frac{9}{11} \approx 80\%$ carbon. This is an underestimation, and therefore the actual value cannot be 62%. Finally, **(D)**, methanol, is $\frac{12 \frac{\text{g}}{\text{mol C}}}{32 \frac{\text{g}}{\text{mol total}}} = \frac{3}{8} = 37.5\%$ carbon.

Note that all four of these compounds are commonly encountered on the MCAT, and you should be familiar with the structure and composition of each, including their common names.

6. **B**

This reaction is a classic example of a neutralization reaction, in which an acid and a base react to form a salt and, usually, water. Although this reaction also fits the criteria for a double-displacement reaction, **(C)**, in which two molecules essentially exchange ions with each other, neutralization is a more specific description of the process.

7. **A**

In this question, you are first given the masses of both reactants used to start the reaction. To figure out what will be left over, we must first determine which species is the limiting reagent. The formula weight of Na_2S is

$$\left(2 \times \frac{23\text{ g}}{\text{mol Na}}\right) + \left(1 \times \frac{32.1\text{ g}}{\text{mol S}}\right) = 78.1\ \frac{\text{g}}{\text{mol}}\ Na_2S.$$

The formula weight of $AgNO_3$ is

$$\left(1 \times \frac{107.9\text{ g}}{\text{mol Ag}}\right) + \left(1 \times \frac{14\text{ g}}{\text{mol N}}\right) + \left(3 \times \frac{16\text{ g}}{\text{mol O}}\right) = 169.9\ \frac{\text{g}}{\text{mol}}\ AgNO_3.$$

From this, we can determine that we are given:

$$\frac{39.05\text{ g }Na_2S}{78.1\ \frac{\text{g}}{\text{mol}}} = 0.5\text{ mol }Na_2S$$

and

$$\frac{85.5\text{ g }AgNO_3}{169.9\ \frac{\text{g}}{\text{mol}}} = 0.5\text{ mol }AgNO_3.$$

Because we need two moles of $AgNO_3$ for every mole of Na_2S, $AgNO_3$ is the limiting reagent, and the correct answer choice will be in grams of Na_2S. If 0.5 mol of $AgNO_3$ are used up, and Na_2S will be consumed at half the rate of $AgNO_3$ (based on their mole ratio), then 0.25 mol Na_2S will be used up. We then have 0.25 mol excess Na_2S, which has a mass of

$$0.25\text{ mol} \times \left(\frac{78.1\text{ g}}{\text{mol}}\right) \approx \frac{1}{4} \times \frac{80}{1} = 20\text{ g (actual value} = 19.5\text{ g)}.$$

8. **A**

This is a question best answered by dimensional analysis. Keeping in mind that molar mass is measured in grams of a substance per moles of that substance, only **(A)** comes out with the units of grams of oxygen. **(B)** has the units of grams per mole of oxygen, not grams of oxygen. **(C)** has the units of moles per gram of oxygen. **(D)** has the units of mol^2 per gram of oxygen.

9. **D**

In the reaction, there is a single displacement, with the silver in silver oxide being replaced by the aluminum to form aluminum oxide. This single-displacement reaction also necessitates a transfer of electrons in an oxidation–reduction reaction; silver, for example, changes from the +2 oxidation state to neutral. Aluminum changes from neutral to the +3 oxidation state.

10. **C**

Typically, both single-displacement and double-displacement reactions have two reactants that swap either one or two components between the two species. Combination reactions, on the other hand, have more reactants than products because the reactants combine together to form the product.

11. **A**

In the unbalanced reaction given in the question stem, zinc is already balanced. Next check carbon. There are 4 carbon atoms in the reactants and 1 in the product, so add a coefficient of 4 to carbon dioxide on the product side. Next, check hydrogen. There are 10 hydrogen atoms in the reactants and 2 in the products, so add a coefficient of 5 to water on the product side. Finally, check oxygen. There are 2 oxygen atoms in the reactants and 14 in the products, so add a coefficient of 7 to molecular oxygen on the reactant side. These alterations yield the balanced reaction

$$Zn(C_2H_5)_2 + 7\ O_2 \rightarrow ZnO + 4\ CO_2 + 5\ H_2O$$

Because of the coefficient of 4 in front of the CO_2 molecule on the product side, the answer is **(A)**.

12. **B**

The equation given is unbalanced, so the first step must be to balance it:

$$6\ CO_2 + 6\ H_2O \xrightarrow{hv} C_6H_{12}O_6 + 6\ O_2$$

The theoretical yield is the amount of product synthesized if the limiting reagent is completely used up. This question therefore asks how much glucose is produced if the limiting reagent is 30 grams of water. Using the three-fraction method discussed in this chapter to solve for the mass of glucose produced gives:

$$30.0\ g\ H_2O \times \left[\frac{1\ mol\ H_2O}{18\ g\ H_2O}\right]\left[\frac{1\ mol\ C_6H_{12}O_6}{6\ mol\ H_2O}\right]\left[\frac{180\ g\ C_6H_{12}O_6}{1\ mol\ C_6H_{12}O_6}\right] = 50\ g\ C_6H_{12}O_6$$

Thus, 50 grams of glucose are produced.

13. **B**

A limiting reagent is by definition a reactant. Because Au and H_2S are products, they cannot act as limiting reagents, eliminating **(C)** and **(D)**. Next, note that the given equation is unbalanced and the first step is to balance it:

$$Au_2S_3\ (s) + 3\ H_2\ (g) \rightarrow 2\ Au\ (s) + 3\ H_2S\ (g)$$

The problem states that 2 moles of gold(III) sulfide and 5 moles of hydrogen gas are available. To use up both moles of gold(III) sulfide, 6 moles of hydrogen gas are needed because there is a 1:3 ratio between these reactants. Since only 5 moles of hydrogen gas are present, that will have to be the limiting reagent.

14. **B**

The best electrolytes dissociate readily (have a high dissociation constant) and are ionic compounds with large amounts of cations and anions. This rules out **(A)** and **(C)**. **(D)** has fewer total ions with a smaller total magnitude of charge and therefore is not as strong an electrolyte as **(B)**.

15. **A**

One approach to answering this question might be to write out an unbalanced equation using the description in the question stem, and then balance that equation. But a faster method is elimination. Three of the given chemical equations are not properly balanced, while one is. Check one element at a time. Observe that in this question, the oxygen atoms in equation **(A)** are balanced, but oxygen is not balanced in **(B)**, **(C)**, and **(D)**. Thus **(A)** must be the correct answer.

GO ONLINE

Consult your online resources for additional practice.

EQUATIONS TO REMEMBER

(4.1) **Moles from mass:** $\text{Moles} = \dfrac{\text{Mass of a sample}}{\text{Molar mass}}$

(4.2) **Gram equivalent weight:** $\text{GEW} = \dfrac{\text{Molar mass}}{n}$

(4.3) **Equivalents from mass:** $\text{Equivalents} = \dfrac{\text{Mass of compound}}{\text{Gram equivalent weight}}$

(4.4) **Molarity from normality:** $\text{Molarity} = \dfrac{\text{Normality}}{n}$

(4.5) **Percent composition:** $\%\ \text{composition} = \dfrac{\text{Mass of element in formula}}{\text{Molar mass}} \times 100\%$

(4.6) **Percent yield:** $\%\ \text{yield} = \dfrac{\text{Actual yield}}{\text{Theoretical yield}} \times 100\%$

SHARED CONCEPTS

General Chemistry Chapter 2
The Periodic Table

General Chemistry Chapter 3
Bonding and Chemical Interactions

General Chemistry Chapter 9
Solutions

General Chemistry Chapter 10
Acids and Bases

General Chemistry Chapter 11
Oxidation–Reduction Reactions

Physics and Math Chapter 5
Electrostatics and Magnetism

CHAPTER 5

CHEMICAL KINETICS

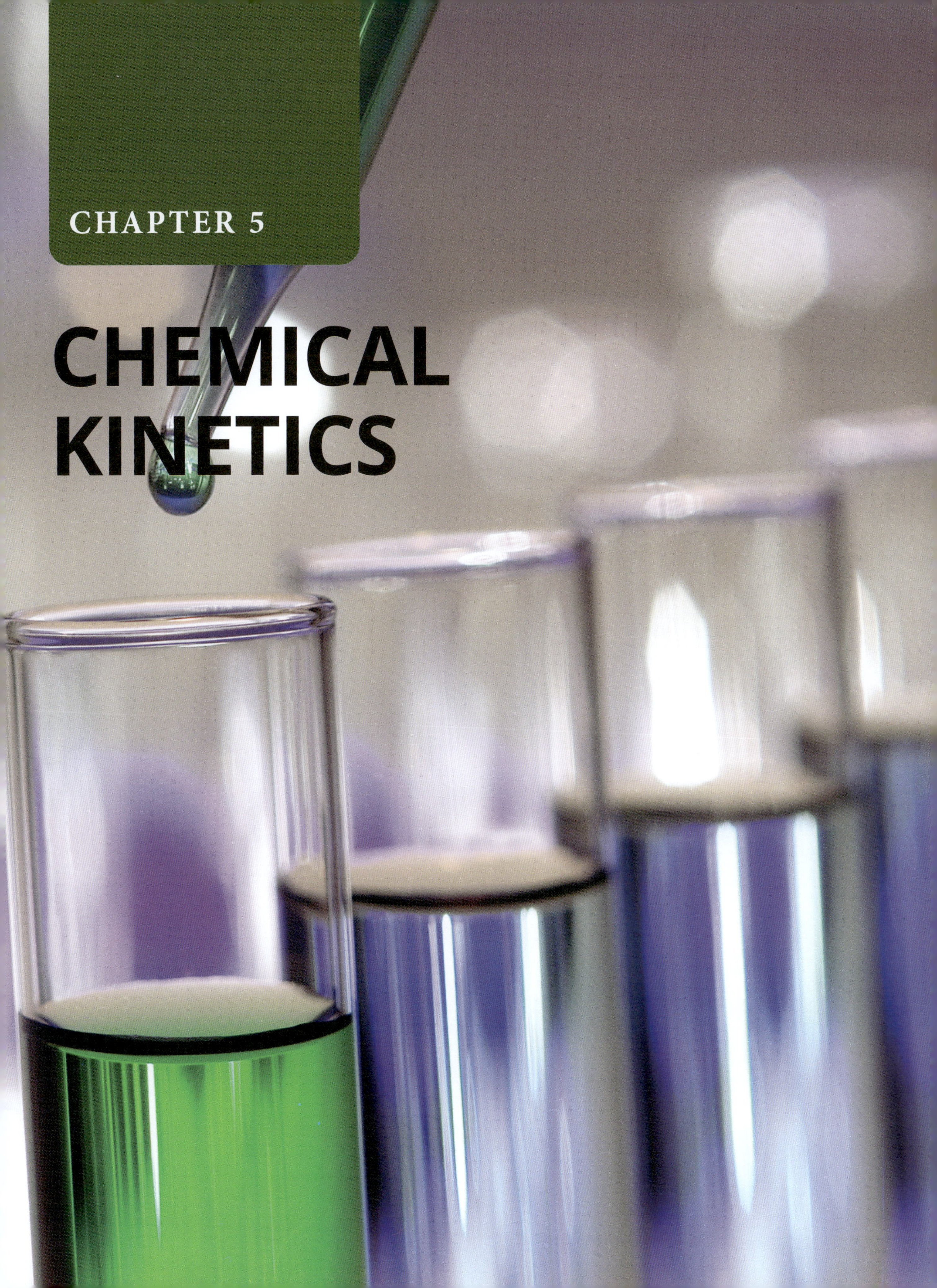

SCIENCE MASTERY ASSESSMENT

Every pre-med knows this feeling: there is so much content I have to know for the MCAT! How do I know what to do first or what's important?

While the high-yield badges throughout this book will help you identify the most important topics, this Science Mastery Assessment is another tool in your MCAT prep arsenal. This quiz (which can also be taken in your online resources) and the guidance below will help ensure that you are spending the appropriate amount of time on this chapter based on your personal strengths and weaknesses. Don't worry though—skipping something now does not mean you'll never study it. Later on in your prep, as you complete full-length tests, you'll uncover specific pieces of content that you need to review and can come back to these chapters as appropriate.

How to Use This Assessment

If you answer 0–7 questions correctly:

Spend about 1 hour to read this chapter in full and take limited notes throughout. Follow up by reviewing **all** quiz questions to ensure that you now understand how to solve each one.

If you answer 8–11 questions correctly:

Spend 20–40 minutes reviewing the quiz questions. Beginning with the questions you missed, read and take notes on the corresponding subchapters. For questions you answered correctly, ensure your thinking matches that of the explanation and you understand why each choice was correct or incorrect.

If you answer 12–15 questions correctly:

Spend less than 20 minutes reviewing all questions from the quiz. If you missed any, then include a quick read-through of the corresponding subchapters, or even just the relevant content within a subchapter, as part of your question review. For questions you answered correctly, ensure your thinking matches that of the explanation and review the Concept Summary at the end of the chapter.

1. In a third-order reaction involving two reactants and two products, doubling the concentration of the first reactant causes the rate to increase by a factor of 2. What will happen to the rate of this reaction if the concentration of the second reactant is cut in half?
   - **A.** It will increase by a factor of 2.
   - **B.** It will increase by a factor of 4.
   - **C.** It will decrease by a factor of 2.
   - **D.** It will decrease by a factor of 4.

2. In a certain equilibrium process, the activation energy of the forward reaction ($\Delta G_f^\ddagger$) is greater than the activation energy of the reverse reaction ($\Delta G_r^\ddagger$). This reaction is:
   - **A.** endothermic.
   - **B.** exothermic.
   - **C.** spontaneous.
   - **D.** nonspontaneous.

3. A reactant in a second-order reaction at a certain temperature is increased by a factor of 4. By how much is the rate of the reaction altered?
   - **A.** It is unchanged.
   - **B.** It is increased by a factor of 4.
   - **C.** It is increased by a factor of 16.
   - **D.** It cannot be determined from the information given.

4. The concentrations of all reactants in a zero-order reaction are increased two-fold. What is the new rate of the reaction?
   - **A.** It is unchanged.
   - **B.** It is decreased by a factor of 2.
   - **C.** It is increased by a factor of 2.
   - **D.** It cannot be determined from the information given.

5. Which of the following experimental methods should NEVER affect the rate of a reaction?
   - **A.** Placing an exothermic reaction in an ice bath.
   - **B.** Increasing the pressure of a reactant in a closed container.
   - **C.** Putting the reactants into an aqueous solution.
   - **D.** Removing the product of an irreversible reaction.

6. What would increasing the concentration of reactants accomplish in a solution containing a saturated catalyst?
   - **A.** It would increase the rate constant but not the reaction rate.
   - **B.** It would decrease the rate constant but increase the reaction rate.
   - **C.** It would increase the rate constant and increase the reaction rate.
   - **D.** The reaction rate would be unaffected.

7. A certain chemical reaction has the following rate law:

$$\text{rate} = k[NO_2][Br_2]$$

Which of the following statements necessarily describe(s) the kinetics of this reaction?
   - **I.** The reaction is second-order.
   - **II.** The amount of NO_2 consumed is equal to the amount of Br_2 consumed.
   - **III.** The rate will not be affected by the addition of a compound other than NO_2 and Br_2.

   - **A.** I only
   - **B.** I and II only
   - **C.** II and III only
   - **D.** I, II, and III

8. The following data shown in the table were collected for the combustion of the theoretical compound XH_4:

$$XH_4 + 2\ O_2 \rightarrow XO_2 + 2\ H_2O$$

Trial	$[XH_4]_{initial}$ (M)	$[O_2]_{initial}$ (M)	$\text{Rate}_{initial}\left(\frac{M}{min}\right)$
1	0.6	0.6	12.4
2	0.6	2.4	49.9
3	1.2	2.4	198.3

What is the rate law for the reaction described here?
   - **A.** $\text{rate} = k[XH_4][O_2]$
   - **B.** $\text{rate} = k[XH_4][O_2]^2$
   - **C.** $\text{rate} = k[XH_4]^2[O_2]$
   - **D.** $\text{rate} = k[XH_4]^2[O_2]^2$

9. Which of the following best describes the purpose of a catalyst?
   A. Catalysts are used up in the reaction, increasing reaction efficiency.
   B. Catalysts increase the rate of the reaction by lowering the activation energy.
   C. Catalysts alter the thermodynamics of the reaction to facilitate the formation of products or reactants.
   D. Catalysts stabilize the transition state by bringing it to a higher energy.

10. If the rate law for a reaction is:

$$\text{rate} = k[A]^0[B]^2[C]^1$$

What is the overall order of the reaction?
   A. 0
   B. 2
   C. 3
   D. 4

For questions 11–13, consider the following energy diagram shown below:

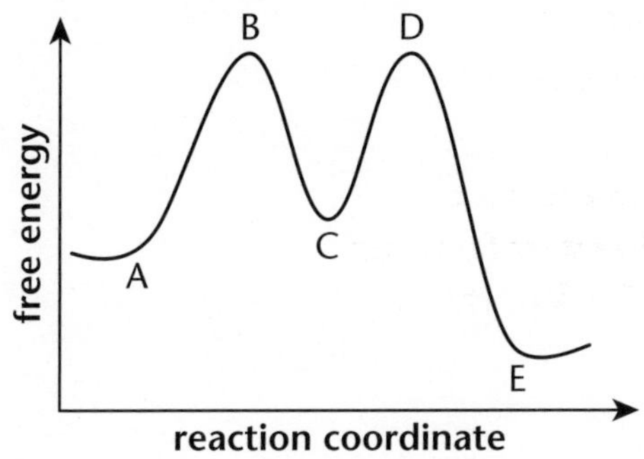

11. The overall reaction depicted by this energy diagram is:
   A. endergonic, because point B is higher than point A.
   B. endergonic, because point C is higher than point A.
   C. exergonic, because point D is higher than point E.
   D. exergonic, because point A is higher than point E.

12. Which process has the highest activation energy?
   A. The first step of the forward reaction
   B. The first step of the reverse reaction
   C. The second step of the forward reaction
   D. The second step of the reverse reaction

13. Point C in this reaction profile refers to the:
   A. reactants.
   B. products.
   C. transition state.
   D. intermediates.

14. The following system obeys second-order kinetics.

$$2\ NO_2 \rightarrow NO_3 + NO \quad \text{(slow)}$$

$$NO_3 + CO \rightarrow NO_2 + CO_2 \quad \text{(fast)}$$

What is the rate law for this reaction?
   A. rate $= k[NO_2][CO]$
   B. rate $= k[NO_2]^2[CO]$
   C. rate $= k[NO_2][NO_3]$
   D. rate $= k[NO_2]^2$

15. The potential energy diagram shown represents four different reactions.

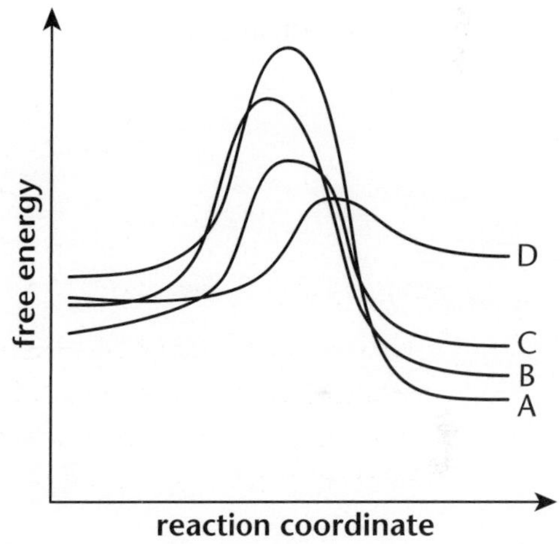

Assuming identical conditions, which of the reactions displayed on the energy diagram proceeds the fastest?
   A. A
   B. B
   C. C
   D. D

Answer Key

1. **D** (See section 5.2)
2. **D** (See section 5.1)
3. **D** (See section 5.2)
4. **A** (See section 5.2)
5. **D** (See section 5.2)
6. **D** (See section 5.1)
7. **A** (See section 5.2)
8. **C** (See section 5.2)
9. **B** (See section 5.1)
10. **C** (See section 5.2)
11. **D** (See section 5.1)
12. **B** (See section 5.1)
13. **D** (See section 5.1)
14. **D** (See section 5.2)
15. **D** (See section 5.1)

The relevant section of the chapter to review for each question is given in parentheses after the correct answer. Detailed explanations can be found at the end of the chapter.

CHAPTER 5

CHEMICAL KINETICS

In This Chapter

CHAPTER PROFILE

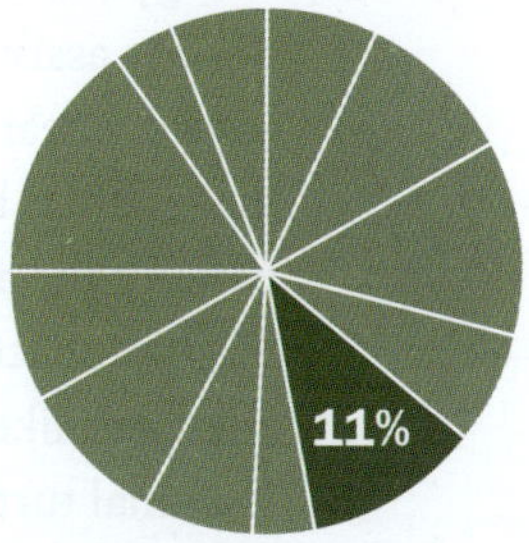

The content in this chapter should be relevant to about 11% of all questions about general chemistry on the MCAT.

This chapter covers material from the following AAMC content categories:

1A: Structure and function of proteins and their constituent amino acids

5E: Principles of chemical thermodynamics and kinetics

Introduction

The following chapters focus on two primary topics: chemical kinetics and chemical equilibrium. As the term suggests, chemical kinetics is the study of reaction rates, the effects of reaction conditions on these rates, and the mechanisms implied by such observations. We start with kinetics because the molecular basis of reactions provides us with a framework of reaction chemistry. Following this, we will explore the equilibria of these reactions, which are related to—but distinct from—the kinetics of the reactions.

You may already have a fairly good understanding of equilibrium and the differences between spontaneous and nonspontaneous reactions. For instance, the utilization of ATP in the body is a spontaneous reaction that can be used to provide thermochemical energy for other reactions. While the equilibrium tells us that ATP will favor dissociation, it tells us nothing about its rate of dissociation. And, in fact, various conditions in the body can alter the rate at which ATP is synthesized and utilized for energy—primarily temperature. Some of the symptoms of hyper- and hypothermia are related to changes in metabolism caused by changes in temperature and reaction kinetics.

More broadly, we will see how multistep reactions, such as those seen in substrate-level and oxidative phosphorylation in biochemistry, have intermediate steps that have crucial kinetic limitations.

5.1 Chemical Kinetics

High Yield

LEARNING OBJECTIVES

After Chapter 5.1, you will be able to:

- Describe the series of events within a multistep mechanism
- Explain the meaning and importance of a rate-determining step
- Describe activation energy
- Compare and contrast transition state theory and collision theory

Reactions can be spontaneous or nonspontaneous; the change in **Gibbs free energy** (**ΔG**) determines whether or not a reaction will occur by itself without outside assistance. However, even if a reaction is spontaneous, this does not necessarily mean that it will run quickly. In fact, nearly every biochemical reaction that enables life to exist, while perhaps spontaneous, proceeds so slowly that, without the aid of enzymes and other catalysts, measurable reaction progress might not actually occur over the course of an average human lifetime. And enzymes, like many other catalyzed reactions, can be saturated and experience a maximal turnover rate, as shown in Figure 5.1. For now, however, let us review reaction mechanisms, rates, rate laws, and the factors that pertain to simple chemical systems.

BRIDGE

Enzymes selectively enhance the rate of certain reactions by a factor of 10^2 to 10^{12} over other thermodynamically feasible reaction pathways. Enzyme function is discussed in Chapter 2 of *MCAT Biochemistry Review.*

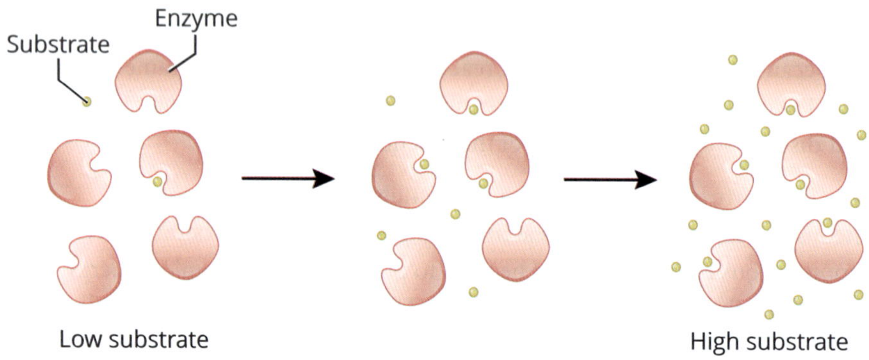

Figure 5.1 Enzymes, as Biological Catalysts, Can Be Saturated
High substrate conditions saturate the active sites of the enzyme, leading to maximal turnover.

Reaction Mechanisms

Very rarely is the balanced reaction equation, used for determining limiting reactants and yields, an accurate representation of the actual steps involved in the chemical process from reactants to products. Many reactions proceed by more than one step, the series of which is known as the **mechanism** of a reaction, and the sum of which gives the overall reaction. Knowing the accepted mechanism of a reaction may help explain the reaction's rate, position of equilibrium, and thermodynamic characteristics. Consider the generic net reaction between molecules A and B as shown in Figure 5.2.

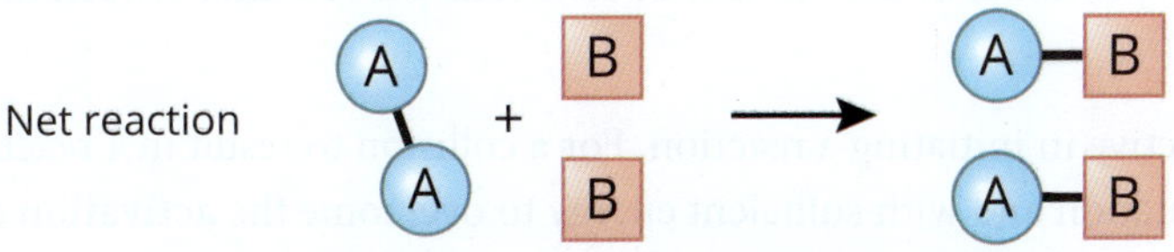

Figure 5.2 Hypothetical Net Reaction
A net reaction does not include intermediate steps.

On its own, this equation seems to imply a mechanism in which two molecules of B collide and react with one molecule of A_2 to form two molecules of AB—but the likelihood of three molecules colliding with the correct orientation and energy at the same time is low. Suppose instead, however, that the hypothetical reaction from Figure 5.2 actually takes place in two steps, as depicted in Figure 5.3.

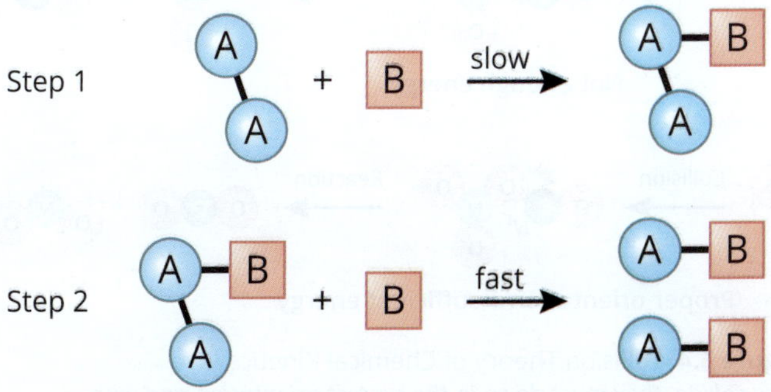

Figure 5.3 Hypothetical Elementary Reactions
Some reactions may contain multiple steps, known as elementary reactions, that sum up to the net reaction when all taken together.

The two steps shown in Figure 5.3 are known as elementary reactions, and together they add up to the overall net reaction. The molecule A_2B, which does not appear in the overall reaction, is called an **intermediate**. Reaction intermediates are often difficult to detect because they may be consumed almost immediately after they are formed, but a proposed mechanism that includes intermediates can be supported through kinetic experiments. One of the most important points to remember is that the slowest step in any proposed mechanism is called the **rate-determining step** because it acts like a kinetic bottleneck, preventing the overall reaction from proceeding any faster than that slowest step. In Figure 5.3, the first step is the rate-determining step since it is slower than the second elementary step.

Molecular Basis of Chemical Reactions

It's one thing to say *A_2 reacts with 2 B to form 2 AB*; it's quite another to be able to describe, as precisely as possible, the actual interactions that occur between A_2 and B to produce AB at some rate. Various theories have been proposed to explain the events that are taking place at the atomic level through the process of a reaction.

BRIDGE

Mechanisms are proposed pathways for a reaction that must coincide with rate data information from experimental observation. Reaction mechanisms are a major topic in organic chemistry and metabolism; Chapters 5 through 10 of *MCAT Organic Chemistry Review* and Chapters 9 through 11 of *MCAT Biochemistry Review* focus almost exclusively on reaction mechanisms in specific contexts.

KEY CONCEPT

The rate of the whole reaction is only as fast as the rate-determining step.

Collision Theory of Chemical Kinetics

The **collision theory of chemical kinetics** states that reactant molecules must collide for a reaction to occur, and that the rate of a reaction is proportional to the number of collisions per second between the reacting molecules.

However, not all collisions are effective in initiating a reaction. For a collision to result in a reaction, molecules must collide with the correct orientation and with sufficient energy to overcome the **activation energy**, E_a. Only a fraction of particles have enough kinetic energy to exceed this energy barrier. An illustration of the collision theory can be seen in Figure 5.4.

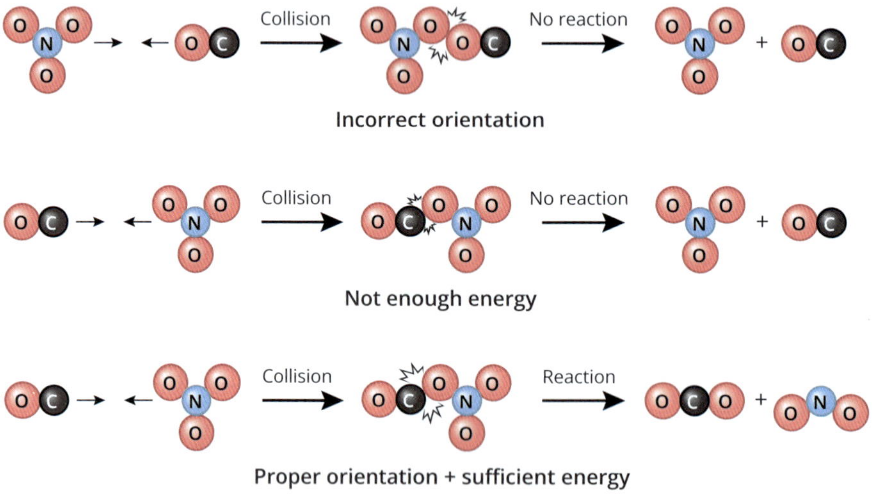

Figure 5.4 Collision Theory of Chemical Kinetics
When molecules collide, they must do so in the correct orientation and with sufficient energy in order to produce a chemical reaction.

The reaction rate is therefore a product of the total number of collisions, Z, and the fraction, f, of those collisions that are effective.

$$\text{rate} = Z \times f$$

Equation 5.1

This concept is more rigorously expressed by the **Arrhenius equation**, which relates the rate constant (k) to the frequency of collisions and the activation energy, as follows:

$$k = Ae^{\frac{-E_a}{RT}}$$

Equation 5.2

In this equation, A is the **frequency factor** (also known as the **attempt frequency**, measuring how often molecules collide and using the units s^{-1}), E_a is the activation energy of the reaction, R is the ideal gas constant, and T is the temperature in kelvin. Activation energy is a subject that will be touched upon briefly in the following subsection and more qualitatively in future chapters.

Overall, what is important here in studying the Arrhenius equation is not the actual calculation (because those involving Euler's number, e, and natural logs, ln, are not commonly found on the MCAT), but rather the relationships between the variables and the exponent rules that govern the equation.

For example, a simple relationship between A and k is evident in the equation. As the frequency factor of the reaction increases, the rate constant of the reaction also increases in a direct relationship. More complex relationships can also be seen in this equation. For example, if the temperature (T) of a chemical system were to increase to infinity, while all other variables are held constant, the value of the exponent would have a magnitude less than 1. However, before assuming that the rate constant is going to decrease as a result, note the presence of the negative sign. As the magnitude of the exponent gets smaller, it actually moves from a more negative value toward zero. The exponent thus becomes less negative (or more positive), which means that the rate constant actually increases. This should make sense conceptually because the rate of a reaction increases with temperature.

The frequency factor can be increased by increasing the number of molecules in a vessel. When there are more molecules, the opportunities for collision are increased, as shown in Figure 5.5.

MCAT EXPERTISE

Low activation energy and high temperatures make the negative exponent of the Arrhenius equation smaller in magnitude and thus increase the rate constant k.

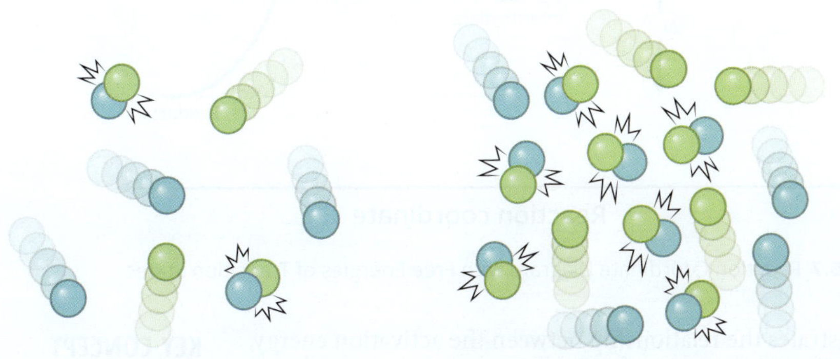

Figure 5.5 Frequency Factor (A) Is Increased by Increasing Concentration

Transition State Theory

When molecules collide with energy equal to or greater than the activation energy, they form a transition state in which the old bonds are weakened and the new bonds begin to form. The transition state then dissociates into products, fully forming the new bonds. For the reaction $A_2 + 2\,B \rightarrow 2\,AB$, the progress along the **reaction coordinate**, which traces the reaction from reactants to products, can be represented as shown in Figure 5.6.

KEY CONCEPT

Relative to reactants and products, transition states have the highest energy. They are only theoretical structures and cannot be isolated. Nevertheless, we can still use the proposed structures to better understand the reactions in which they are involved.

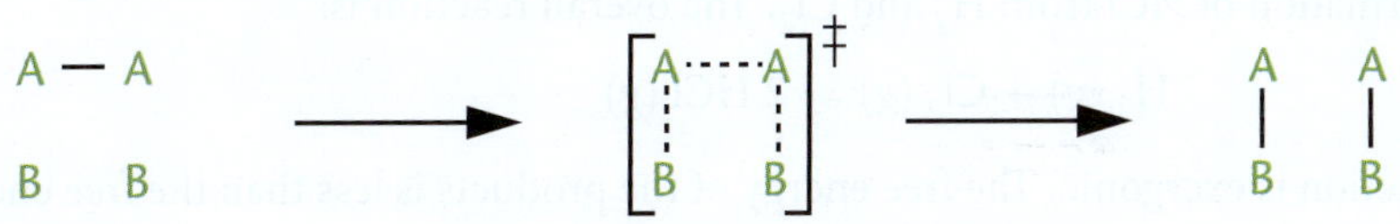

Figure 5.6 The Transition State

The **transition state**, also called the **activated complex**, has greater energy than both the reactants and the products and is denoted by the symbol ‡. The energy required to reach this transition state is the activation energy. Once an activated complex is formed, it can either dissociate into the products or revert to reactants without any additional energy input. Transition states are distinguished from reaction intermediates in that transition states are theoretical constructs that exist at the point of maximum energy, rather than distinct identities with finite lifetimes. An example of transition states can be seen in the free energy diagram in Figure 5.7. This reaction has two different transition states, with each having a higher energy than the reactants, intermediates, or products. The $\Delta G_1^\ddagger$ represents the activation energy of the first transition state. $\Delta G_2^\ddagger$ represents the activation energy of the second transition state.

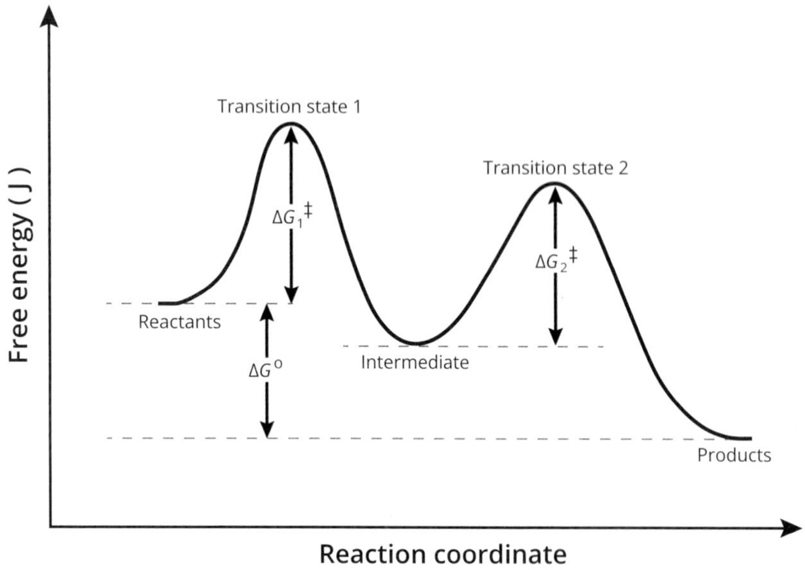

Figure 5.7 Reaction Coordinate Diagram with Free Energies of Transition States

A free energy diagram illustrates the relationship between the activation energy, the free energy of the reaction, and the free energy of the system. The most important features to recognize in such diagrams are the relative energies of all of the products and reactants. The **free energy change of the reaction (ΔG_{rxn})** is the difference between the free energy of the products and the free energy of the reactants. A negative free energy change indicates an **exergonic reaction** (energy is given off), and a positive free energy change indicates an **endergonic reaction** (energy is absorbed). The transition state exists at the peak of the energy diagram. The difference in free energy between the transition state and the reactants is the activation energy of the forward reaction; the difference in free energy between the transition state and the products is the activation energy of the reverse reaction.

KEY CONCEPT

$+\Delta G$ = endergonic = energy absorbed

$-\Delta G$ = exergonic = energy given off

For example, consider the formation of HCl from H_2 and Cl_2. The overall reaction is:

$$H_2\,(g) + Cl_2\,(g) \rightleftharpoons 2\,HCl\,(g)$$

Figure 5.8 shows that the reaction is exergonic. The free energy of the products is less than the free energy of the reactants; energy is released, and the free energy change of the reaction is negative.

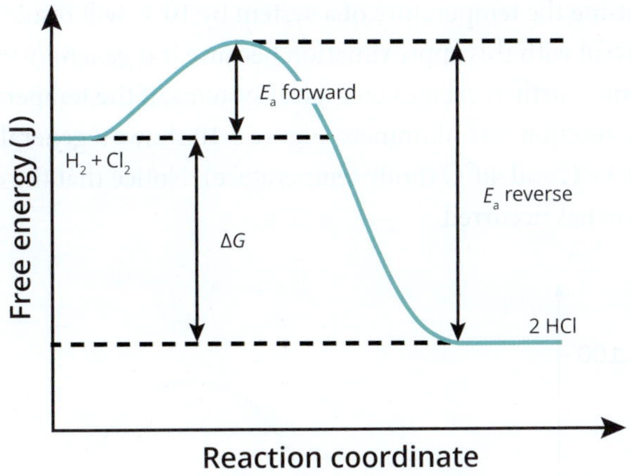

Figure 5.8 Reaction Diagram for the Formation of HCl
On the left are the reactants (H_2 and Cl_2) and on the right are the products (2 HCl); this reaction is exergonic, and forward and reverse activation energies are shown.

MCAT EXPERTISE

Kinetics and thermodynamics should be considered separately. Note that the activation energy can be lowered without affecting the ΔG. In fact, this is how catalysts increase the rate of a reaction.

Factors Affecting Reaction Rate

Before we delve into the specifics of rate calculations, it is helpful to understand the conditions that can alter experimental rates.

Reaction Concentrations

The greater the concentrations of the reactants, the greater the number of effective collisions per unit time. Recall that this leads to an increase in the frequency factor (A) of the Arrhenius equation. Therefore, the reaction rate will increase for all but zero-order reactions, which will be discussed shortly. For reactions occurring in the gaseous state, the partial pressures of the gas reactants serve as a measure of concentration, as discussed in Chapter 8 of *MCAT General Chemistry Review*.

Temperature

For nearly all reactions, the reaction rate will increase as the temperature increases. Because the temperature of a substance is a measure of the particles' average kinetic energy, increasing the temperature increases the average kinetic energy of the molecules. Consequently, the proportion of reactants gaining enough energy to surpass E_a (and thus capable of undergoing reaction) increases with higher temperature. All reactions—even the nuclear reactions shown in Figure 5.9—are temperature-dependent and experience an optimal temperature for activity.

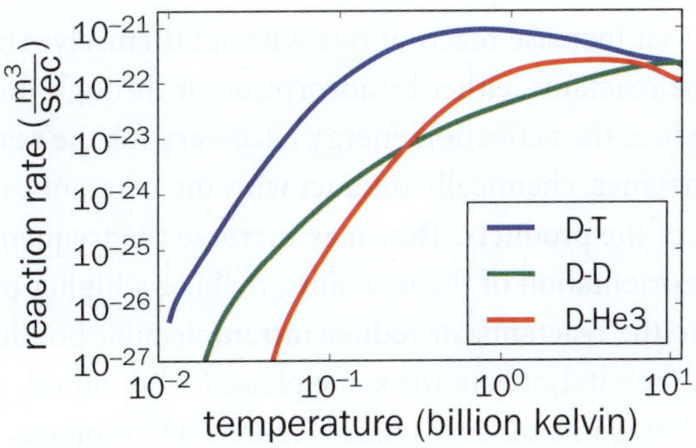

Figure 5.9 All Reactions Are Temperature-Dependent
Examples shown are nuclear fusion reactions; at extreme temperatures, the nucleus itself begins to break down.

You'll often hear that raising the temperature of a system by 10°C will result in an approximate doubling of the reaction rate. Be careful with this approximation because it is *generally* true for biological systems but not so for many other systems. Further, even in biological systems, if the temperature gets too high, a catalyst may denature—and then the reaction rate plummets. Figure 5.10 shows a general curve for an enzymatic reaction that is optimal between 35°C and 40°C (body temperature). Notice that the curve falls sharply after 40°C, at which point denaturation has occurred.

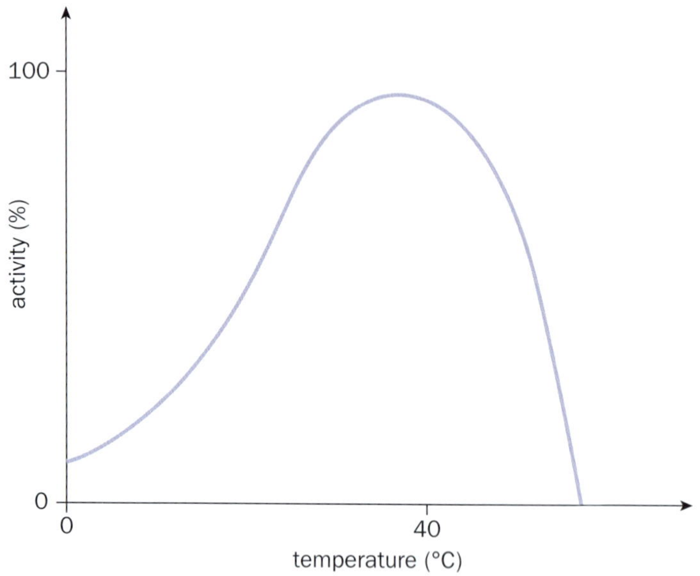

Figure 5.10 An Activity vs. Temperature Curve for a Generic Human Enzyme

Medium

The rate at which a reaction takes place may also be affected by the medium in which it takes place. Some molecules are more likely to react with each other in aqueous environments, while others are more likely to react in nonaqueous solvents, such as in dimethyl sulfoxide (DMSO) or ethanol. Furthermore, the physical state of the medium (liquid, solid, or gas) can also have a significant effect. Generally, polar solvents are preferred because their molecular dipole tends to polarize the bonds of the reactants, thereby lengthening and weakening them, permitting the reaction to occur faster.

Catalysts

Catalysts are substances that increase reaction rate without themselves being consumed in the reaction. Catalysts interact with the reactants, either by adsorption or through the formation of intermediates, and stabilize them so as to reduce the activation energy necessary for the reaction to proceed. While many catalysts, including all enzymes, chemically interact with the reactants, they return to their original chemical state upon formation of the products. They may increase the frequency of collisions between the reactants; change the relative orientation of the reactants, making a higher percentage of the collisions effective; donate electron density to the reactants; or reduce intramolecular bonding within reactant molecules. In **homogeneous catalysis**, the catalyst is in the same phase (solid, liquid, gas) as the reactants. In **heterogeneous catalysis**, the catalyst is in a distinct phase. Figure 5.11 compares the energy profiles of catalyzed and uncatalyzed reactions. Note that, depending on context, reaction profiles can use either Gibbs free energy or enthalpy for the *y*-axis.

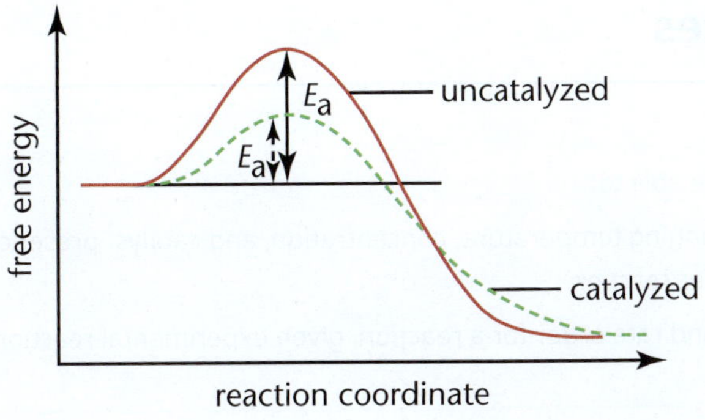

Figure 5.11 Reaction Diagram for a Catalyzed and an Uncatalyzed Reaction

Notice that the only effect of the catalyst is the decrease in the energies of activation, E_a, for both the forward and reverse reactions. The presence of the catalyst has no impact on the free energies of the reactants or the products or the difference between them. This means that catalysts change only the rates of reactions, and in fact, change the forward rate and the reverse rate by the same factor. Consequently, they have no impact whatsoever on the equilibrium position or the measurement of K_{eq}. Remember that, as useful as catalysts are in biological and nonbiological systems, catalysts are not miracle workers: they will not transform a nonspontaneous reaction into a spontaneous one; they only make spontaneous reactions move more quickly toward equilibrium.

BRIDGE

Equilibrium, like biological homeostasis, is a dynamic process that seeks to find balance in all systems. We can use this concept to our advantage on the MCAT in all seven of the basic sciences. Equilibria are dynamic, meaning that they *do* undergo change but their *net* change will be zero.

MCAT CONCEPT CHECK 5.1

Before you move on, assess your understanding of the material with these questions.

1. Describe in words what is occurring in the following two-step mechanism:

   Step 1: $A_2B + A_2B \rightarrow A_4B_2$

   Step 2: $A_4B_2 \rightarrow 2A_2 + B_2$

   ____

2. What does it mean for a step in a mechanism to be the rate-determining step?

   ____

3. What is activation energy?

   ____

4. How does the transition state theory compare with the collision theory of chemical kinetics?

   - Transition state theory:

   ____

   - Collision theory:

   ____

5.2 Reaction Rates

LEARNING OBJECTIVES

After Chapter 5.2, you will be able to:

- Predict the impact of changing temperature, concentration, and catalyst presence on rate of reaction for a zero, first, or second-order reaction
- Determine the rate law and rate order for a reaction, given experimental reaction rate data:

Trial	$[A]_{initial}$ (M)	$[B]_{initial}$ (M)	$rate_{initial}$ $\left(\frac{M}{s}\right)$
1	1.00	1.00	2.0
2	1.00	2.00	8.1
3	2.00	2.00	15.9

Reactions, unfortunately, do not come with handy built-in speedometers. To determine the rate at which a reaction proceeds, we must take measurements of the concentrations of reactants and products and note their change over time.

Definition of Rate

If we consider a generic reaction, $2\text{ A} + \text{B} \rightarrow \text{C}$, in which one mole of C can be produced from two moles of A and one mole of B, we can describe the rate of this reaction in terms of either the disappearance of reactants over time or the appearance of products over time. Because the reactants, by definition, are being consumed in the process of formation of the products, we place a negative sign in front of the rate expression for the reactants. For the above reaction, the rate of the reaction with respect to A is $-\frac{\Delta[\text{A}]}{\Delta t}$, with respect to B is $-\frac{\Delta[\text{B}]}{\Delta t}$, and with respect to C is $+\frac{\Delta[\text{C}]}{\Delta t}$. Notice that the stoichiometric coefficients for the reaction are not equal, which means that the rates of change of concentrations are not equal. Because two moles of A are consumed for every mole of B consumed, the rate of consumption of A is twice the rate of consumption of B. Furthermore, for every two moles of A consumed, only one mole of C is produced; thus, we can say that the rate of consumption of A is twice the rate of production of C. Based on the stoichiometry, we can see that the rate of consumption of B is equal to the rate of production of C. To show a standard rate of reaction in which the rates with respect to all reaction species are equal, the rate of concentration change of each species should be divided by the species' stoichiometric coefficients. Thus, for the general reaction $a\text{A} + b\text{B} \rightarrow c\text{C} + d\text{D}$:

$$\text{rate} = -\frac{\Delta[\text{A}]}{a\Delta t} = -\frac{\Delta[\text{B}]}{b\Delta t} = \frac{\Delta[\text{C}]}{c\Delta t} = \frac{\Delta[\text{D}]}{d\Delta t}$$

Equation 5.3

Rate is expressed in the units of moles per liter per second $\left(\frac{\text{mol}}{\text{L}\cdot\text{s}}\right)$ or molarity per second $\left(\frac{\text{M}}{\text{s}}\right)$.

Determination of Rate Law

In the *Chemical and Physical Foundations of Biological Systems* section of the MCAT, it is unlikely that the testmakers will provide a reaction equation that one can merely look at and write the correct rate law. Therefore, on the MCAT, whenever a question asks to determine the rate law for a reaction, the first thing to look for is experimental data.

MCAT EXPERTISE

Remember that the stoichiometric coefficients for the overall reaction are often different from those for the rate law and will, therefore, not be the same as the order of the reaction.

For nearly all forward, irreversible reactions, the rate is proportional to the concentrations of the reactants, with each concentration raised to some experimentally determined exponent. For the general reaction

$$aA + bB \rightarrow cC + dD$$

the rate is proportional to $[A]^x[B]^y$. By including a proportionality constant, k, we can say that rate is determined according to the following equation:

$$\text{rate} = k[A]^x[B]^y$$

Equation 5.4

where k is the reaction rate coefficient or rate constant and the exponents x and y are the orders of the reaction. This expression is called the **rate law**. Remember that rate is always measured in units of concentration over time; that is, molarity per second. The exponents x and y (or x, y, and z, if there are three reactants) can be used to state the order of the reaction with respect to each reactant or overall: x is the order with respect to reactant A, and y is the order with respect to reactant B. The overall order of the reaction is the sum of x and y. These exponents may be integers or fractions and must be determined experimentally. The MCAT will focus almost exclusively on zero-, first-, second-, and third-order reactions. In most cases, the exponents will be integers.

Before we go any further in our consideration of rate laws, we must offer a few warnings about common traps in chemical kinetics. The first—and most common—is the assumption that the orders of a reaction are the same as the stoichiometric coefficients in the balanced overall equation. Pay close attention: *On the MCAT, the values of* x *and* y *are almost never the same as the stoichiometric coefficients.* The orders of a reaction must be determined experimentally. There are only two cases in which the stoichiometric coefficients match the orders of the reaction. The first is when the reaction mechanism is a single step and the balanced overall reaction is reflective of the entire chemical process. The second is when the complete reaction mechanism is given and the rate-determining step is indicated. The stoichiometric coefficients on the reactant side of the rate-determining step are equal to the orders of the reaction. Occasionally, even this can get a little complicated when the rate-determining step involves an intermediate as a reactant, in which case one must derive the intermediate molecule's concentration by the **law of mass action** (that is, the equilibrium constant expression) for the step that produced the intermediate.

MCAT EXPERTISE

Note that the exponents in the rate law are *not* equal to the stoichiometric coefficients, unless the reaction occurs via a single-step mechanism. Note that product concentrations *never* appear in a rate law. Don't fall into the exceedingly common trap of confusing the rate law with an equilibrium expression!

The second common trap is mistaking the equilibrium constant expression (law of mass action) for the rate law. The expressions for both look similar; if you're not alert on Test Day, you may mistake one for the other or use one when you should be using the other. The expression for equilibrium includes the concentrations of all the species in the reaction, both reactants and products. The expression for chemical kinetics—the rate law expression—includes only the reactants. K_{eq} indicates where the reaction's equilibrium position lies. The rate indicates how quickly the reaction will get there.

The third trap regards the rate constant, k. Technically speaking, k is not a constant because its particular value for any specific chemical reaction will depend on the activation energy for that reaction and the temperature at which the reaction takes place. However, for a specific reaction, at a specific temperature, the rate constant is indeed a constant. For a reversible reaction, the K_{eq} is equal to the ratio of the rate constant for the forward reaction, k, divided by the rate constant for the reverse reaction, k_{-1}.

The fourth and final trap is that the notion and principles of equilibrium apply to the system only at the end of the reaction; that is, after the system has already reached equilibrium. On the other hand, while the reaction rate can theoretically be measured at any time, it is usually measured at or near the beginning of the reaction to minimize the effects of the reverse reaction.

Experimental Determination of Rate Law

This has already been stated a few times, but it bears repeating: The values of k, x, and y in the rate law equation (rate $= k[A]^x[B]^y$) must be determined experimentally for a given reaction at a given temperature. Although rate laws can be quite complex and the orders of the reaction difficult to discern, the MCAT limits its coverage of this topic to fairly straightforward reaction mechanisms, experimental data, and rate laws.

On the MCAT, experimental data for determining rate order is usually provided as a chart that includes the initial concentrations of the reactants and the initial rates of product formation as a function of the reactant concentrations. Often, the data for three or four trials are included in this chart.

To use this data, identify a pair of trials in which the concentration of one of the reactants is changed while the concentrations of all other reactants remain constant. Under these conditions, any change in the rate of product formation from one trial to the other (*if* there is any change) is fully attributable to the change in concentration of that one reactant. Consider a reaction with two reactants, A and B, forming product C. Imagine two trials in which the concentration of A is constant, while the concentration of B doubles. If the rate of the formation of product C has subsequently quadrupled, then the exponent on [B] must be two. Why? Looking at the generic rate law (rate $= k[A]^x[B]^y$), the logic should look something like this: *Doubling [B] has resulted in a quadrupling of the rate, so to determine the order of the reaction, y, with respect to B, I need to calculate the exponent to which the number 2 must be raised to equal 4. Because* $2^y = 4$, $y = 2$.

The next step is to repeat this process for the other reactant, using data from a different pair of trials, making sure that the concentration of only the reactant we are trying to analyze is changed from one trial to the other while the concentrations of all other reactants remain the same. Once the orders of the reaction have been determined with respect to each reactant, we can write the complete rate law, replacing the exponents x and y with actual numbers. To determine the value of the rate constant k, plug in actual values from any one of the trials; pick whichever trial has the most arithmetically convenient numbers.

MCAT EXPERTISE

The testmakers love rate problems. Why? Because solving these questions requires a real understanding of proportionality and variable relationships. With practice, you'll be able to do these quickly in your head with minimal paper-and-pencil calculations. Remember to look for pairs of reaction trials in which the concentration of only one species changes while the others remain constant.

Example: Given the data below, find the rate law for the following reaction at 300 K:

$$A + B \rightarrow C + D$$

Trial	$[A]_{initial}$ (M)	$[B]_{initial}$ (M)	$rate_{initial}$ $\left(\frac{M}{s}\right)$
1	1.00	1.00	2.0
2	1.00	2.00	8.1
3	2.00	2.00	15.9

Solution: First, look for two trials in which the concentrations of all but one of the substances are held constant.

In Trials 1 and 2, the concentration of A is kept constant, while the concentration of B is doubled. The rate increases by a factor of approximately 4. Since k and [A] are constant between the two trials, the rate is proportional to [B] raised to some power (the symbol $\propto$ means "is proportional to"):

$$\text{rate} = k[A]^x[B]^y \xrightarrow{k \text{ and } [A] \text{ are constant}} \text{rate} \propto [B]^y$$

Specifically, the relationship between the change in rate and the change in concentration of B can be written as: $\Delta \text{rate} = \Delta[B]^y$. For this specific set of data, the proportionality becomes: $4 = [2]^y$.

In other words, since the rate was multiplied by 4, and [B] was multiplied by 2, y must be equal to 2. Based on what is known so far, the rate law becomes rate $= k[A]^x[B]^2$.

In Trials 2 and 3, the concentration of B is kept constant, while the concentration of A is doubled. The rate increases by a factor of approximately 2. Since k and [B] are constant between the two trials, rate is proportional to [A] raised to some power:

$$\text{rate} = k[A]^x[B]^2 \xrightarrow{k \text{ and } [B] \text{ are constant}} \text{rate} \propto [A]^x$$

The relationship between the change in rate and the change in concentration of B can be written as: $\Delta\text{rate} = \Delta[A]^x$. For this specific set of data, the proportionality becomes: $2 = [2]^x$.

In other words, since the rate was multiplied by 2, and [A] was multiplied by 2, x must be equal to 1.

Therefore, rate $= k[A]^1[B]^2$, more typically written as rate $= k[A][B]^2$ as raising a value to the first power is equivalent to the value (e.g., $2^1 = 2$). The order of the reaction is 1 with respect to A and 2 with respect to B; the overall reaction order is thus $1 + 2 = 3$.

To calculate k, substitute the values from any one of the trials into the rate law. In this case, trial 1 is chosen because the numbers are straightforward to manipulate:

$$\text{rate} = k[\text{A}][\text{B}]^2$$
$$2.0\,\frac{\text{M}}{\text{s}} = k[1.00\text{ M}][1.00\text{ M}]^2$$
$$k = 2.0\text{ M}^{-2}\,\text{s}^{-1}$$

Therefore, the final rate law is rate $= 2.0\text{ M}^{-2}\,\text{s}^{-1}\,[\text{A}][\text{B}]^2$.

Reaction Orders

We classify chemical reactions as zero-order, first-order, second-order, higher-order, or mixed-order on the basis of kinetics. We will continue to consider the generic reaction $a\text{A} + b\text{B} \rightarrow c\text{C} + d\text{D}$ for this discussion.

Zero-Order Reaction

A **zero-order reaction** is one in which the rate of formation of product C is independent of changes in concentrations of any of the reactants, A and B. These reactions have a constant reaction rate equal to the rate constant (rate coefficient), k. The rate law for a zero-order reaction is:

$$\text{rate} = k[\text{A}]^0[\text{B}]^0 = k$$

where k has units of $\frac{\text{M}}{\text{s}}$. Remember that the rate constant itself is dependent on temperature; thus, it is possible to change the rate for a zero-order reaction by changing the temperature. The only other way to change the rate of a zero-order reaction is by the addition of a catalyst, which lowers the activation energy, thereby increasing the value of k.

Plotting a zero-order reaction on a concentration vs. time curve results in a linear graph, as shown in Figure 5.12. This line shows that the rate of formation of product is independent of the concentration of reactant. The slope of such a line is the opposite of the rate constant, k.

MCAT EXPERTISE

Temperature and the addition of a catalyst are the only factors that can change the rate of a zero-order reaction.

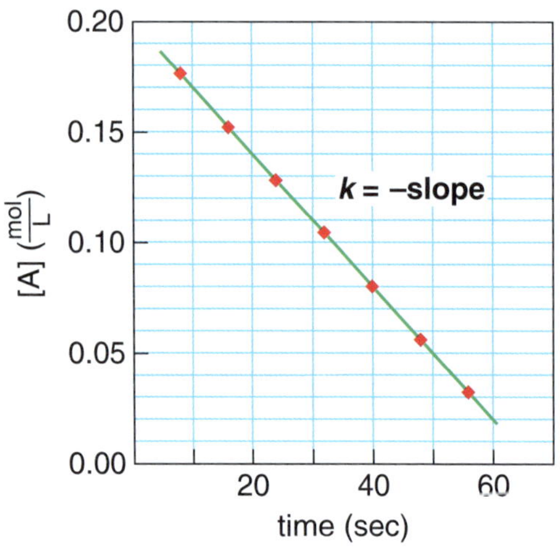

Figure 5.12 Kinetics of a Zero-Order Reaction
Note that the rate of reaction, k, is the opposite of the slope.

First-Order Reaction

A **first-order reaction** has a rate that is directly proportional to only one reactant, such that doubling the concentration of that reactant results in a doubling of the rate of formation of the product. The rate law for a first-order reaction is

$$\text{rate} = k[\text{A}]^1 \text{ or rate} = k[\text{B}]^1$$

where k has units of s^{-1}. A classic example of a first-order reaction is the process of radioactive decay. From the rate law, in which the rate of decrease of the amount of a radioactive isotope A is proportional to the amount of A:

$$\text{rate} = -\frac{\Delta[\text{A}]}{\Delta t} = k[\text{A}]$$

The concentration of radioactive substance A at any time t can be expressed mathematically as:

$$[\text{A}]_t = [\text{A}]_0 e^{-kt}$$

Equation 5.5

where $[\text{A}]_t$ is the concentration of A at time t, $[\text{A}]_0$ is the initial concentration of A, k is the rate constant, and t is time. It is important to recognize that a first-order rate law with a single reactant suggests that the reaction begins when the molecule undergoes a chemical change all by itself, without a chemical interaction, and usually without a physical interaction with any other molecule.

Plotting a first-order reaction on a concentration vs. time curve results in a nonlinear graph, as shown in Figure 5.13. This curve shows that the rate of formation of product is dependent on the concentration of reactant. Plotting ln [A] vs. time reveals a straight line; the slope of such a line is the opposite of the rate constant, k.

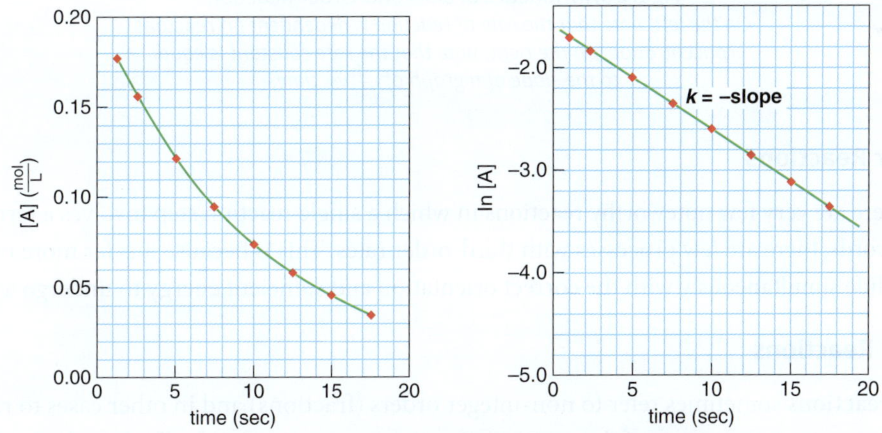

Figure 5.13 Kinetics of a First-Order Reaction
On the left, note that the rate of reaction is dependent on reactant concentration; on the right, note that the rate constant is the opposite of the slope of a graph of ln [A] vs. time.

Second-Order Reaction

A **second-order reaction** has a rate that is proportional to either the concentrations of two reactants or to the square of the concentration of a single reactant. The following rate laws all reflect second-order reactions:

$$\text{rate} = k[A]^1[B]^1 \text{ or rate} = k[A]^2 \text{ or rate} = k[B]^2$$

where k has units of $M^{-1}\ s^{-1}$. It is important to recognize that a second-order rate law often suggests a physical collision between two reactant molecules, especially if the rate law is first-order with respect to each of the two reactants.

Plotting a reaction that is second-order with respect to a single reactant on a concentration vs. time curve results in a nonlinear graph, as shown in Figure 5.14. This curve shows that the rate of formation of product is dependent on the concentration of reactant. Plotting $\frac{1}{[A]}$ vs. time reveals a linear curve; the slope of such a curve is equal to the rate constant, k.

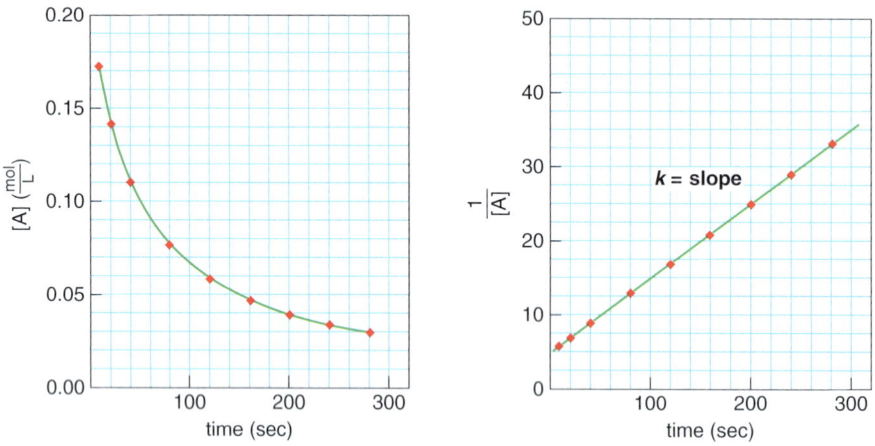

Figure 5.14 Kinetics of a Second-Order Reaction
On the left, note that the rate of reaction is dependent on reactant concentration; on the right, note that the rate constant is equal to the slope of a graph of $\frac{1}{[A]}$ *vs. time.*

Higher-Order Reactions

Fortunately, there are very few noteworthy reactions in which a single reaction step involves a termolecular process; in other words, there are few processes with third-order rates. This is because it is far more rare for three particles to collide simultaneously with the correct orientation and sufficient energy to undergo a reaction.

Mixed-Order Reactions

Mixed-order reactions sometimes refer to non-integer orders (fractions) and in other cases to reactions with rate orders that vary over the course of the reaction. Fractions are more specifically described as **broken-order**. In recent times, the term mixed-order has come to refer solely to reactions that change order over time. Knowing those two definitions will be sufficient for Test Day.

An example of a mixed-order rate law is given by:

$$\text{rate} = \frac{k_1[\text{C}]\,[\text{A}]^2}{k_2 + k_3[\text{A}]}$$

where A represents a single reactant and C, a catalyst. The overall reaction and its mechanism are beyond the relevance and scope of the MCAT, and the derivation of this rate law is even more unnecessary for Test Day; however, understanding what is implied by this equation is important. The result of the large value for [A] at the beginning of the reaction is that $k_3[\text{A}] \gg k_2$, and the reaction will appear to be first-order with respect to A. (Note: The symbol "$\gg$" means "much-greater-than", implying, in this context, that the contribution of k_2 to the denominator "$k_2 + [\text{A}]k_3$" is negligible.) At the end of the reaction, when [A] is low, $k_2 \gg k_3[\text{A}]$, making the reaction appear second-order with respect to A. While the MCAT will not ask you to derive a rate expression for a mixed-order reaction, you are responsible for being able to recognize how the rate order changes as the reactant concentration changes.

MCAT CONCEPT CHECK 5.2

Before you move on, assess your understanding of the material with these questions.

1. Describe the effects the following conditions would have on the initial rate of reaction, given the reaction order: (Examples: rate increased, rate divided by 2, rate unaffected)

Conditions	Zero-Order	First-Order	Second-Order
Temperature lowered			
All reactants' concentrations doubled			
Catalyst added			

2. Determine the rate law and rate order for the following reaction:

$$A + B + C \rightarrow D$$

Trial	$[\text{A}]_{\text{initial}}$ (M)	$[\text{B}]_{\text{initial}}$ (M)	$[\text{C}]_{\text{initial}}$ (M)	$\text{rate}_{\text{initial}} \left(\frac{\text{M}}{\text{s}}\right)$
1	1.00	1.00	1.00	2.0
2	1.00	2.00	1.00	2.1
3	2.00	1.00	1.00	15.9
4	2.00	1.00	2.00	32.2

Conclusion

We began with a consideration of chemical reactions and the mechanisms that illustrate the individual steps necessary to transform reactants into products. We demonstrated the way to derive a reaction's rate law through the analysis of experimental data, and we looked at the factors that can affect the rates of chemical reactions.

After such an overview, you should begin to appreciate that many chemical principles in the human body rely on the principles of chemical kinetics. Why does the body maintain a certain temperature? Primarily to stabilize the enzymes that catalyze the metabolic reactions necessary for life. Why does the body maintain a pH buffer? Altering the concentration of protons affects not only the ability of an enzyme to maintain its secondary, tertiary, and quaternary structure, but can also directly affect the collisions between reactants. You will begin to appreciate these and many other questions from a clinical perspective throughout your medical career. In the next chapter, we will investigate chemical equilibria, which—although related to kinetics—are distinct (and commonly confused!) topics.

GO ONLINE

You've reviewed the content, now test your knowledge and critical thinking skills by completing a test-like passage set in your online resources!

CONCEPT SUMMARY

Chemical Kinetics

- The change in **Gibbs free energy** (ΔG) determines whether or not a reaction is spontaneous.
- **Chemical mechanisms** propose a series of steps that make up the overall reaction.
  - **Intermediates** are molecules that exist within the course of a reaction but are neither reactants nor products overall.
  - The slowest step, also known as the **rate-determining step**, limits the maximum rate at which the reaction can proceed.
- The **collision theory** states that a reaction rate is proportional to the number of effective collisions between the reacting molecules.
  - For a collision to be effective, molecules must be in the proper orientation and have sufficient kinetic energy to exceed the **activation energy**.
  - The **Arrhenius equation** is a mathematical way of representing collision theory.
- The **transition state theory** states that molecules form a **transition state** or **activated complex** during a reaction in which the old bonds are partially dissociated and the new bonds are partially formed.
  - From the transition state, the reaction can proceed toward products or revert back to reactants.
  - The transition state is the highest point on a free energy reaction diagram.
- Reaction rates can be affected by a number of factors.
  - Increasing the concentration of reactant will increase reaction rate (except for zero-order reactions) because there are more effective collisions per time.
  - Increasing the temperature will increase reaction rate because the particles' kinetic energy is increased.
  - Changing the medium can increase or decrease reaction rate, depending on how the reactants interact with the medium.
  - Adding a catalyst increases reaction rate because it lowers the activation energy. **Homogeneous catalysts** are the same phase as the reactants; **heterogeneous catalysts** are a different phase.

Reaction Rates

- Reaction rates are measured in terms of the rate of disappearance of a reactant or appearance of a product.
- **Rate laws** take the form of rate $= k[A]^x[B]^y$.
  - The **rate orders** usually do not match the stoichiometric coefficients.
  - Rate laws must be determined from experimental data.

- The rate order of a reaction is the sum of all individual rate orders in the rate law.
- **Zero-order reactions** have a constant rate that does not depend on the concentration of reactant.
  - The rate of a zero-order reaction can only be affected by changing the temperature or adding a catalyst.
  - A concentration vs. time curve of a zero-order reaction is a straight line; the slope of such a line is equal to $-k$.
- **First-order reactions** have a nonconstant rate that depends on the concentration of reactant.
  - A concentration vs. time curve of a first-order reaction is nonlinear.
  - The slope of a ln [A] vs. time plot is $-k$ for a first-order reaction.
- **Second-order reactions** have a nonconstant rate that depends on the concentration of reactant.
  - A concentration vs. time curve of a second-order reaction is nonlinear.
  - The slope of a $\frac{1}{[A]}$ vs. time plot is k for a second-order reaction.
- **Broken-order reactions** are those with noninteger orders.
- **Mixed-order reactions** are those that have a rate order that changes over time.

ANSWERS TO CONCEPT CHECKS

5.1

1. Two molecules of A_2B come together in a combination reaction to form an intermediate, A_4B_2, which subsequently decomposes to produce the final products, two molecules of A_2 and one molecule of B_2.
2. The rate-determining step is the slowest step of a reaction. It determines the overall rate of the reaction because the reaction can only proceed as fast as the rate at which this step occurs.
3. The activation energy is the minimum energy needed for a chemical reaction to occur.
4. Both theories require a certain activation energy to be overcome in order for a reaction to occur (therefore not all reactions will occur). The transition state theory focuses on forming a high-energy activated complex that can then proceed forward or backward, forming the products or reverting to the reactants, respectively. The collision theory focuses on the energy and orientation of reactants, and considers each potential reaction to be "all-or-nothing" (either there is enough energy to form the products, or there is not).

5.2

1.

Conditions	Zero-Order	First-Order	Second-Order
Temperature lowered	rate decreased	rate decreased	rate decreased
All reactants' concentrations doubled	rate unaffected	rate doubled	rate multiplied by 4
Catalyst added	rate increased	rate increased	rate increased

2. This question asks for the rate law and rate order for the following reaction:

$$A + B + C \rightarrow D$$

Trial	$[A]_{initial}$ (M)	$[B]_{initial}$ (M)	$[C]_{initial}$ (M)	$\text{rate}_{initial}$ $\left(\frac{M}{s}\right)$
1	1.00	1.00	1.00	2.0
2	1.00	2.00	1.00	2.1
3	2.00	1.00	1.00	15.9
4	2.00	1.00	2.00	32.2

Start by writing the generic rate law for the reaction: rate $= k[\text{A}]^x[\text{B}]^y[\text{C}]^z$.

In a complex rate law problem, always check for the possibility of a reagent that has no impact on the rate law. Looking at Trials 1 and 2, the concentration of B is doubled with no change in the rate. Thus, reagent B has no impact on the rate law, and its exponent is zero. The rate law can be updated to rate $= k[\text{A}]^x[\text{B}]^0[\text{C}]^z$.

Next, compare Trials 1 and 3. The concentration of A doubles, the concentrations of B and C remain constant, and the rate increases by a factor of approximately 8. This results in the proportionality $\Delta\text{rate} = \Delta[\text{A}]^x$, so $8 = 2^x$, giving $x = 3$. The rate law can now be updated to rate $= k[\text{A}]^3[\text{B}]^0[\text{C}]^z$.

Finally, compare Trials 3 and 4. The concentration of C doubles, the concentrations of A and B remain constant, and the rate approximately doubles. This results in the proportionality $\Delta\text{rate} = \Delta[\text{C}]^z$, so $2 = 2^z$, giving $z = 1$. The rate law can now be updated to rate $= k[\text{A}]^3[\text{B}]^0[\text{C}]^1$.

Thus, the final rate law is: rate $= k[\text{A}]^3[\text{B}]^0[\text{C}]^1 = k[\text{A}]^3[\text{C}]$. The rate order is $3 + 0 + 1 = 4$.

SCIENCE MASTERY ASSESSMENT EXPLANATIONS

1. **D**

Based on the information given in the question, the rate is first-order with respect to the concentration of the first reactant; when the concentration of that reactant doubles, the rate also doubles. Because the reaction is third-order, the sum of the exponents in the rate law must be equal to 3. Therefore, the reaction order with respect to the other reactant must be $3 - 1 = 2$. If the concentration of this second reactant is multiplied by $\frac{1}{2}$, the rate will be multiplied by $\left(\frac{1}{2}\right)^2 = \frac{1}{4}$.

2. **D**

Before you try to answer this question, you should draw a free energy diagram for the system.

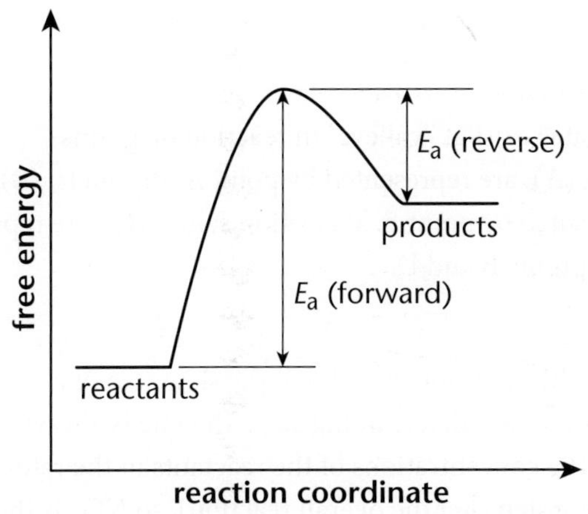

If the activation energy of the forward reaction is greater than the activation energy of the reverse reaction, then the products must have a higher free energy than the reactants. The overall energy of the system is higher at the end than it was in the beginning. The net free energy change is positive, indicating an endergonic (nonspontaneous) reaction. The terms endothermic, **(A)**, and exothermic, **(B)**, are associated with enthalpy. While free energy does depend on enthalpy, it also depends on entropy; there is not enough information in the question stem to reliably determine the sign of the entropy change of the reaction.

3. **D**

A second-order reaction can be second-order with respect to one reactant, or first-order with respect to two different reactants. In this case, one reactant was increased by a factor of 4. If the reaction is second-order with respect to this reactant, the rate law will be rate $= k[A]^2[B]^0$ and the rate will increase by a factor of 16. If it is first-order with respect to this reactant and first-order with respect to another reactant, the rate law will be rate $= k[A]^1[B]^1$, and the rate will increase by a factor of 4. We do not know which of these is the correct rate law and, thus, cannot determine the effect on the rate.

4. **A**

By definition, zero-order reactions are unaffected by the concentrations of any reactants in the reaction. Thus, changing the concentrations of these reactants will not affect the rate.

5. **D**

The question asks which alteration does NOT affect the rate of the reaction. Temperature directly affects the rate constant (k), making **(A)** incorrect. Changing the partial pressure of a gas will affect the number of effective collisions per time. This makes **(B)** incorrect—but note that concentration changes will not affect the rate of zero-order reactions. Solvents affect the rate of reactions depending on how the reactants interact with the solvent, making **(C)** incorrect. Removing the product of an irreversible reaction, **(D)**, should not affect the rate of the reaction because the rate law does not depend on the concentrations of products.

6. **D**

While increasing the concentration of reactants can alter the reaction rate in first- or higher-order reactions, saturated solutions containing a catalyst have a maximum turnover rate and cannot increase the rate constant or the reaction rate any higher by adding more reactant molecules.

7. **A**

If the sum of the exponents (orders) of the concentrations of each species in the rate law is equal to 2, then the reaction is second-order. The exponents in the rate law are unrelated to stoichiometric coefficients, so NO_2 and Br_2 could have any stoichiometric coefficients in the original reaction and still be a second-order reaction, invalidating statement II. Statement III is incorrect because the rate can be affected by a wide variety of compounds. A catalyst, for example, could increase the rate.

8. **C**

Start with the generic rate law: rate $= k[XH_4]^x[O_2]^y$.
In the first two trials, the concentration of XH_4 is held constant while the concentration of O_2 is multiplied by 4, and the rate of the reaction also increases by a factor of approximately 4. This gives the proportion Δrate $= [O_2]^y$, or $4 = 4^y$, meaning $y = 1$. The rate law can be updated to: rate $= k[XH_4]^x[O_2]^1$.

In the last two trials, the concentration of O_2 is held constant while the concentration of XH_4 is doubled, and the rate of the reaction is increased by a factor of approximately 4. This gives Δrate $= [XH_4]^x$, or $4 = 2^x$, and $x = 2$. The rate law can be updated to: rate $= k[XH_4]^2[O_2]^1$. The final version of the rate law is: rate $= k[XH_4]^2[O_2]$.

9. **B**

By definition, a catalyst increases the rate of a reaction by lowering the activation energy, making it easier for both the forward and reverse reactions to overcome this energy barrier. Catalysts are neither used up in the reaction, nor do they alter the equilibrium of a reaction, eliminating **(A)** and **(C)**. Finally, catalysts stabilize the transition state by lowering its energy, not raising it, eliminating **(D)**.

10. **C**

The overall order of a reaction is the sum of the individual orders in the reaction. Therefore, the rate order is $0 + 2 + 1 = 3$.

11. **D**

A system is exergonic if energy is released by the reaction. For exergonic reactions, the net energy change is negative, and the free energy of the final products is lower than the free energy of the initial reactants. Point E, which represents the energy of the final products, is lower on the energy diagram than point A, which represents the energy of initial reactants. Thus, energy must have been given off, and the reaction is exergonic.

12. **B**

The activation energy of a reaction is represented by the distance on the y-axis from the energy of the reactants to the peak energy prior to formation of products. The activation energy of the first step of the forward reaction, for example, is equal to the distance along the y-axis from point A to point B. The largest energy increase on this graph occurs during the progress from point E to point D, which represents the first step of the reverse reaction.

13. **D**

Intermediates exist at "valleys" in reaction diagrams. Reactants, **(A)**, are represented by point A. Products, **(B)**, are represented by point E. Transition states, **(C)**, are represented by points B and D.

14. **D**

To answer this question, recall that the slow step of a reaction is the rate-determining step. The rate is always related to the concentrations of the reactants in the rate-determining step (*not* the overall reaction), so NO_2 is the only compound that should be included in the correct answer. The concentration of NO_2 is squared in the rate law because the question stem tells us that the system obeys second-order kinetics.

15. **D**

The faster a reaction can reach its activation energy, the faster it will proceed to completion. Because this question states that all conditions are equal, the reaction with the lowest activation energy will have the fastest rate. In the diagram, **(D)** has the lowest activation energy.

GO ONLINE

Consult your online resources for additional practice.

EQUATIONS TO REMEMBER

(5.1) **Collision theory:** rate $= Z \times f$

(5.2) **Arrhenius equation:** $k = Ae^{\frac{-E_a}{RT}}$

(5.3) **Definition of rate:** rate $= -\frac{\Delta[A]}{a\Delta t} = -\frac{\Delta[B]}{b\Delta t} = \frac{\Delta[C]}{c\Delta t} = \frac{\Delta[D]}{d\Delta t}$

for the general reaction $aA + bB \rightarrow cC + dD$

(5.4) **Rate law:** rate $= k[A]^x[B]^y$

(5.5) **Radioactive decay:** $[A]_t = [A]_0 e^{-kt}$

SHARED CONCEPTS

Biochemistry Chapter 2
Enzymes

General Chemistry Chapter 3
Bonding and Chemical Interactions

General Chemistry Chapter 6
Equilibrium

General Chemistry Chapter 7
Thermochemistry

Organic Chemistry Chapter 4
Analyzing Organic Reactions

Physics and Math Chapter 3
Thermodynamics

CHAPTER 6

EQUILIBRIUM

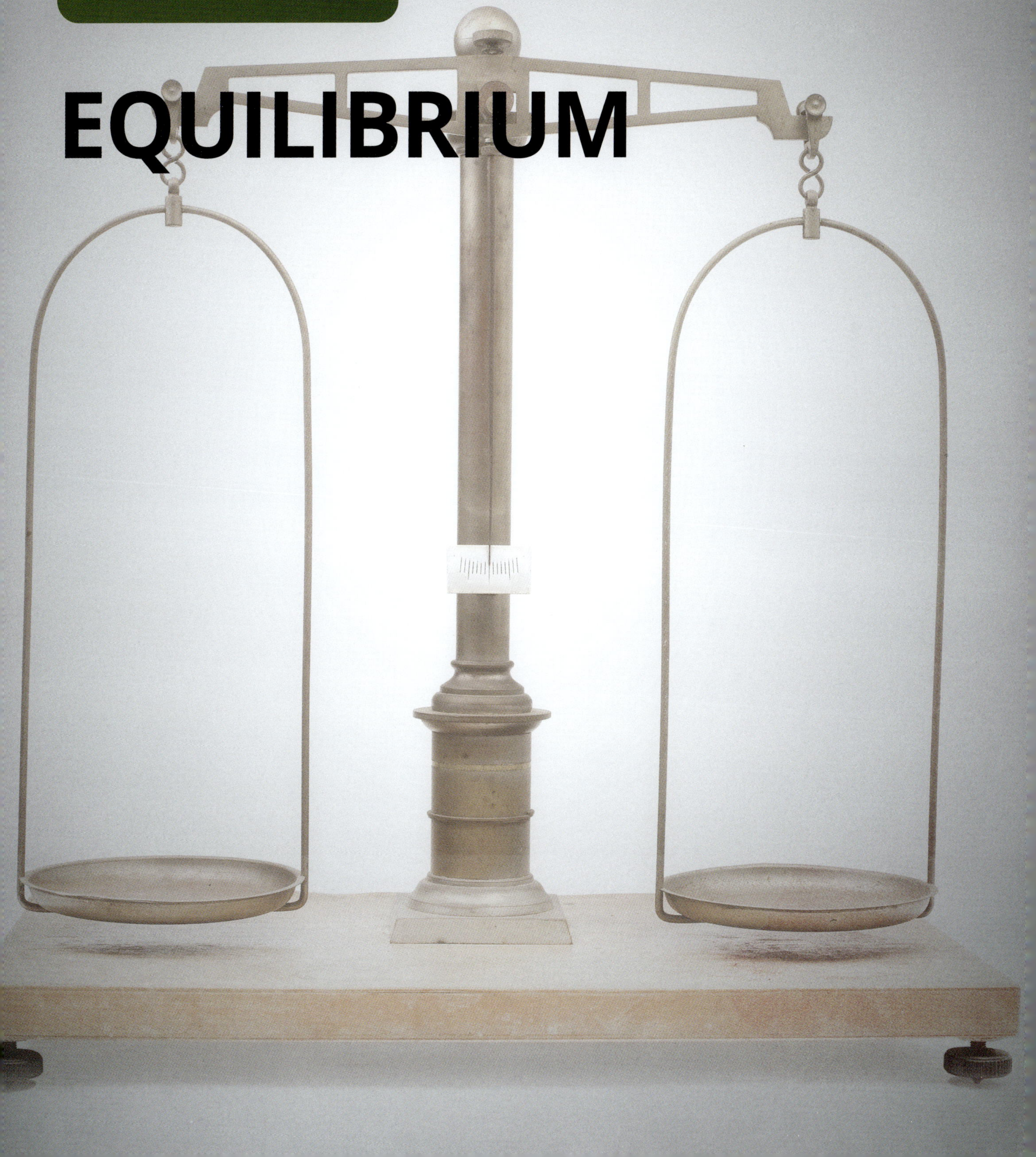

SCIENCE MASTERY ASSESSMENT

Every pre-med knows this feeling: there is so much content I have to know for the MCAT! How do I know what to do first or what's important?

While the high-yield badges throughout this book will help you identify the most important topics, this Science Mastery Assessment is another tool in your MCAT prep arsenal. This quiz (which can also be taken in your online resources) and the guidance below will help ensure that you are spending the appropriate amount of time on this chapter based on your personal strengths and weaknesses. Don't worry though—skipping something now does not mean you'll never study it. Later on in your prep, as you complete full-length tests, you'll uncover specific pieces of content that you need to review and can come back to these chapters as appropriate.

How to Use This Assessment

If you answer 0–7 questions correctly:

Spend about 1 hour to read this chapter in full and take limited notes throughout. Follow up by reviewing **all** quiz questions to ensure that you now understand how to solve each one.

If you answer 8–11 questions correctly:

Spend 20–40 minutes reviewing the quiz questions. Beginning with the questions you missed, read and take notes on the corresponding subchapters. For questions you answered correctly, ensure your thinking matches that of the explanation and you understand why each choice was correct or incorrect.

If you answer 12–15 questions correctly:

Spend less than 20 minutes reviewing all questions from the quiz. If you missed any, then include a quick read-through of the corresponding subchapters, or even just the relevant content within a subchapter, as part of your question review. For questions you answered correctly, ensure your thinking matches that of the explanation and review the Concept Summary at the end of the chapter.

1. A reaction is found to stop just before all reactants are converted to products. Which of the following could be true about this reaction?
   - **A.** The reaction is irreversible, and the forward rate is greater than the reverse rate.
   - **B.** The reaction is irreversible, and the reverse rate is too large for products to form.
   - **C.** The reaction is reversible, and the forward rate is equal to the reverse rate.
   - **D.** The reaction is reversible, and the reverse rate is greater than the forward rate.

2. What is the equilibrium expression for the reaction $Cu_2SO_4\ (s) \rightleftharpoons 2\ Cu^+\ (aq) + SO_4^{2-}\ (aq)$?
   - **A.** $\frac{[Cu^+]^2[SO_4^{2-}]}{[Cu_2SO_4]}$
   - **B.** $\frac{2 \times [Cu^+][SO_4^{2-}]}{[Cu_2SO_4]}$
   - **C.** $[Cu^+][SO_4^{2-}]$
   - **D.** $[Cu^+]^2[SO_4^{2-}]$

3. Carbonated beverages are produced by dissolving carbon dioxide in water to produce carbonic acid:

$$CO_2\ (g) + H_2O\ (l) \rightleftharpoons H_2CO_3\ (aq)$$

When a bottle containing carbonated water is opened, the taste of the beverage gradually changes as the carbonation is lost. Which of the following statements best explains this phenomenon?
   - **A.** The change in pressure and volume causes the reaction to shift to the left, thereby decreasing the amount of aqueous carbonic acid.
   - **B.** The change in pressure and volume causes the reaction to shift to the right, thereby decreasing the amount of gaseous carbon dioxide.
   - **C.** Carbonic acid reacts with environmental oxygen and nitrogen.
   - **D.** Carbon dioxide reacts with environmental oxygen and nitrogen.

4. Which of the following best describes how to favor the production of the kinetic product over the thermodynamic product?
   - **A.** High temperature and short reaction time
   - **B.** Low temperature and short reaction time
   - **C.** High temperature and long reaction time
   - **D.** Low temperature and long reaction time

5. If $K_c \gg 1$:
   - **A.** the equilibrium mixture will favor products over reactants.
   - **B.** the equilibrium mixture will favor reactants over products.
   - **C.** the equilibrium concentrations of reactants and products are equal.
   - **D.** the reaction is essentially irreversible.

6. Acetic acid dissociates in solution according to the following equation:

$$CH_3COOH \rightleftharpoons CH_3COO^- + H^+$$

If sodium acetate is added to a solution of acetic acid in excess water, which of the following effects would be observed in the solution?
   - **A.** Decreased pH
   - **B.** Increased pH
   - **C.** Decreased pK_{eq} (pK_a)
   - **D.** Increased pK_{eq} (pK_a)

Questions 7 and 8 refer to the reaction below:

$$FeI\ (aq) + I_2\ (g) \rightarrow FeI_3\ (aq)$$

7. Which of the following would increase the formation of product?
   - **A.** Decreasing the volume of the container
   - **B.** Decreasing the pressure of the container
   - **C.** Increasing the volume of the container
   - **D.** Decreasing the volume of the container while maintaining a constant pressure

8. If this reaction were exothermic, what effect would decreasing the temperature have on the equilibrium?
   - **A.** The forward reaction rate and the reverse reaction rate both increase.
   - **B.** The forward reaction rate decreases while the reverse reaction rate increases.
   - **C.** The forward reaction rate increases while the reverse reaction rate decreases.
   - **D.** The forward reaction rate and the reverse reaction rate both decrease.

9. Which of the following actions does NOT affect the equilibrium position of a reaction?
   - **A.** Adding or removing heat.
   - **B.** Adding or removing a catalyst.
   - **C.** Increasing or decreasing concentrations of reactants.
   - **D.** Increasing or decreasing volumes of reactants.

10. In a sealed 1 L container, 1 mole of nitrogen gas reacts with 3 moles of hydrogen gas to form 0.05 moles of NH_3 at equilibrium. Which of the following is closest to the K_c of the reaction?
   - **A.** 0.0001
   - **B.** 0.001
   - **C.** 0.01
   - **D.** 0.1

11. Increasing temperature can alter the K_{eq} of a reaction. Why might increasing temperature indefinitely be unfavorable for changing reaction conditions?
   - **A.** The equilibrium constant has a definite limit that cannot be surpassed.
   - **B.** The products or reactants can decompose at high temperatures.
   - **C.** Increasing temperature would decrease pressure, which may or may not alter reaction conditions.
   - **D.** If a reaction is irreversible, its K_{eq} will resist changes in temperature.

12. How does the change in free energy compare between the kinetic and thermodynamic product?
   - **A.** The free energy change for the kinetic product is greater since it is less stable.
   - **B.** The free energy change for the kinetic product is greater since it is more stable.
   - **C.** The free energy change for the thermodynamic product is greater since it is less stable.
   - **D.** The free energy change for the thermodynamic product is greater since it is more stable.

13. Compound A has a K_a (equilibrium constant of acid dissociation) of approximately 10^{-4}. Which of the following compounds is most likely to react with a solution of compound A?
   - **A.** HNO_3
   - **B.** NO_2
   - **C.** NH_3
   - **D.** N_2O_5

14. Consider the following two reactions:

$$3\text{ A} + 2\text{ B} \rightleftharpoons 3\text{ C} + 4\text{ D (Reaction 1)}$$

$$4\text{ D} + 3\text{ C} \rightleftharpoons 3\text{ A} + 2\text{ B (Reaction 2)}$$

If K_{eq} for reaction 1 is equal to 0.1, what is K_{eq} for reaction 2?
   - **A.** 0.1
   - **B.** 1
   - **C.** 10
   - **D.** 100

15. Which of the following statements best describes the effect of lowering the temperature of the following reaction?

$$\text{A} + \text{B} \rightleftharpoons \text{C} + \text{D} \qquad \Delta H = -1.12\ \frac{\text{kJ}}{\text{mol}}$$

   - **A.** [C] and [D] would increase.
   - **B.** [A] and [B] would increase.
   - **C.** ΔH would increase.
   - **D.** ΔH would decrease.

Answer Key

1. **C** (See section 6.1)
2. **D** (See section 6.1)
3. **A** (See section 6.2)
4. **B** (See section 6.3)
5. **A** (See section 6.1)
6. **B** (See section 6.2)
7. **A** (See section 6.2)
8. **C** (See section 6.2)
9. **B** (See section 6.1)
10. **A** (See section 6.1)
11. **B** (See section 6.1)
12. **D** (See section 6.3)
13. **C** (See section 6.1)
14. **C** (See section 6.1)
15. **A** (See section 6.2)

The relevant section of the chapter to review for each question is given in parentheses after the correct answer. Detailed explanations can be found at the end of the chapter.

CHAPTER 6

EQUILIBRIUM

In This Chapter

CHAPTER PROFILE

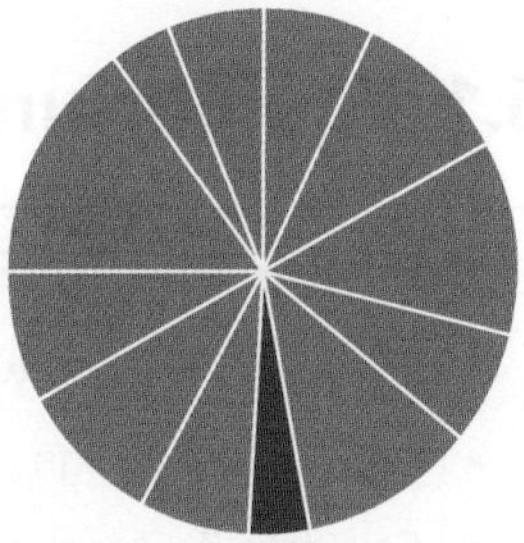

The content in this chapter should be relevant to about 4% of all questions about general chemistry on the MCAT.

This chapter covers material from the following AAMC content categories:

1D: Principles of bioenergetics and fuel molecule metabolism

5A: Unique nature of water and its solutions

5E: Principles of chemical thermodynamics and kinetics

Introduction

You're on the first call of your pediatrics rotation. You get a page: *Come to the emergency room, now,* the resident says. *They just brought in a kid with DKA*. DKA, as you know, stands for diabetic ketoacidosis and is a fairly common way for undiagnosed type I diabetes mellitus to present. You remember from your second-year classes about endocrine pathophysiology that ketoacidosis can arise as a result of the body's metabolism of fatty acids when insulin production shuts down. Fatty acids are metabolized into ketone bodies as an alternative energy source to glucose. Some of the ketones produced are ketoacids, and as the diabetic crisis continues and worsens, the concentration of these ketoacids increases (termed metabolic acidosis), resulting in a plasma pH below 7.35.

As you enter the child's room, the examination is already under way; the child is young, about ten years old, conscious but agitated, and the most obvious sign—which you notice immediately—is rapid, shallow breathing. You ask why the child is hyperventilating, and the resident takes a piece of paper and writes the following:

$$CO_2\ (g) + H_2O\ (l) \rightleftharpoons H_2CO_3\ (aq) \rightleftharpoons H^+\ (aq) + HCO_3^-\ (aq)$$

The child's breathing begins to slow and realization dawns on you. *It's Le Châtelier's principle! The respiratory system is trying to compensate for the metabolic acidosis; the increased breathing rate allows the child to blow off more CO_2, which causes the equilibrium to shift to the left. Hydrogen ions combine with bicarbonate ions to produce carbonic acid, which decomposes into CO_2 gas that's expelled from the lungs. The result is a decrease in the plasma hydrogen ion concentration, which stabilizes the pH and keeps it from getting too low. Wow, chemistry really is essential for medical school!*

Chemical equilibrium is the dynamic state of a chemical reaction in which the concentrations of reactants and products stabilize over time in a low-energy configuration. Pay particular attention to the concepts of chemical equilibrium because we will return to these topics during our review of solutions, acid–base chemistry, and oxidation–reduction reactions.

MCAT EXPERTISE

The AAMC has shown that it will only rarely directly test the details of equilibrium in this chapter. However, you'll need an excellent conceptual understanding of equilibrium to master many other high-yield topics, such as acid-base chemistry (Chapter 10 of *MCAT General Chemistry Review*) and enzymes (Chapter 2 of *MCAT Biochemistry Review*).

6.1 Equilibrium

LEARNING OBJECTIVES

After Chapter 6.1, you will be able to:

- Determine the sign of ΔG and the direction of a reaction given its K_{eq} constant
- Calculate K_{eq} for a reaction
- Write the equilibrium constant expression for a reaction:

$$3\,H_2\,(g) + N_2\,(g) \rightleftharpoons 2\,NH_3\,(g)$$

In the previous chapter, we danced around the term *equilibrium*. We warned you not to confuse the chemical equilibrium expression for the rate expression. We stressed that catalysts make reactions go faster toward their equilibrium position, but that they can't actually change the equilibrium position or alter the value of K_{eq}. The principles and concepts that are the focus of this chapter will direct our discussion in the upcoming chapters about some of the most important general chemistry topics for the MCAT: solutions, acids and bases, and oxidation–reduction reactions.

Dynamic Equilibria and Reversibility

So far, most of the reactions we've covered are **irreversible**; that is, the reaction proceeds in one direction only, the reaction goes to completion, and the maximum amount of product formed is determined by the amount of limiting reagent initially present. **Reversible** reactions are those in which the reaction can proceed in one of two ways: forward (toward the products or "to the right") and reverse (toward the reactants or "to the left"), as seen in Figure 6.1.

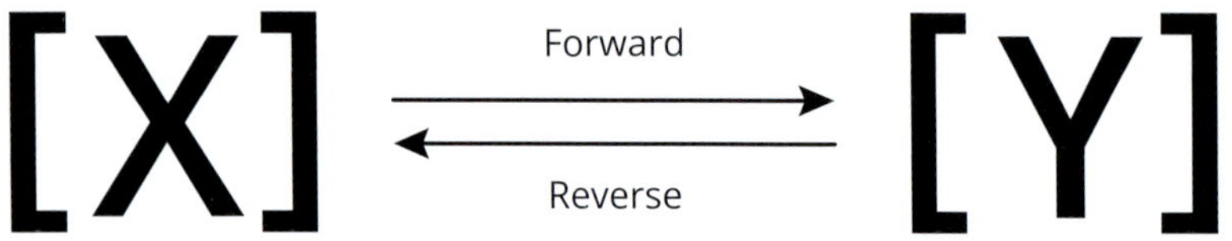

Figure 6.1 Reversible Reaction
[X] represents the concentration of the reactants, and [Y] is the concentration of the products.

BRIDGE

Many biochemical reactions can be classified as reversible, and their activation energies are lowered by enzymes. Irreversible biochemical steps are sometimes termed "committed" because they cannot be reversed in their pathways. These steps also tend to be the rate-limiting steps of metabolic pathways, which are discussed in Chapters 9 through 11 of *MCAT Biochemistry Review.*

Reversible reactions usually do not proceed to completion because the products can react together to reform the reactants. When the reaction system is closed and no reactants or products are added or removed, the system will eventually settle into a state in which the rate of the forward reaction equals the rate of the reverse reaction and the concentrations of the products and reactants remain constant. In this way, equilibrium can be thought of as attempting to climb up an escalator that is going down (see Figure 6.2). If you climb up at the same speed (or rate) that the escalator moves down (that is, in the opposite direction), you will experience no net movement up or down.

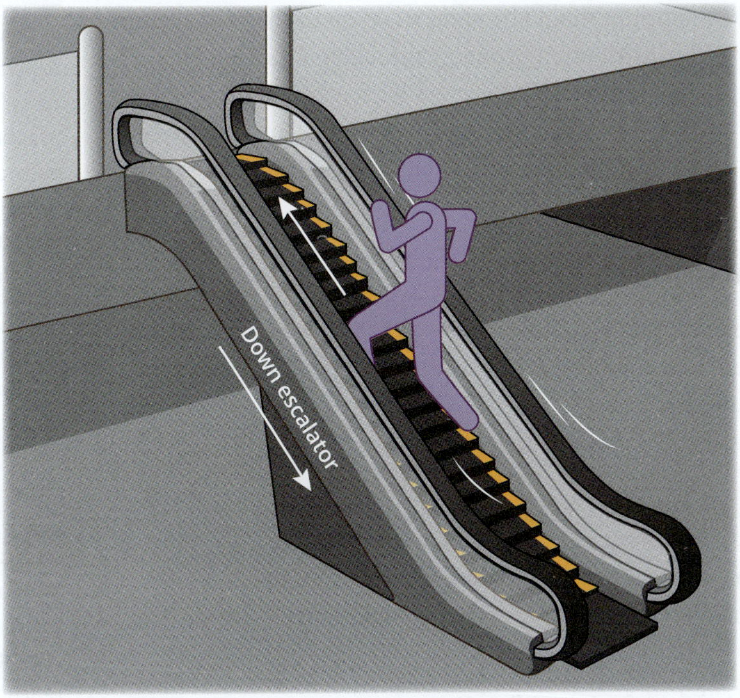

Figure 6.2 Dynamic Equilibrium Escalator Analogy
The rate of the person walking up matches the rate of the escalator moving down, so that the person experiences no net change in position.

In this **dynamic equilibrium**, the forward and reverse reactions are still occurring—they haven't stopped, as they do in a **static equilibrium**—but they are going at the same rate; thus, there is no net change in the concentrations of the products or reactants, as shown in Figure 6.3.

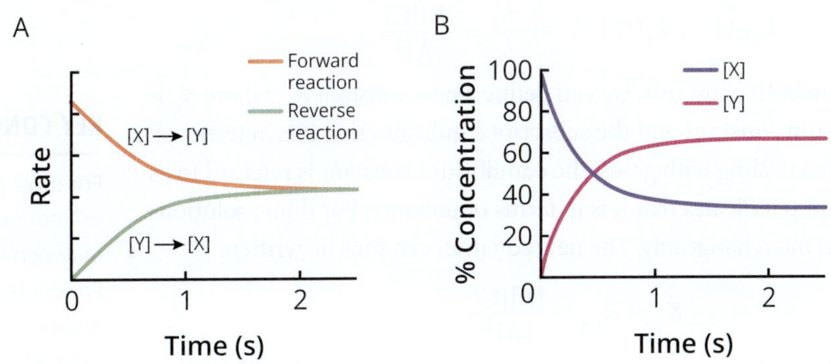

Figure 6.3 Dynamic Equilibrium
Graph A shows the rates of forward and reverse reactions. Graph B shows the resulting changes in concentration of reactants and products, X and Y, respectively, over time. Equilibrium is established when the forward rate matches the reverse rate and the concentration of reactants and products do not change over time.

Consider the generic reversible reaction illustrated in Figure 6.3:

$$X \rightleftharpoons Y$$

At equilibrium, the concentrations of X and Y are constant (although not necessarily equal), and the reactions $X \rightarrow Y$ and $Y \rightarrow X$ continue to occur at equal rates. This occurs roughly at time 2 seconds in the example generic reaction in Figure 6.3.

Equilibrium can be thought of as a balance between the forward and reverse reactions. Better still, equilibrium should be understood on the basis of **entropy**, which is the measure of the distribution of energy throughout a system or between a system and its environment. For a reversible reaction at a given temperature, the reaction will reach equilibrium when the system's entropy—or energy distribution—is at a maximum and the Gibbs free energy of the system is at a minimum.

BRIDGE

In Chapter 7 of *MCAT General Chemistry Review,* we will explore the more "classic" MCAT definition of entropy—a measure of the disorder of a system. It is important to realize, though, that the units of entropy $\left(\frac{\text{J}}{\text{K}\cdot\text{mol}}\right)$ imply a distribution of energy in a system.

Law of Mass Action

For a generic reversible reaction $aA + bB \rightleftharpoons cC + dD$, the **law of mass action** states that, if the system is at equilibrium at a constant temperature, then the following ratio is constant:

$$K_{eq} = \frac{[C]^c [D]^d}{[A]^a [B]^b}$$

Equation 6.1

KEY CONCEPT

At equilibrium, the rate of the forward reaction equals the rate of the reverse reaction, entropy is at a maximum, and Gibbs free energy is at a minimum. This links the concepts of thermodynamics and kinetics.

The law of mass action is actually related to the expressions for the rates of the forward and reverse reactions. Consider the following one-step reversible reaction:

$$2\text{ A} \rightleftharpoons \text{B} + \text{C}$$

Because the reaction occurs in one step, the rates of the forward and reverse reactions are given by:

$$\text{rate}_f = k_f[A]^2 \text{ and rate}_r = k_r[B][C]$$

When $\text{rate}_f = \text{rate}_r$, the system is in equilibrium. Because the rates are equal, we can set the rate expressions for the forward and reverse reactions equal to each other:

$$k_f[A]^2 = k_r[B][C] \rightarrow \frac{k_f}{k_r} = \frac{[B][C]}{[A]^2}$$

Because k_f and k_r are both constants, we can define a new constant K_c, where K_c is called the **equilibrium constant** and the subscript c indicates that it is in terms of concentration. When dealing with gases, the equilibrium constant is referred to as K_p, and the subscript p indicates that it is in terms of pressure. For dilute solutions, K_c and K_{eq} are used interchangeably. The new equation can thus be written:

$$K_c = K_{eq} = \frac{[B][C]}{[A]^2}$$

KEY CONCEPT

For most purposes, you will not need to distinguish between different *K* values. For dilute solutions, $K_{eq} = K_c$ and both are calculated in units of concentration.

While the forward and the reverse reaction rates are equal at equilibrium, the concentrations of the reactants and products are not usually equal. This means that the forward and reverse reaction rate constants, k_f and k_r, respectively, are not usually equal to each other. The ratio of k_f to k_r is K_c:

$$K_c = K_{eq} = \frac{k_f}{k_r}$$

When a reaction occurs in more than one step, the equilibrium constant for the overall reaction is found by multiplying together the equilibrium constants for each step of the reaction. When this is done, the equilibrium constant for the overall reaction is equal to the concentrations of the products divided by the concentrations of the reactants in the overall reaction, with each concentration term raised to the stoichiometric coefficient for the respective species. The forward and reverse rate constants for the nth step are designated k_n and k_{-n}, respectively. For example, if the reaction $a\text{A} + b\text{B} \rightleftharpoons c\text{C} + d\text{D}$ occurs in three steps, each with a forward and reverse rate, then:

$$K_c = \frac{k_1 k_2 k_3}{k_{-1} k_{-2} k_{-3}} = \frac{[\text{C}]^c [\text{D}]^d}{[\text{A}]^a [\text{B}]^b}$$

KEY CONCEPT

Remember the warning in Chapter 5 of *MCAT General Chemistry Review* about confusing equilibrium expressions and rate laws? In equilibrium expressions, the exponents are equal to the coefficients in the balanced equation. In rate laws, the exponents must be determined experimentally and often do not equal the stoichiometric coefficients.

Example: What is the expression for the equilibrium constant for the following reaction?

$$3\ H_2\ (g) + N_2\ (g) \rightleftharpoons 2\ NH_3\ (g)$$

Solution:

$K_c = K_{eq} = \dfrac{[NH_3]^2}{[H_2]^3[N_2]}$. The K_p of this reaction would be: $\dfrac{(P_{NH_3})^2}{(P_{H_2})^3 \times P_{N_2}}$

Reaction Quotient

The law of mass action defines the position of equilibrium; however, equilibrium is a state that is only achieved through time. Depending on the actual rates of the forward and reverse reactions, equilibrium might be achieved in microseconds or millennia. What can serve as a "timer" to indicate how far the reaction has proceeded toward equilibrium? This role is served by the **reaction quotient, *Q***. At any point in time during a reaction, we can measure the concentrations of all of the reactants and products and calculate the reaction quotient according to the following equation:

$$Q_c = \frac{[\text{C}]^c [\text{D}]^d}{[\text{A}]^a [\text{B}]^b}$$

Equation 6.2

This equation looks identical to the equation for K_{eq}. It is the same form, but the information it provides is quite different. While the concentrations used for the law of mass action are equilibrium (constant) concentrations, the concentrations of the reactants and products are not constant when calculating a value for Q of a reaction. Thus, the utility of Q is not the value itself but rather the comparison that can be made between

Q at any given moment in the reaction to the known K_{eq} for the reaction at a particular temperature. Le Châtelier's principle, which will be elaborated upon shortly, will then guide the reaction. For any reaction, if:

- $Q < K_{eq}$, then the forward reaction has not yet reached equilibrium.
  - There is a greater concentration of reactants (and smaller concentration of products) than at equilibrium.
  - The forward rate of reaction is increased to restore equilibrium.
- $Q = K_{eq}$, then the reaction is in dynamic equilibrium.
  - The reactants and products are present in equilibrium proportions.
  - The forward and reverse rates of reaction are equal.
- $Q > K_{eq}$, then the forward reaction has exceeded equilibrium.
  - There is a greater concentration of products (and smaller concentration of reactants) than at equilibrium.
  - The reverse rate of reaction is increased to restore equilibrium.

KEY CONCEPT

- $Q < K_{eq}$: $\Delta G < 0$, reaction proceeds in forward direction
- $Q = K_{eq}$: $\Delta G = 0$, reaction is in dynamic equilibrium
- $Q > K_{eq}$, $\Delta G > 0$: reaction proceeds in reverse direction

Any reaction that has not yet reached the equilibrium state, as indicated by $Q < K_{eq}$, will continue spontaneously in the forward direction (consuming reactants to form products) until the equilibrium ratio of reactants and products is reached. Any reaction in the equilibrium state will continue to react in the forward and reverse directions, but the reaction rates for the forward and reverse reactions will be equal, and the concentrations of the reactants and products will be constant, such that $Q = K_{eq}$. A reaction that is beyond the equilibrium state, as indicated by $Q > K_{eq}$, will proceed in the reverse direction (consuming products to form reactants) until the equilibrium ratio of reactants and products is reached again. Once a reaction is at equilibrium, any further movement in either the forward direction (resulting in an increase in products) or in the reverse direction (resulting in the reformation of reactants) will be nonspontaneous. This trend is illustrated in Figure 6.4.

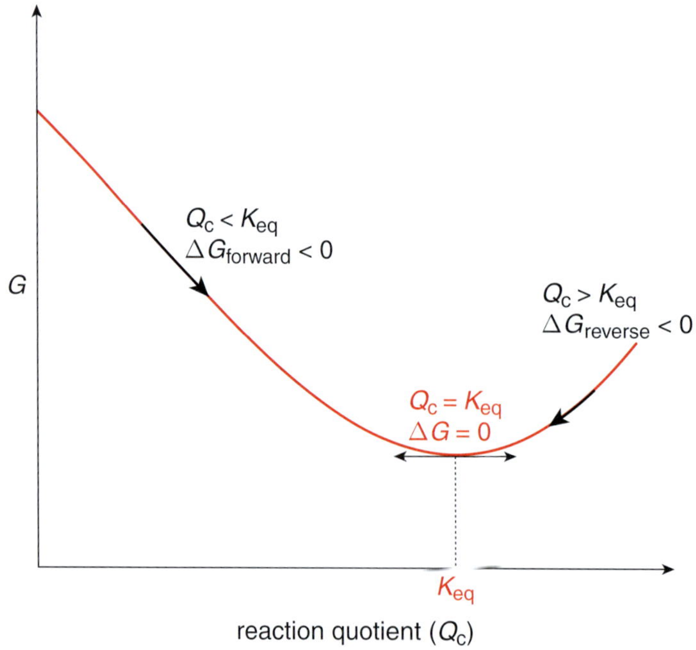

Figure 6.4 Gibbs Free Energy vs. Reaction Quotient

In Chapter 7 of *MCAT General Chemistry Review*, we'll further discuss how the spontaneity of these systems is related to enthalpy and entropy.

Properties of the Law of Mass Action

Make sure to remember the following characteristics of the law of mass action and equilibrium constant expressions:

- The concentrations of pure solids and pure liquids do not appear in the equilibrium constant expression. This is because the equilibrium expression is technically based on the activities of compounds, not concentrations; the activities of pure solids and liquids are defined to be 1. For the purposes of the MCAT, there is a negligible difference between concentration and activity.
- K_{eq} is characteristic of a particular reaction at a given temperature; the equilibrium constant is temperature-dependent.
- The larger the value of K_{eq}, the farther to the right the equilibrium position.
- If the equilibrium constant for a reaction written in one direction is K_{eq}, the equilibrium constant for the reverse reaction is $\frac{1}{K_{eq}}$.

Equilibrium Calculations

Calculations involving the equilibrium constant can take several forms but are also highly repetitive. Although we have discussed K_{eq} in this chapter, equilibrium constants and related calculations appear in solutions (K_{sp}), acids and bases (K_w, K_a, and K_b), and enzyme kinetics (K_d, K_b, and K_a). Thus, learning the "ins and outs" of equilibrium calculations has a large payoff on the MCAT.

One of the first concepts to grasp is the scale of the equilibrium constant. In an ideal situation, the concentrations of products and reactants would all be the same, and regardless of their actual concentrations would reduce to 1:1 ratios. In this case, K_{eq} would equal 1. In the real world, this situation doesn't exist, as it is unlikely that any reaction would have exactly equal concentrations of products and reactants at equilibrium. However, a K_{eq} of 1 can be a valuable reference point, given that $K_{eq} = \frac{[\text{products}]}{[\text{reactants}]}$.

If the concentration of products is greater than the concentration of reactants, K_{eq} becomes a "top heavy" fraction and must be greater than 1. On the other hand, if the concentration of reactants is greater than that of products, K_{eq} becomes a "bottom heavy" fraction and must be less than 1. Keep in mind, however, that K_{eq} is often expressed as a single value using exponents, and the sign and scale of these exponents gives even more information about the relative quantities of reactants and products. A reaction that strongly favors products will have a large, positive exponent, and the larger the exponent, the less reactant that will be present at equilibrium. In other words, a large positive exponent indicates a reaction that goes almost to completion.

On the other hand, a large negative exponent indicates a reaction that strongly favors reactants at equilibrium. In this case, only a small amount of reactant is converted to product. When performing equilibrium calculations, a K_{eq} with a large negative exponent allows a very convenient and very necessary shortcut to be used: the amount that has reacted can be considered negligible compared to the amount of reactant that remains.

Consider the reaction A ↔ B + C, with $K_{eq} = 10^{-12}$ and a starting concentration of $[A] = 1$ M. The K_{eq} expression can be written as:

$$K_{eq} = \frac{[C][B]}{[A]}$$

If x amount of A has reacted, x amount of C and x amount of B have been produced at equilibrium, and the equilibrium concentration of A will be $[1 - x]$ M. Substituting these values into the K_{eq} expression gives:

$$K_{eq} = 10^{-12} = \frac{(x)(x)}{(1 - x)} = \frac{x^2}{1 - x}$$

Unfortunately, performing the calculations required by this equation would give us a polynomial function that would be extremely burdensome to solve. However, the value of K_{eq} has a large negative exponent, allowing us to use the "x is negligible" shortcut. Relative to the 1 M starting concentration, the amount that has reacted is so small, based on $K_{eq} = 10^{-12}$, that we can assume x is negligible and round the denominator to the starting concentration:

$$10^{-12} = \frac{x^2}{1}$$

The problem is much more readily solved, and the value for x is found to be 10^{-6}. This confirms our estimate that x is negligible compared to 1, since $x = 0.000001$, and $[1 - (0.000001)] \approx 1$.

If the value for K_{eq} is within one to two orders of magnitude of one, or if the concentration of reactant that goes to product is within two orders of magnitude of the initial concentration of reactant, this estimation will not be valid. Likewise, if the value of K_{eq} is significantly larger than one, this estimation cannot be used. In both cases, the amount that reacts will be significant compared to the starting concentration of reactant. However, these situations are unlikely to be tested on the MCAT.

MCAT EXPERTISE

You may have been previously taught to solve these types of equilibrium problems using a technique referred to as an ICEbox. On Test Day, generating an entire ICEbox table takes valuable time and effort, and this technique can be shortcut using logic alone. Practice solving equilibrium problems without the ICEbox technique, using the methods described in this chapter, for a faster solution on Test Day.

BRIDGE

Equilibrium constants are calculated for many types of reactions, and go by many different names. For solubility problems (*MCAT General Chemistry Review* Chapter 9), K_{eq} is known as K_{sp}. For acids and bases (*MCAT General Chemistry Review* Chapter 10), K_{eq} is known as K_a, K_b, or K_w. For enzyme kinetics (*MCAT Biochemistry Review* Chapter 2), K_{eq} is known as K_d, K_b, or K_a.

Example: 3 moles of N_2O_4 is placed in a 0.5 L container and allowed to reach equilibrium according to the following reaction:

$$N_2O_4\ (g) \leftrightarrow 2\,NO_2\ (g)$$

What is the equilibrium concentration of NO_2, given K_{eq} for the reaction is 6×10^{-6}?

Solution: Start by writing the expression for K_{eq}: $K_{eq} = \frac{[NO_2]^2}{[N_2O_4]}$

Note that the concentration of NO_2 is squared due to its coefficient of 2 in the balanced reaction. Next, determine the starting concentration of N_2O_4, taking into account that the initial volume is 0.5 L:

$$\frac{3\text{ M}}{0.5\text{ L}} = \frac{[N_2O_4]}{1\text{ L}}$$

$$[N_2O_4] = \frac{(3)(1)}{(0.5)} = 6\text{ M}$$

Thus, the starting concentration of $N_2O_4 = 6$ M. Next, using x to represent the amount of N_2O_4 that reacts, $2x$ to represent the amount of NO_2 that is produced, and 6×10^{-6} for the value of K_{eq}, plug into the expression for the equilibrium constant:

$$K_{eq} = 6 \times 10^{-6} = \frac{[2x]^2}{[6 - x]} \approx \frac{[2x]^2}{[6]}$$

Note that the small negative exponent in the value of K_{eq} indicates that x will be negligible in comparison to 6 M, allowing the K_{eq} expression to be simplified, and x to be determined as follows:

$$6 \times 10^{-6} = \frac{4x^2}{6}$$

$$36 \times 10^{-6} = 4x^2$$

$$x^2 = \frac{36 \times 10^{-6}}{4} = 9 \times 10^{-6}$$

$$x = 3 \times 10^{-3}\text{ M}$$

However, be careful to note that this is the value of x, which represents the amount of N_2O_4 that reacts. The final answer must represent the amount of NO_2 produced, which is twice the amount of N_2O_4 that reacts, or $2x$. Thus the final answer is the concentration of NO_2, which is 6×10^{-3} M.

MCAT CONCEPT CHECK 6.1

Before you move on, assess your understanding of the material with these questions.

1. Given that [product] = 0.075 M and [reactant] = 1.5 M, determine the direction of reaction and the sign of the free energy change for reactions with the following K_{eq} values: (Note: Assume that the reaction has only one product and one reactant, and that the stoichiometric coefficient for each is 1.)

K_{eq}	Direction of Reaction	ΔG
5.0×10^{-2}		
5.0×10^{-3}		
5.0×10^{-1}		

2. Write the equilibrium constant expression for the following reactions:

- $CO\ (g) + 2\ H_2\ (g) \rightleftharpoons CH_3OH\ (g)$:

- $H_3PO_4\ (aq) + H_2O\ (l) \rightleftharpoons H_2PO_4^-\ (aq) + H_3O^+\ (aq)$:

---

3. Consider the hypothetical reaction A ↔ B + C.

For each of the following, determine if the amount of reactant A that has converted to product at equilibrium will be negligible compared to the starting concentration of A.

K_{eq}	Initial Concentration of A (M)	Is the amount reacted negligible?
1.0×10^{-12}	1	
1.0×10^{-2}	0.1	
1.0×10^{-3}	0.001	
1.0×10^{-15}	0.001	

4. The following reaction has a K_{eq} of 2.1×10^{-7}. Given an initial concentration for A equal to 0.1 M and an initial concentration of B equal to 0.2 M, what is the equilibrium concentration of C? Is the approximation that x is negligible valid for this calculation?

$$A\ (aq) + B\ (aq) \leftrightarrow C\ (g) + D\ (s)$$

6.2 Le Châtelier's Principle

LEARNING OBJECTIVES

After Chapter 6.2, you will be able to:

- Use Le Châtelier's principle to determine how changing conditions, including pH, temperature, pressure, and concentration changes, will affect a reaction previously in equilibrium

Le Châtelier's principle states that if a stress is applied to a system, the system shifts to relieve that applied stress. Regardless of the form the stress takes, the reaction is temporarily moved out of its equilibrium state. This is either because the concentrations or partial pressures of the system are no longer in the equilibrium ratio or because the equilibrium ratio itself has changed as a result of a change in the temperature of the system. The reaction then responds by reacting in whichever direction—either forward or reverse—will result in a reestablishment of the equilibrium state.

MCAT EXPERTISE

Le Châtelier's principle applies to a wide variety of systems and, therefore, appears as a fundamental concept in all three MCAT science sections.

Changes in Concentration

Adding or removing reactants or products from a reaction at equilibrium shifts the system from its minimum energy state. This change in concentration makes the reaction quotient (Q_c) unequal to the equilibrium constant (K_{eq}).

- Adding reactants or removing products makes $Q_c < K_{eq}$, causing the reaction to proceed in the forward direction, thus increasing the value of Q_c until equilibrium is restored.
- Removing reactants or adding products makes $Q_c > K_{eq}$, causing the reaction to proceed in the reverse direction, thus decreasing the value of Q_c until equilibrium is restored.

Essentially, the system always reacts in the direction away from the added species and/or toward the removed species to regain equilibrium, as demonstrated in Figure 6.5. Note that equilibrium does not mean that the concentration of the reactants and products are equal; equilibrium is established when the rate of the forward reaction equals the rate of the reverse reaction.

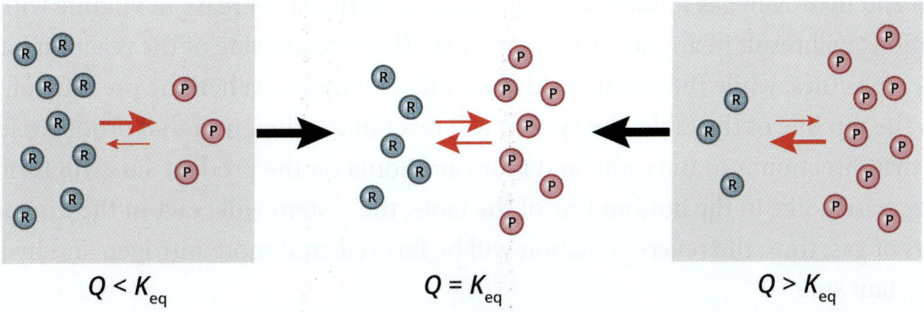

Figure 6.5 Le Châtelier's Principle
When changes in concentration of the reactant (R) or product (P) occur, the system will act to reestablish equilibrium.

We often take advantage of Le Châtelier's principle to improve the yield of chemical reactions. For example, in the industrial production of chemicals, products of reversible reactions are removed as they are formed to prevent the reactions from reaching their equilibrium states. The reaction will continue to react in the forward direction, producing more and more products—assuming reactants are continually replaced as they are consumed. One could also drive a reaction forward by starting with high concentrations of reactants. This will lead to an increase in the absolute quantities of products formed, although the reaction will still eventually reach its equilibrium state unless products are removed as they are formed.

BRIDGE

The bicarbonate buffer system is a classic example of Le Châtelier's principle applied to physiology:

$CO_2\ (g) + H_2O\ (l) \rightleftharpoons H_2CO_3\ (aq) \rightleftharpoons H^+\ (aq) + HCO_3^-\ (aq)$

In the tissues, there is a relatively high concentration of CO_2, and the reaction shifts to the right. In the lungs, CO_2 is lost, and the reaction shifts to the left. Note that blowing off CO_2 (hyperventilation) is used as a mechanism for dealing with acidemia (excess H^+ in the blood). This buffer system plays a key role in the respiratory, circulatory, and excretory systems, discussed in Chapters 6, 7, and 10 of *MCAT Biology Review*, respectively.

Changes in Pressure (and Volume)

Because liquids and solids are essentially incompressible, only chemical reactions that involve at least one gaseous species will be affected by changes in the system's pressure and volume. When a system is compressed, its volume decreases and its total pressure increases. Conversely when the system's volume expands, its total pressure decreases. The change in total pressure is associated with a change in partial pressures of each gas in the system and results in a shift from equilibrium conditions, such that Q_p does not equal K_{eq}. To counteract this, the system will move in such a way to restore equilibrium.

- Increasing pressure shifts the reaction to favor the side with fewer moles of gas to decrease the total pressure.
- Decreasing pressure shifts the reaction to favor the side with more moles of gas to increase the total pressure.

This is a consequence of the ideal gas law, which posits a direct relationship between the number of moles of gas and the pressure of the gas (for example, increasing the pressure on the system results in the system shifting to fewer moles of gas to decrease the pressure).

Consider the following reaction:

$$N_2\,(g) + 3\,H_2\,(g) \rightleftharpoons 2\,NH_3\,(g)$$

Figure 6.6 details how changes in pressure and volume will affect the equilibrium conditions of a reaction between nitrogen and hydrogen gas to form ammonia gas. Note that a decrease in volume with no other changes in conditions will result in an increase in pressure. The reactant side of the reaction has a total of four moles of gas molecules, while the product side has only two moles. When the pressure of this system is increased, like in the top line of the table, the system will react in the direction that produces fewer moles of gas. In this case, that direction is to the right, and more ammonia on the product side will form. However, if the pressure is decreased, like in the bottom line of the table, the system will react in the direction that produces more moles of gas; thus, the reverse reaction will be favored, and more nitrogen and hydrogen gas will reform on the reactant side.

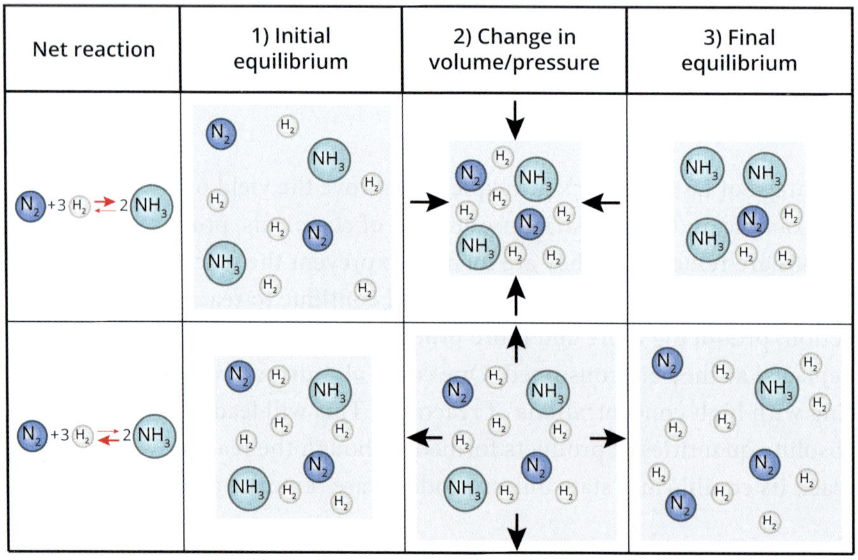

Figure 6.6 Equilibrium Conditions Due to Variations in Pressure and Volume
The top reaction shows the shift in equilibrium due to an increase in pressure/decrease in volume. The bottom reaction shows a shift in equilibrium from a decrease in pressure/increase in volume.

Changes in Temperature

Le Châtelier's principle tells us that changing the temperature of a system will also cause the system to react in a particular way to return to its equilibrium state. However, unlike the effect of changing concentrations or pressures, the result of changing temperature is not a change in the reaction quotient, Q_c or Q_p, but a change in K_{eq}. The change in temperature does not cause the concentrations or partial pressures of the reactants and products to change immediately, so Q immediately after the temperature change is the same as before the temperature change. Thus, because K_{eq} is now a different value, Q no longer equals K_{eq}. The system has to move in whichever direction allows it to reach its new equilibrium state at the new temperature. That direction is determined by the enthalpy of the reaction. If a reaction is endothermic ($\Delta H > 0$), heat functions as a reactant; if a reaction is exothermic ($\Delta H < 0$), heat functions as a product. Thinking about heat as a reactant or product allows us to apply the same principles we used with concentration changes to temperature changes.

For example, consider the following endothermic reaction, shown in Figure 6.7:

$$N_2O_4\ (g) \overset{\Delta}{\rightleftharpoons} 2\ NO_2\ (g)$$

The equilibrium position can be shifted by changing the temperature. When heat is added and the temperature increases, the reaction shifts to the right, and the flask turns reddish-brown due to an increase in $[NO_2]$. When heat is removed and the temperature decreases, the reaction shifts to the left, and the flask turns more transparent due to an increase in N_2O_4. This demonstrates Le Châtelier's principle because the equilibrium shifts in the direction that consumes energy.

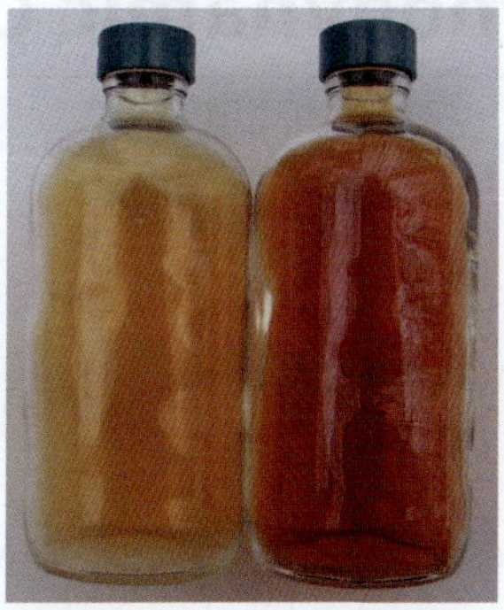

Figure 6.7 Example of a Reversible Endothermic Reaction, $N_2O_4\ (g) \rightleftharpoons 2\ NO_2\ (g)$
Left: As temperature decreases, the equilibrium favors N_2O_4 production, turning the reaction vessel more transparent. Right: As temperature increases, the equilibrium favors NO_2 production, turning the reaction vessel reddish-brown.

KEY CONCEPT

The reaction

A (*aq*) + 2 B (*g*) $\rightleftharpoons$ C (*g*) + heat

Will shift to the right if...	Will shift to the left if...
A or B is added	C is added
C is removed	A or B is removed
the pressure is increased or the volume is reduced	the pressure is reduced or the volume is increased
the temperature is reduced	the temperature is increased

MCAT CONCEPT CHECK 6.2

Before you move on, assess your understanding of the material with this question.

1. Describe what would happen in the following situations:
   - In the reaction $H_2SO_4\ (aq) \rightleftharpoons H^+\ (aq) + HSO_4^-\ (aq)$, the pH has been increased:

   ____

   - In the reaction $2\ C\ (s) + O_2\ (g) \rightleftharpoons 2\ CO\ (g)$, the pressure of the reaction vessel is decreased:

   ____

   - In the reaction $CH_4\ (g) + 2\ O_2\ (g) \rightleftharpoons CO_2\ (g) + 2\ H_2O\ (l)$ + heat, the reaction vessel is warmed:

   ____

   - In the reaction $H_3PO_4\ (aq) + H_2O\ (l) \rightleftharpoons H_3O^+\ (aq) + H_2PO_4^-\ (aq)$, water is removed (without changing temperature):

   ____

6.3 Kinetic and Thermodynamic Control

LEARNING OBJECTIVES

After Chapter 6.3, you will be able to:

- Identify the conditions that will cause a reaction to favor the kinetic or the thermodynamic product
- Distinguish between a kinetic and thermodynamic pathway on a reaction coordinate diagram

Having covered the fundamentals of kinetics and thermodynamics, we come upon a topic that bridges all chemical systems: control of a reaction. In particular, biochemical reactions often require regulation in a precise manner to be useful to an organism. The applications of kinetic and thermodynamic control are common on the MCAT and range from metabolic reactions requiring high-energy phosphate molecules, such as ATP to the effects of temperature and solvents on enzyme activity.

The examples below consider unimolecular systems through the lens of the transition state theory. Figure 6.8 shows starting materials (reactants) at a certain energy level. These reactants can undergo two different sets of reactions. At lower temperatures (with smaller heat transfer), a **kinetic product** is formed. At higher temperatures (with larger heat transfer), a **thermodynamic product** is formed.

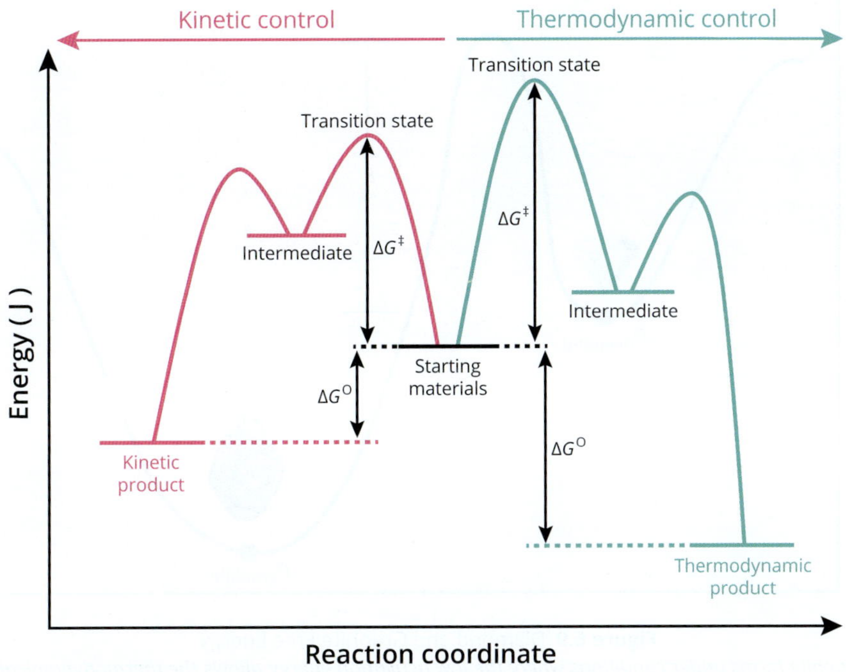

Figure 6.8 Kinetic and Thermodynamic Control of a Reaction
The kinetic pathway requires less free energy to reach the transition state, but results in a higher-energy (less stable) product.

Note that the free energy that must be added for the kinetic pathway is lower than that of the thermodynamic pathway. Therefore, the kinetic products often form faster than the thermodynamic products and are sometimes called "fast" products. On the other hand, the free energy of the thermodynamic product is significantly lower than that of the kinetic product. Thermodynamic products are therefore associated with greater stability, and with a more negative ΔG than kinetic products.

Consider graphite and diamond. Both are composed entirely of carbon but differ in their structure. We can use the concepts from Figure 6.8 to understand their stability at standard temperature and pressure. Graphite has a lower free energy than diamond. This makes graphite the thermodynamically favored form, corresponding to the lowest-energy position on an energy diagram. Based on thermodynamics alone, the higher-energy diamond should spontaneously convert into the lower-energy graphite. However, this does not happen. The reason is kinetic: the conversion from diamond to graphite has an extremely high activation energy barrier (E_a), similar to a very tall transition state peak. Because this barrier is so difficult to overcome under standard conditions, the reaction is extremely slow. Therefore, diamond is kinetically stable (or metastable); it is "trapped" in a higher-energy state, even though it is thermodynamically unstable relative to graphite (Figure 6.9).

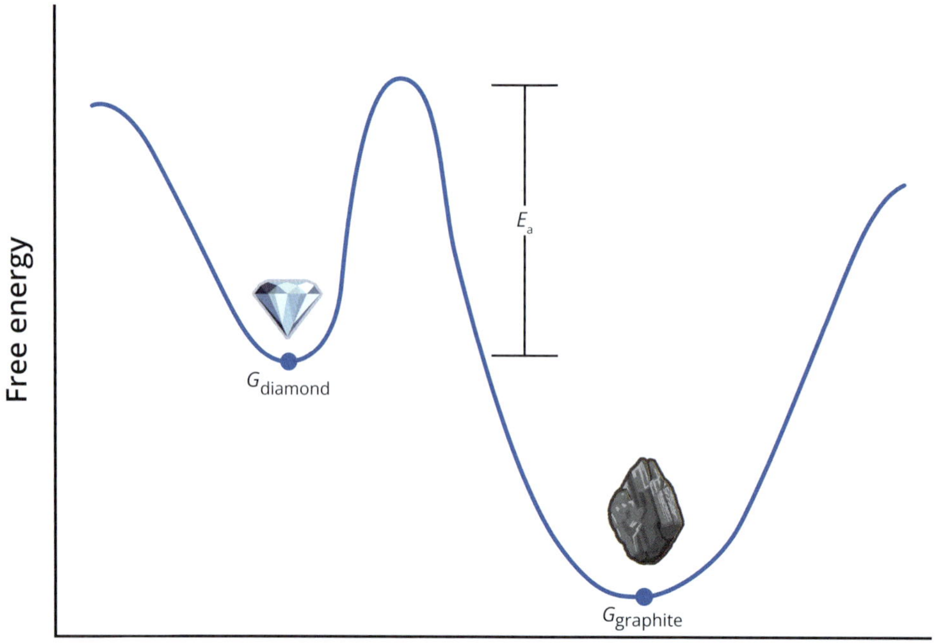

Figure 6.9 Diamond and Graphite Free Energy
Graphite forms under conditions where the low activation energy allows the thermodynamically favored structure to be achieved relatively easily. Diamonds form under extreme high pressure and temperature conditions found deep within Earth, which can overcome the higher energy barrier.

The stability of organic molecules is covered in Chapter 2 of *MCAT Organic Chemistry Review* and is dependent on torsional strain, angle strain, and nonbonded strain. In this example, we consider the conversion of 2-methylcyclohexanone to its thermodynamic product and its kinetic product, as shown in Figure 6.10. Both reactions require a base (B^-) in order to catalyze the conversion, yet two different products are produced.

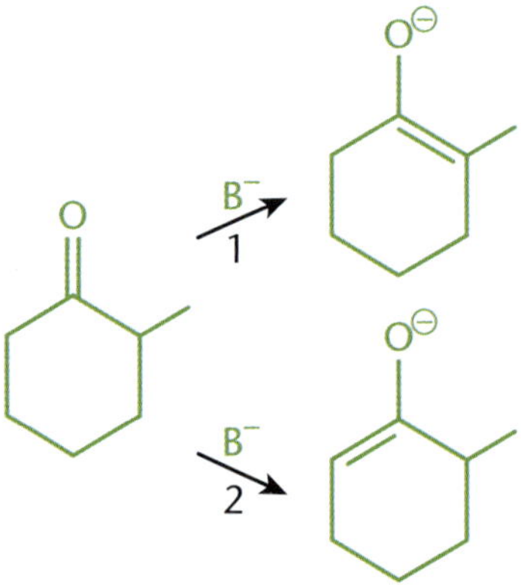

Figure 6.10 Conversion of 2-methylcyclohexanone to (1) Thermodynamic Product and (2) Kinetic Product

For the thermodynamic pathway (**1**), the double bond is located between C-1 and the methyl group. It requires more energy to form the transition state of this reaction because the base must overcome the steric hindrance created by the methyl group. The base squeezes in to reach the carbon with the methyl group attached to abstract a proton. However, because the double bond is more substituted than the other pathway, the product of this reaction is more stable and less likely to react further.

For the kinetic pathway (**2**), the double bond is located between C-1 and C-6. This pathway is preferred when there is little heat available because less energy is needed to reach the transition state. The base can more easily reach C-6 to remove a proton, and the resulting enolate can form. This product has a less substituted double bond, which reduces its stability. This lack of stability may leave the ring susceptible to further attack.

MCAT CONCEPT CHECK 6.3

Before you move on, assess your understanding of the material with these questions.

1. What conditions favor formation of a kinetic product? A thermodynamic product?
   - Kinetic product:

   ____

   - Thermodynamic product:

   ____

2. On a reaction coordinate diagram, how would the kinetic pathway appear as compared to the thermodynamic pathway?

   ____

Conclusion

We've discussed some very important concepts and principles in the past two chapters related to the studies of reaction rates and chemical equilibria. In this chapter, we began with the law of mass action and the significance of the equilibrium state of a chemical reaction. With our understanding of the significance of K_{eq} and Q, we are able to predict the direction that a reaction will go in response to various stresses—concentration, pressure, or temperature changes—that might be applied to a system.

The concept of homeostasis in biology is a direct result of the energy associated with disturbing equilibria in the body. Reactions are often held slightly out of the equilibrium state to generate energy. Many pathologies you will encounter in your future career in medicine will have a fundamental basis in disturbed chemical equilibria—just wait until you start ordering metabolic panels on your patients!

GO ONLINE

You've reviewed the content, now test your knowledge and critical thinking skills by completing a test-like passage set in your online resources!

CONCEPT SUMMARY

Equilibrium

- **Reversible** reactions eventually reach a state in which energy is minimized and entropy is maximized.
  - Chemical equilibria are **dynamic**—the reactions are still occurring, just at a constant rate.
  - The concentrations of reactants and products remain constant because the rate of the forward reaction equals the rate of the reverse reaction.
- The **law of mass action** gives the expression for the equilibrium constant, K_{eq}. The reaction quotient, Q, has the same form but can be calculated at any concentrations of reactants and products.
  - Q is a calculated value that relates the reactant and product concentrations at any given time during a reaction.
  - K_{eq} is the ratio of products to reactants at equilibrium, with each species raised to its stoichiometric coefficient. K_{eq} for a reaction is constant at a constant temperature.
  - Pure solids and liquids do not appear in the law of mass action; only gases and aqueous species do.
- Comparison of Q to K_{eq} provides information about where the reaction is with respect to its equilibrium state.
  - If $Q < K_{eq}$, $\Delta G < 0$, and the reaction proceeds in the forward direction.
  - If $Q = K_{eq}$, $\Delta G = 0$, and the reaction is in dynamic equilibrium.
  - If $Q > K_{eq}$, $\Delta G > 0$, and the reaction proceeds in the reverse direction.
- Equilibrium calculations are broadly applicable to many areas of chemistry but are often formulaic in their application. The magnitude of K_{eq} determines the balance of a reaction and whether the amount that has reacted can be treated as negligible when compared to other concentrations.
  - If $K_{eq} > 1$, the products are present in greater concentration at equilibrium.
  - If $K_{eq} \approx 1$, products and reactants are both present at equilibrium at reasonably similar levels.
  - If $K_{eq} < 1$, the reactants are present in greater concentration at equilibrium.
  - If $K_{eq} \lll 1$, the amount of reactants that have been converted to products can be considered negligible in comparison to the initial concentration of reactants.

Le Châtelier's Principle

- **Le Châtelier's principle** states that when a chemical system experiences a stress, it will react so as to restore equilibrium.
- There are three main types of stresses applied to a system: changes in concentration, pressure and volume, and temperature.
  - Increasing the concentration of reactants or decreasing the concentration of products will shift the reaction to the right. Increasing the concentration of products or decreasing the concentration of reactants will shift the reaction to the left.
  - Increasing pressure on a gaseous system (decreasing its volume) will shift the reaction toward the side with fewer moles of gas. Decreasing pressure on a gaseous system (increasing its volume) will shift the reaction toward the side with more moles of gas.

- Increasing the temperature of an endothermic reaction or decreasing the temperature of an exothermic reaction will shift the reaction to the right. Decreasing the temperature of an endothermic reaction or increasing the temperature of an exothermic reaction will shift the reaction to the left.

Kinetic and Thermodynamic Control

- Reactions may have both kinetic and thermodynamic products that can be regulated by temperature and the presence of a catalyst.
  - **Kinetic products** are higher in free energy than thermodynamic products and can form at lower temperatures. These are sometimes termed "fast" products because they can form more quickly under such conditions.
  - **Thermodynamic products** are lower in free energy than kinetic products and are therefore more stable. Despite proceeding more slowly than the kinetic pathway, the thermodynamic pathway is more spontaneous (more negative ΔG).

ANSWERS TO CONCEPT CHECKS

6.1

1. First calculate the value of Q from the given concentrations:
$Q = \frac{[\text{products}]}{[\text{reactants}]} = \frac{0.075}{1.5} = \frac{7.5 \times 10^{-2}}{1.5} = 5 \times 10^{-2}$.
Q can now be compared to each value of K_{eq} to predict the direction of the reaction.

K_{eq}	Direction of Reaction	ΔG
5.0×10^{-2}	At equilibrium: no net reaction	0
5.0×10^{-3}	$Q_c > K_{eq}$: proceeds toward reactants (left)	Positive
5.0×10^{-1}	$Q_c < K_{eq}$: proceeds toward products (right)	Negative

2. $K_p = \frac{P_{CH_3OH}}{P_{CO} \times (P_{H_2})^2}$

$K_c = K_a = \frac{[H_2PO_4^-][H_3O^+]}{[H_3PO_4]}$

3. The concentration of a reactant that converts to product can be considered negligible if it is two or more orders of magnitude less than the initial concentration of the reactant.

K_{eq}	Initial Concentration of A (M)	Is the amount reacted negligible?
1×10^{-12}	1	Yes
1×10^{-2}	0.1	No
1×10^{-3}	0.001	No
1×10^{-15}	0.001	Yes

4. The first step in solving is to write the equation for K_{eq} for the reaction: A (aq) + B (aq) ↔ C (g) + D (s).

$$K_{eq} = \frac{[C]}{[A][B]} = 2.1 \times 10^{-7}$$

Note that the equation for K_{eq} does not include product D because D is a solid.

Next, using the initial concentrations for A and B and x for the amount that has reacted, plug into the equation for K_{eq}:

$$K_{eq} = \frac{[C]}{[A][B]} = \frac{[x]}{[0.1 - x][0.2 - x]}$$

Given that $K_{eq} = 2.1 \times 10^{-7}$, the concentrations of A and B are sufficiently large that x can be considered negligible in comparison to both. This allows the equation for K_{eq} to be simplified and solved:

$$K_{eq} = 2.1 \times 10^{-7} \approx \frac{x}{[0.1][0.2]}$$
$$x = (2.1 \times 10^{-7})(0.1)(0.2) = 4.2 \times 10^{-9}$$

The value of $x = 4.2 \times 10^{-9}$ is equal to both the equilibrium concentration of C and the amount of A and B that have reacted. The approximation that x is negligible compared to the initial concentrations of A and B is valid.

6.2

1. • Increasing pH of $H_2SO_4\ (aq) \rightleftharpoons H^+\ (aq) + HSO_4^-\ (aq)$: $[H^+]$ decreases, shifting reaction to the right.
   - Decreasing pressure of $2\ C\ (s) + O_2\ (g) \rightleftharpoons 2\ CO\ (g)$: Reaction shifts right, favoring the side with more moles of gas.
   - Warming $CH_4\ (g) + 2O_2\ (g) \rightleftharpoons CO_2\ (g) + 2\ H_2O\ (l)$ + heat: Reaction shifts left, using the additional heat energy to produce more reactants.
   - Removing water from $H_3PO_4\ (aq) + H_2O\ (l) \rightleftharpoons H_3O^+\ (aq) + H_2PO_4^-\ (aq)$: Reaction shifts left. All concentrations would increase proportionately; because there are more products than reactants (and the stoichiometric coefficient is 1 for each reactant and product), the value of Q will increase.

6.3

1. Kinetic products are favored at low temperatures with low heat transfer. Thermodynamic products are favored at high temperatures with high heat transfer.
2. Kinetic pathways require a smaller gain in free energy to reach the transition state. They also have a higher free energy of the products, with a smaller difference in free energy between the transition state and the products.

SCIENCE MASTERY ASSESSMENT EXPLANATIONS

1. **C**

This scenario likely describes a situation in which a reaction has reached equilibrium very far to the right (with high product concentration and low reactant concentration). This reaction must be reversible because the reaction did not proceed all the way to the right. Any reaction in equilibrium has equal forward and reverse rates of reaction.

2. **D**

Recall that pure solids and liquids do not appear in the equilibrium expression; thus, this K_{eq} has no denominator because the only reactant is a solid, cuprous sulfate. This could also be called K_{sp} because a solid is dissociating into ions in solution. The correct K_{eq} should have $[Cu^{+}]$ squared because its stoichiometric coefficient is 2.

3. **A**

Carbon dioxide gas evolves and leaves the bottle, which decreases the total pressure of the reactants. Le Châtelier's principle explains that a decrease in pressure shifts the equilibrium to increase the number of moles of gas present. This particular reaction will shift to the left, which in turn will decrease the amount of carbonic acid and increase the amount of carbon dioxide and water. Oxygen and nitrogen are not highly reactive and are unlikely to combine spontaneously with carbon dioxide or carbonic acid, as in **(C)** and **(D)**.

4. **B**

Recall that when multiple products are possible and an equilibrium exists between these multiple products, one product will be called the kinetic product and the other the thermodynamic product. The transition state leading to the kinetic product is lower in energy, so that the kinetic product is formed more rapidly in solution. However, the kinetic product is less stable than the thermodynamic product. The end result is that the equilibrium of products initially favors the kinetic product, but eventually favors the more stable thermodynamic product. Taking these factors together, to favor the kinetic product, conduct the reaction for a short duration, so that the thermodynamic product does not have much chance to form. Also, the reaction should be conducted at a lower temperature to help stabilize the otherwise less stable kinetic product. These factors—low temperature and short reaction time—justify choice **(B)**.

5. **A**

The larger the value of K_{eq} (whether K_c or K_p), the larger the ratio of products to reactants. Therefore, if $K_c \gg 1$, there are significantly larger concentrations of products than reactants at equilibrium. Even with a large K_{eq}, the reaction will ultimately reach equilibrium far toward the products side and is therefore reversible, eliminating **(D)**.

6. **B**

Adding sodium acetate increases the number of acetate ions present. According to Le Châtelier's principle, this change will push this reaction to the left, resulting in a decrease in the number of free H^+ ions. Because pH is determined by the hydrogen ion concentration, a decrease in the number of free protons will increase the pH. An acid's K_a (which is simply the K_{eq} for acid dissociation) will remain constant under a given temperature and pressure, eliminating **(C)** and **(D)**.

7. **A**

Both increasing the pressure of the container and decreasing the volume would favor the side with fewer moles of gas, which is the product side. This makes **(B)** and **(C)** incorrect. **(D)** would not disturb the equilibrium—the significance of decreasing the volume of the container in most equilibria is that there is an increase in pressure; in this case, however, the pressure remains constant despite the change in volume.

8. **C**

An exothermic reaction produces heat. Decreasing the temperature favors product formation, resulting in an increase in the forward reaction rate with a concomitant decrease in the reverse reaction rate.

9. **B**

The equilibrium of a reaction can be changed by several factors. Adding or subtracting heat, **(A)**, would shift the equilibrium based on the enthalpy change of the reaction. Increasing reactant concentrations would shift the equilibrium in the direction of the product, and the opposite would occur if reactant concentrations were decreased, eliminating **(C)**. Changing the volume of a reactant would affect any reaction with gaseous reactants or products, eliminating **(D)**. While adding or removing a catalyst would change the reaction rates, it would not change where the equilibrium lies.

10. **A**

Start with the balanced equation for the reaction of H_2 and N_2 to produce NH_3: $N_2 + 3\,H_2 \rightleftharpoons 2\,NH_3$.

Next, write out $K_c = K_{eq} = \frac{[NH_3]^2}{[N_2]\,[H_2]^3}$. Because the volume is 1 L, the amount of each gas in moles is equal to the value of the concentration of each gas in moles per liter (*M*). The relatively small amount of NH_3 produced indicates that it will be possible to consider the amount of N_2 and H_2 that reacts to be negligible compared to their starting concentrations. Putting the amounts of each reactant and product into the K_{eq} expression gives:

$$K_{eq} = \frac{[NH_3]^2}{[N_2]\,[H_2]^3} = \frac{[0.05]^2}{[1-x][3-x]^3} \approx \frac{[0.05]^2}{[1][3]^3} = \frac{\left[5 \times 10^{-2}\right]^2}{27}$$

$$K_{eq} = \frac{25 \times 10^{-4}}{27} \approx \frac{25 \times 10^{-4}}{25} = 1 \times 10^{-4} = 0.0001$$

11. **B**

At extremely high temperatures, reactants or products may decompose, which will affect the equilibrium and potentially destroy the desired products. **(A)** implies that reactions have limits, which is true; however, this does not make increasing temperature unfavorable. **(C)** is false because increasing temperature would also increase pressure, assuming constant volume. **(D)** is incorrect because it refers to properties of irreversible reactions, which would not be involved in an equilibrium between products and reactants.

12. **D**

The thermodynamic product is more stable than the kinetic product, making the thermodynamic product lower in energy. Because the energy of the product is lower, the *change* in free energy is greater for the thermodynamic product compared to the kinetic product. Thus, **(D)** is correct.

13. **C**

K_a is equal to the ratio of products to reactants, with each species raised to its stoichiometric coefficient. A compound with a K_a greater than 10^{-7} contains more H^+ cations than HA^- anions at equilibrium, which makes it an acid. This means that the compound in question is likely to react with a compound that is basic. Of the four answer choices, NH_3 is the only base.

14. **C**

Reaction 2 is the reverse of reaction 1. This means that K_{eq} for reaction 2 is the inverse of K_{eq} of reaction 1, so the answer is $\frac{1}{0.1} = \frac{1}{\frac{1}{10}} = 10$.

15. **A**

A negative ΔH value indicates an exothermic reaction, meaning that the forward reaction produces heat. Visualize this as follows:

$$A + B \rightleftharpoons C + D + \text{heat}$$

This means that removing heat by decreasing the temperature is similar to removing any other product of the reaction. To compensate for this loss, the reaction will shift to the right, causing an increase in the concentrations of C and D, as well as a decrease in the concentrations of A and B.

GO ONLINE

Consult your online resources for additional practice.

EQUATIONS TO REMEMBER

(6.1) **Equilibrium constant:** $K_{eq} = \frac{[C]^c[D]^d}{[A]^a[B]^b}$

(6.2) **Reaction quotient:** $Q_c = \frac{[C]^c[D]^d}{[A]^a[B]^b}$

SHARED CONCEPTS

Biochemistry Chapter 2
Enzymes

General Chemistry Chapter 5
Chemical Kinetics

General Chemistry Chapter 7
Thermochemistry

General Chemistry Chapter 9
Solutions

General Chemistry Chapter 10
Acids and Bases

Organic Chemistry Chapter 2
Isomers

CHAPTER 7

THERMOCHEMISTRY

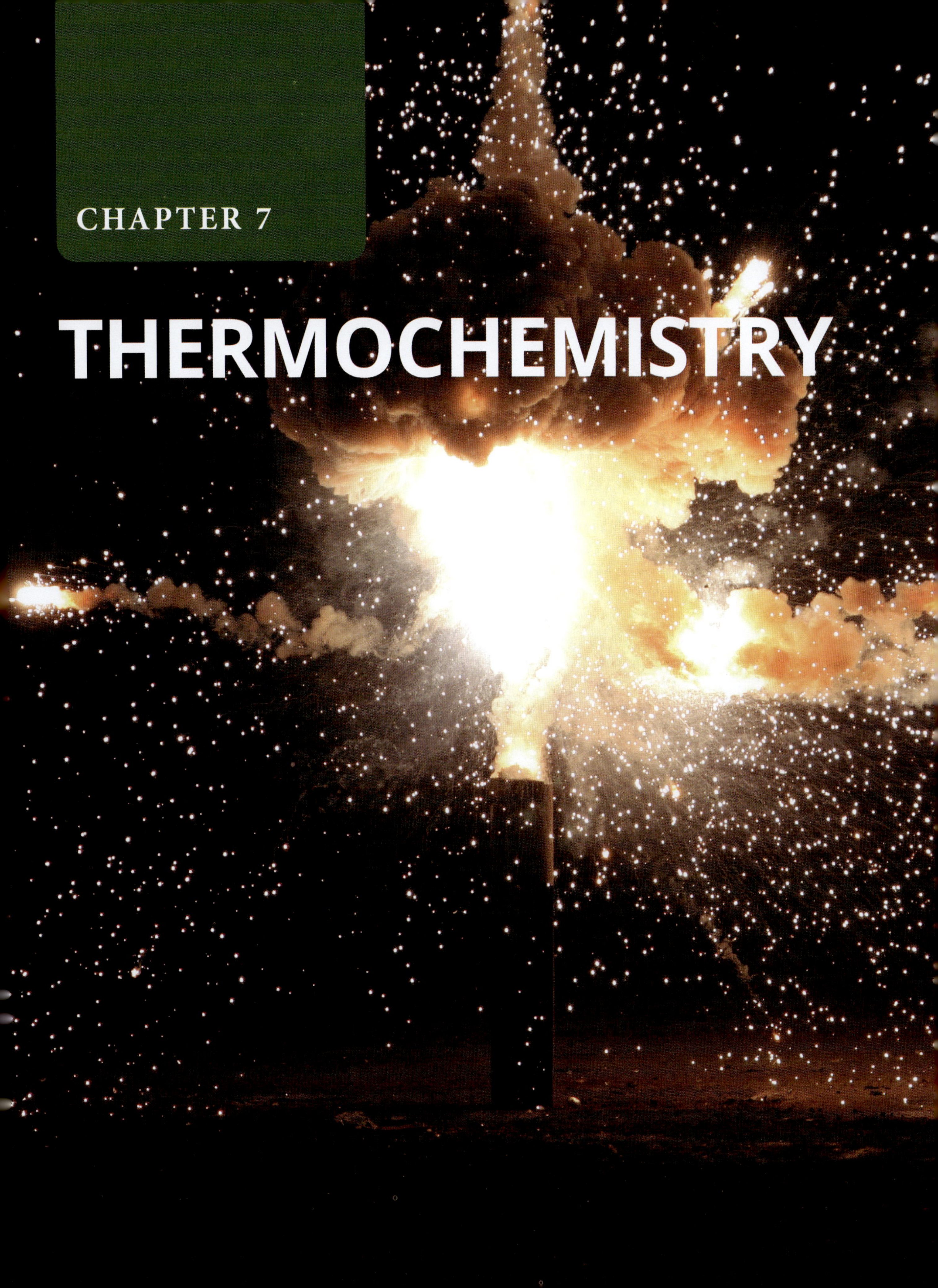

SCIENCE MASTERY ASSESSMENT

Every pre-med knows this feeling: there is so much content I have to know for the MCAT! How do I know what to do first or what's important?

While the high-yield badges throughout this book will help you identify the most important topics, this Science Mastery Assessment is another tool in your MCAT prep arsenal. This quiz (which can also be taken in your online resources) and the guidance below will help ensure that you are spending the appropriate amount of time on this chapter based on your personal strengths and weaknesses. Don't worry though—skipping something now does not mean you'll never study it. Later on in your prep, as you complete full-length tests, you'll uncover specific pieces of content that you need to review and can come back to these chapters as appropriate.

How to Use This Assessment

If you answer 0–7 questions correctly:

Spend about 1 hour to read this chapter in full and take limited notes throughout. Follow up by reviewing **all** quiz questions to ensure that you now understand how to solve each one.

If you answer 8–11 questions correctly:

Spend 20–40 minutes reviewing the quiz questions. Beginning with the questions you missed, read and take notes on the corresponding subchapters. For questions you answered correctly, ensure your thinking matches that of the explanation and you understand why each choice was correct or incorrect.

If you answer 12–15 questions correctly:

Spend less than 20 minutes reviewing all questions from the quiz. If you missed any, then include a quick read-through of the corresponding subchapters, or even just the relevant content within a subchapter, as part of your question review. For questions you answered correctly, ensure your thinking matches that of the explanation and review the Concept Summary at the end of the chapter.

1. Consider the cooling of an ideal gas in a closed system. This process is illustrated in the pressure–volume graph shown in the following figure.

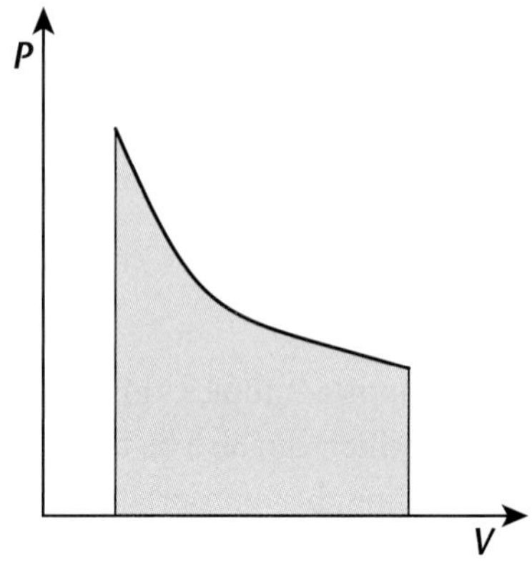

Based on this information, the process may be:
   A. adiabatic.
   B. isobaric.
   C. isothermal.
   D. isochoric.

2. A pot of water at 100°C sits on a heating element and boils. Which of the following best characterizes this phase change process?
   A. Isothermal expansion
   B. Adiabatic expansion
   C. Isovolumetric heating
   D. Adiabatic compression

3. Pure sodium metal spontaneously combusts upon contact with room temperature water. What is true about the equilibrium constant of this combustion reaction at 25°C?
   A. $K_{eq} < 0$
   B. $0 < K_{eq} < 1$
   C. $K_{eq} = 1$
   D. $K_{eq} > 1$

4. Which of the following processes has the most exothermic standard heat of combustion?
   A. Combustion of ethane
   B. Combustion of propane
   C. Combustion of *n*-butane
   D. Combustion of *n*-pentane

5. Methanol reacts with acetic acid to form methyl acetate and water.

Type of Bond	Bond Dissociation Energy $\left(\frac{kJ}{mol}\right)$
C–C	348
C–H	415
C=O	805
O–H	463
C–O	360

Based on the values in the table above, what is the heat of reaction in $\frac{kJ}{mol}$?
   A. 0
   B. 464
   C. 824
   D. 1288

6. Which of the following refers to the temperature and pressure at which all three phases exist in equilibrium?
   A. Critical point
   B. Triple point
   C. Deposition
   D. State function

7. A 10 g sample of water is brought from 40°C to boiling and is completely boiled to the gas phase. Which of the following expressions represents the total amount of energy required if the final temperature of the vapor is 100°C? (The heat of vaporization of water is 2,260 J/g.)
   A. (10 g)(40°C)(4.2 J/g°C) + (2,260 J/g)(10 g)
   B. (10 g)(40°C)(4.2 J/g°C) + (2,260 J/°C)(60°C)
   C. (10 g)(60°C)(4.2 J/g°C) + (2,260 J/g)(10 g)
   D. (10 g)(60°C)(4.2 J/g°C) + (2,260 J/°C)(60°C)

8. Consider the chemical reaction in the vessel depicted in the following diagram.

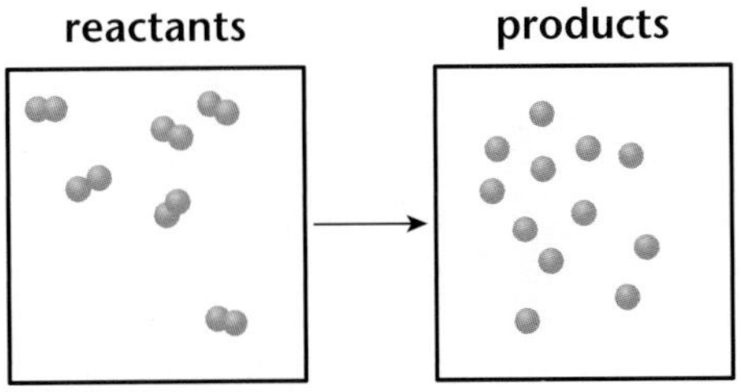

A. The reaction is spontaneous.
B. The reaction is nonspontaneous.
C. The reaction is at equilibrium.
D. There is not enough information to determine if the reaction is spontaneous.

9. Suppose $\Delta G^{\circ}_{rxn} = -2000 \frac{\text{J}}{\text{mol}}$ for a chemical reaction. At 300 K, what is the change in Gibbs free energy in $\frac{\text{J}}{\text{mol}}$?

A. $\Delta G = -2000 + (300\text{ K})(8.314)(\ln Q)$
B. $\Delta G = -2000 - (300\text{ K})(8.314)(\ln Q)$
C. $\Delta G = -2000 + (300\text{ K})(8.314)(\log Q)$
D. $\Delta G = -2000 - (300\text{ K})(8.314)(\log Q)$

10. A chemical reaction has a negative enthalpy and a negative entropy. Which of the following terms necessarily describes this reaction?
A. Exothermic
B. Endothermic
C. Exergonic
D. Endergonic

11. Which of the following statements is true of a process that is spontaneous in the forward direction?
A. $\Delta G > 0$ and $K_{eq} > Q$
B. $\Delta G > 0$ and $K_{eq} < Q$
C. $\Delta G < 0$ and $K_{eq} > Q$
D. $\Delta G < 0$ and $K_{eq} < Q$

12. Which of the following reactions has the greatest decrease in entropy?
A. $2\ NH_3\ (g) \rightarrow 3\ H_2\ (g) + N_2\ (g)$
B. $2\ Na\ (s) + Cl_2\ (g) \rightarrow 2\ NaCl\ (s)$
C. $2\ H_2O_2\ (l) \rightarrow 2\ H_2O\ (l) + O_2\ (g)$
D. $Zn\ (s) + CuSO_4\ (aq) \rightarrow ZnSO_4\ (aq) + Cu\ (s)$

13. A reaction coordinate for a chemical reaction is displayed in the graph below.

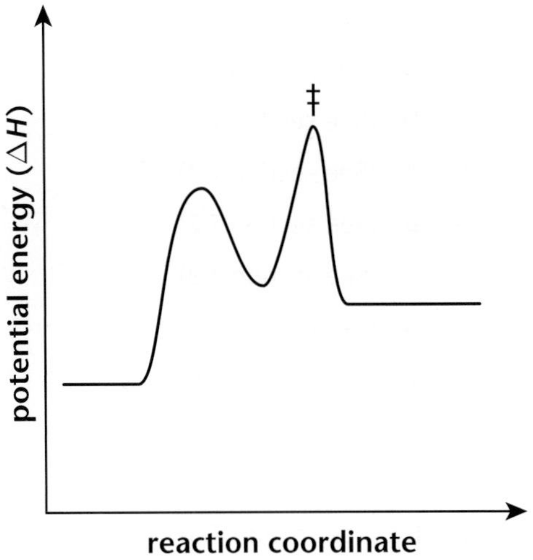

Which of the following terms describes the energy of this reaction?
A. Endothermic
B. Exothermic
C. Endergonic
D. Exergonic

14. The process of melting NaCl requires a large amount of energy due to the strong attraction between ions. A researcher finds that 58 g of salt melts at 1060 K and requires a heat input of 30,000 J. What is the change in entropy?
A. 28 J/K
B. 1,580 J/K
C. 61,000 J/K
D. Not enough information is provided

15. Explosions are necessarily characterized by:
A. $\Delta G < 0$.
B. $\Delta H > 0$.
C. $\Delta S < 0$.
D. $T < 0$.

Answer Key

1. **A** (See section 7.1)
2. **A** (See section 7.1)
3. **D** (See section 7.6)
4. **D** (See section 7.4)
5. **A** (See section 7.4)
6. **B** (See section 7.2)
7. **C** (See section 7.3)
8. **D** (See section 7.6)
9. **A** (See section 7.6)
10. **A** (See section 7.6)
11. **C** (See section 7.6)
12. **B** (See section 7.5)
13. **A** (See section 7.6)
14. **A** (See section 7.5)
15. **A** (See section 7.6)

The relevant section of the chapter to review for each question is given in parentheses after the correct answer. Detailed explanations can be found at the end of the chapter.

CHAPTER 7

THERMOCHEMISTRY

In This Chapter

CHAPTER PROFILE

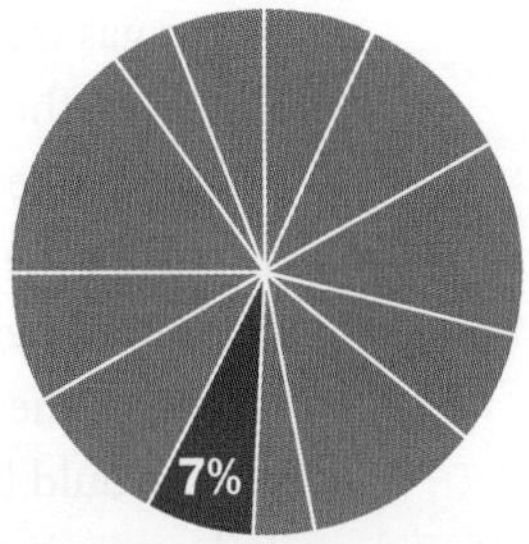

The content in this chapter should be relevant to about 7% of all questions about general chemistry on the MCAT.

This chapter covers material from the following AAMC content categories:

1D: Principles of bioenergetics and fuel molecule metabolism

5E: Principles of chemical thermodynamics and kinetics

Introduction

Styrofoam cups are such good insulators that they can be used as holding containers for certain calorimetry experiments. Coffee-cup calorimetry, which uses Styrofoam cups to measure heats of solution and specific heats of metals and other materials, is low-tech, yet it can produce remarkably accurate results as long as care has been taken to calibrate the calorimeter and to minimize heat loss through the top of the container. The next time you are at your favorite coffee chain, think about what occurs when cold cream is added to hot coffee. If we took the time to measure the masses and temperatures of the hot coffee and the cold cream before mixing them, measured the drink's temperature after it had been stirred, and looked up the specific heats of water and cream, we would have enough information to calculate the amount of heat exchanged between the hot coffee and the cold cream.

This chapter will review the basic principles of thermochemistry, which is the study of the energy changes that accompany chemical and physical processes. Starting with the first law of thermodynamics, which states that energy is never created nor destroyed but—at most—simply changed from one form to another, we will quantify the various exchanges in energy as a system moves from some initial state to a final state. As we go along, we will define what is meant by system and surroundings, state functions, heat, enthalpy, entropy, and Gibbs free energy.

7.1 Systems and Processes

LEARNING OBJECTIVES

After Chapter 7.1, you will be able to:

- Identify the system and its surroundings given a situation involving transfer of heat
- Recall the features of isothermal, adiabatic, isobaric, and isovolumetric processes

Students often have some anxiety over what constitutes a *system* and what—by exclusion from the system—constitutes the *surroundings* or *environment*. Perhaps the problem isn't so much the definitions themselves but the way in which the boundary between the two can be shifted to suit the needs of the experimenter or observer. Simply put, the **system** is the matter that is being observed—the total amount of reactants and products in a chemical reaction. It could be the amount of solute and solvent used to create a solution. It could be the gas inside a balloon. Then, the **surroundings**, or **environment**, are everything outside of that system. However, the boundary between system and surroundings is not permanently fixed and can be moved. For example, one might consider the mass of coffee in a coffee cup to be the system and the cup containing it to be part of the environment. This setup would likely be used if someone was interested in determining the amount of heat transferred from the hot coffee to the cooler coffee cup. Alternatively, one might define the system as the hot coffee and the cup together, and the environment as the air surrounding the coffee cup. This setup would likely be used if someone was interested in calculating the heat exchange between the hot coffee and cup system and the cooler surrounding air. The boundary can be extended out farther and farther, until the entire mass of the universe is ultimately included in the system. At this point, there are no surroundings. Again, where the boundary is placed is a decision based on what phenomenon one is interested in studying.

Thermodynamic Terminology

Systems can be characterized by whether or not they can exchange heat or matter with the surroundings. Simple examples of all three types of systems are shown in Figure 7.1. A system may be characterized as follows:

- **Open:** The system can exchange both energy (heat and work) and matter with the surroundings; for example, a human body or an uncovered pot of boiling water.
- **Closed:** The system can exchange energy (heat and work) but not matter with the surroundings; for example, a steam radiator or a pot of boiling water with a lid on it.
- **Isolated:** The system cannot exchange energy (heat and work) or matter with the surroundings; for example, an insulated bomb calorimeter or a double-wall insulated coffee thermos.

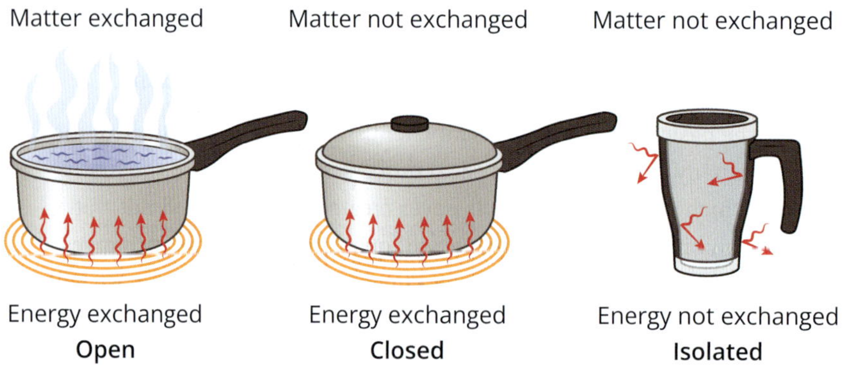

Figure 7.1 Open, Closed, and Isolated Systems

When a system experiences a change in one or more of its properties (such as concentrations of reactants or products, temperature, or pressure), it undergoes a **process**.

While processes, by definition, are associated with a change of the state of a system, some processes are uniquely identified by some property that is constant throughout the process. Many of these processes create special conditions because they allow us to simplify the **first law of thermodynamics**:

$$\Delta U = Q - W$$

Equation 7.1

where ΔU is the change in internal energy of the system, Q is the heat added to the system, and W is the work done by the system.

For example, **isothermal processes** occur when the system's temperature is constant. Constant temperature implies that the total internal energy of the system (U) is constant throughout the process. This is because temperature and internal energy are directly proportional. When U is constant, $\Delta U = 0$ and the first law simplifies to $Q = W$ (the heat added to the system equals the work done by the system). An example of an isothermal process is boiling water, as seen in Figure 7.2. Heat energy added to the liquid water is used to break intermolecular bonds and convert to steam without a change in temperature, which is a type of phase change. All phase changes are isothermal.

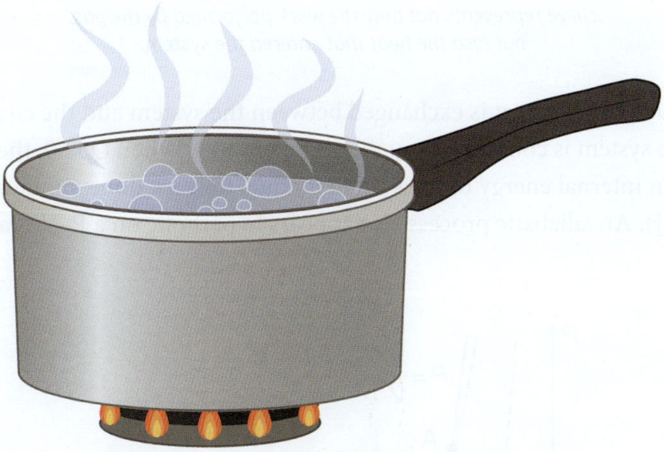

Figure 7.2 Boiling Water as Isothermal Process
During a phase change, the temperature remains constant even as heat energy is added to break intermolecular bonds.

An isothermal process appears as a hyperbolic curve on a pressure–volume graph (P–V graph). Work is represented by the area under such a curve, as shown in Figure 7.3.

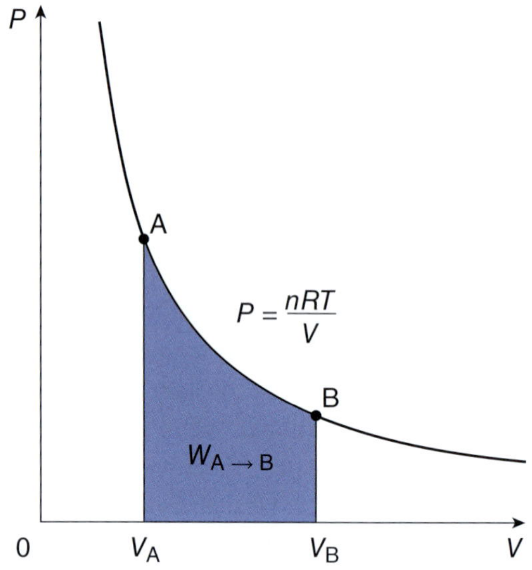

Figure 7.3 Graph of an Isothermal Expansion
Temperature is constant in an isothermal process; thus, the area under the curve represents not only the work performed by the gas, but also the heat that entered the system.

Adiabatic processes occur when no heat is exchanged between the system and the environment; thus, the thermal energy of the system is constant throughout the process. When $Q = 0$, the first law simplifies to $\Delta U = -W$ (the change in internal energy of the system is equal to work done *on* the system [the opposite of work done *by* the system]). An adiabatic process also appears hyperbolic on a P–V graph, as shown in Figure 7.4.

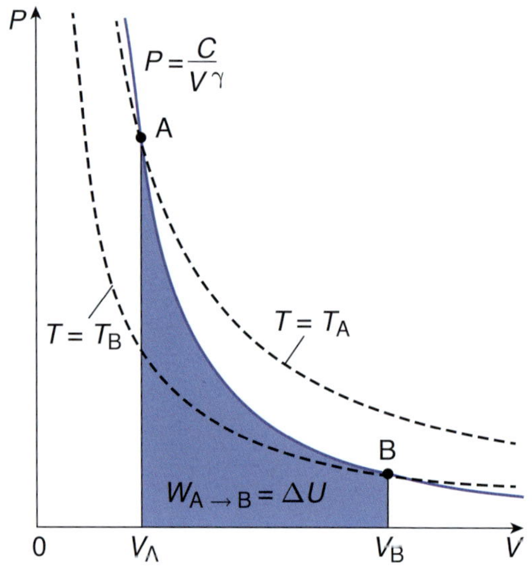

Figure 7.4 Graph of an Adiabatic Expansion
Heat exchange is zero in an adiabatic process; temperature is not constant (as shown by the dotted lines).

Since heat energy takes time to transfer, a key component of an adiabatic process is that it occurs rapidly. This means that the temperature of an adiabatic process is a function of the work done by or on the system. In the case of an air compressor, gas is heavily pressurized inside a fixed volume tank. When the release valve is opened, the pressurized gas rapidly escapes and expands into the new environment. During this adiabatic expansion, the temperature of an ideal gas decreases because the gas performs work on its surroundings without any heat transfer, causing its internal energy to decrease and thus its temperature to drop. This can be seen in Figure 7.5, where the gas's temperature as it escaped from the release valve decreased enough to cause the humidity in the atmosphere to form ice at the valve.

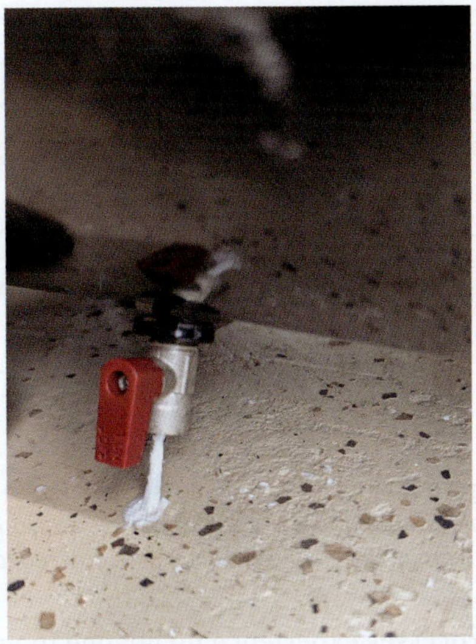

Figure 7.5 Compressed Air Release as Adiabatic Process
Compressed pressurized air escapes from a release valve under adiabatic conditions. The gas does work to expand and, in the absence of heat transfer, its temperature drops.

Isobaric processes occur when the pressure of the system is constant. Isothermal and isobaric processes are common because it is usually easy to control temperature and pressure. Isobaric processes do not alter the first law, but note that an isobaric process appears as a flat line on a P–V graph, as shown in Figure 7.6.

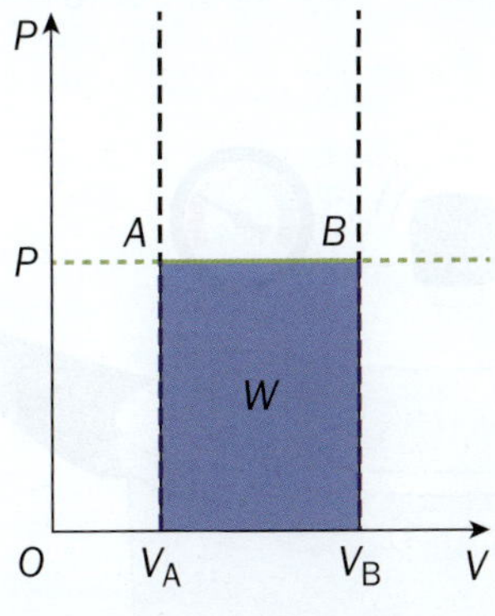

Figure 7.6 Graph of an Isobaric Expansion
Pressure is constant in an isobaric process; the slope of the line is therefore zero.

An example of an isobaric process is that of a steam powered engine, shown in Figure 7.7. In this example, water is heated and turned into steam. As the steam heats and its volume expands, it flows into a cylinder and pushes on a piston, which drives a crankshaft to turn the wheels. After powering the piston, the steam is then cooled, condensed back to water, and reheated to repeat the process. In real world applications, the pressure will fluctuate slightly, but is held as close to constant as possible. Note that the steam engine contains other special processes other than an isobaric expansion since it's a cyclic process.

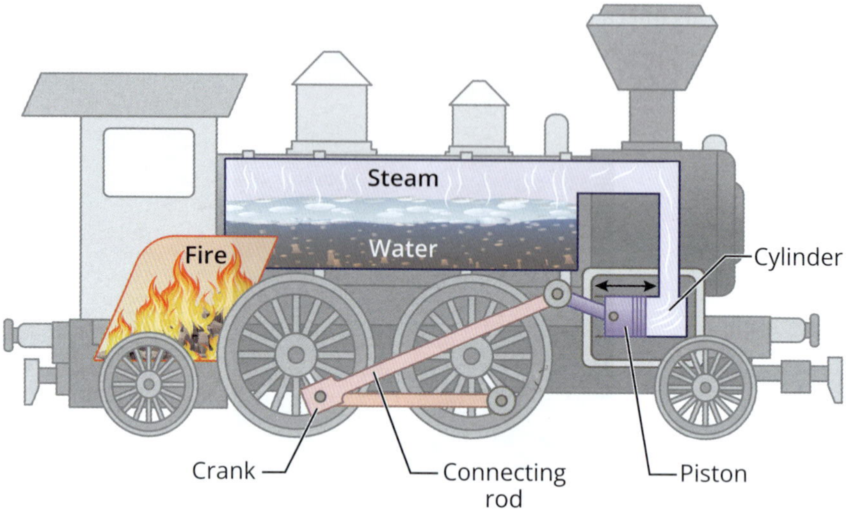

Figure 7.7 Steam Engine as Isobaric Process
Isobaric expansion of steam drives a piston outward via work done by the gas. The steam is then cooled, condensed, and reheated.

Finally, **isovolumetric (isochoric) processes** experience no change in volume. Because the gas neither expands nor compresses, no work is performed in such a process. Thus, the first law simplifies to $\Delta U = Q$ (the change in internal energy is equal to the heat added to the system). An isovolumetric process is a vertical line on a P–V graph; the area under the curve, which represents the work done by the gas, is zero.

An example of an isochoric process is a pressure cooker, shown in Figure 7.8, where heat is added to a gas in a fixed volume container, resulting in an increase in pressure without a change in volume.

BRIDGE

The terms isothermal, adiabatic, isobaric, and isovolumetric (isochoric) may seem familiar because they are also discussed in Chapter 3 of *MCAT Physics and Math Review.*

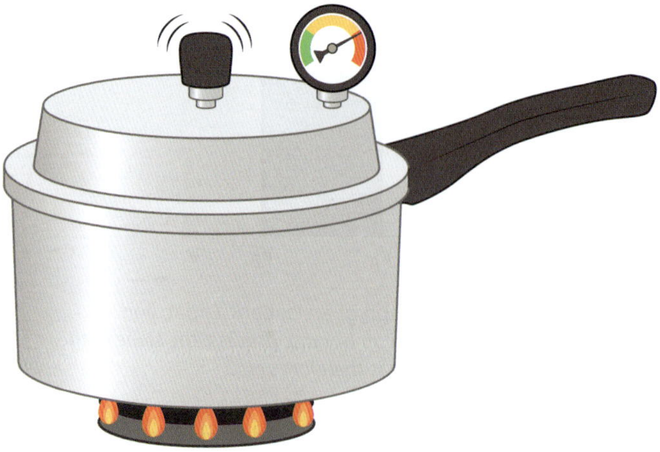

Figure 7.8 Pressure Cooker as Isochoric Process
Gas inside the pot is heated in a fixed-volume container.

Processes themselves can also be classified as spontaneous or nonspontaneous. A **spontaneous process** is one that can occur by itself without having to be driven by energy from an outside source. Calculating the change in the Gibbs free energy (ΔG) for a process, such as a chemical reaction, allows us to predict whether the process will be spontaneous or nonspontaneous. As discussed later in the chapter, the same quantities that are used to calculate the change in the Gibbs free energy, ΔH and ΔS, can also tell us whether the process will be temperature dependent; that is, spontaneous at some temperatures and nonspontaneous at others.

Spontaneous reactions, as mentioned in Chapters 5 and 6 of *MCAT General Chemistry Review*, will not necessarily happen quickly and may not go to completion. Many spontaneous reactions have very high activation energies and, therefore, rarely take place. For example, when was the last time you saw a match ignite itself? However, providing a quantity of thermal energy (generated by the friction associated with striking the match) that equals or exceeds the activation energy will allow the match to light and burn spontaneously. At this point, the combustion of the chemical components of the match using molecular oxygen in the air will not need any additional external energy once the activation energy has been supplied.

Some spontaneous reactions proceed very slowly. The role of enzymes—biological catalysts—is to selectively enhance the rate of certain spontaneous (but slow) chemical reactions so that the biologically necessary products can be formed at a rate sufficient for sustaining life. As we discussed in Chapter 6 of *MCAT General Chemistry Review*, some reactions do not go to completion but settle into a low-energy state called equilibrium. Spontaneous reactions may go to completion, but many simply reach equilibrium with dynamically stable concentrations of reactants and products. A common method for supplying energy for nonspontaneous reactions is by **coupling** nonspontaneous reactions to spontaneous ones, as shown in Figure 7.9.

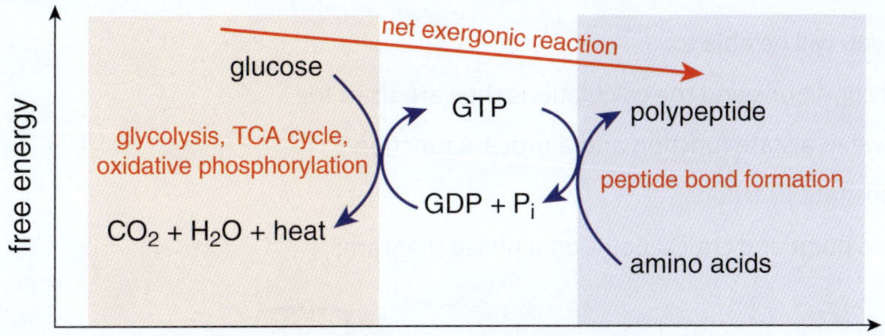

Figure 7.9 Coupling of Reactions
The combustion of glucose is exergonic; the formation of peptide bonds is endergonic. Energy from the combustion of glucose can be stored in the bonds in GTP, which are then lysed to provide the energy for forming peptide bonds.

MCAT CONCEPT CHECK 7.1

Before you move on, assess your understanding of the material with these questions.

1. A person snaps an ice pack and places it on one leg. In terms of energy transfer, what would be considered the system and what would be the surroundings in this scenario?
   - System:

   ___

   - Surroundings:

   ___

2. What is unique about each of the following types of processes?
   - Isothermal:

   ___

   - Adiabatic:

   ___

   - Isobaric:

   ___

   - Isovolumetric (isochoric):

   ___

7.2 States and State Functions

LEARNING OBJECTIVES

After Chapter 7.2, you will be able to:

- Recall standard conditions and the calculations they are used for
- Distinguish between a state function and a process function
- List the common state functions
- Identify the triple point and critical point on a phase diagram:

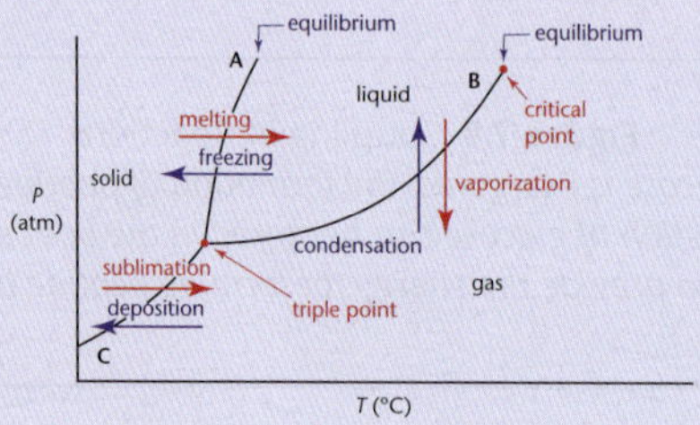

The state of a system can be described by certain macroscopic properties. These properties, or **state functions**, describe the system in an equilibrium state. They cannot describe the process of the system; that is, how the system got to its current equilibrium. They are useful only for comparing one equilibrium state to another. The pathway taken from one equilibrium state to another is described quantitatively by the **process functions**, the most important of which are work (W) and heat (Q).

Overview

The state functions include pressure (P), density (ρ), temperature (T), volume (V), enthalpy (H), internal energy (U), Gibbs free energy (G), and entropy (S). When the state of a system changes from one equilibrium to another, one or more of these state functions will change. In addition, while state functions are independent of the path (process) taken, they are not necessarily independent of one another. For example, Gibbs free energy is related to enthalpy, temperature, and entropy.

Because systems can be in different equilibrium states at different temperatures and pressures, a set of **standard conditions** has been defined for measuring the enthalpy, entropy, and Gibbs free energy changes of a reaction. The standard conditions are defined as 25°C (298 K), 1 atm pressure, and 1 M concentrations of each reactant and each product. Don't confuse standard conditions with **standard temperature and pressure** (**STP**), for which the temperature is 0°C (273 K) and pressure is 1 atm. Standard conditions are used for kinetics, equilibrium, and thermodynamics problems; STP is used for ideal gas calculations.

Under standard conditions, the most stable form of a substance is called the **standard state** of that substance. You should recognize the standard states for some elements and compounds commonly encountered on the MCAT. For example, H_2 (*g*), H_2O (*l*), NaCl (*s*), O_2 (*g*), and C (*s*, graphite) are the most stable forms of these substances under standard conditions. Recognizing whether or not a substance is in its standard state is important for thermochemical calculations, such as heats of reactions and—in particular—heats of formation. The changes in enthalpy, entropy, and free energy that occur when a reaction takes place under standard conditions are called the **standard enthalpy**, **standard entropy**, and **standard free energy changes**, respectively, and are symbolized by ΔH°, ΔS°, and ΔG°. The degree sign in these variables represents zero, as the standard state is used as the "zero point" for all thermodynamic calculations.

MNEMONIC

State functions: When I'm under **pressure** and feeling **dense**, all I want to do is watch **TV** and get **HUGS**.

Pressure (P), density (ρ), temperature (T), volume (V), enthalpy (H), internal energy (U), Gibbs free energy (G), and entropy (S).

MCAT EXPERTISE

On the MCAT, be sure that you do not confuse standard conditions in thermodynamics with standard temperature and pressure (STP), which is used in gas law calculations:

- Standard conditions: 25°C (298 K), 1 atm pressure, 1 M concentrations
- STP: 0°C (273 K), 1 atm pressure

Phase Changes

Phase diagrams (see Figure 7.10 below) are graphs that show the standard and nonstandard states of matter for a given substance in an isolated system, as determined by temperatures and pressures. **Phase changes** (solid $\rightleftharpoons$ liquid $\rightleftharpoons$ gas) are reversible, and an equilibrium of phases will eventually be reached at any given combination of temperature and pressure. For example, at 0°C and 1 atm in an isolated system, ice and water exist in an equilibrium. In other words, some of the ice may absorb heat (from the liquid water) and melt, but because that heat is being removed from the liquid water, an equal amount of the liquid water will freeze and form ice. Thus, the relative amounts of ice and water remain constant. Equilibrium between the liquid and gas states of water will be established in a closed container at room temperature and atmospheric pressure, such as a plastic water bottle with the cap screwed on tightly. Most of the water in the bottle will be in the liquid phase, but a small number of molecules at the surface will gain enough kinetic energy to escape into the gas phase; likewise, a small number of gas molecules will lose sufficient kinetic energy to reenter the liquid phase. After a while, equilibrium is established, and the relative amounts of water in the liquid and gas phases become constant—at standard conditions, equilibrium occurs when the air above the water has about 3 percent water vapor by mass. Phase equilibria are analogous to the dynamic equilibria of reversible chemical reactions: the concentrations of reactants and products are constant because the rates of the forward and reverse reactions are equal.

KEY CONCEPT

As with all equilibria, the rates of the forward and reverse processes will be the same when considering phase changes.

Gas–Liquid Equilibrium

The temperature of any substance in any phase is related to the average kinetic energy of the molecules that make up the substance. However, not all of the molecules have exactly the same instantaneous speeds. Therefore, the molecules possess a range of instantaneous kinetic energy values. In the liquid phase, the molecules are relatively free to move around one another. Some of the molecules near the surface of the liquid may have enough kinetic energy to leave the liquid phase and escape into the gaseous phase. This process is known as **evaporation** or **vaporization**. Each time the liquid loses a high-energy particle, the temperature of the remaining liquid decreases. Evaporation is an endothermic process for which the heat source is the liquid water. Of course, the liquid water itself may be receiving thermal energy from some other source, as in the case of a puddle of water drying up under the hot summer sun or a pot of water on the stovetop. Given enough energy, the liquid will completely evaporate.

Boiling is a specific type of vaporization that occurs only under certain conditions. Any liquid will lose some particles to the vapor phase over time; however, boiling is the rapid bubbling of the entire liquid with rapid release of the liquid as gas particles. While evaporation happens in all liquids at all temperatures, boiling can only occur above the boiling point of a liquid and involves vaporization through the entire volume of the liquid.

In a covered or closed container, the escaping molecules are trapped above the solution. These molecules exert a countering pressure, which forces some of the gas back into the liquid phase; this process is called **condensation**. Condensation is facilitated by lower temperature or higher pressure. Atmospheric pressure acts on a liquid in a manner similar to that of an actual physical lid. As evaporation and condensation proceed, the respective rates of the two processes become equal, and equilibrium is reached. The pressure that the gas exerts over the liquid at equilibrium is the vapor pressure of the liquid. Vapor pressure increases as temperature increases because more molecules have sufficient kinetic energy to escape into the gas phase. The temperature at which the vapor pressure of the liquid equals the ambient (also known as external, applied, or incident) pressure is called the **boiling point**.

Liquid–Solid Equilibrium

We've already illustrated the equilibrium that can exist between the liquid and the solid phases of water at 0°C. Even though the atoms or molecules of a solid are confined to specific locations, each atom or molecule can undergo motions about some equilibrium position. These vibrational motions increase when heat is applied. From our understanding of entropy, we can say that the availability of energy **microstates** increases as the temperature of the solid increases. In basic terms, this means that the molecules have greater freedom of movement, and energy disperses. If atoms or molecules in the solid phase absorb enough energy, the three-dimensional structure of the solid will break down, and the atoms or molecules will escape into the liquid phase. The transition from solid to liquid is called **fusion** or **melting**. The reverse process, from liquid to solid, is called **solidification**, **crystallization**, or **freezing**. The temperature at which these processes occur is called the **melting point** or **freezing point**, depending on the direction of the transition. Whereas pure crystalline solids have distinct, very precise melting points, amorphous solids, such as glass, plastic, chocolate, and candle wax, tend to melt (or solidify) over a larger range of temperatures due to their less-ordered molecular structure.

Gas–Solid Equilibrium

The final phase equilibrium is that which exists between the gaseous and solid phases. When a solid goes directly into the gas phase, the process is called **sublimation**. Dry ice (solid CO_2) sublimes at room temperature and atmospheric pressure; the absence of the liquid phase makes it a convenient dry refrigerant. The reverse transition, from the gaseous to the solid phase, is called **deposition**. In organic chemistry laboratories, a device known as a **cold finger** may be used to purify a product that is heated under reduced pressure, causing it to sublime. The desired product is usually more volatile than the impurities, so the gas is purer than the original product and the impurities are left in the solid state. The gas then deposits onto the cold finger, which has cold water flowing through it, yielding a purified solid product that can be collected.

Phase Diagrams

Phase diagrams are graphs that show the temperatures and pressures at which a substance will be thermodynamically stable in a particular phase. They also show the temperatures and pressures at which phases will be in equilibrium.

The lines on a phase diagram are called the **lines of equilibrium** or the **phase boundaries** and indicate the temperature and pressure values for the equilibria between phases. The lines of equilibrium divide the diagram into three regions corresponding to the three phases—solid, liquid, and gas—and they themselves represent the phase transformations. The phase diagram for a single compound is shown in Figure 7.10.

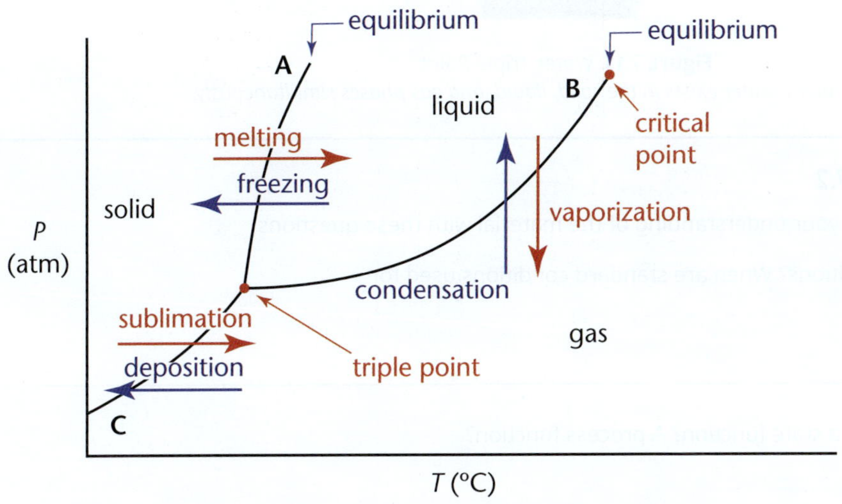

Figure 7.10 Phase Diagram for a Single Compound

MCAT EXPERTISE

On the MCAT, you should be able to identify and understand each area and every line of a phase diagram.

Line **A** represents the solid–liquid interface, line **B** the liquid–gas interface, and line **C** the solid–gas interface. In general, the gas phase is found at high temperatures and low pressures, the solid phase is found at low temperatures and high pressures, and the liquid phase is found at moderate temperatures and moderate pressures. The point at which the three phase boundaries meet is called the **triple point**. This is the temperature and pressure at which the three phases exist in equilibrium. Figure 7.11 shows a beaker of water at its triple point. In the same beaker, water exists as a gas, a liquid, and as solid ice. The phase boundary that separates the solid and the liquid phases extends indefinitely from the triple point. The phase boundary between the liquid and gas phases, however, terminates at a point called the **critical point**. This is the temperature and pressure above which there is no distinction between the phases. Although this may seem to be an impossibility—after all, it's always possible to distinguish between the liquid and the solid phase—such **supercritical fluids** are perfectly logical. As a liquid is heated in a closed system its

REAL WORLD

Because of water's unique properties, ice floats and skates flow smoothly over ice rinks. This all "boils" down to the negative slope of the solid–liquid equilibrium line in its phase diagram. Because the density of ice is less than that of liquid water, an increase in pressure (at a constant temperature) will actually melt ice (the opposite of what is seen for the substance in Figure 7.10).

density decreases and the density of the vapor sitting above it increases. The critical point is the temperature and pressure at which the two densities become equal and there is no distinction between the two phases. The heat of vaporization at this point and for all temperatures and pressures above the critical point values is zero.

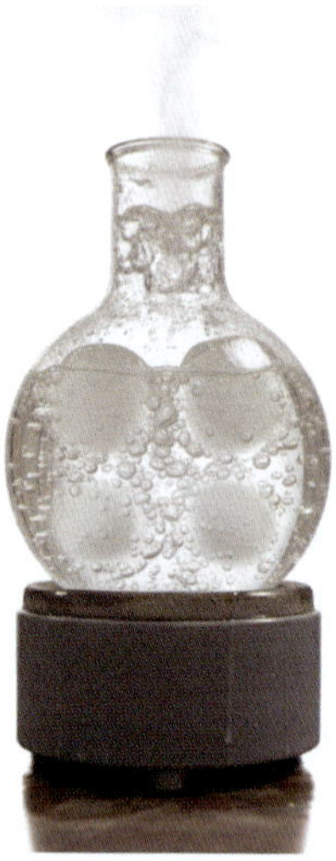

Figure 7.11 Water Triple Point
At its triple point, water exists in the solid, liquid, and gas phases simultaneously.

MCAT CONCEPT CHECK 7.2

Before you move on, assess your understanding of the material with these questions.

1. What are standard conditions? When are standard conditions used for calculations?

____

2. What is the definition of a state function? A process function?
   - State function:

____

   - Process function:

____

3. List at least five common state functions:
   -

____

   -

____

   -

____

-

-

4. Identify the triple point and critical point on the diagram below. What is the definition of the triple point? The critical point?

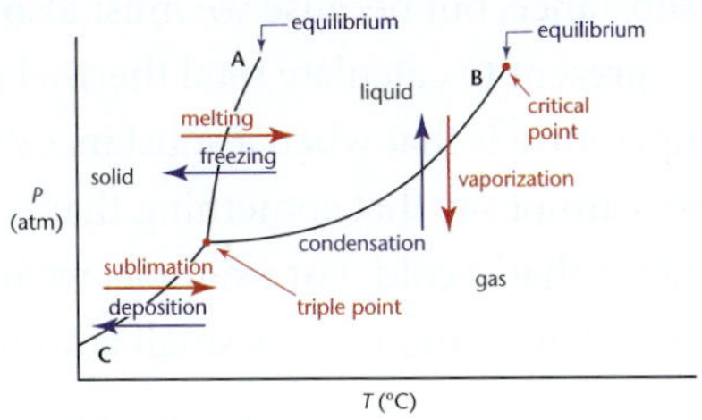

- Triple point:

- Critical point:

7.3 Heat

LEARNING OBJECTIVES

After Chapter 7.3, you will be able to:

- Differentiate between temperature and heat
- Compare specific heat and heat capacity
- Recall the specific heat of water
- Describe the processes for constant-volume and constant-pressure calorimetry:

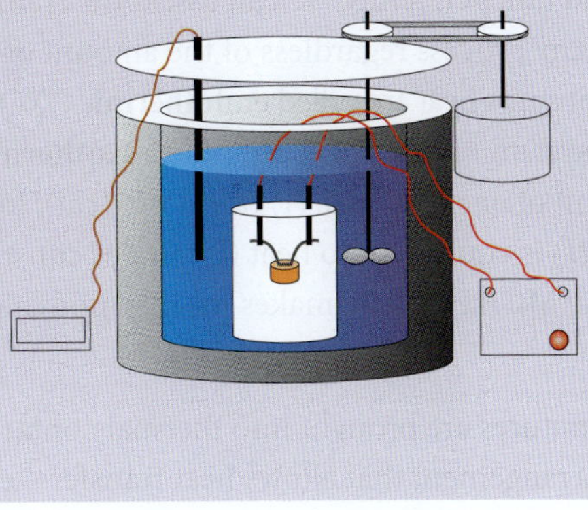

Before we can examine the first of the four state functions that are the focus of this chapter, we must address the topic of heat, which is a source of confusion for many students. Perhaps the greatest barrier to a proper understanding of heat is the semantic conflation of the terms *heat* and *temperature*. Many people use these terms interchangeably in everyday conversation, but this obscures the lexicon of thermodynamics. **Temperature** (*T*) is related to the average kinetic energy of the particles of a substance. Temperature is the way that we scale how hot or cold something is. We are familiar with a few temperature scales: Fahrenheit, Celsius, and Kelvin. The average kinetic energy of the particles in a substance is related to the **thermal energy** (**enthalpy**) of the substance, but because we must also include consideration of how much substance is present to calculate total thermal energy content, the most we can say about temperature is that when a substance's thermal energy increases, its temperature also increases. Nevertheless, we cannot say that something that is hot necessarily has greater thermal energy (in absolute terms) than a substance that is cold. For example, we might determine that a large amount of lukewarm water has a greater *total* heat content than a very small amount of hot water.

KEY CONCEPT

Remember that heat and temperature are different. Heat is a specific form of energy that can enter or leave a system, while temperature is a measure of the average kinetic energy of the particles in a system.

The absolute temperature scale, Kelvin, was determined via the third law of thermodynamics, which elucidated that there is a finite limit to temperature below which nothing can exist. There can be no temperature below 0 K because, by definition, the system is said to be unable to lose any more heat energy. Quantum mechanics describes a state of molecular motions possible below absolute zero, but this is beyond the scope of the MCAT.

REAL WORLD

One of the most important ways that the body works to prevent overheating is through the production of sweat—an exocrine secretion of water, electrolytes, and urea. However, it is not the *production* of sweat that is the cooling mechanism. It's the *evaporation* of the sweat that helps cool the body. Evaporation (vaporization) from the liquid to gas phase is an endothermic process: energy must be absorbed from the body for the particles of the liquid to gain enough kinetic energy to escape into the gas phase. Hot, arid desert air has a lower partial pressure of water vapor than humid, tropical air, so sweat vaporizes more readily in the dry air than it does in the humid air. Accordingly, most people will feel more comfortable in dry heat than in humid heat.

Overview

Heat (***Q***) is the transfer of energy from one substance to another as a result of their differences in temperature. In fact, the **zeroth law of thermodynamics** implies that objects are in thermal equilibrium only when their temperatures are equal. Heat is therefore a process function, not a state function: we can quantify how much thermal energy is transferred between two or more objects as a result of their difference in temperatures by measuring the heat transferred.

Remember that the first law of thermodynamics states that the change in the total internal energy (ΔU) of a system is equal to the amount of heat (Q) transferred to the system minus the amount of work (W) done by the system: $\Delta U = Q - W$.

Because heat and work are measured independently, we can assess the transfer of energy in the form of heat through any process regardless of the amount of work done. Processes in which the system absorbs heat are called **endothermic** ($\Delta Q > 0$), while those processes in which the system releases heat are called **exothermic** ($\Delta Q < 0$). The unit of heat is the unit of energy: joule (J) or calorie (cal), for which 1 cal = 4.184 J. **Enthalpy** ($\boldsymbol{\Delta H}$) is equivalent to heat (Q) under constant pressure, which is an assumption the MCAT usually makes for thermodynamics problems.

When substances of different temperatures are brought into thermal contact with each other—that is, some physical arrangement that allows heat transfer—energy will move from the warmer substance to the cooler substance. When a substance undergoes an endothermic or exothermic reaction, heat energy will be exchanged between the system and the environment.

The process of measuring transferred heat is called **calorimetry**. Two basic types of calorimetry include constant-pressure calorimetry and constant-volume calorimetry. The coffee-cup calorimeter, introduced at the beginning of this chapter, is a low-tech example of a constant-pressure calorimeter, while a bomb calorimeter is an example of a constant-volume calorimeter.

The heat (q) absorbed or released in a given process is calculated via the equation:

$$q = mc\Delta T$$

Equation 7.2

where m is the mass, c is the specific heat of the substance, and ΔT is the change in temperature (in kelvin or degrees Celsius). **Specific heat** is defined as the amount of energy required to raise the temperature of one gram of a substance by one degree Celsius (or one kelvin). Specific heat values will generally be provided on Test Day, but one constant to remember is the specific heat of $H_2O(l) : c_{H_2O} = 1 \frac{\text{cal}}{\text{g} \cdot \text{K}}$.

It requires less heat to raise the temperature of a glass of water the same amount as a swimming pool. While these two items have the same specific heat, c, they have different **heat capacities**—the product mc (mass times specific heat).

MNEMONIC

The equation for heat transfer, given a specific heat, is the same as the test you're studying for! $q = mc\Delta T$ looks a lot like "q equals MCAT."

REAL WORLD

When walking barefoot, a blacktop *feels* much hotter than a wooden walkway even when they are the same temperature. This is because they have different specific heats.

Constant-Pressure and Constant-Volume Calorimetry

To picture the setup of a **constant-pressure calorimeter**, just think of the coffee-cup calorimeter: an insulated container covered with a lid and filled with a solution in which a reaction or some physical process, such as dissolution, is occurring. The incident pressure, which is atmospheric pressure, remains constant throughout the process, and the temperature can be measured as the reaction progresses. There should be sufficient thermal insulation (such as Styrofoam) to ensure that the heat being measured is an accurate representation of the reaction, without gain or loss of heat to the environment. Other commercial applications of these same principles include home insulation, padded clothing, and certain food containers such as thermoses.

REAL WORLD

Tests looking at plasma proteins or cancer diagnostics in medicine have utilized differential scanning calorimetry (DSC), which is a constant-pressure device, to identify blood components. Such results have shown that thermal properties of major plasma proteins are altered from early- to late-stage tumors.

The term **bomb calorimeter** may sound rather ominous, but a more accurate descriptive term is **decomposition vessel**. This better reflects what is actually taking place in **constant-volume calorimetry**. As shown in Figure 7.12, a sample of matter, typically a hydrocarbon, is placed in the steel decomposition vessel, which is then filled with almost pure oxygen gas. The decomposition vessel is then placed in an insulated container holding a known mass of water. The contents of the decomposition vessel are ignited by an electric ignition mechanism. The material combusts (burns) in the presence of the oxygen, and the heat that evolves is the heat of the combustion reaction. Because $W = P\Delta V$, no work is done in an isovolumetric process ($\Delta V = 0$), so $W_{\text{calorimeter}} = 0$. Furthermore, because of the insulation, the whole calorimeter can be considered isolated from the rest of the universe, so we can identify the system as the sample plus the oxygen and steel vessel, and the surroundings as the water.

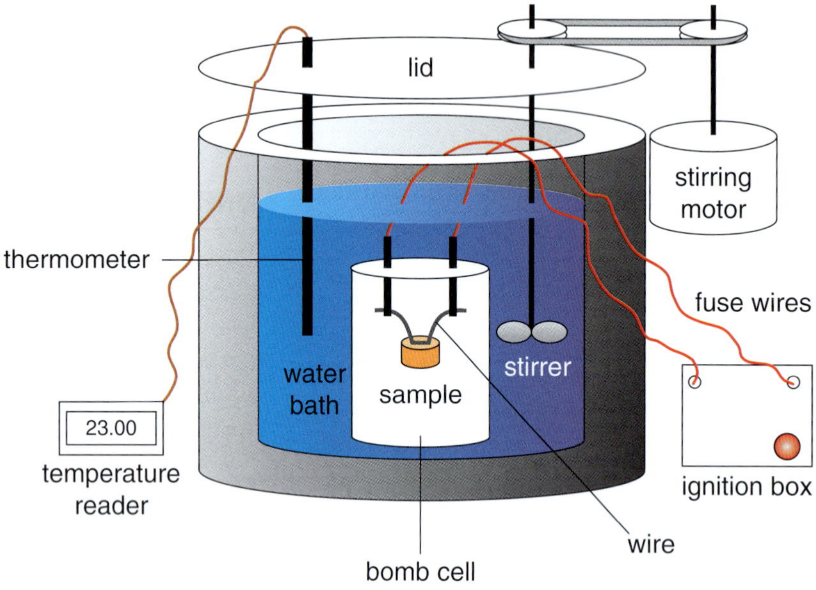

Figure 7.12 Diagram of a Bomb Calorimeter

Because no heat is exchanged between the calorimeter and the rest of the universe, $Q_{\text{calorimeter}}$ is 0. So,

$$\Delta U_{\text{system}} + \Delta U_{\text{surroundings}} = \Delta U_{\text{calorimeter}} = Q_{\text{calorimeter}} - W_{\text{calorimeter}} = 0$$

Therefore,

$$\Delta U_{\text{system}} = -\Delta U_{\text{surroundings}}$$

and because no work is done,

$$q_{\text{system}} = -q_{\text{surroundings}}$$

$$m_{\text{steel}} c_{\text{steel}} \Delta T + m_{\text{oxygen}} c_{\text{oxygen}} \Delta T = -m_{\text{water}} c_{\text{water}} \Delta T$$

Note that by using the layer of insulation to isolate the entire calorimeter from the rest of the universe, we've created an adiabatic process. This means that no heat is exchanged between the calorimeter and the rest of the universe, but it *is* exchanged between the steel decomposition vessel and the surrounding water. As the previous derivation shows, heat exchange between the system and its surroundings makes it possible for us to calculate the heat of combustion.

REAL WORLD

Bomb calorimeters have helped elucidate the thermodynamic properties of various chemical compounds, including food additives, to determine nutritional value (the caloric content of the additive).

MCAT EXPERTISE

Knowing that heat can transfer energy from a system to the surroundings is a key concept tested on calorimetry questions. Whenever you are asked about equilibrium questions regarding the final temperature of a two-liquid (or liquid–solid) system, remember that the colder object gains thermal energy and the hotter object loses it. You should instinctively realize that a metal bar at 1000 K is hotter than a bath of water at 298 K even though water has a high specific heat. Thus, set up the equation as $q_{\text{cold}} = -q_{\text{hot}}$. This form of the equation avoids the pesky sign notation issues in the ΔT equation encountered in most general chemistry texts.

Example: One cup containing 100 grams of water at 300 K is mixed into another cup containing 200 g of water at 450 K. What is the equilibrium temperature of the system? (Note: Assume that the pressure is sufficiently high to avoid boiling.)

Solution: The two liquids undergo thermal exchange; thus, the heat given off by one liquid will be equal to the heat absorbed by the other.

$$q_{\text{cold}} = -q_{\text{hot}}$$
$$m_{\text{cold}} c_{H_2O} \Delta T_{\text{cold}} = m_{\text{hot}} c_{H_2O}(-\Delta T_{\text{hot}})$$

Now plug in the values from the question. Because we are solving for final (equilibrium) temperature of a mixture, we can use any value of c so long as we are consistent for both liquids (in this case we have two quantities of water and will use $c_{H_2O} = 1 \frac{\text{cal}}{\text{g} \cdot \text{K}}$).

$$m_{\text{cold}} c_{H_2O} \Delta T_{\text{cold}} = m_{\text{hot}} c_{H_2O}(-\Delta T_{\text{hot}})$$
$$(100 \text{ g})\left(1 \frac{\text{cal}}{\text{g} \cdot \text{K}}\right)(T_f - 300 \text{ K}) = (200 \text{ g})\left(1 \frac{\text{cal}}{\text{g} \cdot \text{K}}\right)(450 \text{ K} - T_f)$$
$$100\, T_f - 30{,}000 \text{ cal} = 90{,}000 \text{ cal} - 200\, T_f$$
$$300\, T_f = 120{,}000$$
$$T_f = \frac{120{,}000}{300} = 400 \text{ K}$$

Heating Curves

When a compound is heated, the temperature rises until the melting or boiling point is reached. Then, the temperature remains constant as the compound is converted to the next phase (liquid or gas, respectively). Once the entire sample is converted, then the temperature begins to rise again. This is depicted in the heating curves in Figure 7.13.

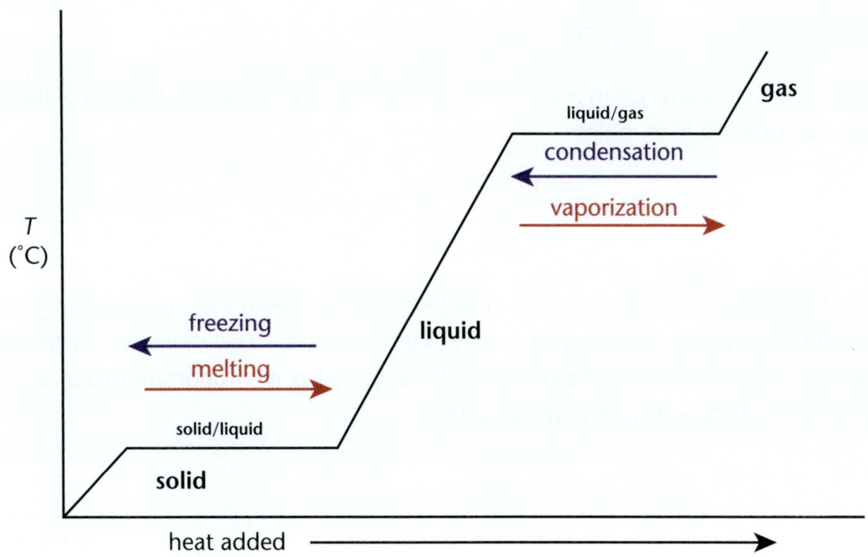

Figure 7.13 Heating Curve for a Single Compound

Heating curves show that phase change reactions do not undergo changes in temperature. For this reason, we cannot use $q = mc\Delta T$ during this interval because $\Delta T = 0$. We know intuitively that heat must continue to be added in order for the whole solid to melt, so where does this heat go? The solid absorbs energy, which allows particles to overcome the attractive forces that hold them in a rigid, three-dimensional arrangement. When melting an ice cube, all of the heat added during the process is used to overcome the intermolecular forces between water molecules in ice, forming liquid water. Once all of the ice has been turned into liquid water, the temperature of the liquid water can then increase again. The converse is also true: removing heat from a liquid at the solid–liquid phase transition temperature will cause the formation of a rigid lattice of water molecules.

During phase changes, we must use values based on enthalpy. When transitioning at the solid–liquid boundary, the **enthalpy** (or **heat**) **of fusion** (**ΔH_{fus}**) must be used to determine the heat transferred during the phase change. When transitioning from solid to liquid, the change in enthalpy will be positive because heat must be added; when transitioning from a liquid to a solid, the change in enthalpy will be negative because heat must be removed. At the liquid–gas boundary, the **enthalpy** (or **heat**) **of vaporization** (**ΔH_{vap}**) must be used, and its sign convention also follows a similar pattern. These are utilized in the equation

$$q = mL$$

Equation 7.3

where m is the mass and L is the **latent heat**, a general term for the enthalpy of an isothermal process, given in the units $\frac{\text{cal}}{\text{g}}$.

The total amount of heat needed to cross multiple phase boundaries is simply a summation of the heats for changing the temperature of each of the respective phases and the heats associated with phase changes.

KEY CONCEPT

We need a different formula to calculate q during phase changes when $\Delta T = 0$. If we used $q = mc\Delta T$, we'd erroneously think $q = 0$.

Example: What amount of energy is required to change a 90 gram ice cube at −10°C to vapor at 110°C? (Note:

$c_{H_2O\,(l)} = 4.18\,\frac{\text{J}}{\text{g}\cdot\text{K}}$, $c_{H_2O\,(s)} = 2.18\,\frac{\text{J}}{\text{g}\cdot\text{K}}$, $c_{H_2O\,(g)} = 2.00\,\frac{\text{J}}{\text{g}\cdot\text{K}}$,

$\Delta H_{fus} = 6.02\,\frac{\text{kJ}}{\text{mol}}$, $\Delta H_{vap} = 40.67\,\frac{\text{kJ}}{\text{mol}}$)

Solution: Some of the constants given are in terms of mass (g), and some are in terms of moles, so we should convert the mass (90 g) to moles:

$$n = \frac{90\text{ g } H_2O}{18\,\frac{\text{g}}{\text{mol}}} = \frac{10}{2} = 5\text{ moles } H_2O$$

Because we are beginning in the ice phase, we must heat the ice cube to the solid–liquid phase transition, which occurs at 0°C. This first step involves a change in temperature, so we must use the heat formula that contains ΔT and all the pertinent variables for ice (solid water). Also, it is important to match all results in terms of J and kJ for the different steps of the calculation.

$$q_1 = m_{ice} c_{ice} \Delta T_1$$

$$q_1 = (90\text{ g})\left(2.18 \frac{\text{J}}{\text{g}\cdot\text{K}}\right)(10\text{ K}) \approx 90 \times 2 \times 10 = 1800\text{ J} = 1.8\text{ kJ}$$

In step 2, we must convert the ice into liquid form. During this phase change, there will be no temperature change.

$$q_2 = mL = n_{H_2O} \Delta H_{fus}$$

$$q_2 = (5\text{ mol})\left(6.02 \frac{\text{kJ}}{\text{mol}}\right) \approx 5 \times 6 = 30\text{ kJ}$$

In step 3, we heat the water to its liquid–gas phase transition temperature at 100°C.

$$q_3 = m_{water} c_{water} \Delta T_3$$

$$q_3 = (90\text{ g})\left(4.18 \frac{\text{J}}{\text{g}\cdot\text{K}}\right)(100\text{ K}) \approx 90 \times 4 \times 100 = 36{,}000\text{ J} = 36\text{ kJ}$$

In step 4, we vaporize the water. Again, no temperature change will occur during this phase change.

$$q_4 = mL = n_{H_2O} \Delta H_{vap}$$

$$q_4 = (5\text{ mol})\left(40.67 \frac{\text{kJ}}{\text{mol}}\right) \approx 5 \times 40 = 200\text{ kJ}$$

In step 5, we must finally heat the water to the target temperature of 110°C.

$$q_5 = m_{steam} c_{steam} \Delta T_5$$

$$q_5 = (90\text{ g})\left(2.00 \frac{\text{J}}{\text{g}\cdot\text{K}}\right)(10\text{ K}) = 90 \times 2 \times 10 = 1800\text{ J} = 1.8\text{ kJ}$$

The total heat required for this whole phase change from beginning to end is:

$$q_{tot} = q_1 + q_2 + q_3 + q_4 + q_5$$

$$q_{tot} = 1.8 + 30 + 36 + 200 + 1.8$$

$$q_{tot} \approx 2 + 30 + 36 + 200 + 2 = 270\text{ kJ (actual value} = 274.8\text{ kJ)}$$

A question *this* involved is unlikely to be seen on the MCAT because so many steps must be calculated. However, understanding the significance and rationale of this calculation is definitely within the scope of the test.

MCAT EXPERTISE

It is not in your best interest to memorize all the possible values for c and ΔH for Test Day. The MCAT will provide constants as needed, especially if the system is not water. That being said, practicing with heat calculations for water solutions and gaining familiarity with the heat capacities of water will help on Test Day.

MCAT CONCEPT CHECK 7.3

Before you move on, assess your understanding of the material with these questions.

1. Contrast temperature and heat.
   - Temperature:

   - Heat:

   ---

2. Contrast specific heat and heat capacity.
   - Specific heat:

   - Heat capacity:

   ---

3. Contrast constant-volume and constant-pressure calorimetry.
   - Constant-volume:

   - Constant-pressure:

   ---

4. What is the specific heat of liquid water (in calories)?

7.4 Enthalpy

LEARNING OBJECTIVES

After Chapter 7.4, you will be able to:

- Distinguish between endothermic and exothermic reactions
- Determine the enthalpy of a molecule or atom given reaction data:

$$C\,(s,\text{graphite}) + 2\,H_2\,(g) \rightarrow CH_4\,(g)$$

$$CH_4(g) + 2\,O_2\,(g) \rightarrow CO_2(g) + 2\,H_2O\,(l) \qquad \Delta H_a = -890.4\,\frac{\text{kJ}}{\text{mol}}$$

$$C\,(s,\text{graphite}) + O_2(g) \rightarrow CO_2\,(g) \qquad \Delta H_b = -393.5\,\frac{\text{kJ}}{\text{mol}}$$

$$2 \times \left[H_2(g) + \tfrac{1}{2}\,O_2(g) \rightarrow H_2O\,(l)\right] \qquad \Delta H_g = 2 \times -285.8\,\frac{\text{kJ}}{\text{mol}}$$

Most reactions in the laboratory occur under constant pressure (at 1 atm) in closed thermodynamic systems. To express heat changes at constant pressure, chemists use the term **enthalpy** (***H***). Enthalpy is a state function, so we can calculate the change in enthalpy (ΔH) for a system that has undergone a process—for example, a chemical reaction—by comparing the enthalpy of the final state to the enthalpy of the initial state, irrespective of the path taken. The change in enthalpy is equal to the heat transferred into or out of the system at constant pressure. To find the enthalpy change of a reaction, ΔH_{rxn}, one must subtract the enthalpy of the reactants from the enthalpy of the products:

$$\Delta H_{\text{rxn}} = H_{\text{products}} - H_{\text{reactants}}$$

Equation 7.4

A positive ΔH_{rxn} corresponds to an endothermic process, and a negative ΔH_{rxn} corresponds to an exothermic process. It is not possible to measure enthalpy directly; only ΔH can be measured, and only for certain fast and spontaneous processes. Thus, several methods have been developed to calculate ΔH for any process.

Standard Heat of Formation

The **standard enthalpy of formation** of a compound, ΔH_f°, is the enthalpy required to produce one mole of a compound from its elements in their standard states. Remember that *standard state* refers to the most stable physical state of an element or compound at 298 K and 1 atm. Note that ΔH_f° of an element in its standard state, by definition, is zero. The ΔH_f° values of most known substances are tabulated. You do not need to memorize these values because they will be provided for you.

Standard Heat of Reaction

The **standard enthalpy of a reaction**, ΔH_{rxn}°, is the enthalpy change accompanying a reaction being carried out under standard conditions. This can be calculated by taking the difference between the sum of the standard heats of formation for the products and the sum of the standard heats of formation of the reactants:

$$\Delta H_{\text{rxn}}^\circ = \Sigma\, \Delta H_{\text{f,products}}^\circ - \Sigma\, \Delta H_{\text{f,reactants}}^\circ$$

Equation 7.5

Hess's Law

Enthalpy is a state function and is a property of the equilibrium state, so the pathway taken for a process is irrelevant to the change in enthalpy from one equilibrium state to another. As a consequence of this, **Hess's law** states that enthalpy changes of reactions are additive. When thermochemical equations (chemical equations for which energy changes are known) are added to give the net equation for a reaction, the corresponding heats of reaction are also added to give the net heat of reaction, as shown in Figure 7.14.

KEY CONCEPT

State functions are always path independent.

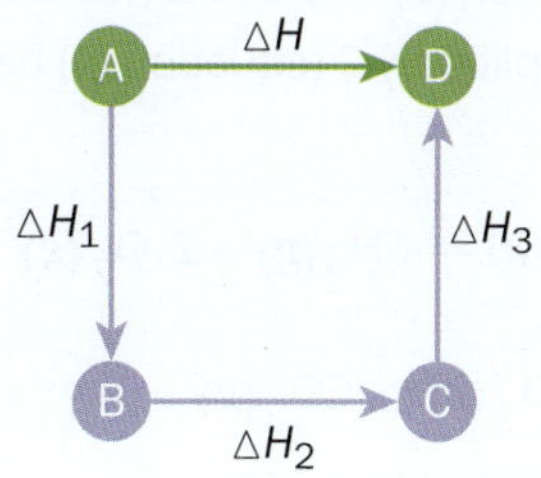

Figure 7.14 Illustration of Hess's Law: Forming Product (D) from Reactant (A)
Because enthalpy is a state function, $\Delta H = \Delta H_1 + \Delta H_2 + \Delta H_3$

Hess's law is embodied in the enthalpy equations we've already introduced. For example, we can describe any reaction as the result of breaking down the reactants into their component elements, then forming the products from these elements. The enthalpy change for the reverse of any reaction has the same magnitude, but the opposite sign, as the enthalpy change for the forward reaction. Therefore,

$$\Delta H_{\text{reactants} \rightarrow \text{elements}} = -\Delta H_{\text{elements} \rightarrow \text{reactants}}$$

The ΔH_{rxn} can be written as:

$$\Delta H_{\text{rxn}} = \Delta H_{\text{reactants} \rightarrow \text{elements}} + \Delta H_{\text{elements} \rightarrow \text{products}}$$

which is another way of writing

$$\Delta H^\circ_{\text{rxn}} = \Sigma\, \Delta H^\circ_{\text{f,products}} - \Sigma\, \Delta H^\circ_{\text{f,reactants}}$$

Consider the following phase change:

$$Br_2(l) \rightarrow Br_2(g) \qquad \Delta H^\circ_{\text{rxn}} = 31\ \frac{\text{kJ}}{\text{mol}}$$

The enthalpy change for the phase change is called the heat of vaporization ($\Delta H^\circ_{\text{vap}}$). As long as the initial and final states exist at standard conditions, the $\Delta H^\circ_{\text{rxn}}$ will always equal the $\Delta H^\circ_{\text{vap}}$, irrespective of the particular pathway that the process takes. For example, it's possible that Br_2 (l) could first decompose to Br atoms, which then recombine to form Br_2 (g), rather than simply boiling from the liquid to gaseous state. However, because the net reaction is the same, the change in enthalpy will be the same.

MCAT EXPERTISE

When doing a problem like this on the MCAT, make sure to switch signs when you reverse the equation. Also, make sure to multiply by the correct stoichiometric coefficients when performing your calculations.

Example: Given the following thermochemical equations:

(a) $CH_4\,(g) + 2\,O_2\,(g) \rightarrow CO_2\,(g) + 2\,H_2O\,(l)$ $\quad \Delta H_a = -890.4\ \frac{\text{kJ}}{\text{mol}}$

(b) $C\,(s, \text{graphite}) + O_2\,(g) \rightarrow CO_2\,(g)$ $\quad \Delta H_b = -393.5\ \frac{\text{kJ}}{\text{mol}}$

(c) $H_2\,(g) + \frac{1}{2}\,O_2\,(g) \rightarrow H_2O\,(l)$ $\quad \Delta H_c = -285.8\ \frac{\text{kJ}}{\text{mol}}$

Calculate ΔH for this reaction:

(d) $C\,(s, \text{graphite}) + 2\,H_2\,(g) \rightarrow CH_4\,(g)$

Solution: Equations (a), (b), and (c) must be combined to obtain equation (d). Because equation (d) contains only C, H_2, and CH_4, we must eliminate O_2, CO_2, and H_2O from the first three equations. Equation (a) is reversed to move CH_4 to the product side (equation (e) below). Next, equation (b) is left as is (we will call this equation (f) for consistency below) and (c) is multiplied by 2 (equation (g) below). Then, (d) can be calculated from (e) + (f) + (g):

(e) $CO_2\,(g) + 2\,H_2O\,(l) \rightarrow CH_4\,(g) + 2\,O_2\,(g)$ $\quad \Delta H_e = 890.4\ \frac{\text{kJ}}{\text{mol}}$

(f) $C\,(s, \text{graphite}) + O_2\,(g) \rightarrow CO_2\,(g)$ $\quad \Delta H_f = -393.5\ \frac{\text{kJ}}{\text{mol}}$

(g) $2 \times \left[H_2(g) + \frac{1}{2}O_2(g) \rightarrow H_2O(l)\right]$ $\qquad \Delta H_g = 2 \times -285.8 \frac{\text{kJ}}{\text{mol}}$

$C(s, \text{graphite}) + 2H_2(g) \rightarrow CH_4(g)$ $\qquad \Delta H_d = \Delta H_e + \Delta H_f + \Delta H_g$

$\Delta H_d = 890.4 + (-393.5) + [2 \times (-285.8)] \approx 900 + (-400) - (2 \times 285)$

$\Delta H_d = 900 - 400 - 570 = -70 \frac{\text{kJ}}{\text{mol}} \left(\text{actual value} = -74.7 \frac{\text{kJ}}{\text{mol}}\right)$

It is important to realize that Hess's law applies to *any* state function, including entropy and Gibbs free energy.

Bond Dissociation Energy

Hess's law can also be expressed in terms of **bond enthalpies**, also called **bond dissociation energies**. Bond dissociation energy is the average energy that is required to break a particular type of bond between atoms in the gas phase—remember, bond dissociation is an endothermic process. Bond dissociation energy is given in the units $\frac{\text{kJ}}{\text{mol of bonds broken}}$ and is often given in tables on the MCAT in a format similar to Table 7.1.

Bond	Enthalpy $\left(\Delta H, \frac{\text{kJ}}{\text{mol}}\right)$
O=O	498
C–H	415
H–H	436

Table 7.1 Sample Bond Enthalpies

Bond enthalpies are the averages of the bond energies for the same bond in many different compounds. For example, the C–H bond enthalpy $\left(415 \frac{\text{kJ}}{\text{mol}}\right)$ is averaged from measurements of the individual C–H bond enthalpies of thousands of different organic compounds. Note that bond formation, the opposite of bond breaking, has the same magnitude of energy but is negative rather than positive; that is, energy is released when bonds are formed. Remember that atoms generally form bonds to become more stable (often by completing an octet). Thus, it makes sense that bond formation is exothermic and bond dissociation is endothermic. The enthalpy change associated with a reaction is given by

KEY CONCEPT

Because it takes energy to pull two atoms apart, bond breakage is generally endothermic. The reverse process, bond formation, is generally exothermic.

$$\Delta H^\circ_{\text{rxn}} = \Sigma\, \Delta H_{\text{bonds broken}} - \Sigma\, \Delta H_{\text{bonds formed}} = \text{total energy absorbed} - \text{total energy released}$$

Equation 7.6

Example: Calculate the enthalpy change for the following reaction:

$$C\,(s) + 2\,H_2\,(g) \rightarrow CH_4\,(g) \qquad \Delta H = ?$$

Bond dissociation energies of H–H and C–H bonds are $436\,\frac{kJ}{mol}$ and $415\,\frac{kJ}{mol}$, respectively. The ΔH_f of C (g) is $715\,\frac{kJ}{mol}$.

Solution: CH_4 is formed from free elements in their standard states (C in solid state and H_2 in gaseous state). Thus, here $\Delta H_{rxn} = \Delta H_f$. The reaction can be written in three steps:

$$\text{(a) } C\,(s) \rightarrow C\,(g) \qquad \Delta H_1$$

$$\text{(b) } 2[H_2\,(g) \rightarrow 2\,H\,(g)] \qquad 2 \times \Delta H_2$$

$$\text{(c) } C\,(g) + 4\,H\,(g) \rightarrow CH_4\,(g) \qquad \Delta H_3$$

with $\Delta H_f = \Delta H_1 + (2 \times \Delta H_2) + \Delta H_3$.

$\Delta H_1 = \Delta H_f$ of C(g) $= 715\,\frac{kJ}{mol}$

ΔH_2 is the energy required to break the H–H bond of one mole of H_2, so ΔH_2 = bond enthalpy of H_2 = $436\,\frac{kJ}{mol}$. Note that reaction (b) is doubled in order to produce 4 atoms of H from two molecules of H_2.

ΔH_3 is the energy released when 4 C–H bonds are formed. Because energy is released when bonds are formed, ΔH_3 is negative.

$$\Delta H_3 = -(4 \times \text{bond energy of C–H}) = -\left(4 \times 415\,\frac{kJ}{mol}\right) = -1660\,\frac{kJ}{mol}$$

Therefore, for the entire reaction,

$$\Delta H_{rxn} = \Delta H_f = 715\,\frac{kJ}{mol} + \left(2 \times 436\,\frac{kJ}{mol}\right) - 1660\,\frac{kJ}{mol}$$

$$\Delta H_{rxn} \approx 700 + (2 \times 450) - 1660 = 700 + 900 - 1660 = -60\,\frac{kJ}{mol}$$

$$\left(\text{actual value} = -73\,\frac{kJ}{mol}\right)$$

Standard Heat of Combustion

As the name implies, the **standard heat of combustion, ΔH°_{comb}**, is the enthalpy change associated with the combustion of a fuel. Because measurements of enthalpy change require a reaction to be spontaneous and fast, combustion reactions are the ideal processes for such measurements. Most combustion reactions presented on the MCAT occur in the presence of atmospheric oxygen, but keep in mind that there are other combustion reactions in which oxygen is not the oxidant. Diatomic fluorine, for example, can be used as an oxidant. In addition, hydrogen gas will combust with chlorine gas to form gaseous hydrochloric acid and, in the process, will evolve a large amount of heat and light as is characteristic of combustion reactions. The reactions listed in the CH_4 (g) example shown earlier are combustion reactions with O_2 (g) as the oxidant. Therefore, the enthalpy change listed for each of the three reactions is the ΔH_{comb} for each of the reactions.

The glycolytic pathway, described in Chapter 9 of *MCAT Biochemistry Review*, is also a combustion reaction that utilizes a fuel (glucose) mixed with an oxidant (oxygen) to produce carbon dioxide and water.

$$C_6H_{12}O_6 + 6\ O_2 \rightarrow 6\ CO_2 + 6\ H_2O$$

The heat of combustion for this reaction is found in a similar fashion to that of Hess's Law. Given the numerous reactions and pathways involved, we can determine the overall enthalpy of the reaction, as shown in Figure 7.15.

KEY CONCEPT

The larger the alkane reactant, the more numerous the combustion products.

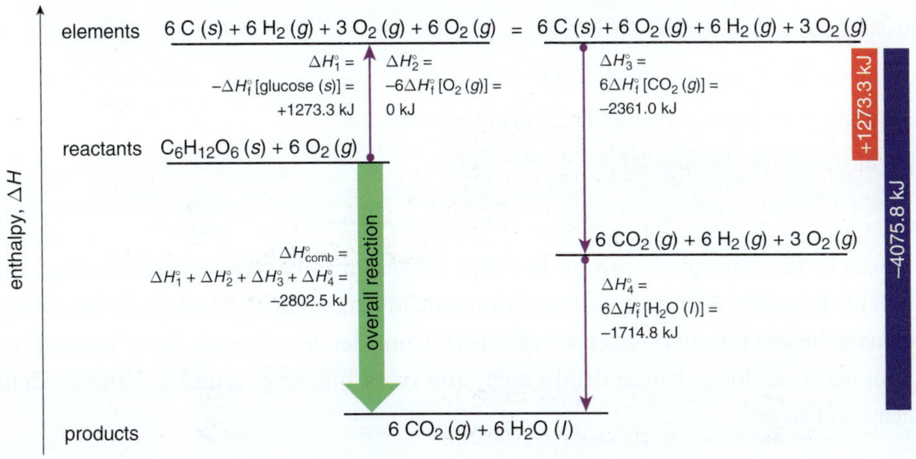

Figure 7.15 Determining the Enthalpy of Glycolysis

MCAT CONCEPT CHECK 7.4

Before you move on, assess your understanding of the material with these questions.

1. Define endothermic and exothermic processes.
   - Endothermic:

   ___

   - Exothermic:

   ___

2. Given the following reactions, determine the enthalpy of:

   $C\ (s, \text{graphite}) + \frac{1}{2}\ O_2 \rightarrow CO.$

   $C\ (s, \text{graphite}) + O_2 \rightarrow CO_2 \qquad \Delta H = -393.5\ \frac{kJ}{mol}$

   $CO + \frac{1}{2}\ O_2 \rightarrow CO_2 \qquad \Delta H = -283\ \frac{kJ}{mol}$

   ___

3. What is the enthalpy of reaction for the reaction: $2\ H_2O\ (g) \rightarrow 2\ H_2\ (g) + O_2\ (g)$, given the following and bond enthalpies: $H{-}H = 436\ \frac{kJ}{mol}$, $O{=}O = 498\ \frac{kJ}{mol}$, $O{-}O = 146\ \frac{kJ}{mol}$, and $O{-}H = 463\ \frac{kJ}{mol}$

7.5 Entropy

LEARNING OBJECTIVES

After Chapter 7.5, you will be able to:

- Order the phases of matter from lowest to highest entropy
- Define entropy in terms of its relation to energy distribution and disorder
- Predict the direction of change in entropy within a given reaction

Many students are perplexed by the concept of entropy. Enthalpy makes intuitive sense, especially when the energy change from reactants to products is large, fast, and dramatic (as in combustion reactions involving explosions). Entropy seems to be less intuitive—except that it isn't. Consider, for example, how "normal" each of the following seems: hot tea cools down, frozen drinks melt, iron rusts, buildings crumble, balloons deflate, living things die and decay, and so on.

These examples have a common denominator: in each of them, energy of some form is going from being localized or concentrated to being spread out or dispersed. The thermal energy in the hot tea is spreading out to the cooler air that surrounds it. The thermal energy in the warmer air is spreading out to the cooler frozen drink. The chemical energy in the bonds of elemental iron and oxygen is released and dispersed as a result of the formation of the more stable, lower-energy bonds of iron oxide (rust). The potential energy of the building is released and dispersed in the form of light, sound, and heat as the building crumbles and falls. The energy of the pressurized air is released to the surrounding atmosphere as the balloon deflates. The chemical energy of all the molecules and atoms in living flesh is released into the environment during the process of death and decay.

The **second law of thermodynamics** states that energy spontaneously disperses from being localized to becoming spread out if it is not hindered from doing so. Pay attention to this: *the usual way of thinking about entropy as "disorder" must not be taken too literally, a trap that many students fall into. Be very careful in thinking about entropy as disorder.* The old analogy between a messy (disordered) room and entropy is deficient and may not only hinder understanding but actually increase confusion.

Entropy is the measure of the spontaneous dispersal of energy at a specific temperature: *how much* energy is spread out, or *how widely* spread out energy becomes, in a process. The equation for calculating the change in entropy is:

$$\Delta S = \frac{Q_{\text{rev}}}{T}$$

Equation 7.7

where ΔS is the change in entropy, Q_{rev} is the heat that is gained or lost in a reversible process, and T is the temperature in kelvin. The units of entropy are usually $\frac{\text{J}}{\text{mol}\cdot\text{K}}$. When energy is distributed into a system at a given temperature, its entropy increases. When energy is distributed out of a system at a given temperature, its entropy decreases.

KEY CONCEPT

Entropy changes that accompany phase changes can be easily estimated, at least qualitatively. For example, freezing is accompanied by a decrease in entropy, as the relatively disordered liquid becomes a well-ordered solid. Meanwhile, boiling is accompanied by a large increase in entropy, as the liquid becomes a much more disordered gas. For any substance, sublimation will be the phase transition with the greatest increase in entropy.

Notice that the second law states that energy will spontaneously disperse; it does not say that energy can never be localized or concentrated. However, the concentration of energy will rarely happen spontaneously in a closed system. Work usually must be done to concentrate energy. For example, refrigerators work against the direction of spontaneous heat flow (that is, they counteract the flow of heat from the "warm" exterior of the refrigerator to the "cool" interior), thereby "concentrating" energy outside of the system in the surroundings. As a result, refrigerators consume a lot of energy to accomplish this movement of energy against the temperature gradient.

The second law has been described as *time's arrow* because there is a unidirectional limitation on the movement of energy by which we recognize *before and after* or *new and old*, as shown in Figure 7.16. For example, you would instantly recognize whether a video recording of an explosion was running forward or backward. Another way of understanding this is to say that energy in a closed system will spontaneously spread out, and entropy will increase if it is not hindered from doing so. Remember that a system can be variably defined to include the entire universe; in fact, the second law ultimately claims that the entropy of the universe is increasing.

$$\Delta S_{\text{universe}} = \Delta S_{\text{system}} + \Delta S_{\text{surroundings}} > 0$$

Equation 7.8

Entropy is a state function, so a change in entropy from one equilibrium state to another is pathway independent and only depends upon the difference in entropies of the final and initial states. Further, the standard entropy change for a reaction, $\Delta S^\circ_{\text{rxn}}$, can be calculated using the standard entropies of the reactants and products—much like enthalpy:

$$\Delta S^\circ_{\text{rxn}} = \Sigma\, \Delta S^\circ_{\text{f,products}} - \Sigma\, \Delta S^\circ_{\text{f,reactants}}$$

Equation 7.9

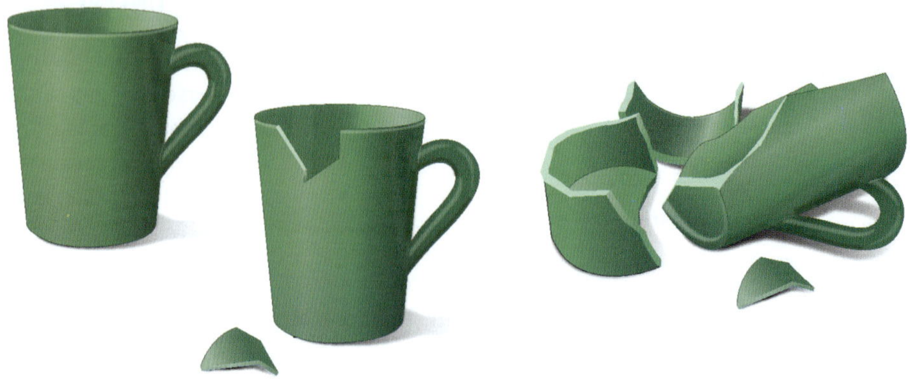

Figure 7.16 Entropy in the Kitchen
A new coffee mug can break if dropped, but a broken mug cannot put itself back together, one example of the asymmetry of time. The broken mug's entropy is higher than the new mug's.

MCAT CONCEPT CHECK 7.5

Before you move on, assess your understanding of the material with these questions.

1. Rank the phases of matter from lowest to highest entropy.

____

2. Describe entropy in terms of energy dispersal and disorder.

____

3. Do the following situations result in an increase or decrease in entropy?

Reaction	ΔS
$H_2O\ (l) \rightarrow H_2O\ (s)$	
Dry ice sublimates into carbon dioxide	
$NaCl\ (s) \rightarrow NaCl\ (aq)$	
$N_2\ (g) + 3\ H_2\ (g) \rightarrow 2\ NH_3\ (g)$	
An ice pack is placed on a wound	

7.6 Gibbs Free Energy

LEARNING OBJECTIVES

After Chapter 7.6, you will be able to:

- Determine the Gibbs free energy for a reaction at varying temperatures
- Predict the temperature necessary for a temperature-dependent reaction to be at equilibrium
- Identify how changing concentrations of reactant or product will alter the progress of a reaction

The final state function that we will examine in this chapter is **Gibbs free energy**, ***G***. This state function is a combination of the three that we've just examined: temperature, enthalpy, and entropy. The change in Gibbs free energy, ΔG, is a measure of the change in the enthalpy and the change in entropy as a system undergoes a process, and it indicates whether a reaction is spontaneous or nonspontaneous. The change in the free energy is the maximum amount of energy released by a process—occurring at constant temperature and pressure—that is available to perform useful work. The change in Gibbs free energy is defined as follows:

$$\Delta G = \Delta H - T\Delta S$$

Equation 7.10

where T is the temperature in kelvin and $T\Delta S$ represents the total amount of energy that is absorbed by a system when its entropy increases reversibly.

MNEMONIC

Gibbs free energy:
$\Delta G = \Delta H - T\Delta S$

Goldfish are (equals sign) Horrible without (minus sign) Tartar Sauce.

Overview

A helpful visual aid for conceptualizing Gibbs free energy is to think of it as a valley between two hills. Just as a ball would tend to roll down the hill into the valley and eventually come to rest at the lowest point in the valley, any system—including chemical reactions—will move in whichever direction results in a reduction of the free energy of the system. The bottom of the valley represents equilibrium, and the sides of the hill represent the various points in the pathway toward or away from equilibrium. This is shown graphically in Figure 7.17 and was also discussed in the previous chapter.

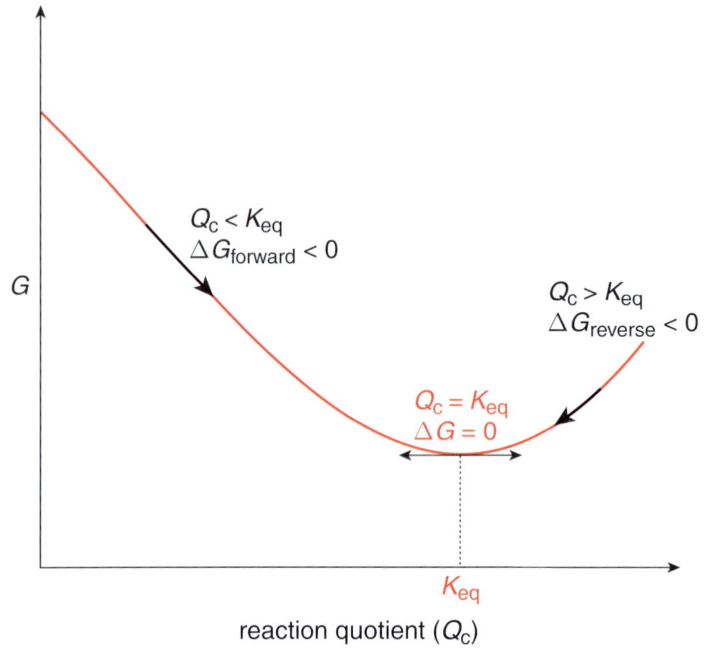

Figure 7.17 Gibbs Free Energy and Spontaneity
A decrease in Gibbs free energy indicates that a reaction is spontaneous. When an equilibrated system is disturbed, it will spontaneously act to restore equilibrium.

Movement toward the equilibrium position is associated with a decrease in Gibbs free energy ($\Delta G < 0$) and is spontaneous. When a system releases energy, it is said to be **exergonic**, as shown in Figure 7.18.

MCAT EXPERTISE

Be careful not to confuse endergonic/exergonic (describing Gibbs free energy) with endothermic/exothermic (describing enthalpy).

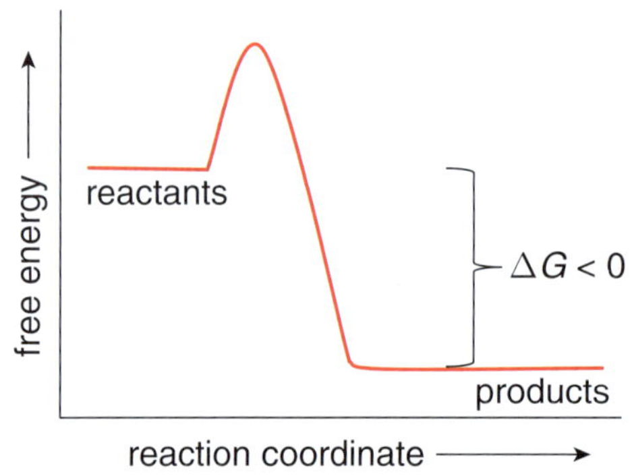

Figure 7.18 Exergonic Reaction Profile
Exergonic reactions release energy and are spontaneous ($\Delta G_{rxn} < 0$).

On the other hand, movement away from the equilibrium position is associated with an increase in Gibbs free energy ($\Delta G > 0$) and is nonspontaneous. Such a reaction is said to be **endergonic**, as shown in Figure 7.19.

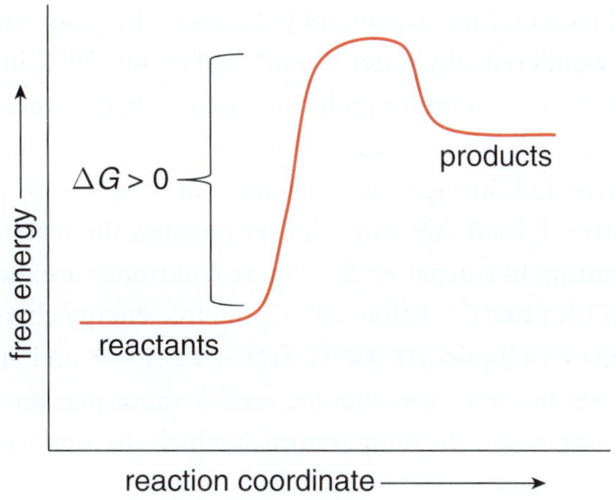

Figure 7.19 Endergonic Reaction Profile
Endergonic reactions absorb energy and are nonspontaneous ($\Delta G_{rxn} > 0$).

Once at the energy minimum state—equilibrium—the system will resist any changes to its state, and the change in free energy is zero. To summarize:

1. If ΔG is negative, the reaction is spontaneous.
2. If ΔG is positive, the reaction is nonspontaneous.
3. If ΔG is zero, the system is in a state of equilibrium; $\Delta H = T\Delta S$.

You should recall that phase equilibria are states in which more than one phase exists. As with all equilibria, the change in Gibbs free energy must be equal to zero ($\Delta G = 0$). For an equilibrium between a gas and a solid,

$$\Delta G = G\,(g) - G\,(s) = 0$$

Therefore,

$$G\,(g) = G\,(s)$$

Because the temperature in Gibbs free energy is in kelvin, it is always positive. Therefore, the effects of the signs of ΔH and ΔS on the spontaneity of a process can be summarized as in Table 7.2.

ΔH	ΔS	Outcome
+	+	Spontaneous at high *T*
+	−	Nonspontaneous at all *T*
−	+	Spontaneous at all *T*
−	−	Spontaneous at low *T*

Table 7.2 Effects of ΔH, ΔS, and T on Spontaneity

KEY CONCEPT

Recall that thermodynamics and kinetics are separate topics. When a reaction is thermodynamically spontaneous, it has no bearing on how fast it goes. It only means that it will proceed *eventually* without external energy input.

KEY CONCEPT

ΔG is temperature dependent when ΔH and ΔS have the same sign.

Phase changes are examples of temperature-dependent processes. The phase changes of water should be familiar to you; have you ever wondered why water doesn't boil at, say, 20°C instead of 100°C? When water boils, hydrogen bonds are broken, and the water molecules gain sufficient energy to escape into the gas phase. Thus, boiling is an endothermic process, and ΔH is positive. As thermal energy is transferred to the water molecules, energy is distributed through the molecules entering the gas phase. Thus, entropy is positive and the term $T\Delta S$ is positive. If both ΔH and $T\Delta S$ are positive, the reaction will only be spontaneous if $T\Delta S$ is greater than ΔH, resulting in a negative ΔG. These conditions are met only when the temperature of the system is greater than 373 K (100°C). Below 100°C, the free energy change is positive, and boiling is nonspontaneous; the water remains a liquid. At 100°C, $\Delta H - T\Delta S = 0$, and an equilibrium is established between the liquid and gas phases in such a way that the water's vapor pressure equals the ambient pressure. This is the definition of the boiling point: the temperature at which the vapor pressure equals the ambient pressure.

It is important to remember that the rate of a reaction depends on the activation energy E_a, not ΔG. Spontaneous reactions may be fast or slow. Sometimes a reversible reaction may produce two products that differ both in their stability (as measured by the change in the free energy associated with their production) and in their kinetics (as measured by their respective activation energies). Sometimes, the thermodynamically more stable product will have the slower kinetics due to higher activation energy. In this situation, we talk about kinetic vs. thermodynamic reaction control, which is discussed in Chapter 6 of *MCAT General Chemistry Review*. For a period of time after the reaction begins, the major product will be the one that is produced more quickly as a result of its lower activation energy. The reaction can be said to be under kinetic control at this time. Given enough time, however, and assuming a reversible reaction, the dominant product will be the thermodynamically more stable product as a result of its lower free energy value. The reaction can then be said to be under thermodynamic control. Eventually, the reaction will reach equilibrium, as defined by its K_{eq}.

Standard Gibbs Free Energy

The free energy change of reactions can be measured under standard state conditions to yield the **standard free energy, ΔG°_{rxn}**. For standard free energy determinations, the concentrations of any solutions in the reaction are 1 *M*. The standard free energy of formation of a compound, ΔG°_f, is the free energy change that occurs when 1 mole of a compound in its standard state is produced from its respective elements in their standard states under standard state conditions. The standard free energy of formation for any element under standard state conditions is, by definition, zero. The standard free energy of a reaction, ΔG°_{rxn}, is the free energy change that occurs when that reaction is carried out under standard state conditions; that is, when the reactants are converted to the products at standard conditions of temperature (298 K) and pressure (1 atm). Like enthalpy and entropy, the free energy of the reaction can be calculated from the free energies of formation of the reactants and products:

$$\Delta G^\circ_{rxn} = \sum \Delta G^\circ_{f,\text{products}} - \sum \Delta G^\circ_{f,\text{reactants}}$$

Equation 7.11

Free Energy, K_{eq}, and Q

We can derive the standard free energy change for a reaction from the equilibrium constant K_{eq} for the reaction using the equation:

$$\Delta G^\circ_{rxn} = -RT \ln K_{eq}$$

Equation 7.12

where R is the ideal gas constant, T is the temperature in kelvin, and K_{eq} is the equilibrium constant. This equation allows us to make not only quantitative evaluations of the free energy change of a reaction, but also qualitative assessments of the spontaneity of the reaction. The greater the value of K_{eq}, the more positive the value of its natural logarithm. The more positive the natural logarithm, the more negative the standard free energy change. The more negative the standard free energy change, the more spontaneous the reaction.

Once a reaction begins, however, the standard state conditions (specifically 1 M solutions) no longer apply. The value of the equilibrium constant must be replaced with another number that is reflective of where the reaction is in its path toward equilibrium. To determine the free energy change for a reaction that is in progress, we relate ΔG_{rxn} (not ΔG°_{rxn}) to the reaction quotient, Q:

$$\Delta G_{rxn} = \Delta G^\circ_{rxn} + RT \ln Q = RT \ln \frac{Q}{K_{eq}}$$

Equation 7.13

KEY CONCEPT

Note that the right side of this equation is similar to Equation 7.12. The use of the Q indicates that the system is not at equilibrium.

As described in Chapter 6 of *MCAT General Chemistry Review*, if the ratio of $\frac{Q}{K_{eq}}$ is less than one ($Q < K_{eq}$), then the natural logarithm will be negative, and the free energy change will be negative, so the reaction will spontaneously proceed forward until equilibrium is reached. If the ratio of $\frac{Q}{K_{eq}}$ is greater than one ($Q > K_{eq}$), then the natural logarithm will be positive, and the free energy change will be positive. In that case, the reaction will spontaneously move in the reverse direction until equilibrium is reached. Of course, if the ratio is equal to one, the reaction quotient is equal to the equilibrium constant; the reaction is at equilibrium, and the free energy change is zero ($\ln 1 = 0$).

Reaction profiles of free energy can be altered by the presence of catalysts. While the overall free energy change of the reaction is not altered, the activation energy required to accomplish the reaction is reduced significantly in the presence of a catalyst, as shown in Figure 7.20.

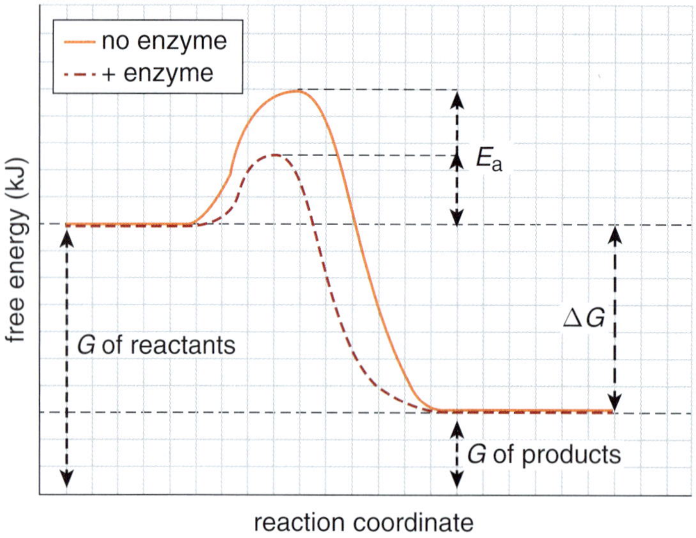

Figure 7.20 Catalysts Alter Kinetics but Not Equilibrium or Free Energy Change

MCAT CONCEPT CHECK 7.6

Before you move on, assess your understanding of the material with these questions.

1. The Haber–Bosch process creates ammonia through several reactions, the final step of which is

$$N_2 + 3\,H_2 \rightarrow 2\,NH_3 \left(\Delta H_{rxn} = -93\,\frac{kJ}{mol},\ \Delta S_{rxn} = -198\,\frac{J}{mol \cdot K}\right)$$

   Determine what the Gibbs free energy of this reaction is at standard conditions and at 500 K:

   - At standard conditions:

___

   - At 500 K:

___

2. At what temperature would the reaction described above be at equilibrium?

___

3. If you were to suddenly flood the reaction vessel with significant amounts of ammonia, what would occur?

___

Conclusion

We began our discussion of thermochemistry with a review of different ways in which we characterize systems (open, closed, and isolated) and processes (isothermal, adiabatic, isobaric, and isovolumetric). We then further classified systems according to their state functions—system properties such as pressure, density, temperature, volume, enthalpy, internal energy, Gibbs free energy, and entropy that describe the equilibrium state. We examined the equilibria that exist between the different phases and noted that the change in Gibbs free energy for each phase change in equilibrium is zero, as is the case for all equilibria. We defined enthalpy as the heat content of the system and the change in enthalpy as the change in heat content of the system as it moves from one equilibrium state to another. Enthalpy is defined as the energy found in the intermolecular interactions and bonds of the compounds in the system. We explored the various ways Hess's law can be applied to calculate the total enthalpy change for a series of reactions. Moving on to entropy, we described this property as a measure of the degree to which energy in a system becomes spread out through a process. There is danger in thinking too literally about entropy as "disorder" because a system's entropy may be increasing even if there is no observable change in the system's macroscopic disorder (such as ice warming from $-10°C$ to $-5°C$). Gibbs free energy combines the effects of temperature, enthalpy, and entropy, and the change in Gibbs free energy determines whether a process will be spontaneous or nonspontaneous. When the change in Gibbs free energy is negative, the process is spontaneous, but when the change in Gibbs free energy is positive, the process is nonspontaneous.

Many reactions in the body must be spontaneous in order for cells to function. While there are some nonspontaneous reactions in our body, we are able to couple them to thermodynamically favorable (exergonic) reactions that allow the cell to perform even more complex functions.

▶ GO ONLINE

You've reviewed the content, now test your knowledge and critical thinking skills by completing a test-like passage set in your online resources!

CONCEPT SUMMARY

Systems and Processes

- Systems are classified based on what is or is not exchanged with the surroundings.
  - **Isolated systems** exchange neither matter nor energy with the environment.
  - **Closed systems** can exchange energy but not matter with the environment.
  - **Open systems** can exchange both energy and matter with the environment.
- Processes can be characterized based on a single constant property.
  - **Isothermal** processes occur at a constant temperature.
  - **Adiabatic** processes exchange no heat with the environment.
  - **Isobaric** processes occur at a constant pressure.
  - **Isovolumetric** (**isochoric**) processes occur at a constant volume.

States and State Functions

- **State functions** describe the physical properties of an equilibrium state; they are pathway independent and include pressure, density, temperature, volume, enthalpy, internal energy, Gibbs free energy, and entropy.
- **Standard conditions** are defined as 298 K, 1 atm, and 1 *M* concentrations.
- The **standard state** of an element is its most prevalent form under standard conditions; **standard enthalpy**, **standard entropy**, and **standard free energy** are all calculated under standard conditions.
- **Phase changes** exist at characteristic temperatures and pressures.
  - **Fusion** (**melting**) and **freezing** (**crystallization** or **solidification**) occur at the boundary between the solid and the liquid phases.
  - **Vaporization** (**evaporation** or **boiling**) and **condensation** occur at the boundary between the liquid and the gas phases.
  - **Sublimation** and **deposition** occur at the boundary between the solid and gas phases.
  - At temperatures above the **critical point**, the liquid and gas phases are indistinguishable.
  - At the **triple point**, all three phases of matter exist in equilibrium.
- The **phase diagram** for a system graphs the phases and phase equilibria as a function of temperature and pressure.

Heat

- Temperature and heat are not the same thing.
  - **Temperature** is a scaled measure of the average kinetic energy of a substance.
  - **Heat** is the transfer of energy that results from differences of temperature between two substances.
- The heat content of a system undergoing heating, cooling, or phase changes is the sum of all the respective energy changes.

Enthalpy

- **Enthalpy** is a measure of the potential energy of a system found in intermolecular attractions and chemical bonds.
- **Hess's law** states that the total change in potential energy of a system is equal to the changes of potential energies of the individual steps of the process.
- Enthalpy can also be calculated using heats of formation, heats of combustion, or bond dissociation energies.

Entropy

- **Entropy**, while often thought of as disorder, is a measure of the degree to which energy has been spread throughout a system or between a system and its surroundings.
  - Entropy is a ratio of heat transferred per mole per unit kelvin.
  - Entropy is maximized at equilibrium.

Gibbs Free Energy

- **Gibbs free energy** is derived from both enthalpy and entropy values for a given system.
- The change in Gibbs free energy determines whether a process is spontaneous or nonspontaneous.
  - $\Delta G < 0$: reaction proceeds in forward direction (spontaneous)
  - $\Delta G = 0$: reaction is in dynamic equilibrium
  - $\Delta G > 0$: reaction proceeds in reverse direction (nonspontaneous)
- Gibbs free energy depends on temperature; temperature-dependent processes change between spontaneous and nonspontaneous, depending on the temperature.

ANSWERS TO CONCEPT CHECKS

7.1

1. The boundary between system and surroundings could be placed anywhere. Most commonly, the ice pack would be considered the chemical system using up energy, and the person (and the remainder of the universe) constitutes the surroundings that are providing the heat for the ice pack to function.
2. • Isothermal: no change in temperature; $\Delta U = 0$, $Q = W$
   • Adiabatic: no heat exchange; $Q = 0$, $\Delta U = -W$
   • Isobaric: no change in pressure; line appears flat in a P–V graph
   • Isovolumetric (isochoric): no change in volume; $W = 0$, $\Delta U = Q$

7.2

1. Kinetics, equilibrium, and thermodynamics calculations use standard conditions, which are 25°C (298 K), 1 atm pressure, and 1 *M* concentrations.
2. State functions are properties of a system at equilibrium and are independent of the path taken to achieve the equilibrium; they may be dependent on one another. Process functions define the path between equilibrium states and include Q (heat) and W (work).
3. State functions include pressure (P), density (ρ), temperature (T), volume (V), enthalpy (H), internal energy (U), Gibbs free energy (G), and entropy (S).
4. The triple point is the specific combination of temperature and pressure at which all three phases are in equilibrium. The critical point is the temperature and pressure above which the liquid and gas phases are indistinguishable and the heat of vaporization is zero.

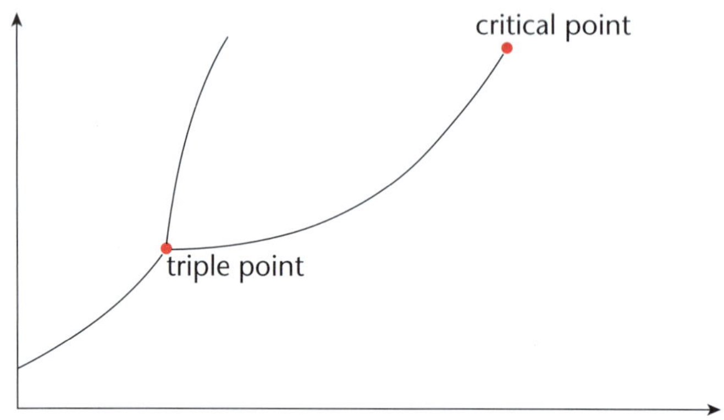

7.3

1. Temperature is an indirect measure of the thermal content of a system that looks at average kinetic energy of particles in a sample. Heat is the thermal energy transferred between objects as a result of differences in their temperatures.
2. Specific heat (c) is the energy required to raise the temperature of one gram of a substance by one degree Celsius. Heat capacity (mc) is the product of mass and specific heat and is the energy required to raise any given amount of a substance one degree Celsius.
3. A constant-pressure calorimeter (coffee cup calorimeter) is exposed to constant (atmospheric) pressure. As the reaction proceeds, the temperature of the contents is measured to determine the heat of the reaction. A constant-volume calorimeter (bomb calorimeter) is one in which heats of certain reactions (like combustion) can be measured indirectly by assessing temperature change in a water bath around the reaction vessel.
4. $c_{H_2O\ (l)} = 1\ \frac{\text{cal}}{\text{g} \cdot \text{K}}$

7.4

1. Endothermic reactions involve an increase in heat content of a system from the surroundings ($\Delta H > 0$), while exothermic reactions involve a release of heat content from a system ($\Delta H < 0$).
2. To reach the net equation C (s, graphite) $+ \frac{1}{2}O_2 \rightarrow CO$, the second reaction must be reversed along with the sign of its enthalpy of reaction.

$$\text{C }(s, \text{graphite}) + O_2 \rightarrow CO_2 \qquad \Delta H = -393.5\ \frac{\text{kJ}}{\text{mol}}$$

$$CO_2 \rightarrow CO + \frac{1}{2}O_2 \qquad \Delta H = +283\ \frac{\text{kJ}}{\text{mol}}$$

Adding the enthalpies gives:

$$-393.5\ \frac{\text{kJ}}{\text{mol}} + 283\ \frac{\text{kJ}}{\text{mol}} \approx -400 + 285 = -115\ \frac{\text{kJ}}{\text{mol}}$$

$$\left(\text{actual value} = -110.5\ \frac{\text{kJ}}{\text{mol}}\right)$$

3. Enthalpy of reaction = bonds broken − bonds formed. There are four O–H bonds broken, two H–H bonds formed, and one O=O bond formed. Therefore,

$$\Delta H_{rxn} = \text{bonds broken} - \text{bonds formed}$$

$$\Delta H_{rxn} = (4 \times \text{O} - \text{H}) - [(2 \times \text{H} - \text{H}) + (1 \times \text{O} = \text{O})]$$

$$\Delta H_{rxn} = \left(4 \times 463\ \frac{\text{kJ}}{\text{mol}}\right) - \left[\left(2 \times 436\ \frac{\text{kJ}}{\text{mol}}\right) + \left(1 \times 498\ \frac{\text{kJ}}{\text{mol}}\right)\right]$$

$$\Delta H_{rxn} \approx (4 \times 450) - [(2 \times 435) + (500)] = 1800 - (870 + 500)$$

$$\Delta H_{rxn} = 1800 - 1370 = 430\ \frac{\text{kJ}}{\text{mol}} \left(\text{actual value} = 482\ \frac{\text{kJ}}{\text{mol}}\right)$$

7.5

1. Solids have the lowest entropy, followed by liquids, with gases having the highest entropy.
2. Entropy increases as a system has more disorder or freedom of movement, and energy is dispersed in a spontaneous system. Entropy of the universe can never be decreased spontaneously.
3.

Reaction	ΔS
H_2O (*l*) → H_2O (*s*)	Decrease (freezing)
Dry ice sublimates into carbon dioxide	Increase (sublimation)
NaCl (*s*) → NaCl (*aq*)	Increase (dissolution)
N_2 (*g*) + 3 H_2 (*g*) → 2 NH_3 (*g*)	Decrease (fewer moles of gas)
An ice pack is placed on a wound	Increase (heat is transferred)

7.6

1. At standard conditions:

$$\Delta G = \Delta H - T\Delta S = -93{,}000\ \frac{\text{J}}{\text{mol}} - (298\ \text{K})\left(-198\ \frac{\text{J}}{\text{mol}\cdot\text{K}}\right) \approx$$

$$-93{,}000 - (300 \times -200) = -93{,}000 + 60{,}000 = -33{,}000\ \frac{\text{J}}{\text{mol}} = -33\ \frac{\text{kJ}}{\text{mol}}$$

$$\left(\text{actual} = -34.0\ \frac{\text{kJ}}{\text{mol}}\right)$$

At 500 K:

$$\Delta G = \Delta H - T\Delta S = -93{,}000\ \frac{\text{J}}{\text{mol}} - (500\ \text{K})\left(-198\ \frac{\text{J}}{\text{mol}\cdot\text{K}}\right) \approx$$

$$-93{,}000 - (500 \times -200) = -93{,}000 + 100{,}000 = 7{,}000\ \frac{\text{J}}{\text{mol}} = 7\ \frac{\text{kJ}}{\text{mol}}$$

$$\left(\text{actual} = 6\ \frac{\text{kJ}}{\text{mol}}\right)$$

2. The system is at equilibrium when $\Delta G = 0$:

$$\Delta G = \Delta H - T\Delta S$$

$$0 = -93{,}000\ \frac{\text{J}}{\text{mol}} - \left[(T)\left(-198\ \frac{\text{J}}{\text{mol}\cdot\text{K}}\right)\right]\ 93{,}000 \approx 200\ T$$

$$T = \frac{93{,}000}{200} = \frac{930}{2} = 465\ \text{K}\ (\text{actual} = 470\ \text{K}).$$

3. The value of Q would increase significantly, causing the system to shift left, forming more reactants until the system again reached equilibrium.

SCIENCE MASTERY ASSESSMENT EXPLANATIONS

1. **A**

This process may be adiabatic. Given that the gas was cooled, it did not maintain constant temperature, eliminating **(C)**. Isobaric and isovolumetric processes appear as horizontal and vertical lines in pressure–volume graphs, respectively, eliminating **(B)** and **(D)**. Adiabatic processes appear hyperbolic on pressure–volume graphs, as illustrated here.

2. **A**

Since the temperature during a phase change is constant, all phase changes are isothermal processes. During boiling, heat is added to the system to break the intermolecular attractions between the water molecules. As the water molecules vaporize, they expand outward, occupying a larger volume. Thus, boiling is an isothermal expansion, consistent with **(A)**.

3. **D**

Solve this question using the equation $\Delta G^\circ_{rxn} = -RT \ln K_{eq}$. ΔG°_{rxn} is negative (as it must be for a spontaneous reaction), and R and T are always positive. Therefore, $\ln K_{eq}$ must also be positive for the sign convention to work out correctly. Since $\ln(1) = 0$, the natural logarithm of any number greater than 1 will be positive, and the natural logarithm of any number less than 1 will be negative. In order for $\ln K_{eq}$ to be a positive number, K_{eq} must be greater than 1.

4. **D**

Combustion often involves the reaction of a hydrocarbon with oxygen to produce carbon dioxide and water. Longer hydrocarbon chains yield greater amounts of combustion products and release more heat in the process—that is, the reaction is more exothermic. Of the hydrocarbons listed here, n-pentane is the longest chain.

5. **A**

At first glance, this might seem like a math-heavy problem, but it really doesn't require any calculations at all. We just have to keep track of which bonds are broken and which bonds are formed. Remember, breaking bonds requires energy, while forming bonds releases energy. Two bonds are broken: a C–O bond between the carbonyl carbon and oxygen of acetic acid 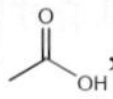, and an O–H bond between the hydroxyl oxygen and hydrogen of methanol 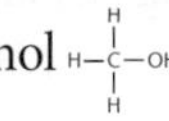. Two bonds are also formed: a C–O bond between the carbonyl carbon and the oxygen of methyl acetate 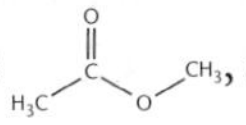, and an O–H bond between a hydroxyl group and a hydrogen to form water 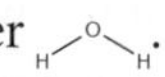. Given that the same two bonds are broken and formed in this reaction, the energy change must be $0 \frac{\text{kJ}}{\text{mol}}$.

6. **B**

At the triple point (triple for three phases), the solid, liquid, and gas phases exist in equilibrium, consistent with **(B)**. On the other hand, the critical point refers to the temperature and pressure above which gases and liquids are indistinguishable, so **(A)** can be eliminated.

7. **C**

There are two parts to this computation. First, the water must be heated from 40°C to 100°C, then it must be vaporized. To calculate the energy required to heat the water, use the formula $q = mc\Delta T$. Plugging in values yields (10 g)(60°C)(4.2 J/g°C). Next, calculate the energy required to vaporize using the equation $q = mL$. Plugging in values yields (2,260 J/g)(10 g). Finally combine the two energies together: (10 g)(60°C)(4.2 J/g°C) + (2,260 J/g)(10 g), matching **(C)**.

8. **D**

There is not enough information available to determine the free energy of this reaction. While the entropy is clearly increasing (there are more particles in the system), it is unclear what the enthalpy change is. Because bonds are breaking, the reaction should be endothermic, meaning that both ΔS and ΔH are positive. In this case, it is a temperature-dependent process, and—without a temperature given—we cannot determine the sign on ΔG.

9. **A**

This problem asks for the free energy of a reaction at nonstandard conditions, which can be determined with the equation $\Delta G = \Delta G^\circ + RT \ln Q$.

10. **A**

A reaction with a negative enthalpy is, by definition, exothermic. Because both enthalpy and entropy are negative, this is a temperature-dependent process, and the reaction will be both endergonic and exergonic—but only at particular temperatures, eliminating **(C)** and **(D)**.

11. **C**

For a process to progress forward spontaneously, Q must be less than K_{eq} and will therefore have a tendency to move in the direction toward equilibrium. A spontaneous reaction's free energy is negative by convention.

12. **B**

This question is asking for a reaction with the greatest decrease in entropy, so the phases of the reactants and products must be evaluated. In general, the entropy of gases is the highest, while the entropy of solids is the lowest. Thus, a reaction in which gases react to produce solids will have a significant entropy decrease. In reaction **(B)**, a gaseous reactant forms a solid product, so the entropy decreases, making **(B)** correct. By contrast, the other reactions have either a minimal change or increase in entropy. In reaction **(A)**, two moles of gaseous reactants become four moles of gaseous product, so the entropy increases. In **(C)**, a liquid reactant forms a gaseous product, so entropy likewise increases. In reaction **(D)**, each side of the equation has a solid and an aqueous component, so there is approximately no change in entropy.

13. **A**

Eliminate **(C)** and **(D)**, which describe the free energy of reaction and cannot be determined from this graph. While most reaction coordinate graphs we've explored in this book use free energy for the y-axis, this one uses potential energy (enthalpy). If the heat of formation of the products is greater than that of the reactants, the reaction is endothermic. We can determine this information from their relative positions on the graph: because the products are higher than the reactants, this is an endothermic reaction.

14. **A**

The entropy change can be calculated using the formula $\Delta S = q/T$. Note that more information is given in the question than is necessary, so ignore the mass. Plugging in values yields: $\Delta S = 30{,}000\ \text{J} / 1{,}060\ \text{K} = 28\ \text{J/K}$. Thus, **(A)** is correct.

15. **A**

In an explosion, a significant amount of heat energy is released, meaning that the reaction is exothermic ($\Delta H < 0$), eliminating **(B)**. The entropy change associated with an explosion is positive because energy is dispersed over a much larger area, eliminating **(C)**. If this is true, the expression $\Delta H - T\Delta S$ must be negative, indicating that this is an exergonic process ($\Delta G < 0$). Absolute temperature can never be negative, eliminating **(D)**.

GO ONLINE

Consult your online resources for additional practice.

EQUATIONS TO REMEMBER

(7.1) **First law of thermodynamics:** $\Delta U = Q - W$

(7.2) **Heat transfer (no phase change):** $q = mc\Delta T$

(7.3) **Heat transfer (during phase change):** $q = mL$

(7.4) **Generalized enthalpy of reaction:** $\Delta H_{\text{rxn}} = H_{\text{products}} - H_{\text{reactants}}$

(7.5) **Standard enthalpy of reaction:** $\Delta H^{\circ}_{\text{rxn}} = \Sigma\ \Delta H^{\circ}_{\text{f,products}} - \Sigma\ \Delta H^{\circ}_{\text{f,reactants}}$

(7.6) **Bond enthalpy:** $\Delta H^{\circ}_{\text{rxn}} = \Sigma\ \Delta H_{\text{bonds broken}} - \Sigma\ \Delta H_{\text{bonds formed}} =$ total energy absorbed $-$ total energy released

(7.7) **Entropy:** $\Delta S = \dfrac{Q_{\text{rev}}}{T}$

(7.8) **Second law of thermodynamics:** $\Delta S_{\text{universe}} = \Delta S_{\text{system}} + \Delta S_{\text{surroundings}} > 0$

(7.9) **Standard entropy of reaction:** $\Delta S^{\circ}_{\text{rxn}} = \Sigma\ \Delta S^{\circ}_{\text{f,products}} - \Sigma\ \Delta S^{\circ}_{\text{f,reactants}}$

(7.10) **Gibbs free energy:** $\Delta G = \Delta H - T\Delta S$

(7.11) **Standard Gibbs free energy of reaction:**
$\Delta G^{\circ}_{\text{rxn}} = \Sigma\ \Delta G^{\circ}_{\text{f,products}} - \Sigma\ \Delta G^{\circ}_{\text{f,reactants}}$

(7.12) **Standard Gibbs free energy from equilibrium constant:**
$\Delta G^{\circ}_{\text{rxn}} = -RT \ln K_{\text{eq}}$

(7.13) **Gibbs free energy from reaction quotient:**

$$\Delta G_{\text{rxn}} = \Delta G^{\circ}_{\text{rxn}} + RT \ln Q = RT \ln \frac{Q}{K_{\text{eq}}}$$

SHARED CONCEPTS

General Chemistry Chapter 3
Bonding and Chemical Interactions

General Chemistry Chapter 4
Compounds and Stoichiometry

General Chemistry Chapter 5
Chemical Kinetics

General Chemistry Chapter 6
Equilibrium

Physics and Math Chapter 2
Work and Energy

Physics and Math Chapter 3
Thermodynamics

CHAPTER 8

THE GAS PHASE

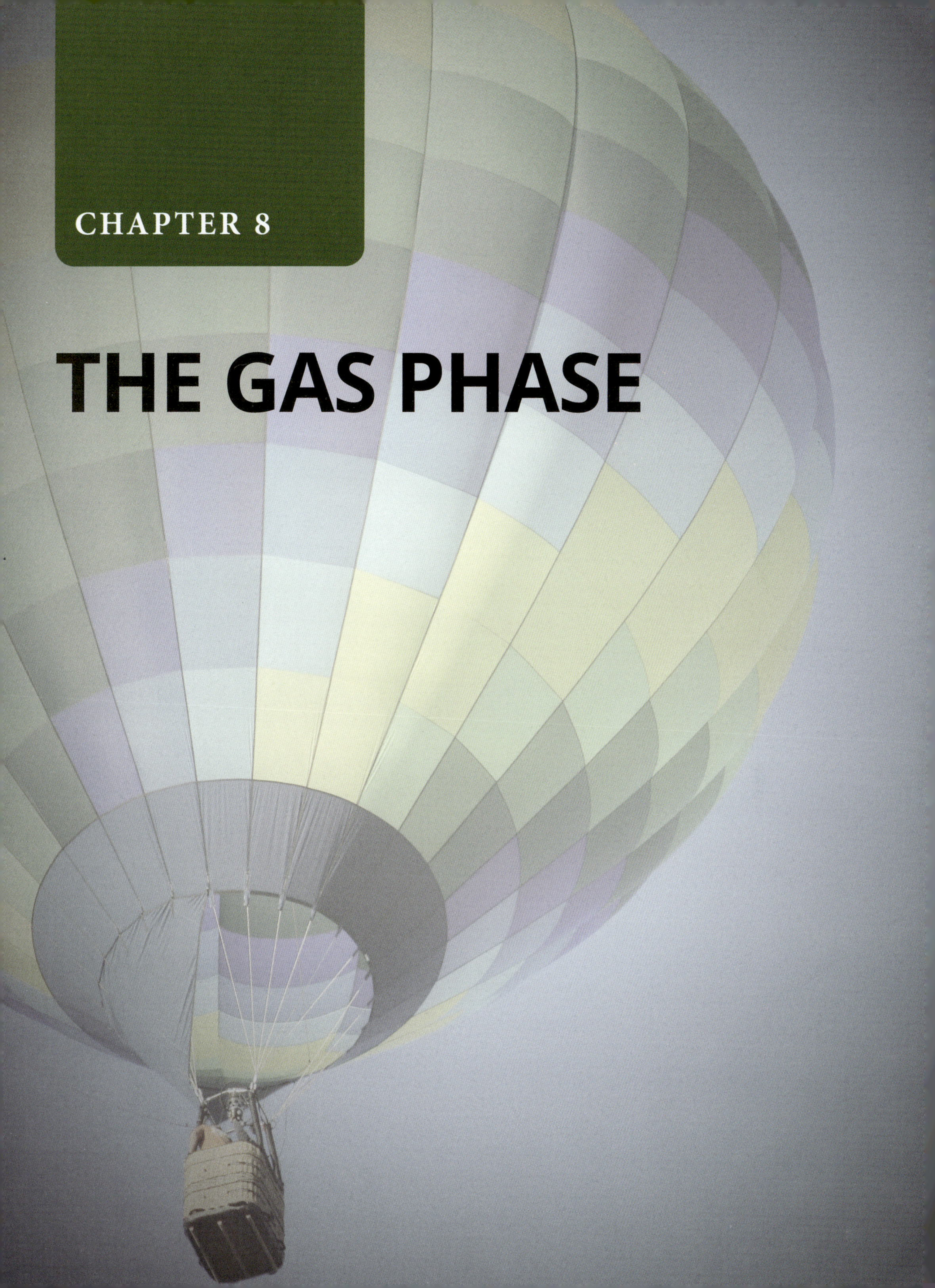

SCIENCE MASTERY ASSESSMENT

Every pre-med knows this feeling: there is so much content I have to know for the MCAT! How do I know what to do first or what's important?

While the high-yield badges throughout this book will help you identify the most important topics, this Science Mastery Assessment is another tool in your MCAT prep arsenal. This quiz (which can also be taken in your online resources) and the guidance below will help ensure that you are spending the appropriate amount of time on this chapter based on your personal strengths and weaknesses. Don't worry though—skipping something now does not mean you'll never study it. Later on in your prep, as you complete full-length tests, you'll uncover specific pieces of content that you need to review and can come back to these chapters as appropriate.

How to Use This Assessment

If you answer 0–7 questions correctly:

Spend about 1 hour to read this chapter in full and take limited notes throughout. Follow up by reviewing **all** quiz questions to ensure that you now understand how to solve each one.

If you answer 8–11 questions correctly:

Spend 20–40 minutes reviewing the quiz questions. Beginning with the questions you missed, read and take notes on the corresponding subchapters. For questions you answered correctly, ensure your thinking matches that of the explanation and you understand why each choice was correct or incorrect.

If you answer 12–15 questions correctly:

Spend less than 20 minutes reviewing all questions from the quiz. If you missed any, then include a quick read-through of the corresponding subchapters, or even just the relevant content within a subchapter, as part of your question review. For questions you answered correctly, ensure your thinking matches that of the explanation and review the Concept Summary at the end of the chapter.

1. Which of the following sets of conditions would be LEAST likely to result in ideal gas behavior?
   - **A.** High pressure and low temperature
   - **B.** Low temperature and large volume
   - **C.** High pressure and large volume
   - **D.** Low pressure and high temperature

2. What is the density of neon gas in $\frac{g}{L}$ at STP?
   - **A.** 452.3
   - **B.** 226.0
   - **C.** 1.802
   - **D.** 0.9018

3. A leak of helium gas through a small hole occurs at a rate of $3.22 \times 10^{-5}\ \frac{mol}{s}$. How will the leakage rates of neon and oxygen gases compare to helium at the same temperature and pressure?
   - **A.** Neon will leak faster than helium; oxygen will leak faster than helium.
   - **B.** Neon will leak faster than helium; oxygen will leak slower than helium.
   - **C.** Neon will leak slower than helium; oxygen will leak faster than helium.
   - **D.** Neon will leak slower than helium; oxygen will leak slower than helium.

4. A 0.10 g piece of magnesium is placed in a beaker of hydrochloric acid. Hydrogen gas is generated according to the following equation:

   $$Mg\ (s) + 2\ HCl\ (aq) \rightarrow MgCl_2\ (aq) + H_2\ (g)$$

   The gas is collected over water at 25°C, and the gauge pressure during the experiment reads 784 mmHg.

   The gas displaces a volume of 100 mL. The vapor pressure of water at 25°C is approximately 24.0 mmHg. Based on this data, how many moles of hydrogen are produced in this reaction? (Note: $R = 0.0821\ \frac{L \cdot atm}{mol \cdot K} = 8.314\ \frac{J}{K \cdot mol}$.)
   - **A.** 4.04×10^{-5} moles hydrogen
   - **B.** 4.09×10^{-3} moles hydrogen
   - **C.** 3.07×10^{-2} moles hydrogen
   - **D.** 3.11 moles hydrogen

5. Ideal gases:
   - **I.** have no volume.
   - **II.** have particles with no attractive forces between them.
   - **III.** have no mass.

   - **A.** I only
   - **B.** II only
   - **C.** I and II only
   - **D.** I, II, and III

6. Which of the following best explains the difference in ideal behavior between nitrogen and fluoromethane gas?
   - **A.** Nitrogen gas is more ideal because it is smaller and forms stronger intermolecular interactions.
   - **B.** Nitrogen gas is more ideal because it is smaller and forms weaker intermolecular interactions.
   - **C.** Fluoromethane is more ideal because it is larger and forms stronger intermolecular interactions.
   - **D.** Fluoromethane is more ideal because it is smaller and forms weaker intermolecular interactions.

7. The kinetic molecular theory states that:
   - **A.** the average kinetic energy of a molecule of gas is directly proportional to the temperature of the gas in kelvin.
   - **B.** collisions between gas molecules are inelastic.
   - **C.** gas particles occupy discrete areas of space.
   - **D.** all gas molecules have the same kinetic energy at the same temperature.

8. The plots of two gases at STP are shown below. One of the gases is 1.0 L of helium, and the other is 1.0 L of bromine. Which plot corresponds to each gas and why?

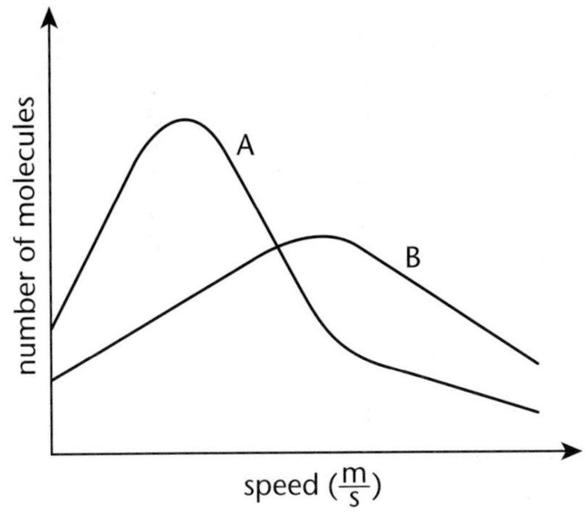

A. Curve A is helium and curve B is bromine because helium has a smaller molar mass than bromine.
B. Curve A is helium and curve B is bromine because the average kinetic energy of bromine is greater than the average kinetic energy of helium.
C. Curve A is bromine and curve B is helium because helium has a smaller molar mass than bromine.
D. Curve A is bromine and curve B is helium because the average kinetic energy of bromine is greater than the average kinetic energy of helium.

9. At sea level and 25°C, the solubility of oxygen gas in water is 1.25×10^{-3} M. In Denver, a city in the United States that lies high above sea level, the atmospheric pressure is 0.800 atm. What is the solubility of oxygen in water in Denver?
A. 1.00×10^{-3} M
B. 1.05×10^{-3} M
C. 1.50×10^{-3} M
D. 2.56×10^{-3} M

10. Given that the gases at the center of the sun have an average molar mass of 2.00 $\frac{g}{mol}$, compressed to a density of 1.20 $\frac{g}{cm^3}$ under 1.30×10^9 atm of pressure, what is the temperature at the center of the sun?
A. 2.6×10^4 K
B. 2.6×10^6 K
C. 2.6×10^7 K
D. 2.6×10^{10} K

11. The gaseous state of matter is characterized by which of the following properties?
I. Gases are compressible.
II. Gases assume the volume of their containers.
III. Gas particles exist as diatomic molecules.

A. I only
B. I and II only
C. II and III only
D. I, II, and III

12. A gas at a temperature of 27°C has a volume of 60.0 mL. What temperature change is needed to increase this gas to a volume of 90.0 mL?
A. A reduction of 150°C
B. An increase of 150°C
C. A reduction of 13.5°C
D. An increase of 13.5°C

13. How do a significant decrease in temperature and volume affect ideal gas behavior, respectively?
A. Both lead to more ideal behavior.
B. A lower temperature leads to deviations from ideal behavior, while lower volume causes more ideal behavior.
C. A lower temperature leads to more ideal behavior, while lower volume causes deviations from ideal behavior.
D. Both lead to deviations from ideal behavior.

14. In which of the following situations is it impossible to predict how the pressure will change for a gas sample?
A. The gas is cooled at a constant volume.
B. The gas is heated at a constant volume.
C. The gas is heated, and the volume is simultaneously increased.
D. The gas is cooled, and the volume is simultaneously increased.

15. Experimenters notice that the molar concentration of dissolved oxygen in an enclosed water tank has decreased to one-half its original value. In an attempt to counter this decrease, they quadruple the partial pressure of oxygen in the container. What is the final concentration of the gas?
A. Half of the original concentration
B. The same as the original concentration
C. Double the original concentration
D. Quadruple the original concentration

Answer Key

1. **A** (See section 8.2)
2. **D** (See section 8.1)
3. **D** (See section 8.3)
4. **B** (See section 8.2)
5. **B** (See section 8.2)
6. **B** (See section 8.4)
7. **A** (See section 8.3)
8. **C** (See section 8.3)
9. **A** (See section 8.2)
10. **C** (See section 8.2)
11. **B** (See section 8.1)
12. **B** (See section 8.2)
13. **D** (See section 8.4)
14. **C** (See section 8.2)
15. **C** (See section 8.2)

The relevant section of the chapter to review for each question is given in parentheses after the correct answer. Detailed explanations can be found at the end of the chapter.

CHAPTER 8

THE GAS PHASE

In This Chapter

CHAPTER PROFILE

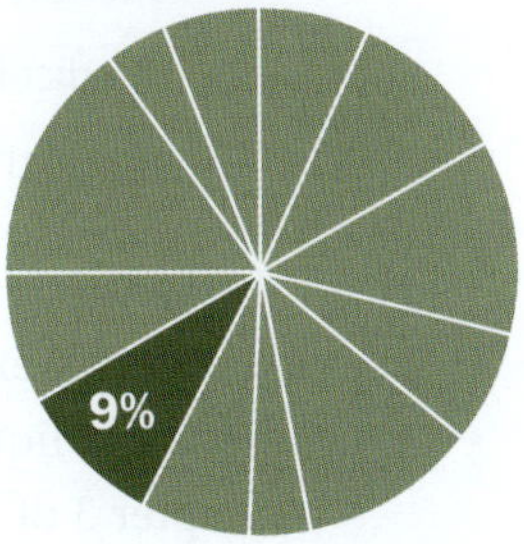

The content in this chapter should be relevant to about 9% of all questions about general chemistry on the MCAT.

This chapter covers material from the following AAMC content categories:

3B: Structure and integrative functions of the main organ systems

4B: Importance of fluids for the circulation of blood, gas movement, and gas exchange

Introduction

Let's start this chapter with a thought experiment. Imagine a helium balloon tied to the gearshift lever between the seats of a car and allowed to float freely. What do you think will happen to the balloon as the car accelerates forward? You might think, based on how you feel when you are in an accelerating vehicle, that the balloon will be pushed backwards due to its inertia. However, the balloon's movement isn't what we might predict: the balloon shifts forward as the car accelerates!

The molar mass of helium is $4 \frac{\text{g}}{\text{mol}}$, while that of air, which is mostly nitrogen and oxygen, is about $29 \frac{\text{g}}{\text{mol}}$. This means that air is about seven times denser than helium. Because the air in which the balloon is floating is more dense than the balloon itself, the air has greater inertia. Therefore, as the car accelerates forward, everything that has significant mass, including the air in the car, resists the forward motion (has inertia) and shifts toward the back of the car (even though, of course, everything in the car is accelerating forward, just not as quickly as the car itself). As the air shifts toward the back, a pressure gradient builds up such that there is greater air pressure in the back of the car than in the front, and this pressure difference results in a pushing force against the balloon that is directed from the back toward the front. Responding to this force, the balloon shifts forward in the direction of the car's acceleration. Who would have thought that general chemistry and physics could be so much fun?

In this chapter, we will discuss some MCAT favorites—the gas phase and the ideal gas laws. We will begin our discussion with ideal gases and the laws that govern their behavior. We will then examine the kinetic molecular theory that describes ideal gases and conclude with an evaluation of the ways in which the behavior of real gases deviates from that predicted by the ideal gas law.

8.1 The Gas Phase

LEARNING OBJECTIVES

After Chapter 8.1, you will be able to:

- Identify the unique characteristics of the gas phase
- Predict how pressure will change in different positions and locations, including underwater
- Recall the conditions at STP and standard conditions

Matter can exist in three different physical forms, called **phases** or **states**: gas, liquid, and solid. We have discussed liquids in the context of intermolecular forces and solids in the context of organized crystals in Chapter 3 of *MCAT General Chemistry Review*. The gaseous phase may be the simplest to understand because all gases display similar behavior and follow similar laws regardless of their particular chemical identities. Like liquids, gases are classified as fluids because they can flow and take on the shapes of their containers. However, the atoms or molecules in a gaseous sample move rapidly and are far apart from each other. In addition, only very weak intermolecular forces exist between gas particles; this results in certain characteristic physical properties, such as the ability to expand to fill any volume. Gases are also easily—although not infinitely—compressible, which distinguishes them from liquids.

Variables

We can define the state of a gaseous sample by four variables: **pressure (*P*)**, **volume (*V*)**, **temperature (*T*)**, and number of **moles (*n*)**.

Gas pressures are usually expressed in units of **atmospheres (atm)** or in **millimeters of mercury (mmHg)**, which are equivalent to **torr**. The SI unit for pressure, however, is the **pascal (Pa)**. The mathematical relationships among all of these units are as follows:

$$1 \text{ atm} = 760 \text{ mmHg} \equiv 760 \text{ torr} = 101.325 \text{ kPa}$$

Medical devices that measure blood pressure are termed **sphygmomanometers**, and the most clinically relevant unit of measurement for them is mmHg. In fact many medical devices utilize the same conceptual design of a **barometer**, shown in Figure 8.1, to continuously monitor blood pressure.

REAL WORLD

Blood pressure is measured by a sphygmomanometer, which uses units of mmHg. A normal adult blood pressure is considered less than 120 mmHg systolic and 80 mmHg diastolic (<120/80). Hypertension (high blood pressure) is defined as having at least two blood pressure readings >140 mmHg systolic or >90 mmHg diastolic.

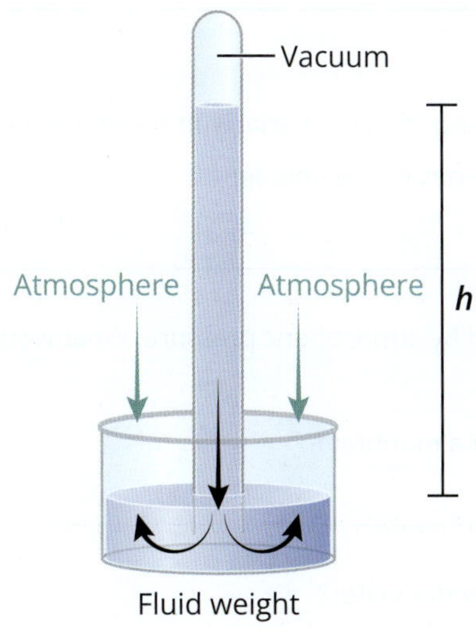

Figure 8.1 Schematic of a Simple Mercury Barometer
*The height (*h*) of the mercury column is proportional to the atmospheric pressure.*

In order to explain why the mercury rises in a barometer, we must summarize the forces at play here. **Atmospheric pressure** creates a downward force on the pool of mercury at the base of the barometer while the mercury in the column exerts an opposing force (its weight) based on its density. The weight of the mercury creates a vacuum in the top of the tube. When the external air exerts a higher force than the weight of the mercury in the column, the column rises. When the external air exerts a lower force than the weight of the mercury, the column falls. Thus, a reading can be obtained by measuring the height of the mercury column (in mm), which will be directly proportional to the atmospheric pressure being applied.

BRIDGE

Fluid dynamics is an important concept discussed in Chapter 4 of *MCAT Physics and Math Review* that applies to multiple aspects of the gas laws covered here, including the functionality of a mercury barometer.

It is important to mention here that atmospheric pressure is not the only external pressure that can exert this force. For instance, a clinical blood pressure cuff creates a force that is opposed by the person's systolic and diastolic arterial blood pressure.

The volume of a gas is generally expressed in liters (L) or milliliters (mL). Temperature is usually given in kelvin (K), although degrees Celsius (°C) may be used instead. Many processes involving gases take place under **standard temperature and pressure (STP)**, which refers to conditions of 273 K (0°C) and 1 atm.

A note of caution: **STP conditions** are not identical to **standard state conditions**. The two standards involve different temperatures and are used for different purposes. STP (273 K and 1 atm) is generally used for gas law calculations; standard state conditions (298 K, 1 atm, 1 M concentrations) are used when measuring standard enthalpy, entropy, free energy changes, and electrochemical cell voltage.

MCAT EXPERTISE

On the MCAT, remember that STP is different from standard state. Temperature at STP is 0°C (273 K). Temperature at standard state is 25°C (298 K).

MCAT CONCEPT CHECK 8.1

Before you move on, assess your understanding of the material with these questions.

1. Name some characteristics that make the gas phase unique:

____

2. A mercury barometer is primarily affected by atmospheric pressure. What would happen to the level of the mercury in the column if:
   - the barometer was moved to the top of a mountain?

   ____

   - the barometer was placed ten meters under water?

   ____

3. What are the conditions for STP?

____

4. What are the standard conditions?

____

8.2 Ideal Gases High Yield

LEARNING OBJECTIVES

After Chapter 8.2, you will be able to:

- Apply the ideal gas equation to calculations of pressure, temperature, volume, or number of moles
- Calculate the density of a substance given its molecular formula, current pressure, and current temperature
- Apply Avogadro's principle, Boyle's law, Charles's law, Gay–Lussac's law, and the combined ideal gas law to given scenarios
- Solve problems using Dalton's law of partial pressures and Henry's law

When we examine the behavior of gases under varying conditions of temperature and pressure, we assume that the gases are ideal. An **ideal gas** represents a hypothetical gas with molecules that have no **intermolecular forces** and occupy no volume. Although **real gases** deviate from this ideal behavior at high pressures (low volumes) and low temperatures, many compressed real gases demonstrate behavior that is close to ideal.

KEY CONCEPT

An ideal gas follows the gas laws we will discuss at all pressures and temperatures. A real gas deviates from these laws at high pressures (low volumes) and low temperatures because of intermolecular forces or volume effects.

Ideal Gas Law

The ideal gas law was first stated in 1834 by Benoît Paul Émile Clapeyron, more than 170 years after Sir Robert Boyle performed his experimental studies on the relationship between pressure and volume in the gas state. In fact, by the time the ideal gas law found its expression, Boyle's law, Charles's law, and Dalton's law had already been well-established. Historical considerations aside, it will benefit us to examine the ideal gas law first so that we can then understand the other laws, which had been identified earlier, to be only special cases of the ideal gas law.

The ideal gas law shows the relationship among four variables that define a sample of gas:

$$PV = nRT$$

Equation 8.1

where P is the pressure, V is the volume, n is the number of moles, and T is the temperature. R represents the **ideal gas constant**, which has a value of $8.21 \times 10^{-2} \frac{\text{L} \cdot \text{atm}}{\text{mol} \cdot \text{K}}$. Be aware that the gas constant can be expressed in other units. On the MCAT, you may also encounter R given as $8.314 \frac{\text{J}}{\text{K} \cdot \text{mol}}$, which is derived when SI units of pascal (for pressure) and cubic meters (for volume) are substituted into the ideal gas law. Although the relevant values for R will be provided on Test Day if needed, it is important to recognize the appropriate value for R based on the units of the variables given in a passage or question stem.

The ideal gas law is used to determine the missing term when given all of the others. It can also be used to calculate the change in a term while holding two of the others constant. It is most commonly used to solve for volume or pressure at any given temperature and number of moles; Figure 8.2 shows graphs of P-V relationships at different temperatures, where T_1 is the highest temperature, and T_4 is the lowest temperature.

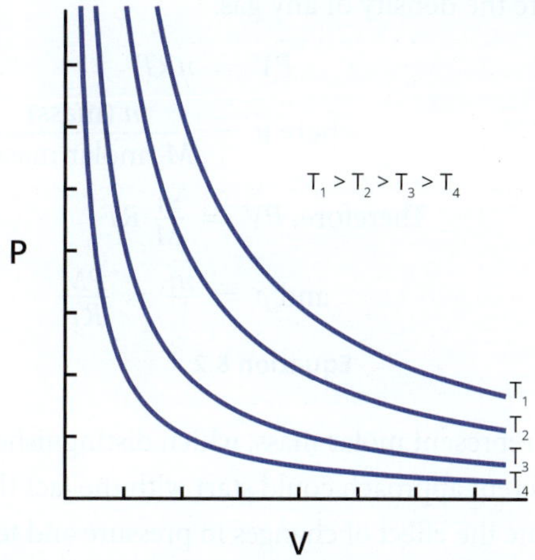

Figure 8.2 Ideal Gas Isothermal Curves
When number of moles of gas is held constant at a given temperature, the relationship between pressure and volume can be traced.

The ideal gas law is useful not only for standard calculations of pressure, volume, or temperature of a gas under a given set of conditions, but also for determinations of gas density and molar mass.

BRIDGE

Round numbers to speed up your arithmetic on Test Day. For instance, constants such as 0.0821 can be rounded to 0.08. Choices will be sufficiently different so that your estimated answer will be nearly identical to the true answer choice. Arithmetic and math strategies are discussed in Chapter 10 of *MCAT Physics and Math Review*.

Example: What volume would 12 g of helium occupy at 27°C and a pressure of 380 mmHg?

Solution: The ideal gas law can be used, but first, all of the variables must be converted to units that will correspond to the expression of the gas constant as $8.21 \times 10^{-2} \frac{\text{L} \cdot \text{atm}}{\text{mol} \cdot \text{K}}$.

$$P = 380 \text{ mmHg} \left[\frac{1 \text{ atm}}{760 \text{ mmHg}}\right] = 0.5 \text{ atm}$$

$$T = 27^\circ\text{C} + 273 = 300 \text{ K}$$

$$n = 12 \text{ g He} \left[\frac{1 \text{ mol}}{4.0 \text{ g}}\right] = 3 \text{ mol He}$$

$$PV = nRT$$

$$(0.5 \text{ atm})(V) = (3 \text{ mol He})\left(0.0821 \frac{\text{L} \cdot \text{atm}}{\text{mol} \cdot \text{K}}\right)(300 \text{ K})$$

$$0.5\,V \approx 3 \times 8 \times 3$$

$$V = 144 \text{ L (actual} = 148 \text{ L)}$$

Density

We define **density** (ρ) as the ratio of the mass per unit volume of a substance. The densities of gases are usually expressed in units of grams per liter. The ideal gas law contains variables for volume and number of moles, so we can rearrange the law to calculate the density of any gas:

$$PV = nRT$$

$$\text{where } n = \frac{m \text{ (mass)}}{M \text{ (molar mass)}}$$

$$\text{Therefore, } PV = \frac{m}{M} RT$$

$$\text{and } \rho = \frac{m}{V} = \frac{PM}{RT}$$

Equation 8.2

Note that the italicized M is used to represent molar mass, which distinguishes it from the unitalicized M used to represent units of molarity. A different approach could start with the fact that a mole of an ideal gas at STP occupies 22.4 L. We can then calculate the effect of changes in pressure and temperature when they differ from STP conditions, predicting the volume of the gas. Finally, we'll calculate the density by dividing the mass by the predicted volume. The following equation, the **combined gas law**, is an amalgam of some of the special cases we will discuss in the following section. It can be used to relate changes in temperature, volume, and pressure of a gas:

$$\frac{P_1 V_1}{T_1} = \frac{P_2 V_2}{T_2}$$

Equation 8.3

where the subscripts 1 and 2 refer to the two states of the gas (at STP and at the conditions of actual temperature and pressure, for example). This equation assumes the number of moles stays constant.

To calculate a change in volume, the equation is rearranged as follows:

$$V_2 = V_1\left[\frac{P_1}{P_2}\right]\left[\frac{T_2}{T_1}\right]$$

V_2 is then used to find the density of the gas under nonstandard conditions:

$$\rho = \frac{m}{V_2}$$

On Test Day, it may be helpful to visualize how the changes in pressure and temperature affect the volume of the gas, and this can serve as a check to avoid accidentally switching the values of pressure and temperature in the numerator and denominator. For example, one could predict that doubling the temperature of a gas would result in doubling its volume, and doubling the pressure of a gas would result in halving the volume, so doubling both the temperature and pressure at the same time results in a final volume that is equal to the original volume.

Example: What is the density of CO_2 gas at 2 atm and 273°C?

Solution: At STP, a mole of gas occupies 22.4 L. Because the increase in pressure to 2 atm decreases volume proportionally, 22.4 L must be multiplied by $\frac{1\text{ atm}}{2\text{ atm}} = 0.5$. Because the increase in temperature increases volume proportionally, the temperature factor will be $\frac{546\text{ K}}{273\text{ K}} = 2$.

$$V_2 = \left[\frac{22.4\text{ L}}{\text{mol}}\right]\left[\frac{1\text{ atm}}{2\text{ atm}}\right]\left[\frac{546\text{ K}}{273\text{ K}}\right] = 22.4\frac{\text{L}}{\text{mol}}$$

$$\rho = \frac{44\frac{\text{g}}{\text{mol}}}{22.4\frac{\text{L}}{\text{mol}}} \approx 2\frac{\text{g}}{\text{L}}\left(\text{actual} = 1.96\ \frac{\text{g}}{\text{L}}\right).$$

Molar Mass

Sometimes the identity of a gas is unknown, and the molar mass, discussed in Chapter 4 of *MCAT General Chemistry Review*, can be determined in order to identify it. Using the equation for density derived from the ideal gas law, we can calculate the molar mass of a gas experimentally in the following way:

The pressure and temperature of a gas contained in a bulb of a given volume are measured, and the mass of the bulb with the sample is measured. Then, the bulb is evacuated—the gas is removed—and the mass of the empty bulb is determined. The mass of the bulb with the sample minus the mass of the evacuated bulb gives the mass of the sample. Finally, the density of the sample is determined by dividing the mass of the sample by the volume of the bulb. This gives the density at the given temperature and pressure.

Using $V_2 = V_1\left[\frac{P_1}{P_2}\right]\left[\frac{T_2}{T_1}\right]$, we then calculate the volume of the gas at STP, substituting 273 K for T_2 and 1 atm for P_2. The ratio of the sample mass divided by V_2 gives the density of the gas at STP. The molar mass can then be calculated as the product of the gas's density at STP and the STP volume of one mole of gas, $22.4\ \frac{\text{L}}{\text{mol}}$:

$$M = (\rho_{\text{STP}})\left(22.4\ \frac{\text{L}}{\text{mol}}\right)$$

Example: What is the molar mass of a 22.4 L sample of gas that has a mass of 225 g at a temperature of 273°C and a pressure of 10 atm?

Solution: Determine how the current conditions compare to STP, and use this to set up a proportional relationship. Be careful to note the differences between degrees C and K, and current versus STP conditions.

$$\frac{P_1V_1}{T_1} = \frac{P_2V_2}{T_2} \text{ giving } V_2 = V_1\left[\frac{P_1}{P_2}\right]\left[\frac{T_2}{T_1}\right]$$

$$V_{STP} = V_1\left[\frac{P_1}{P_{STP}}\right]\left[\frac{T_{STP}}{T_1}\right] = 22.4\text{ L}\left[\frac{10\text{ atm}}{1\text{ atm}}\right]\left[\frac{273\text{ K}}{546\text{ K}}\right] = 22.4 \times 10 \times \frac{1}{2} = 112\text{ L}$$

$$\frac{225\text{ g}}{112\text{ L}} \approx 2\frac{\text{g}}{\text{L}} \text{ at STP}$$

$$M = 2\frac{\text{g}}{\text{L}}\left[\frac{22.4\text{ L}}{\text{mol}}\right] \approx 44.8\frac{\text{g}}{\text{mol}}$$

Special Cases

Now that we have considered the ideal gas law as the mathematical relationship between four variables that define the state of a gas (pressure, volume, temperature, and moles of gas), we can examine the other laws that preceded its discovery. Even though the following laws were developed before the ideal gas law, it is conceptually helpful to think of them as special cases of the more general ideal gas law.

Avogadro's Principle

One important discovery that preceded Clapeyron's formulation of the ideal gas law was **Avogadro's principle**, which states that all gases at a constant temperature and pressure occupy volumes that are directly proportional to the number of moles of gas present. Equal amounts of all gases at the same temperature and pressure will occupy equal volumes. As discussed above, one mole of any gas, irrespective of its chemical identity, will occupy 22.4 liters at STP.

$$\frac{n}{V} = k \text{ or } \frac{n_1}{V_1} = \frac{n_2}{V_2}$$

Equation 8.4

where k is a constant, n_1 and n_2 are the number of moles of gas 1 and gas 2, respectively, and V_1 and V_2 are the volumes of the gases, respectively. This can be summarized in the following statement: *as the number of moles of gas increases, the volume increases in direct proportion.*

Example: A 2.0 L sample at 100°C and 20 atm contains 5 moles of a gas. If an additional 25 moles of gas at the same pressure and temperature are added, what is the final volume of the gas?

Solution: If pressure and temperature are held constant, the ideal gas law reduces to Avogadro's principle:

$$\frac{n_1}{V_1} = \frac{n_2}{V_2}$$

$$\frac{5\text{ mol}}{2.0\text{ L}} = \frac{5\text{ mol} + 25\text{ mol}}{V_2}$$

$$V_2 = \frac{30\text{ mol} \times 2.0\text{ L}}{5\text{ mol}} = 12.0\text{ L}$$

Boyle's Law

Robert Boyle conducted a series of experimental studies in 1660 that led to his formulation of a law that now bears his name: **Boyle's law**. His work showed that, for a given gaseous sample held at constant temperature (isothermal conditions), the volume of the gas is inversely proportional to its pressure:

$$PV = k \text{ or } P_1V_1 = P_2V_2$$

Equation 8.5

where k is a constant, and the subscripts 1 and 2 represent two different sets of pressure and volume conditions. Careful examination of Boyle's law shows that it is, indeed, simply the special case of the ideal gas law in which n and T are constant.

A plot of volume vs. pressure for a gas—with axes swapped from the curves in Figure 8.2—is shown in Figure 8.3.

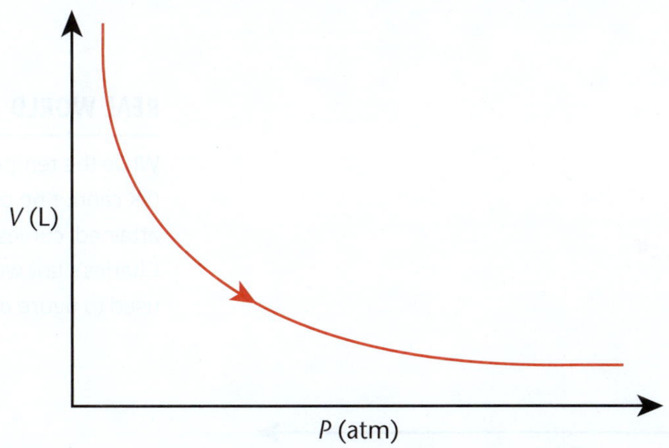

Figure 8.3 Boyle's Law (Isothermal Compression)
As pressure increases, volume decreases.

KEY CONCEPT

Boyle's law is a derivation of the ideal gas law and states that pressure and volume are inversely related: when one increases, the other decreases.

MCAT EXPERTISE

Sometimes it is easier to remember the shape of the graph to help you recall the variables' relationship on Test Day. Here we can see that, as pressure increases, the volume decreases, and vice-versa. These ratios and relationships will often allow you to answer questions on the MCAT without having to do much math.

Example: What would be the volume of a 1 L sample of helium if its pressure is changed from 12 atm to 4 atm under isothermal conditions?

Solution: If the number of moles of gas and temperature are held constant, the ideal gas law reduces to Boyle's law:

$$P_1V_1 = P_2V_2$$

$$(12 \text{ atm})(1 \text{ L}) = (4 \text{ atm})(V_2)$$

$$V_2 = \frac{12 \text{ atm} \times 1 \text{ L}}{4 \text{ atm}} = 3 \text{ L}$$

Charles's Law

In the early 19th century, Joseph Louis Gay-Lussac published findings based, in part, on earlier unpublished work by Jacques Charles; hence, the law of Charles and Gay-Lussac is more commonly known simply as **Charles's law.** The law states that, at constant pressure, the volume of a gas is proportional to its absolute temperature, expressed in kelvin. Expressed mathematically, Charles's law is

$$\frac{V}{T} = k \text{ or } \frac{V_1}{T_1} = \frac{V_2}{T_2}$$

Equation 8.6

KEY CONCEPT

Charles's law is also a derivation of the ideal gas law and states that volume and temperature are directly proportional: when one increases, the other increases in direct proportion.

where, again, k is a proportionality constant and the subscripts 1 and 2 represent two different sets of temperature and volume conditions. Careful examination of Charles's law shows that it is another special case of the ideal gas law in which n and P are constant.

A plot of temperature vs. volume is shown in Figure 8.4. Note that if one extrapolates the V vs. T plot for a gas back to where $T = 0$ (absolute zero), we find that $V = 0$!

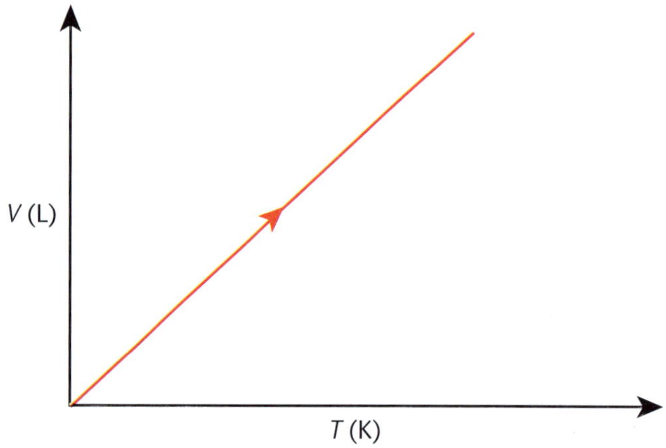

Figure 8.4 Charles's Law (Isobaric Expansion)
As temperature increases, volume increases.

REAL WORLD

While the temperature of 0 K cannot be physically attained, curves such as Charles's law were originally used to figure out its value.

Example: If the temperature of 2 L of gas at constant pressure is changed from 290 K to 580 K, what would be its final volume?

Solution: If the number of moles of gas and pressure are held constant, the ideal gas law reduces to Charles's law:

$$\frac{V_1}{T_1} = \frac{V_2}{T_2}$$

$$\frac{2\text{ L}}{290\text{ K}} = \frac{V_2}{580\text{ K}}$$

$$V_2 = \frac{2\text{ L} \times 580\text{ K}}{290\text{ K}} = 4\text{ L}$$

Gay-Lussac's Law

Gay-Lussac's law is complementary to Charles's Law. It utilizes the same derivation from the ideal gas law, but it relates pressure to temperature instead. Expressed mathematically, Gay-Lussac's law is

$$\frac{P}{T} = k \text{ or } \frac{P_1}{T_1} = \frac{P_2}{T_2}$$

Equation 8.7

where, again, k is a proportionality constant, and the subscripts 1 and 2 represent two different sets of temperature and pressure conditions. Careful examination of Gay-Lussac's law shows that it is another special case of the ideal gas law in which n and V are constant.

Figure 8.5 graphs this concept, which is nearly identical to Charles's law. Again, an increase in temperature will increase the pressure in direct proportion.

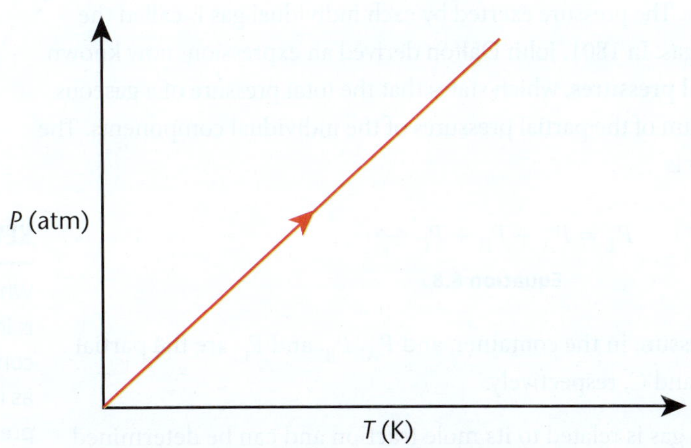

Figure 8.5 Gay-Lussac's Law (Isovolumetric Heating)
As temperature increases, pressure increases.

Example: If the pressure of a sample of gas with a temperature of 300 K changes from 2 atm to 5 atm during heating, what would be the final temperature if volume is held constant?

Solution: If the number of moles of gas and volume are held constant, the ideal gas law reduces to Gay-Lussac's law:

$$\frac{P_1}{T_1} = \frac{P_2}{T_2}$$

$$\frac{2\text{ atm}}{300\text{ K}} = \frac{5\text{ atm}}{T_2}$$

$$T_2 = \frac{5\text{ atm} \times 300\text{ K}}{2\text{ atm}} = 750\text{ K}$$

Combined Gas Law

As discussed earlier, the **combined gas law** (Equation 8.3) was a combination of many of the preceding laws. This law relates pressure and volume (Boyle's law) in the numerator, and relates the variations in temperature to both volume (Charles's law) and pressure (Gay-Lussac's law) simultaneously. When using this equation, take care to place all of the variables in the right place.

Dalton's Law of Partial Pressures

When two or more gases that do not chemically interact are found in one vessel, each gas will behave independently of the others. That is, each gas will behave as if it were the only gas in the container. Therefore, the pressure exerted by each gas in the mixture will be equal to the pressure that the gas would exert if it were the only one in the container. The pressure exerted by each individual gas is called the **partial pressure** of that gas. In 1801, John Dalton derived an expression, now known as **Dalton's law of partial pressures**, which states that the total pressure of a gaseous mixture is equal to the sum of the partial pressures of the individual components. The equation for Dalton's law is

$$P_T = P_A + P_B + P_C + \cdots$$

Equation 8.8

where P_T is the total pressure in the container, and P_A, P_B, and P_C are the partial pressures of gases A, B, and C, respectively.

The partial pressure of a gas is related to its mole fraction and can be determined using the following equation:

$$P_A = X_A P_T$$

$$\text{where } X_A = \frac{\text{moles of gas A}}{\text{total moles of gas}}$$

Equation 8.9

MCAT EXPERTISE

Understanding how the combined gas law functions helps avoid the need to memorize every other special case of the ideal gas law. Read the question stem or passage with an eye toward the quantities that remain constant to know when assumptions can be made.

KEY CONCEPT

When more than one gas is in a container, each contributes to the whole as if it were the only gas present. Add up all of the pressures of the individual gases and you get the whole pressure of the system.

Example: A vessel contains 0.75 mol of nitrogen, 0.20 mol of hydrogen, and 0.05 mol of fluorine at a total pressure of 2.5 atm. What is the partial pressure of each gas?

Solution: First calculate the mole fraction of each gas.

$$X_{N_2} = \frac{0.75\text{ mol}}{1.00\text{ mol}} = 0.75 \quad X_{H_2} = \frac{0.20\text{ mol}}{1.00\text{ mol}} = 0.20 \quad X_{F_2} = \frac{0.05\text{ mol}}{1.00\text{ mol}} = 0.05$$

Then calculate the partial pressure.

$$P_A = X_A P_T$$

$$P_{N_2} = (0.75)(2.5\text{ atm}) = 1.875\text{ atm}$$

$$P_{H_2} = (0.20)(2.5\text{ atm}) = 0.5\text{ atm}$$

$$P_{F_2} = (0.05)(2.5\text{ atm}) = 0.125\text{ atm}$$

Henry's Law

The difference in gas solubility between fluids was explained by William Henry in 1803. What Henry noticed was that, at various applied pressures, the concentration of a gas in a liquid increased or decreased. This was a characteristic of a gas's vapor pressure. **Vapor pressure** is the pressure exerted by evaporated particles above the surface of a liquid. Evaporation, as discussed in Chapter 7 of *MCAT General Chemistry Review*, is a dynamic process that requires the molecules at the surface of a liquid to gain enough energy to escape into the gas phase.

Vapor pressure from the evaporated molecules forces some of the gas back into the liquid phase, and equilibrium is reached between evaporation and condensation. Mathematically, this is expressed as:

$$[A] = k_H \times P_A \text{ or } \frac{[A]_1}{P_1} = \frac{[A]_2}{P_2} = k_H$$

Equation 8.10

where [A] is the concentration of A in solution, k_H is Henry's constant, and P_A is the partial pressure of A. The value of Henry's constant depends on the identity of the gas.

KEY CONCEPT

The solubility of a gas will increase with increasing partial pressure of the gas.

According to this relationship, solubility (concentration) and pressure are directly related. In biology, this is a critically important relationship for gas and nutrient exchange. As discussed in Chapter 6 of *MCAT Biology Review*, lung tissue—at the microscopic level—is organized into grapelike clusters of sacs called alveoli. These sacs are perfused by capillaries that allow for the exchange of carbon dioxide and oxygen, as shown in Figure 8.6. Venous blood is largely deoxygenated with a low partial pressure of oxygen and carries large amounts of carbon dioxide as a waste product of respiration. The relatively high pressure of oxygen in the alveoli allows for unidirectional movement of oxygen from the lungs into the blood; pressure differences for carbon dioxide in venous blood compared to the alveolus are small but enough to move carbon dioxide from blood to lungs. If the atmospheric pressure changes, as it does from sea level to high altitude, then the partial pressure of oxygen in the atmosphere also changes (as explained by Dalton's law), and the amount of gas exchanged is altered accordingly; if the partial pressure of a particular gas is elevated, such as when giving hyperbaric oxygen, the amount of that gas dissolved in the blood is also elevated.

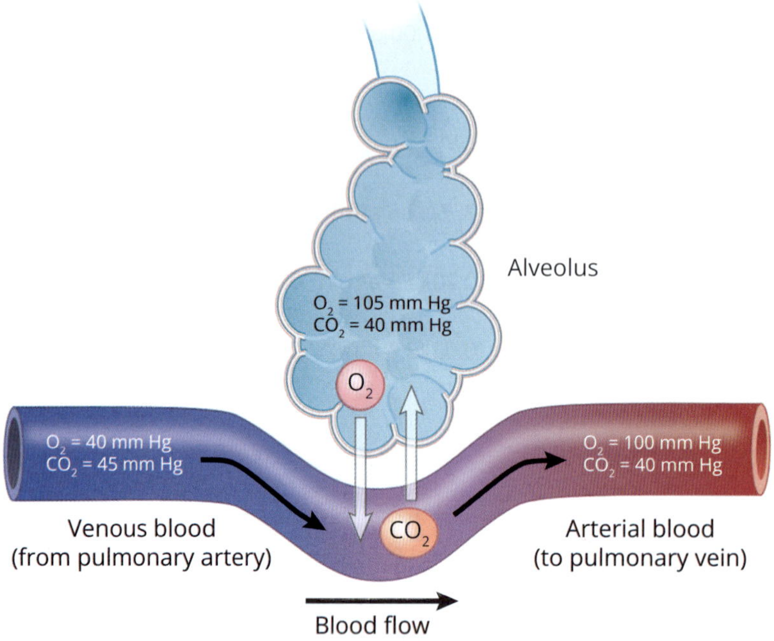

Figure 8.6 Alveolar Capillary Gas Exchange
Differences in partial pressure of oxygen and carbon dioxide in the alveolus and blood results in oxygen flowing into the blood and carbon dioxide moving into the alveolus.

Example: If 4×10^{-4} moles of gas are dissolved in 2 L of solution under an ambient pressure of 2 atm, what will be the molar concentration of the gas under 10 atm?

Solution: Start by determining the initial concentration of the gas in solution.

$$[A]_1 = \frac{4 \times 10^{-4}\ \text{mol}}{2\ \text{L}} = 2 \times 10^{-4}\ \text{M}$$

Next, utilize the direct relationship between solubility and pressure according to Henry's law.

$$\frac{[A]_1}{P_1} = \frac{[A]_2}{P_2}$$

$$\frac{2 \times 10^{-4}\ \text{M}}{2\ \text{atm}} = \frac{[A]_2}{10\ \text{atm}}$$

$$[A]_2 = \frac{(2 \times 10^{-4}\ \text{M})(10\ \text{atm})}{2\ \text{atm}} = 10^{-3}\ \text{M}$$

MCAT CONCEPT CHECK 8.2

Before you move on, assess your understanding of the material with these questions.

1. A container with 4 moles of a gas at a pressure of 8 atm has a volume of 12 liters. What is its temperature? (Note: $R = 8.21 \times 10^{-2} \frac{\text{L} \cdot \text{atm}}{\text{mol} \cdot \text{K}}$)

___

2. What is the density of argon gas at 4 atm and 127°C?

___

3. A 20 L sample at 300°C and 5 atm of pressure contains 2 moles of a gas. If an additional 3 moles of gas at the same pressure and temperature are added, what is the final total volume of the gas?

___

4. What would be the volume of a 2 L sample of neon if its pressure is changed from 1 atm to 40 atm under isothermal conditions?

___

5. If the temperature of 6 L of gas at constant pressure is changed from 27°C to 127°C, what would be its final volume?

___

6. If the pressure of a sample of gas with a temperature of 227°C is changed from 5 atm to 2 atm during cooling, what would be the final temperature?

___

7. A vessel contains 8 mol O_2, 3 mol CH_4, and 1 mol CO_2 at a total pressure of 240 atm. What is the partial pressure of each gas?

___

8. How can the concentration of carbon dioxide in sodas or other carbonated beverages be so much higher than that of atmospheric carbon dioxide?

___

8.3 Kinetic Molecular Theory

LEARNING OBJECTIVES

After Chapter 8.3, you will be able to:

- Recall the assumptions made by kinetic molecular theory
- Calculate the average speed of a gas, given its temperature
- Compare the relative speeds of two different gases at the same temperature
- Apply Graham's law to situations involving gas effusion:

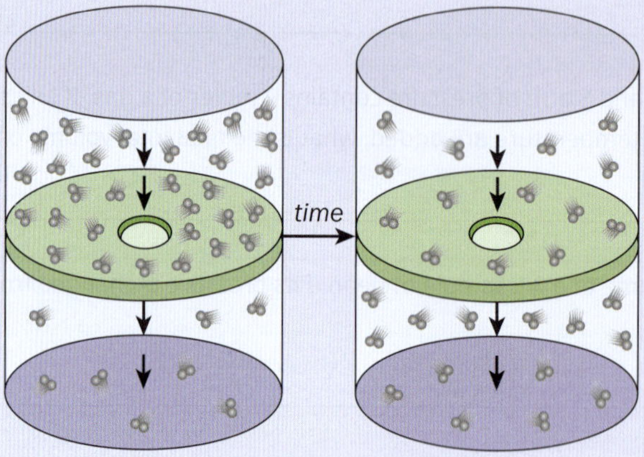

The **kinetic molecular theory** was developed in the second half of the 19th century, well after the laws describing gas behavior had been developed. The kinetic molecular theory was used to *explain* the behavior of gases, which the other laws merely *described*. The gas laws demonstrate that all gases show similar physical characteristics and behavior irrespective of their particular chemical identity. The behavior of real gases deviates from the ideal behavior predicted under the assumptions of this theory, but these deviations can be corrected for in calculations. The combined efforts of James Maxwell, Ludwig Boltzmann, and others led to a simple explanation of gaseous molecular behavior based on the motion of individual molecules. Like the gas laws, the kinetic molecular theory was developed in reference to ideal gases, although it can be applied with reasonable accuracy to real gases as well.

Assumptions

To simplify the model proposed by the kinetic molecular theory, certain assumptions are made:

1. Gases are made up of particles with volumes that are negligible compared to the container volume.
2. Gas atoms or molecules exhibit no intermolecular attractions or repulsions.
3. Gas particles are in continuous, random motion, undergoing collisions with other particles and the container walls.
4. Collisions between any two gas particles (or between particles and the container walls) are elastic, meaning that there is conservation of both momentum and kinetic energy.
5. The average kinetic energy of gas particles is proportional to the absolute temperature of the gas (in kelvins), and it is the same for all gases at a given temperature, irrespective of chemical identity or atomic mass.

Applications

It is fairly straightforward to imagine gas particles as little rubber balls bouncing off each other and off the walls of the container. Of course, rubber balls, like real gas particles, have measurable mass and volume, and not even the bounciest rubber balls will collide in a completely elastic manner. Still, this provides an apt visualization of the behaviors described by the kinetic molecular theory.

Average Molecular Speeds

According to the kinetic molecular theory of gases, the average kinetic energy of a gas particle is proportional to the absolute temperature of the gas:

$$\text{KE} = \frac{1}{2} m v^2 = \frac{3}{2} k_\text{B} T$$

Equation 8.11

where k_B is the **Boltzmann constant** $\left(1.38 \times 10^{-23} \frac{\text{J}}{\text{K}}\right)$, which serves as a bridge between the macroscopic and microscopic behaviors of gases (that is, as a bridge between the behavior of the gas as a whole and the individual gas molecules). This equation shows that the speed of a gas particle is related to its absolute temperature. However, because of the large number of rapidly and randomly moving gas particles, which may travel only nanometers before colliding with another particle or the container wall, the speed of an individual gas molecule is nearly impossible to define. Therefore, the speeds of gases are defined in terms of their average molecular speed. One way to define an average speed is to determine the average kinetic energy per particle and then calculate the speed to which this corresponds. The resultant quantity, known as the **root-mean-square speed** ($\boldsymbol{u_{\text{rms}}}$), is given by the following equation:

MCAT EXPERTISE

Understanding concepts will be much more fruitful on Test Day than memorizing all of the facts. The higher the temperature, the faster the molecules move. The larger the molecules, the slower they move.

$$u_{\text{rms}} = \sqrt{\frac{3RT}{M}}$$

Equation 8.12

where R is the ideal gas constant, T is the temperature, and M is the molar mass.

A **Maxwell–Boltzmann distribution curve** shows the distribution of gas particle speeds at a given temperature. Figure 8.7 shows a distribution curve of molecular speeds at two temperatures, T_1 and T_2, where T_2 is greater than T_1. Notice that the bell-shaped curve flattens and shifts to the right as the temperature increases, indicating that at higher temperatures, more molecules are moving at higher speeds.

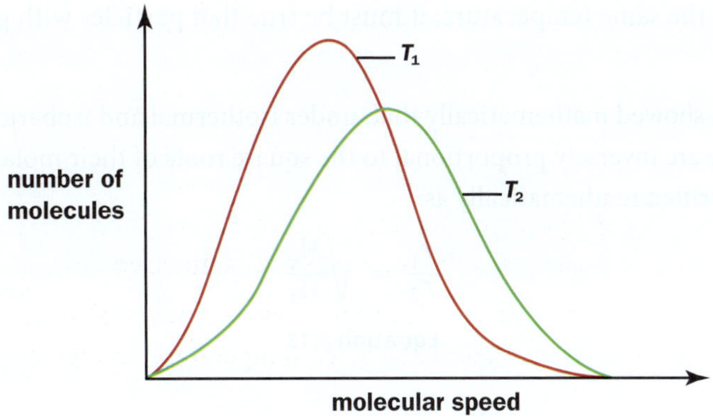

Figure 8.7 Maxwell–Boltzmann Distribution Curves of Molecular Speeds at Two Different Temperatures

Example: What is the average speed of xenon difluoride molecules at 20°C?

Solution: The ideal gas constant $R = 8.314 \frac{\text{J}}{\text{K} \cdot \text{mol}}$ should be used, and the molar mass of xenon difluoride is $169.3 \frac{\text{g}}{\text{mol}}$. M must be expressed in $\frac{\text{kg}}{\text{mol}}$ because joules are also derived from kilograms.

$$u_{\text{rms}} = \sqrt{\frac{3RT}{M}}$$

$$u_{\text{rms}} = \sqrt{\frac{(3)\left(8.314 \frac{\text{J}}{\text{K} \cdot \text{mol}}\right)(293 \text{ K})}{0.17 \frac{\text{kg}}{\text{mol}}}}$$

$$u_{\text{rms}} \approx \sqrt{\frac{(3)(8)(300)}{0.18}} = \sqrt{\frac{(8)(300)}{0.06}} = \sqrt{(8)(5{,}000)} = \sqrt{40{,}000}$$

$$u_{\text{rms}} \approx 200 \frac{\text{m}}{\text{s}} \left(\text{actual} = 208 \frac{\text{m}}{\text{s}}\right)$$

Graham's Law of Diffusion and Effusion

The movement of molecules from high concentration to low concentration through a medium (such as air or water) is called **diffusion**, as shown in Figure 8.8.

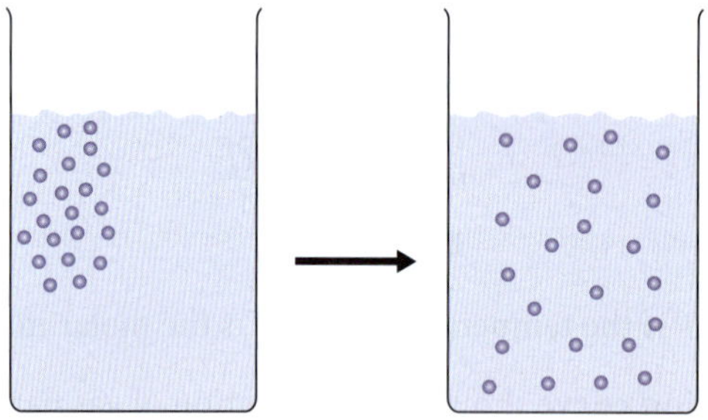

Figure 8.8 Diffusion of Solutes in a Solvent

The kinetic molecular theory of gases predicts that heavier gases diffuse more slowly than lighter ones because of their differing average speeds, as shown in Figure 8.9. Because all gas particles have the same average kinetic energy at the same temperature, it must be true that particles with greater mass travel at a slower average speed.

In 1832, Thomas Graham showed mathematically that, under isothermal and isobaric conditions, the rates at which two gases diffuse are inversely proportional to the square roots of their molar masses. This is called **Graham's law**, which is written mathematically as:

$$\frac{r_1}{r_2} = \sqrt{\frac{M_2}{M_1}}$$

Equation 8.13

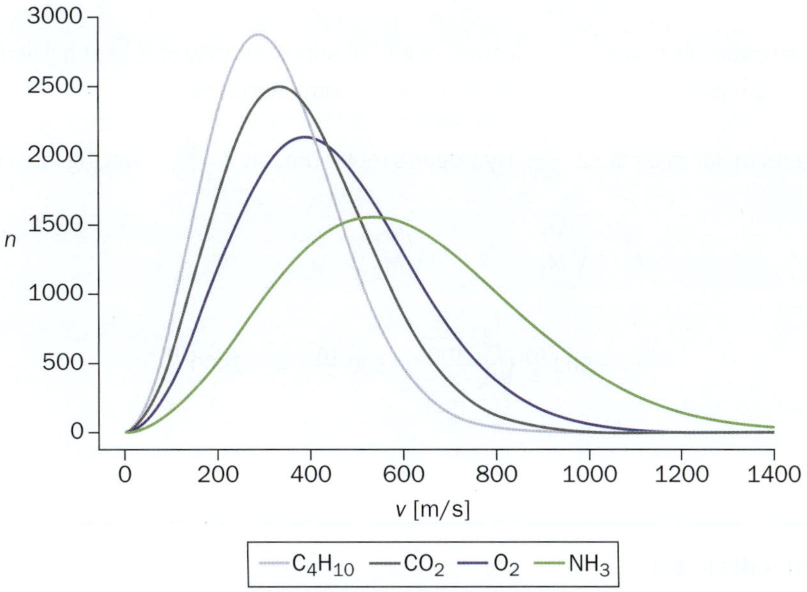

Figure 8.9 Maxwell–Boltzmann Distribution Curves of Molecular Speeds for Gases with Different Molar Masses
The more massive the gas particles, the slower their average speed.

where r_1 and r_2 are the diffusion rates of gas 1 and gas 2, respectively, and M_1 and M_2 are the molar masses of gas 1 and gas 2, respectively. From this equation, we can see that a gas that has a molar mass four times that of another gas will travel half as fast as the lighter gas.

Effusion is the flow of gas particles under pressure from one compartment to another through a small opening, as shown in Figure 8.10. Graham used the kinetic molecular theory of gases to show that, for two gases at the same temperature, the rates of effusion are proportional to the average speeds. He then expressed the rates of effusion in terms of molar mass and found that the relationship is the same as that for diffusion.

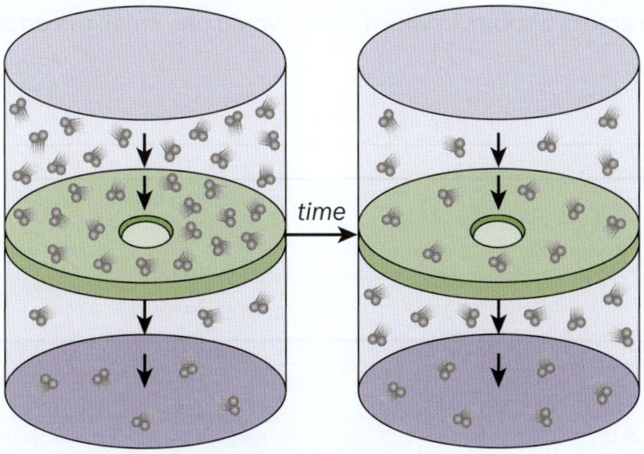

Figure 8.10 Effusion of Gas Particles
Effusion is the flow of gas particles under pressure from one compartment to another through a small opening.

REAL WORLD

Clinically, a pleural effusion is a condition in which fluid enters the intrapleural space through small openings in the capillaries or lymphatic vessels. This causes a pressure buildup around the lungs that hinders breathing.

KEY CONCEPT

Diffusion—When gases mix with one another.

Effusion—When a gas moves through a small hole under pressure.

Both will be slower for larger molecules.

Both conditions use the same equation.

Example: Oxygen molecules travel at an average speed of approximately 500 $\frac{\text{m}}{\text{s}}$ at a given temperature. Calculate the average speed of hydrogen molecules at the same temperature.

Solution: Oxygen's molar mass is 32 $\frac{\text{g}}{\text{mol}}$. Hydrogen's molar mass is 2 $\frac{\text{g}}{\text{mol}}$. Plugging into Graham's law, we get:

$$\frac{r_1}{r_2} = \sqrt{\frac{M_2}{M_1}} \rightarrow r_2 = r_1\sqrt{\frac{M_1}{M_2}}$$

$$r_2 = 500\,\frac{\text{m}}{\text{s}}\sqrt{\frac{32\,\frac{\text{g}}{\text{mol}}}{2\,\frac{\text{g}}{\text{mol}}}} = 500\,\frac{\text{m}}{\text{s}} \times 4 = 2000\,\frac{\text{m}}{\text{s}}$$

MCAT CONCEPT CHECK 8.3

Before you move on, assess your understanding of the material with these questions.

1. What are the assumptions made by the kinetic molecular theory?

---

2. What is the average speed of helium atoms at −173°C?

---

3. If neon gas travels at 400 $\frac{\text{m}}{\text{s}}$ at a given temperature, calculate the average speed of krypton at the same temperature.

---

4. Hydrogen sulfide (H_2S) has a very strong rotten egg odor. Methyl salicylate (C_8H_8O) has a wintergreen odor, and benzaldehyde (C_7H_6O) has a pleasant almond odor. If the vapors for these three substances were released at the same time from across a room, in which order would one smell the odors? Explain your answer.

8.4 Real Gases

LEARNING OBJECTIVES

After Chapter 8.4, you will be able to:

- Distinguish between real gases and ideal gases
- Predict how differences in attractive forces or volumes will affect real gas behavior

Throughout our discussions of the laws and theory that describe and explain the behaviors of gases, we have stressed that the fundamental assumption is a gas that behaves ideally. However, our world is not one of ideal gases but rather real ones.

MNEMONIC

Just like an ideal beach vacation (Figure 8.11), ideal gas conditions are approximated with high temperature and low pressure (high volume); good approximations can still be made using the ideal gas law.

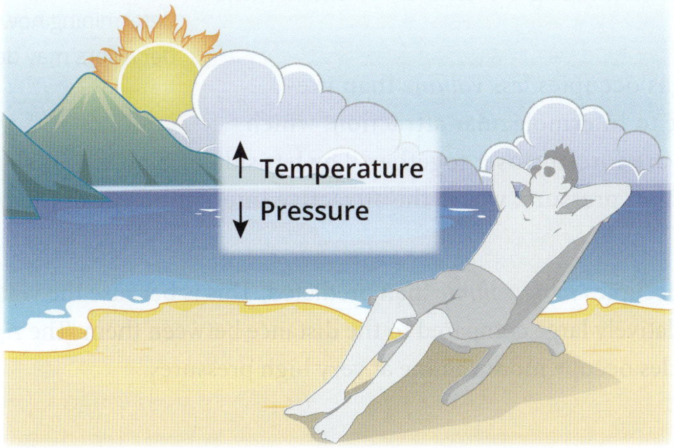

Figure 8.11 Ideal Gas Conditions
Just like an ideal beach day, ideal gas conditions are high temperature and low pressure.

The ideal gas law assumes particles have no volume and no intermolecular forces, but real gases have particles that occupy non-negligible volumes and that interact with each other in measurable ways. In reality, all real gases deviate from ideal behavior to some degree, but it is more pronounced under conditions that force particles into close proximity, such as high pressure and low temperature. These effects are implied by Figure 8.12, which shows isothermal lines on a pressure-volume graph for a real gas compared to the lines for ideal gas isotherms. Theoretically, according to the ideal gas law, gases stay in the gas phase in all conditions, but in reality, low volume, high pressure, and low temperature forces a phase change so that the behavior of the particles is not predicted anymore by the ideal gas law.

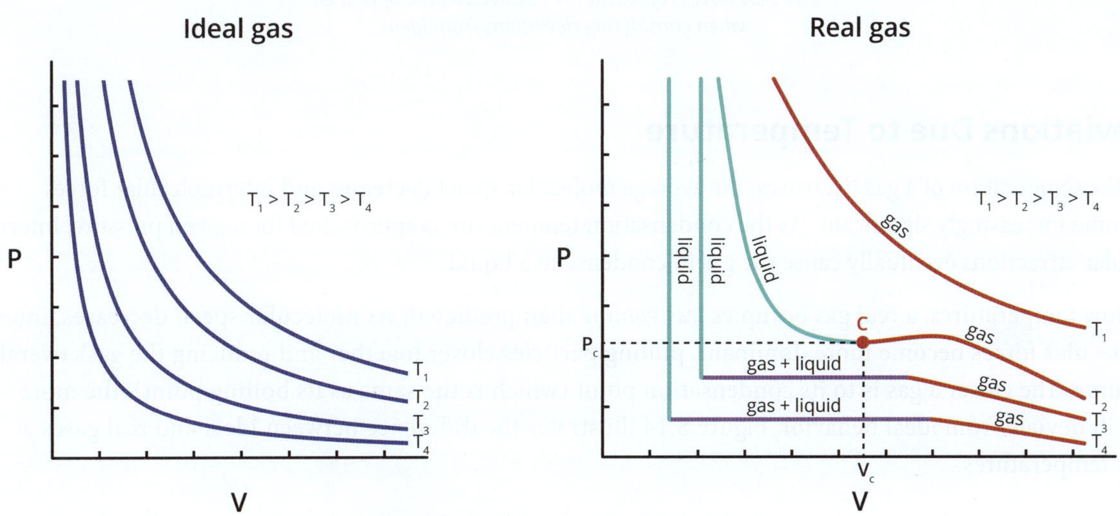

Figure 8.12 Ideal vs. Real Gas Isothermal Lines
Real gases deviate from ideal gases in that real gas particles occupy non-negligible volume and interact via intermolecular forces.

Deviations Due to Pressure

As the pressure of a gas increases, the particles are pushed closer together. As the condensation pressure for a given temperature is approached, intermolecular attraction forces become more significant until the gas eventually condenses into a liquid.

MCAT EXPERTISE

On the MCAT, an understanding of nonideal conditions will help with determining how gases' behaviors may deviate.

At moderately high pressures, a real gas occupies *less volume* than predicted by the ideal gas law. This is due to intermolecular attraction, which becomes more significant as particles are forced closer together. The left side of Figure 8.13 shows how gas particles react under moderately high pressure, where the attractive interactions push the particles closer together.

At extremely high pressures, a real gas occupies *more volume* than predicted. This is because the volume of the gas particles themselves becomes relatively large compared to the distance between them. The right side of Figure 8.13 shows how real gas particles occupy more volume at very high pressures.

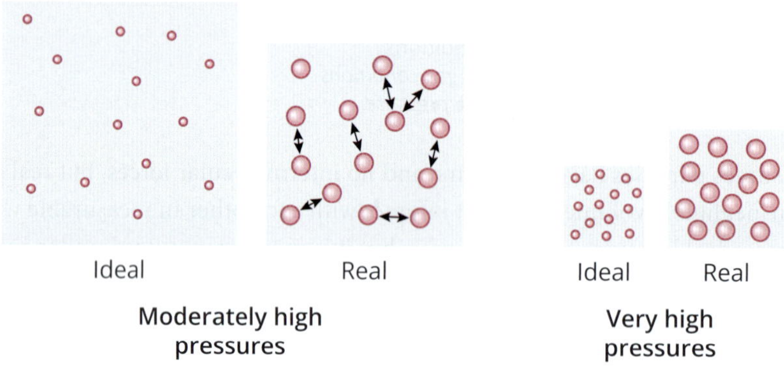

Figure 8.13 Deviations from Ideal Gas Law at High Pressure
Ideal gas particles do not have volume or intermolecular interactions, while real gases have both size and intermolecular interactions. The gray boxes represent the relative volume of real gas when considering deviations from ideal.

Deviations Due to Temperature

As the temperature of a gas decreases, the average molecular speed decreases and intermolecular forces become increasingly significant. As the condensation temperature is approached for a given pressure, intermolecular attractions eventually cause the gas to condense to a liquid.

At low temperatures, a real gas occupies *less volume* than predicted. As molecular speed decreases, intermolecular forces become more dominant, pulling particles closer together and reducing the gas's overall volume. The closer a gas is to its condensation point (which is the same as its boiling point), the more it will deviate from ideal behavior. Figure 8.14 illustrates the difference between ideal and real gases at low temperatures.

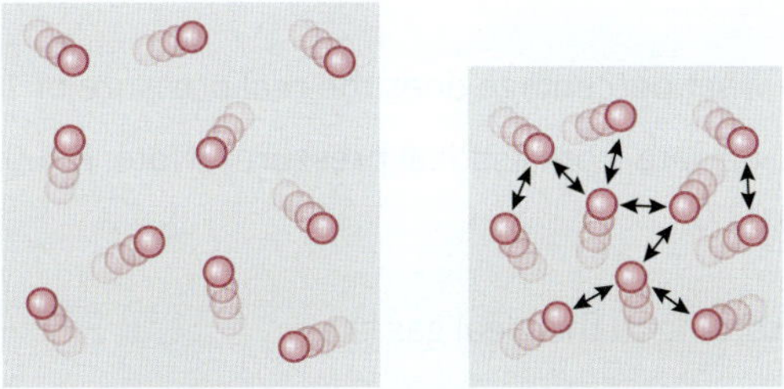

Figure 8.14 Deviations from Ideal Gas Law at Low Temperature
Low temperature decreases the molecular speed of particles, resulting in greater intermolecular attraction, effectively decreasing the volume of the gas (illustrated by the gray box) compared to an ideal gas.

At extremely low temperatures, as also occurs at extremely high pressures, the volume of the gas particles themselves causes the real gas to occupy *more volume* than predicted by the ideal gas law, since the particles cannot be compressed to zero volume.

van der Waals Equation of State

There are several gas equations that attempt to correct for the deviations from ideality that occur when a gas does not closely follow the ideal gas law. The van der Waals equation of state is one such equation:

$$\left(P + \frac{n^2 a}{V^2}\right)(V - nb) = nRT$$

Equation 8.14

where a and b are physical constants experimentally determined for each gas. The a term corrects for the attractive forces between molecules and, as such, will be smaller for gases that are small and less polarizable (such as helium), larger for gases that are larger and more polarizable (such as Xe or N_2), and largest for polar molecules such as HCl and NH_3. The b term corrects for the volume of the molecules themselves. Larger molecules thus have larger values of b. Numerical values for a are generally much larger than those for b.

KEY CONCEPT

Note that if a and b are both zero, the van der Waals equation of state reduces to the ideal gas law.

MNEMONIC

a is the van der Waals term for the **a**ttractive forces.

b is the van der Waals term for **b**ig particles.

MCAT EXPERTISE

Be familiar with the concepts embodied by this equation but do not bother memorizing it; if the testmakers want you to apply the equation, it will be provided in a passage or question stem.

Example: By what percentage does the real pressure of 1 mole of ammonia in a 1 liter flask at 227°C deviate from its ideal pressure? (Note: $R = 0.0821 \frac{\text{L} \cdot \text{atm}}{\text{mol} \cdot \text{K}}$; for NH_3, $a = 4.2$, $b = 0.037$)

Solution: According to the ideal gas law,

$$P = \frac{nRT}{V} = \frac{(1\text{ mol})\left(0.0821 \frac{\text{L} \cdot \text{atm}}{\text{mol} \cdot \text{K}}\right)(500\text{ K})}{1\text{ L}} = \frac{(0.0821)(1000)}{2}$$

$$= \frac{82.1}{2} = 41.5\text{ atm}$$

According to the van der Waals equation of state,

$$P = \frac{nRT}{V - nb} - \frac{n^2 a}{V^2} = \left[\frac{(1\text{ mol})\left(0.0821 \frac{\text{L} \cdot \text{atm}}{\text{mol} \cdot \text{K}}\right)(500\text{ K})}{1\text{ L} - (1\text{ mol})(0.037)}\right] - \left[\frac{(1\text{ mol})^2(4.2)}{(1\text{ L})^2}\right]$$

$$P = \frac{41.5}{0.963} - 4.2 \approx [41.5 + 4\%(41.5)] \approx 43 - 4 \approx 39\text{ atm (actual} = 38.8\text{ atm)}$$

The pressure is thus approximately $41.5 - 38.8 = 2.7$ atm less than would be predicted from the ideal gas law, representing an error of

$$\frac{2.7\text{ atm}}{41.5\text{ atm}} \times 100\% \approx \frac{3}{40} \times 100\% = 7.5\text{ percent.}$$

MCAT CONCEPT CHECK 8.4

Before you move on, assess your understanding of the material with these questions.

1. In what ways do real gases differ from ideal gases?

___

2. Which gas will exert a higher pressure under the same, nonideal conditions: methane or chloromethane?

___

3. If methane and isobutane are placed in the same size container under the same conditions, which will exert the higher pressure (consider both as having negligible attractive forces)?

___

Conclusion

In this chapter, we reviewed the basic characteristics and behaviors of gases. The ideal gas law shows the mathematical relationship among four variables associated with gases: pressure, volume, temperature, and number of moles. We examined special cases of the ideal gas law in which temperature (Boyle's law), pressure (Charles's law), or volume (Gay-Lussac's law) is held constant. Henry's law helped explain the principles behind dissolution of gases in liquids and gas exchange in biological systems. We also examined Dalton's law, which relates the partial pressure of a gas to its mole fraction and the sum of the partial pressures of all the gases in a system to the total pressure of the system. The kinetic molecular theory of gases provided the explanation for the behaviors of ideal gases as described by the ideal gas law. Finally, we examined the ways in which real gases deviate from the predicted behaviors of ideal gases. The van der Waals equation of state is a useful equation for correcting deviations caused by molecular interactions and volumes.

From helium-filled balloons to the bubbles of carbon dioxide in a glass of soda, from the pressurized gases used for scuba diving to the air we breathe on land, gases are all around us. And yet, all the different gases that bubble, flow, and settle in and through our daily living experiences behave in remarkably similar ways. Human life is dependent on the exchange of two gases: oxygen and carbon dioxide—to that end, expect that the MCAT will frequently test gases because of their importance in our everyday lives.

GO ONLINE

You've reviewed the content, now test your knowledge and critical thinking skills by completing a test-like passage set in your online resources!

CONCEPT SUMMARY

The Gas Phase

- Gases are the least dense phase of matter.
- Gases are fluids and therefore conform to the shapes of their containers.
- Gases are easily compressible.
- Gas systems are described by the variables **temperature** (*T*), **pressure** (*P*), **volume** (*V*), and **number of moles** (*n*).
- Important pressure equivalencies include
  1 atm = 760 mmHg ≡ 760 torr = 101.325 kPa.
- A **simple mercury barometer** measures incident (usually atmospheric) pressure. As pressure increases, more mercury is forced into the column, increasing its height. As pressure decreases, mercury flows out of the column under its own weight, decreasing its height.

Ideal Gases

- **Standard temperature and pressure (STP)** is 273 K (0°C) and 1 atm.
- Equations for ideal gases assume negligible mass and volume of gas molecules.
- Regardless of the identity of the gas, equimolar amounts of two gases will occupy the same volume at the same temperature and pressure. At STP, one mole of an ideal gas occupies 22.4 L.
- The **ideal gas law** describes the relationship between the four variables of the gas state for an ideal gas.
- **Avogadro's principle** is a special case of the ideal gas law for which the pressure and temperature are held constant; it shows a direct relationship between the number of moles of gas and volume.
- **Boyle's law** is a special case of the ideal gas law for which temperature and number of moles are held constant; it shows an inverse relationship between pressure and volume.
- **Charles's law** is a special case of the ideal gas law for which pressure and number of moles are held constant; it shows a direct relationship between temperature and volume.
- **Gay-Lussac's law** is a special case of the ideal gas law for which volume and number of moles are held constant; it shows a direct relationship between temperature and pressure.
- The **combined gas law** is a combination of Boyle's, Charles's, and Gay-Lussac's laws; it shows an inverse relationship between pressure and volume along with direct relationships between pressure and volume with temperature.
- **Dalton's law of partial pressures** states that individual gas components of a mixture of gases will exert individual pressures in proportion to their **mole fractions**. The total pressure of a mixture of gases is equal to the sum of the partial pressures of the component gases.
- **Henry's law** states that the amount of gas dissolved in solution is directly proportional to the partial pressure of that gas at the surface of a solution.

Kinetic Molecular Theory

- The **kinetic molecular theory** attempts to explain the behavior of gas particles. It makes a number of assumptions about the gas particles:
  - Gas particles have negligible volume.
  - Gas particles do not have intermolecular attractions or repulsions.
  - Gas particles undergo random collisions with each other and the walls of the container.
  - Collisions between gas particles (and with the walls of the container) are elastic.
  - The average kinetic energy of the gas particles is directly proportional to temperature.
- **Graham's law** describes the behavior of gas diffusion or effusion, stating that gases with lower molar masses will diffuse or effuse faster than gases with higher molar masses at the same temperature.
  - **Diffusion** is the spreading out of particles from high to low concentration.
  - **Effusion** is the movement of gas from one compartment to another through a small opening under pressure.

Real Gases

- **Real gases** deviate from ideal behavior under high pressure (low volume) and low temperature conditions.
  - At moderately high pressures, low volumes, or low temperatures, real gases will occupy less volume than predicted by the ideal gas law because the particles have intermolecular attractions.
  - At extremely high pressures, low volumes, or low temperatures, real gases will occupy more volume than predicted by the ideal gas law because the particles occupy physical space.
  - The **van der Waals equation of state** is used to correct the ideal gas law for intermolecular attractions (a) and molecular volume (b).

ANSWERS TO CONCEPT CHECKS

8.1

1. Gases are compressible fluids with rapid molecular motion, large intermolecular distances, and weak intermolecular forces.
2. At the top of the mountain, atmospheric pressure is lower, causing the column to fall. Under water, hydrostatic pressure is exerted on the barometer in addition to atmospheric pressure, causing the column to rise.
3. STP: $T = 273$ K (0°C), $P = 1$ atm
4. Standard conditions: $T = 298$ K (25°C), $P = 1$ atm, concentrations = 1 M

8.2

1. $PV = nRT \rightarrow T = \frac{PV}{nR} = \frac{(8\text{ atm})(12\text{ L})}{(4\text{ mol})\left(0.0821\ \frac{\text{L}\cdot\text{atm}}{\text{mol}\cdot\text{K}}\right)} \approx \frac{8\times 3}{0.08} = \frac{3}{0.01} = 300\text{ K}$

   (actual = 292.3K)

2. $\rho = \frac{m}{V} = \frac{PM}{RT} = \frac{(4\text{ atm})\left(39.9\ \frac{\text{g}}{\text{mol}}\right)}{\left(0.0821\ \frac{\text{L}\cdot\text{atm}}{\text{mol}\cdot\text{K}}\right)(400\text{ K})} \approx 5\ \frac{\text{g}}{\text{L}}$

   $\left(\text{actual} = 4.85\ \frac{\text{g}}{\text{L}}\right)$

3. $\frac{n_1}{V_1} = \frac{n_2}{V_2} \rightarrow V_2 = \frac{n_2 \times V_1}{n_1} = \frac{(2+3\text{ mol})(20\text{ L})}{2\text{ mol}} = 50\text{ L}$

4. $P_1V_1 = P_2V_2 \rightarrow V_2 = \frac{P_1V_1}{P_2} = \frac{(1\text{ atm})(2\text{ L})}{40\text{ atm}} = 0.05\text{ L}$

5. $\frac{V_1}{T_1} = \frac{V_2}{T_2} \rightarrow V_2 = \frac{V_1 \times T_2}{T_1} = \frac{(6\text{ L})(400\text{ K})}{300\text{ K}} = 8\text{ L}$

6. $\frac{P_1}{T_1} = \frac{P_2}{T_2} \rightarrow T_2 = \frac{P_2 \times T_1}{P_1} = \frac{(2\text{ atm})(500\text{ K})}{5\text{ atm}} = 200\text{ K}$

7. There are twelve total moles of gas, so the mole fractions of each gas are:

   $X_{O_2} = \frac{8\text{ mol }O_2}{12\text{ mol}} = \frac{2}{3} = 0.67;\ X_{CH_4} = \frac{3\text{ mol }CH_4}{12\text{ mol}} = \frac{1}{4} = 0.25;$

   $X_{CO_2} = \frac{1\text{ mol }CO_2}{12\text{ mol}} = 0.083$

   Then multiply each mole fraction by the total pressure to get the partial pressures (this is typically simpler with fractions than with decimals):

   $P_{O_2} = \frac{2}{3}(240\text{ atm}) = 160\text{ atm};\ P_{CH_4} = \frac{1}{4}(240\text{ atm}) = 60\text{ atm};$

   $P_{CO_2} = \frac{1}{12}(240\text{ atm}) = 20\text{ atm}$

8. High pressures of carbon dioxide gas are forced on top of the liquid in sodas, increasing its concentration in the liquid.

8.3

1. Assumptions in the kinetic molecular theory include: negligible volume of gas particles, no intermolecular forces, random motion, elastic collisions, and proportionality between absolute temperature and energy.

2. $$u_{\text{rms}} = \sqrt{\frac{3\,RT}{M}} = \sqrt{\frac{3\left(8.314\,\frac{\text{J}}{\text{mol}\cdot\text{K}}\right)(100\text{ K})}{0.004\,\frac{\text{kg}}{\text{mol}}}} \approx \sqrt{\frac{(3)(8)(100)}{4\times10^{-3}}}$$

$$= \sqrt{(3)(8)(25)(10^3)}$$

$$u_{\text{rms}} = \sqrt{(3)(200)(10^3)} = \sqrt{600\times10^3} = \sqrt{60\times10^4}$$

$$\approx \sqrt{64}\times\sqrt{10^4}$$

$$u_{\text{rms}} = 8\times10^2 = 800\,\frac{\text{m}}{\text{s}}\ \left(\text{actual} = 790\,\frac{\text{m}}{\text{s}}\right)$$

3. $$\frac{r_1}{r_2} = \sqrt{\frac{M_2}{M_1}} \rightarrow r_2 = r_1\sqrt{\frac{M_1}{M_2}} = 400\,\frac{\text{m}}{\text{s}}\sqrt{\frac{20.2\,\frac{\text{g}}{\text{mol}}}{83.8\,\frac{\text{g}}{\text{mol}}}} \approx 400\times\frac{1}{2} = 200\,\frac{\text{m}}{\text{s}}$$

$$\left(\text{actual} = 196.4\,\frac{\text{m}}{\text{s}}\right)$$

4. The rotten egg odor (hydrogen sulfide) first, almond (benzaldehyde) next, and wintergreen (methyl salicylate) last. Because all of the gases have the same temperature, they have the same kinetic energy; thus, the lightest molecules travel the fastest.

8.4

1. Real gas molecules have nonnegligible volume and attractive forces. Real gases deviate from ideal gases at high pressure (low volume) and low temperature.
2. According to the van der Waals equation, if a is increased while b remains negligible, the correction term $\left(\frac{n^2a}{V^2}\right)$ gets larger, and the pressure drops to compensate. Therefore, methane will behave more ideally than chloromethane because a is smaller for methane. The real pressure of methane will thus be higher (closer to ideal).
3. Isobutane is larger and will thus have a larger correction term for the size of the molecule, b. This makes the term $V - nb$ smaller. The pressure or volume must rise to compensate. Because the two gases are in the same size container, isobutane must exert a higher pressure.

SCIENCE MASTERY ASSESSMENT EXPLANATIONS

1. **A**

Gases deviate from ideal behavior at higher pressures and lower volumes and temperatures, all of which force molecules closer together. The closer they are, the more they can participate in intermolecular forces, which violates the definition of an ideal gas. At low temperatures, the kinetic energy of the particles is reduced, so collisions with other particles or the walls of the container are more likely to result in significant changes in kinetic energy.

2. **D**

Density equals mass divided by volume. The mass of 1 mole of neon gas equals 20.2 grams. At STP, 1 mole of neon occupies 22.4 L.

$$\text{density} = \rho = \frac{\text{mass}}{\text{volume}} = \frac{20.2\text{ g}}{22.4\text{ L}} \approx \frac{10}{11} < 1\ \frac{\text{g}}{\text{L}}$$

$$\left(\text{actual} = 0.902\ \frac{\text{g}}{\text{L}}\right)$$

3. **D**

Graham's law of effusion states that the relative rates of effusion of two gases at the same temperature and pressure are given by the inverse ratio of the square roots of the masses of the gas particles. In other words, a gas with a higher molar mass will leak more slowly than a gas with a lower molar mass. Both neon and oxygen gases will leak at slower rates than helium because they both have more mass than helium.

4. **B**

The pressure of the gas is calculated by subtracting the vapor pressure of water from the measured pressure during the experiment: 784 mmHg − 24 mmHg = 760 mmHg, or 1 atm. This is because the reaction is carried out in an aqueous environment; the water present will contribute to the partial pressures of the gas over the liquid. The ideal gas law can be used to calculate the moles of hydrogen gas. The volume of the gas is 0.100 L, the temperature is 298 K, and $R = 0.0821\ \frac{\text{L}\cdot\text{atm}}{\text{mol}\cdot\text{K}}$. Plugging in gives:

$$n = \frac{PV}{RT} = \frac{(1\text{ atm})(0.1\text{ L})}{\left(0.0821\ \frac{\text{L}\cdot\text{atm}}{\text{mol}\cdot\text{K}}\right)(298\text{ K})} \approx \frac{1}{0.8 \times 300}$$

$$= \frac{1}{240} \approx \frac{1}{250} = 0.004$$

(A) incorrectly substitutes 8.314 into the gas law, rather than 0.0821. Remember that the value of *R* depends on the other variables in the equation; using 1 atm in the numerator necessitates using 0.0821. **(C)** incorrectly substitutes the wrong *R* and keeps the pressure in mmHg. **(D)** also keeps the pressure in mmHg.

5. **B**

Ideal gases are said to have no attractive forces between molecules. While each particle within the gas is considered to have negligible volume, ideal gases as a whole certainly do have a measurable volume, thus option I is eliminated. Gases have molar masses, thus option III is eliminated.

6. **B**

Deviations from ideal behavior are due either to large particle size and/or strong intermolecular forces between molecules. Nitrogen gas consists of two nitrogen atoms triple bonded. This molecule is therefore relatively small and its nonpolar triple bond leads to very weak intermolecular forces. Together, these observations support **(B)** as the correct answer. By contrast, fluoromethane consists of all single bonds, making this molecule somewhat larger. Furthermore, due to the polarity of the carbon-fluorine bond, this molecule can participate in dipole-dipole interactions. Fluoromethane would therefore exhibit greater deviations from ideal behavior.

7. **A**

The average kinetic energy is directly proportional to the temperature of a gas in kelvin. The kinetic molecular theory states that collisions between molecules are elastic and thus do not result in a loss of energy, eliminating **(B)**. Gas particles are assumed to take up negligible space in kinetic molecular theory, eliminating **(C)**. While the average kinetic energy of any gas as a whole is the same at a given temperature, the particles themselves have a distribution of speeds (as seen in the Maxwell–Boltzmann distribution curve), eliminating **(D)**.

8. **C**

At STP, the difference between the distribution of speeds for helium and bromine gas is due to the difference in molar mass. Helium has a smaller molar mass than bromine. Particles with small masses travel faster than those with large masses, so the helium gas corresponds to curve B, which has a higher average speed. Because the gases are at the same temperature (273 K), they have the same average kinetic energy, eliminating **(B)** and **(D)**.

9. **A**

The solubility of gases in liquids is directly proportional to the atmospheric pressure, as shown by Henry's law.

$$\frac{[O_2]_1}{P_1} = \frac{[O_2]_2}{P_2}$$

$$\frac{1.25 \times 10^{-3}\,\text{M}}{1.000\ \text{atm}} = \frac{[O_2]_2}{0.8000\ \text{atm}}$$

$$[O_2]_2 = \frac{0.8 \times 1.25 \times 10^{-3}}{1} = \frac{8}{10} \times \frac{5}{4} \times 10^{-3}$$

$$= 1 \times 10^{-3}\,\text{M}$$

Note that the use of fractions allows this problem to be simplified more readily than it would be with decimals.

10. **C**

The ideal gas law can be modified to include density (ρ) because the number of moles of gas, n, is equal to the mass divided by the molar mass. Thus, $PV = nRT = \frac{m}{M}RT \rightarrow P = \frac{m}{V} \times \frac{RT}{M} = \frac{\rho RT}{M}$. Isolating for temperature gives:

$$T = \frac{PM}{\rho R}$$

$$T = \frac{(1.3 \times 10^9\ \text{atm})\left(2.00\ \frac{\text{g}}{\text{mol}}\right)}{\left(1.2\ \frac{\text{g}}{\text{cm}^3}\right)\left(1000\ \frac{\text{cm}^3}{\text{L}}\right)\left(0.0821\ \frac{\text{L}\cdot\text{atm}}{\text{mol}\cdot\text{K}}\right)}$$

$$\approx \frac{(1.3 \times 2 \times 10^9)}{(1)(1000)(0.1)} \approx \frac{2.6 \times 10^9}{100}$$

$$\approx 2.6 \times 10^7\ \text{K}$$

11. **B**

Gases are easily compressible because they travel freely with large amounts of space between molecules. Because gas particles are far apart from each other and in rapid motion, they tend to take up the volume of their container. Many gases exist as diatomic molecules, but this is not a property that characterizes all gases, eliminating option III.

12. **B**

We will use Charles's law. First, we must convert the temperature to kelvin by adding 273 to get 300 K as the initial temperature. Think of this as a proportionality: If the volume is multiplied by $\frac{3}{2}$, the temperature will also have to be multiplied by $\frac{3}{2}$. Thus the final temperature is 450 K, which represents a 150 K increase (which is equivalent to an increase of 150°C).

13. **D**

A decrease in temperature leads to a decrease in the kinetic energy of the particles so intermolecular interactions become more significant. This change leads to deviations from ideal behavior. Similarly, decreases in volume cause the volume of the particles themselves to become significant. This change also leads to deviations from ideal behavior. Thus, **(D)** is correct.

14. **C**

Both a change in temperature and a change in volume can affect a gas's pressure. So if one of those two variables is kept constant, as in **(A)** and **(B)**, we'll definitely be able to predict which way the pressure will change. At a constant volume, heating the gas will increase its pressure, and cooling the gas will decrease it. What about when both temperature and volume are changing? If both changes have the same effect on pressure, then we can still predict which way it will change. This is the case in **(D)**. Cooling the gas and increasing its volume both decrease pressure. **(C)**, on the other hand, presents too vague a scenario for us to predict definitively the change in pressure. Heating the gas would amplify the pressure, while increasing the volume would decrease it. Without knowing the magnitude of each influence, it's impossible to say whether the pressure would increase, decrease, or stay the same.

15. **C**

Initially the concentration of the gas is decreased to one-half its original value. Recall that concentration (solubility) and partial pressure are directly related—as one increases, the other increases. If the experimenters then quadruple the partial pressure of oxygen in the vessel, the solubility is also increased by a factor of four. One-half times four gives twice the original concentration value. Misreading the answer choices as being related to the concentration before the experimenters increased the partial pressure leads to **(D)**.

GO ONLINE

Consult your online resources for additional practice.

EQUATIONS TO REMEMBER

(8.1) **Ideal gas law:** $PV = nRT$

(8.2) **Density of a gas:** $\rho = \frac{m}{V} = \frac{PM}{RT}$

(8.3) **Combined gas law:** $\frac{P_1V_1}{T_1} = \frac{P_2V_2}{T_2}$

(8.4) **Avogadro's principle:** $\frac{n}{V} = k$ or $\frac{n_1}{V_1} = \frac{n_2}{V_2}$

(8.5) **Boyle's law:** $PV = k$ or $P_1V_1 = P_2V_2$

(8.6) **Charles's law:** $\frac{V}{T} = k$ or $\frac{V_1}{T_1} = \frac{V_2}{T_2}$

(8.7) **Gay-Lussac's law:** $\frac{P}{T} = k$ or $\frac{P_1}{T_1} = \frac{P_2}{T_2}$

(8.8) **Dalton's law (total pressure from partial pressures):** $P_T = P_A + P_B + P_C + \cdots$

(8.9) **Dalton's law (partial pressure from total pressure):** $P_A = X_AP_T$

(8.10) **Henry's law:** $[A] = k_H \times P_A$ or $\frac{[A]_1}{P_1} = \frac{[A]_2}{P_2} = k_H$

(8.11) **Average kinetic energy of a gas:** $KE = \frac{1}{2}mv^2 = \frac{3}{2}k_BT$

(8.12) **Root-mean-square speed:** $u_{rms} = \sqrt{\frac{3RT}{M}}$

(8.13) **Graham's law:** $\frac{r_1}{r_2} = \sqrt{\frac{M_2}{M_1}}$

(8.14) **van der Waals equation of state:** $\left(P + \frac{n^2a}{V^2}\right)(V - nb) = nRT$

SHARED CONCEPTS

Biology Chapter 6
The Respiratory System

General Chemistry Chapter 3
Bonding and Chemical Interactions

General Chemistry Chapter 6
Equilibrium

Physics and Math Chapter 2
Work and Energy

Physics and Math Chapter 3
Thermodynamics

Physics and Math Chapter 4
Fluids

CHAPTER 9

SOLUTIONS

SCIENCE MASTERY ASSESSMENT

Every pre-med knows this feeling: there is so much content I have to know for the MCAT! How do I know what to do first or what's important?

While the high-yield badges throughout this book will help you identify the most important topics, this Science Mastery Assessment is another tool in your MCAT prep arsenal. This quiz (which can also be taken in your online resources) and the guidance below will help ensure that you are spending the appropriate amount of time on this chapter based on your personal strengths and weaknesses. Don't worry though—skipping something now does not mean you'll never study it. Later on in your prep, as you complete full-length tests, you'll uncover specific pieces of content that you need to review and can come back to these chapters as appropriate.

How to Use This Assessment

If you answer 0–7 questions correctly:

Spend about 1 hour to read this chapter in full and take limited notes throughout. Follow up by reviewing **all** quiz questions to ensure that you now understand how to solve each one.

If you answer 8–11 questions correctly:

Spend 20–40 minutes reviewing the quiz questions. Beginning with the questions you missed, read and take notes on the corresponding subchapters. For questions you answered correctly, ensure your thinking matches that of the explanation and you understand why each choice was correct or incorrect.

If you answer 12–15 questions correctly:

Spend less than 20 minutes reviewing all questions from the quiz. If you missed any, then include a quick read-through of the corresponding subchapters, or even just the relevant content within a subchapter, as part of your question review. For questions you answered correctly, ensure your thinking matches that of the explanation and review the Concept Summary at the end of the chapter.

SOLUTIONS

1. An aqueous solution was prepared by mixing 70 g of an unknown nondissociating solute into 100 g of water. The solution has a boiling point of 101.0°C. What is the molar mass of the solute? (Note: $K_b = 0.512 \frac{\text{K} \cdot \text{kg}}{\text{mol}}$)
   - **A.** $358.4 \frac{\text{g}}{\text{mol}}$
   - **B.** $32.3 \frac{\text{g}}{\text{mol}}$
   - **C.** $123.2 \frac{\text{g}}{\text{mol}}$
   - **D.** $233.6 \frac{\text{g}}{\text{mol}}$

2. Which phases of solvent and solute can form a solution?
   - **I.** Solid solvent, gaseous solute
   - **II.** Solid solvent, solid solute
   - **III.** Gaseous solvent, gaseous solute

   - **A.** I and II only
   - **B.** I and III only
   - **C.** II and III only
   - **D.** I, II, and III

3. Two organic liquids, pictured in the figure below, are combined to form a solution. Based on their structures, will the solution closely obey Raoult's law?

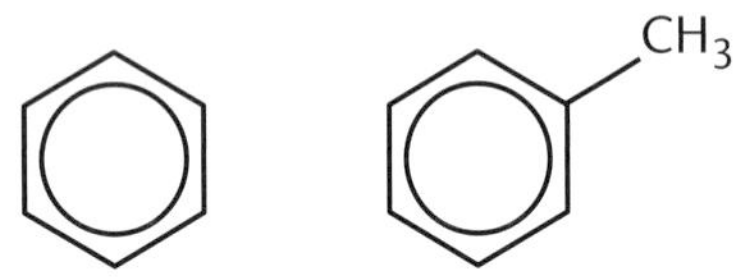

   - **A.** Yes; the liquids differ due to the additional methyl group on toluene and, therefore, will not deviate from Raoult's law.
   - **B.** Yes; the liquids are very similar and, therefore, will not deviate from Raoult's law.
   - **C.** No; the liquids differ due to the additional methyl group on toluene and, therefore, will deviate from Raoult's law.
   - **D.** No; the liquids both contain benzene rings, which will interact with each other and cause deviation from Raoult's law.

4. Which of the following explanations best describes the mechanism by which solute particles affect the melting point of ice?
   - **A.** Melting point is elevated because the kinetic energy of the substance increases.
   - **B.** Melting point is elevated because the kinetic energy of the substance decreases.
   - **C.** Melting point is depressed because solute particles interfere with lattice formation.
   - **D.** Melting point is depressed because solute particles enhance lattice formation.

5. The process of formation of a salt solution can be better understood by breaking the process into three steps:
   1. Breaking the solute into its individual components
   2. Making room for the solute in the solvent by overcoming intermolecular forces in the solvent
   3. Allowing solute–solvent interactions to occur to form the solution

   Which of the following correctly lists the enthalpy changes for these three steps, respectively?
   - **A.** Endothermic, exothermic, endothermic
   - **B.** Exothermic, endothermic, endothermic
   - **C.** Exothermic, exothermic, endothermic
   - **D.** Endothermic, endothermic, exothermic

6. The entropy change when a solution forms can be expressed by the term ΔS°_{soln}. When water molecules become ordered around an ion as it dissolves, the ordering would be expected to make a negative contribution to ΔS°_{soln}. An ion that has more charge density will have a greater hydration effect, or ordering of water molecules. In an experiment, an equimolar amount of each of the following aqueous soluble compounds is dissolved in its own test tube containing 100 mL of water. Which will have the most negative contribution to ΔS°_{soln}? (Assume that the charge density of each ion is equal to its actual charge.)
   - **A.** KCl
   - **B.** CsI
   - **C.** BeF_2
   - **D.** NaCl

7. When ammonia, NH_3, is used as a solvent, it can form complex ions. For example, dissolving AgCl in NH_3 will result in the complex ion $[Ag(NH_3)]^{2+}$. What effect would the formation of complex ions have on the solubility of a compound like AgCl in NH_3?
   - **A.** The solubility of AgCl will increase because complex ion formation will cause more ions to exist in solution, which interact with AgCl to cause it to dissociate.
   - **B.** The solubility of AgCl will increase because complex ion formation will consume Ag^+ ions and cause the equilibrium to shift away from solid AgCl.
   - **C.** The solubility of AgCl will decrease because Ag^+ ions are in complexes, and the Ag^+ ions that are not complexed will associate with Cl^- to form solid AgCl.
   - **D.** The solubility of AgCl will decrease because complex ion formation will consume Ag^+ ions and cause the equilibrium to shift toward the solid AgCl.

8. One hundred grams of sucrose are dissolved in a cup of hot water at 80°C. The cup of water contains 300.00 mL of water. What is the percent composition by mass of sugar in the resulting solution? (Note: Sucrose $= C_{12}H_{22}O_{11}$, density of water at $80°C = 0.975\ \frac{g}{mL}$)
   - **A.** 25.0%
   - **B.** 25.5%
   - **C.** 33.3%
   - **D.** 34.2%

9. Which of the following combinations of liquids would be expected to have a vapor pressure higher than the vapor pressure that would be predicted by Raoult's law?
   - **A.** Ethanol and hexane
   - **B.** Acetone and water
   - **C.** Isopropanol and methanol
   - **D.** Nitric acid and water

10. The salt KCl is dissolved in a beaker. To an observer holding the beaker, the solution begins to feel colder as the KCl dissolves. From this observation, one could conclude that:
    - **A.** ΔS°_{soln} is large enough to overcome the unfavorable ΔH°_{soln}.
    - **B.** KCl is mostly insoluble in water.
    - **C.** ΔS°_{soln} must be negative when KCl dissolves.
    - **D.** boiling point depression will occur in this solution.

11. Which of the following will cause the greatest increase in the boiling point of water when it is dissolved in 1.00 kg H_2O?
    - **A.** 0.4 mol calcium sulfate
    - **B.** 0.5 mol iron(III) nitrate
    - **C.** 1.0 mol acetic acid
    - **D.** 1.0 mol sucrose

12. Reverse osmosis is a process that allows fresh water to be obtained by using pressure to force an impure water source through a semi-permeable membrane that only allows water molecules to pass. What is the minimum pressure that would be required to purify seawater at 25°C that has a total osmolarity of 1,000 mOsm/L?
    - **A.** 23.5 atm
    - **B.** 24.5 atm
    - **C.** 24,000 atm
    - **D.** 24,500 atm

13. Lead is a toxic element that can cause many symptoms, including intellectual disabilities in children. If a body of water is polluted with lead ions at 200 ppb (parts per billion), what is the concentration of lead expressed as molarity? (Note: The density of water is $1\ \frac{g}{mL}$, and ppb = grams per 10^9 grams of solution)
    - **A.** 9.7×10^{-10} M Pb^{2+}
    - **B.** 9.7×10^{-7} M Pb^{2+}
    - **C.** 6.2×10^{-7} M Pb^{2+}
    - **D.** 6.2×10^{-6} M Pb^{2+}

14. A saturated solution of aqueous cobalt(III) hydroxide ($K_{sp} = 1.6 \times 10^{-44}$) is added to a saturated solution of aqueous thallium(III) hydroxide ($K_{sp} = 6.3 \times 10^{-46}$). What is likely to occur?

A. Both cobalt(III) hydroxide and thallium(III) hydroxide remain stable in solution.
B. Thallium(III) hydroxide precipitates and cobalt(III) hydroxide remains stable in solution.
C. Cobalt(III) hydroxide precipitates and thallium(III) hydroxide remains stable in solution.
D. Both thallium(III) hydroxide and cobalt(III) hydroxide precipitate.

15. The following equilibrium exists when AgBr ($K_{sp} = 5.35 \times 10^{-13}$) is in solution:

$$AgBr\ (s) \rightleftharpoons Ag^{+}\ (aq) + Br^{-}\ (aq)$$

What is the solubility of AgBr in a solution of 0.0010 M NaBr?

A. $5.35 \times 10^{-13}\ \frac{g}{L}$
B. $1.04 \times 10^{-12}\ \frac{g}{L}$
C. $5.35 \times 10^{-10}\ \frac{g}{L}$
D. $1.04 \times 10^{-7}\ \frac{g}{L}$

Answer Key follows on next page.

Answer Key

1. **A** (See section 9.4)
2. **D** (See section 9.1)
3. **B** (See section 9.4)
4. **C** (See section 9.4)
5. **D** (See section 9.1)
6. **C** (See section 9.1)
7. **B** (See section 9.1)
8. **B** (See section 9.2)
9. **A** (See section 9.4)
10. **A** (See section 9.1)
11. **B** (See section 9.4)
12. **B** (See section 9.3)
13. **B** (See section 9.2)
14. **A** (See section 9.3)
15. **D** (See section 9.3)

The relevant section of the chapter to review for each question is given in parentheses after the correct answer. Detailed explanations can be found at the end of the chapter.

CHAPTER 9

SOLUTIONS

In This Chapter

CHAPTER PROFILE

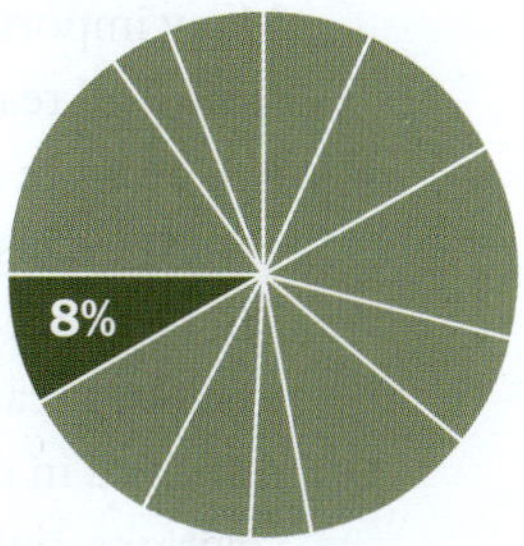

The content in this chapter should be relevant to about 8% of all questions about general chemistry on the MCAT.

This chapter covers material from the following AAMC content categories:

2A: Assemblies of molecules, cells, and groups of cells within single cellular and multicellular organisms

5A: Unique nature of water and its solutions

Introduction

What do first aid instant cold packs and sweet tea have in common? Not much, you might think—but both, in fact, demonstrate the same principles of solution chemistry. Instant cold packs contain two compartments, one holding water and the other ammonium nitrate. When the barrier between the two compartments is broken, it allows the ammonium nitrate to dissolve into the water. Sweet tea is made by dissolving a large amount of sugar into strongly brewed tea.

The creation of both the ammonium nitrate and sugar solutions is an endothermic process. However, the formation of the ammonium nitrate solution is much more endothermic than the formation of the sugar solution. This is why ammonium nitrate is useful in instant cold packs. When it dissolves in water, the system must absorb an amount of energy equal to $6.14\,\frac{\text{kcal}}{\text{mol}}$ of ammonium nitrate. The heat is absorbed from the surrounding environment, so the pack feels cool to the touch.

Although the dissolution of sugar into water is not as strongly endothermic, we nevertheless have an intuitive understanding that the process is endothermic because we all know that the easiest way to dissolve lots of sugar into water (such as in tea or coffee) is to heat up the water and then add the sugar. Because heating the water increases the solubility of sugar, it must be that the dissolution of sugar into water is an endothermic process—think of Le Châtelier's principle and changes in temperature from Chapter 6.

In this chapter, our focus will be on the characteristics and behaviors of solutions, the nature of solutions, the formation of aqueous solutions, the measurements of solution concentration, and finally the qualitative and quantitative evaluation of solution equilibria.

9.1 Nature of Solutions High Yield

LEARNING OBJECTIVES

After Chapter 9.1, you will be able to:

- Describe the process of solvation
- Define key terms involved in solutions, such as complex, solubility, and saturation
- Explain how to increase solubility of a compound
- Recall the solubility rules and apply them to predict solubility of a compound

Many important chemical reactions, both in the laboratory and in nature, take place in solutions, including almost all reactions in living organisms. **Solutions** are homogeneous (the same throughout) mixtures of two or more substances that combine to form a single phase, usually the liquid phase. The MCAT will focus almost exclusively on solids dissolved into aqueous solutions, but it's important to remember that solutions can be formed from different combinations of the three phases of matter. For example, gases can be dissolved in liquids (carbonating soda); liquids can be dissolved in other liquids (ethanol in water); solids can even be dissolved in other solids (metal alloys). Incidentally, gases "dissolved" into other gases can be thought of as solutions, but are more properly defined only as **mixtures** because gas molecules do not interact all that much chemically, as described by the kinetic molecular theory of gases. As a point of clarification: all solutions are considered mixtures, but not all mixtures are considered solutions.

A solution consists of a **solute** (such as NaCl, NH_3, $C_6H_{12}O_6$, or CO_2) dissolved (dispersed) in a solvent (such as H_2O, benzene, or ethanol). The **solvent** is the component of the solution that remains in the same phase after mixing. If the two substances are already in the same phase (for example, a solution of two liquids), the solvent is the component present in greater quantity. If the two same-phase components are in equal proportions in the solution, then the component that is more commonly used as a solvent in other contexts is considered the solvent. Solute molecules move about freely in the solvent and interact with it by way of intermolecular forces such as ion–dipole, dipole–dipole, or hydrogen bonding. Dissolved solute molecules are also relatively free to interact with other dissolved molecules of different chemical identities; consequently, chemical reactions occur easily in solution.

Solvation

Solvation is the electrostatic interaction between solute and solvent molecules. This is also known as **dissolution**, and when water is the solvent, it can be called **hydration**. Solvation involves breaking intermolecular interactions between solute molecules and between solvent molecules and forming new intermolecular interactions between solute and solvent molecules together, as shown in Figure 9.1.

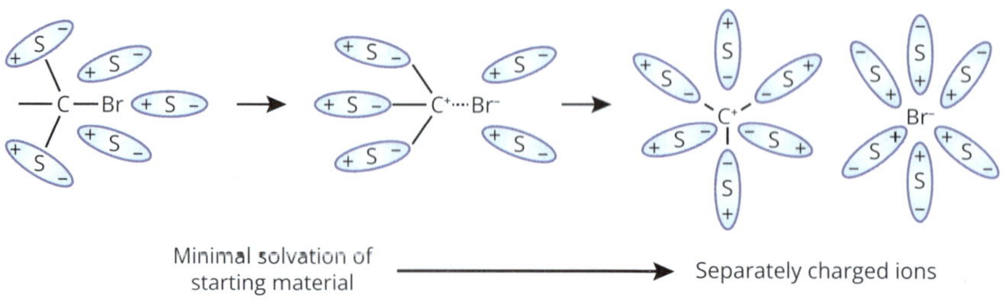

Figure 9.1 Solvation of a Polar Covalent Compound
S indicates a solvent particle.

When the new interactions are stronger than the original ones, solvation is exothermic, and the process is favored at low temperatures. For example, the dissolution of carbon dioxide into water is shown Figure 9.2. Minimal intermolecular interactions exist between carbon dioxide molecules, and breaking those interactions (as well as the interactions between water particles) leads to the initial increase in energy required in the reaction coordinate diagram. The product, which is solvated carbon dioxide molecules, has a lower free energy than the reactants, and that difference in energy is released as heat, making this an exothermic process. Le Châtelier's principle tells us this is the reason that lowering the temperature of a liquid favors solubility of a gas in the liquid.

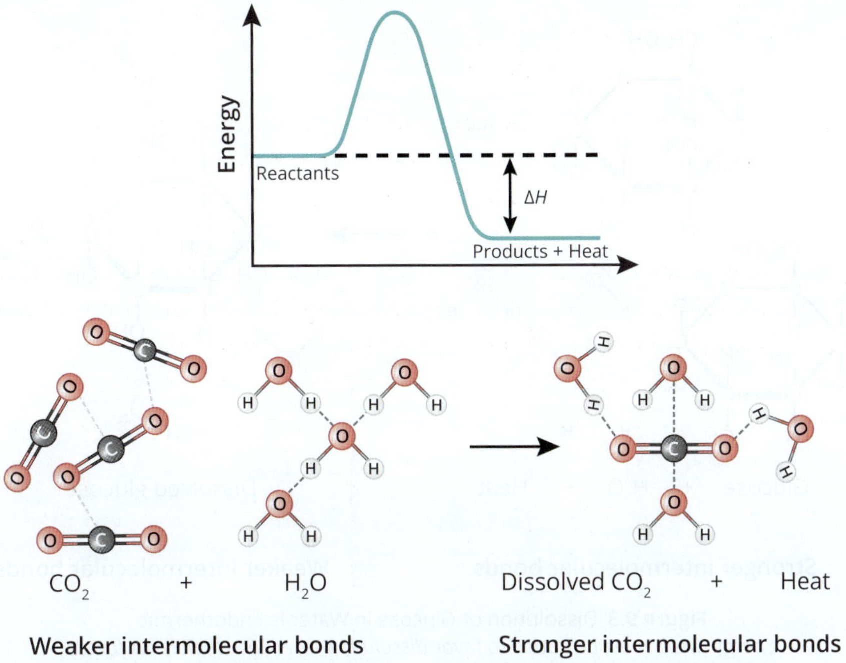

Figure 9.2 Dissolution of Carbon Dioxide in Water is Exothermic
Hydrogen bonding between water and CO_2 produces stronger intermolecular forces than CO_2 gas alone and the reaction is favorable.

When the new interactions are weaker than the original ones, solvation is endothermic and the process is favored at high temperatures. Most dissolutions are of this type. Two such examples have already been given: dissolving ammonium nitrate or, as depicted in Figure 9.3, sugar into water. Because the new interactions between the glucose and water are weaker than the original interactions between the glucose molecules and between the water molecules, energy (heat) must be supplied to facilitate the formation of these weaker, less stable interactions. Sometimes the overall strength of the new interactions is approximately equal to the overall strength of the original interactions. In this case, the overall enthalpy change for the dissolution is close to zero. These types of solutions approximate the formation of an **ideal solution**, for which the enthalpy of dissolution is equal to zero.

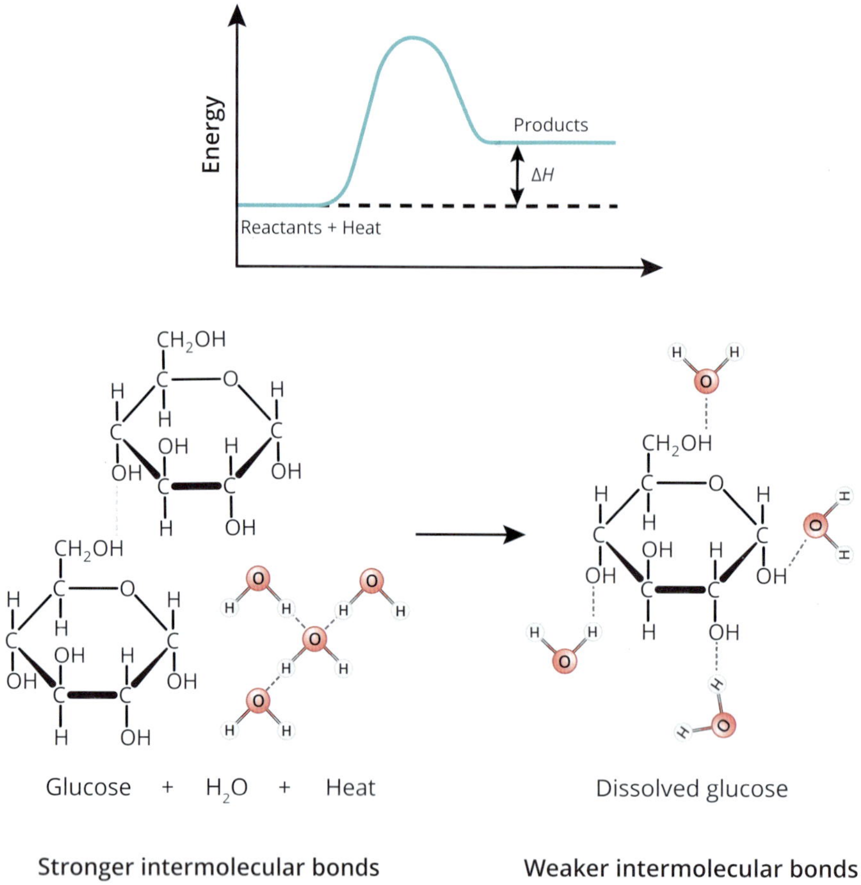

Figure 9.3 Dissolution of Glucose in Water is Endothermic
Energy (heat) must be added to favor dissolution when intermolecular forces in the products are similar or weaker in strength than in the reactants.

The spontaneity of dissolution is dependent not only on the enthalpy change; solutions may form spontaneously for both endothermic and exothermic dissolutions. The second property that contributes to the spontaneity of dissolution is the entropy change that occurs in the process. At constant temperature and pressure, entropy always increases upon dissolution. As with any process, the spontaneity of dissolution depends on the change in Gibbs free energy: spontaneous processes are associated with a decrease in free energy, while nonspontaneous processes are associated with an increase in free energy. Thus, whether or not dissolution will happen spontaneously depends on both the change in enthalpy and the change in entropy for the solute and solvent of the system.

BRIDGE

Proteins dissolve in solution with their most hydrophilic amino acids on the outside and hydrophobic amino acids on the inside because this maximizes the increase in entropy during dissolution. As described in Chapter 1 of *MCAT Biochemistry Review*, a protein dissolves by forming a solvation layer.

Consider, for example, the formation of another common solution: sodium chloride dissolved in water. When NaCl dissolves in water, its component ions dissociate from each other and become surrounded by water molecules. For this new interaction to occur, ionic bonds between Na^+ and Cl^- must be broken, and hydrogen bonds between water molecules must also be broken. This step requires energy and is therefore endothermic. Because water is polar, it can interact with each of the component ions through ion–dipole interactions: the partially positive hydrogen end of the water molecules will surround the Cl^- ions, and the partially negative oxygen end of the water molecules will surround the Na^+ ions, as shown in Figure 9.4. The formation of these ion–dipole bonds is exothermic, but the magnitude is slightly less than the energy required to break the ionic bonds and hydrogen bonds. As a result, the overall dissolution of table salt into water is endothermic $\left(+3.87\ \frac{\text{kJ}}{\text{mol}}\right)$ and favored at high temperatures.

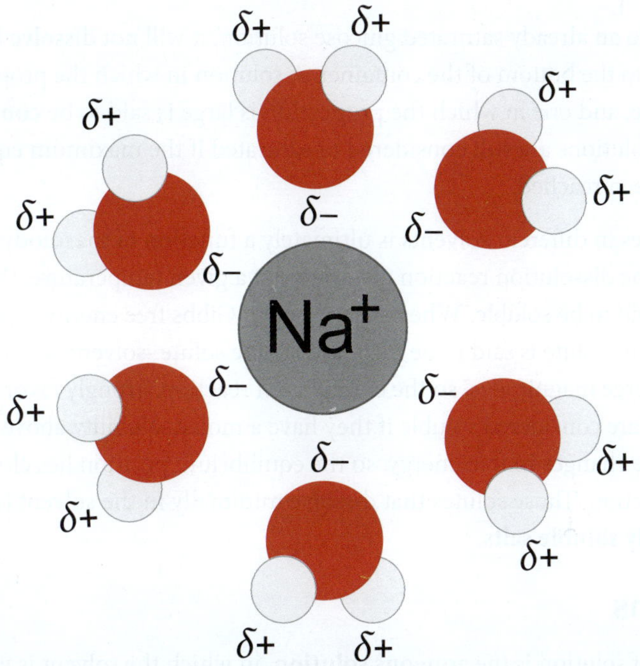

Figure 9.4 Solvation of Na^+ Ions in Aqueous Solutions

We've considered the enthalpy change for the formation of a sodium chloride solution, and now we need to examine the entropy change. Remember that entropy can be thought of as the degree to which energy is dispersed throughout a system or the amount of energy distributed from the system to the surroundings at a given temperature. Another way to understand entropy is the measure of molecular disorder, or the number of energy **microstates** available to a system at a given temperature. When solid sodium chloride dissolves into water, the rigidly ordered arrangement of the sodium and chloride ions is broken up as the ion–ion interactions are disrupted and new ion–dipole interactions with the water molecules are formed. The ions, freed from their lattice arrangement, have a greater number of energy microstates available to them (in simpler terms, they are freer to move around in different ways), and consequently, their energy is more distributed and their entropy increases. The water, however, becomes more restricted in its movement because it is now interacting with the ions. The number of energy microstates available to it (that is, the water molecules' ability to move around in different ways) is reduced, so the entropy of the water decreases. In the end, the increase in the entropy experienced by the dissolved sodium chloride is greater than the decrease in the entropy experienced by the water, so the overall entropy change is positive—energy is, overall, dispersed by the dissolution of sodium chloride in water. Because of the relatively low endothermicity and relatively large positive change in entropy, sodium chloride will spontaneously dissolve in liquid water ($\Delta G = \Delta H - T\Delta S$).

Solubility

We often want to know more than just whether or not dissolution of a solute into a solvent will be spontaneous or nonspontaneous—we also want to know how much solute will dissolve into a given solvent. The **solubility** of a substance is the maximum amount of that substance that can be dissolved in a particular solvent at a given temperature. When this maximum amount of solute has been added, the dissolved solute is in equilibrium with its undissolved state, and we say that the solution is **saturated.** If more solute is added, it will not dissolve. For example, at 25°C, a maximum of 90.9 g glucose will dissolve in 100 mL H_2O. Thus, the solubility of glucose is 909 $\frac{g}{L}$.

If more glucose is added to an already saturated glucose solution, it will not dissolve but rather will remain in solid form, **precipitating** to the bottom of the container. A solution in which the proportion of solute to solvent is small is said to be **dilute**, and one in which the proportion is large is said to be **concentrated.** Note that both dilute and concentrated solutions are still considered unsaturated if the maximum equilibrium concentration (saturation) has not yet been reached.

The solubility of substances in different solvents is ultimately a function of thermodynamics. When the change in Gibbs free energy for the dissolution reaction is negative at a given temperature, the process will be spontaneous, and the solute is said to be soluble. When the change in Gibbs free energy is positive, the process will be nonspontaneous, and the solute is said to be insoluble. Some solute–solvent systems have negative changes in free energy with very large magnitudes, so the equilibrium reaction strongly favors the dissolution of the solute. In general, solutes are considered soluble if they have a molar solubility above 0.1 M in solution. Others have only slightly negative changes in free energy, so the equilibrium position lies closer to the undissociated (reactants) side of the reaction. Those solutes that dissolve minimally in the solvent (molar solubility under 0.1 M) are called **sparingly soluble salts.**

Aqueous Solutions

The most common type of solution is the **aqueous solution**, in which the solvent is water. The aqueous state is denoted by the symbol (*aq*). Aqueous solutions rely on the interactions between water molecules and solutes in solutions. We have mentioned previously that hydration is often the process through which dissolution occurs. It is also important to note that in some solutions, such as acids, the formation of a complex called the **hydronium ion (H_3O^+)** can occur. This is facilitated by the transfer of a hydrogen ion (H^+) from a molecule in solution to a water molecule (H_2O). The reaction of acetic acid (H^+ donor) with water is shown in Figure 9.5.

$$CH_3COOH\ (aq) + H_2O\ (l) \rightleftharpoons CH_3COO^-\ (aq) + H_3O^+\ (aq)$$

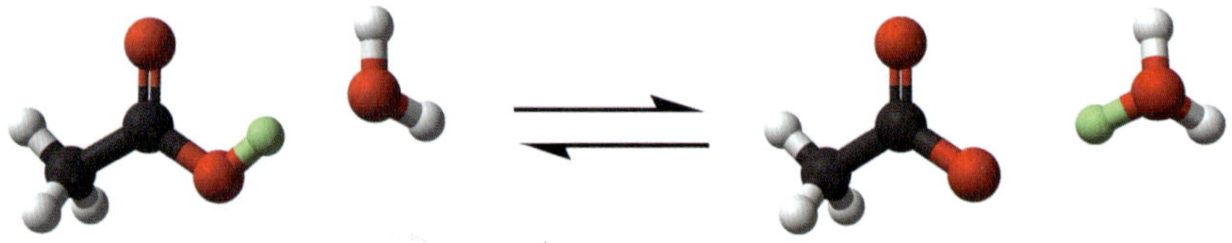

Figure 9.5 Transfer of a Proton in Solution, Forming the Hydronium Ion
The transferred proton is highlighted in green.

It is important to realize that H^+ is never found alone in solution because a free proton is difficult to isolate; rather, it is found bonded to an electron pair donor (carrier) molecule such as a water molecule. This is an example of a coordinate covalent bond. The hydronium ion and its effects on the solubilities of other compounds using Le Châtelier's principle will be described further in Chapter 10 of *MCAT General Chemistry Review.*

Because aqueous solutions are so common and so important to biological systems, the MCAT focuses on them above all others. In aqueous solutions, there are seven general solubility rules:

1. All salts containing ammonium (NH_4^+) and alkali metal (Group 1) cations are water-soluble.
2. All salts containing nitrate (NO_3^-) and acetate (CH_3COO^-) anions are water-soluble.

3. Halides (Cl^-, Br^-, I^-), excluding fluorides, are water-soluble, with the exceptions of those formed with Ag^+, Pb^{2+}, and Hg_2^{2+}.
4. All salts of the sulfate ion (SO_4^{2-}) are water-soluble, with the exceptions of those formed with Ca^{2+}, Sr^{2+}, Ba^{2+}, and Pb^{2+}.
5. All metal oxides are insoluble, with the exception of those formed with the alkali metals, ammonium, and CaO, SrO, and BaO, all of which hydrolyze to form solutions of the corresponding metal hydroxides.
6. All hydroxides are insoluble, with the exception of those formed with the alkali metals, ammonium, and Ca^{2+}, Sr^{2+}, and Ba^{2+}.
7. All carbonates (CO_3^{2-}), phosphates (PO_4^{3-}), sulfides (S^{2-}), and sulfites (SO_3^{2-}) are insoluble, with the exception of those formed with the alkali metals and ammonium.

MCAT EXPERTISE

Because most solutions in the real world involve water as the solvent, it is not a surprise that solutions are common on the MCAT. These solubility rules are not bad to know, but memorizing them all may be a little excessive. It is never a bad thing to know facts, but being able to apply them is more important. Know rules 1 and 2 for sure, and be aware of some of the more common insoluble exceptions, like Pb^{2+} and Ag^+.

The MCAT will not expect memorization of all of the solubility rules, but it is worth knowing two absolutes: all salts of Group 1 metals, and all nitrate salts are soluble. Otherwise, *familiarity* with rules listed above will suffice—the MCAT generally supplies solubility information for most compounds. Sodium and nitrate ions are generally used as counterions to what is actually chemically important; for example, if a pH problem gives a sodium formate concentration of 0.10 M, it is *really* indicating that the concentration of the formate ion is 0.10 M because the sodium ion concentration does not affect pH. The only time one needs to worry about the nitrate ion concentration is in an oxidation–reduction reaction, for the nitrate ion can function—although only weakly—as an oxidizing agent. In all other cases with nitrate ions, only focus on the cation as the chemically reacting species.

Complex Ion Formation

We have mentioned the hydronium ion as a complex that forms in acidic solutions, but it is worthwhile to mention that there are even more varied forms of complex ions that can appear in solution. By definition, a **complex ion**—or **coordination compound**—refers to a molecule in which a cation is bonded to at least one electron pair donor (which could include the water molecule). The electron pair donor molecules are called **ligands**. An example of such a **complexation reaction** is shown for the *tetraaquadioxouranyl* cation, which has water (*aqua–*) and oxygen (*oxo–*) ligands, in Figure 9.6.

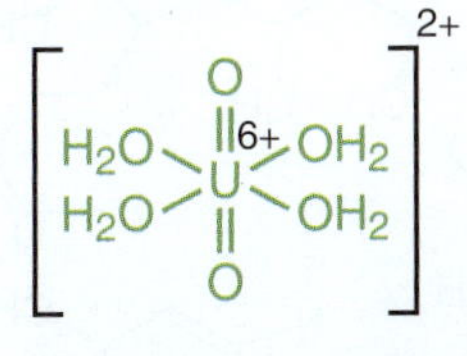

Figure 9.6 Structure of the Tetraaquadioxouranyl Complex Cation
Water and oxygen act as ligands with a U^{6+} cation.

Complexes are held together with **coordinate covalent bonds**, in which an electron pair donor (a Lewis base) and an electron pair acceptor (a Lewis acid) form very stable Lewis acid–base adducts. Most general chemistry courses do not stress the biological importance of coordination compounds. However, complex ions have profound biological applications in macromolecules such as proteins. For instance, many active sites of proteins utilize complex ion binding and transition metal complexes to carry out their function. One classic example is the iron cation in hemoglobin, which can carry oxygen, carbon dioxide, and carbon monoxide as ligands, as shown in Figure 9.7.

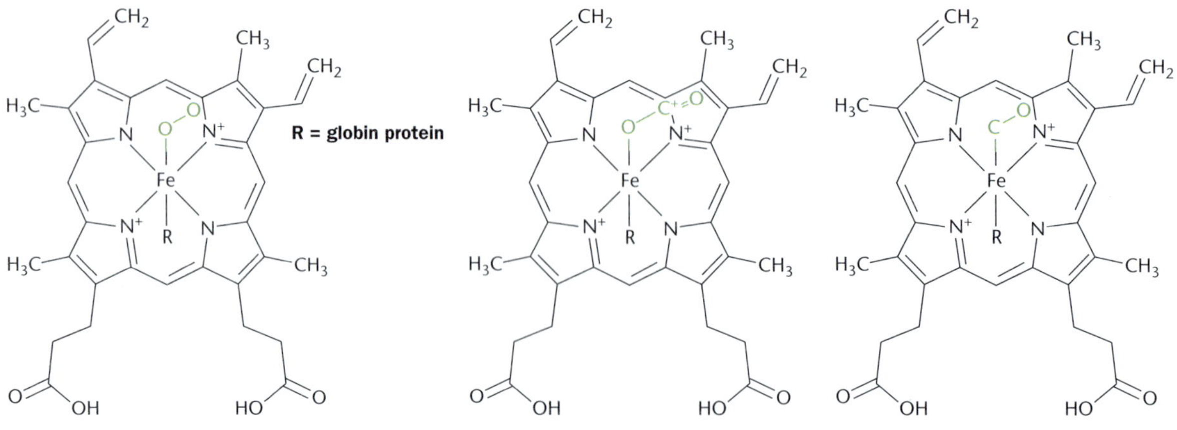

oxyhemoglobin **carbaminohemoglobin** **carboxyhemoglobin**

Figure 9.7 Hemoglobin Is a Classic Example of Biochemical Complex Formation
The iron in hemoglobin can bind various gases, leading to the formation of oxyhemoglobin (O_2), carbaminohemoglobin (CO_2), and carboxyhemoglobin (CO).

Many coenzymes (vitamins) and cofactors also contain complexes of transition metals, such as cobalamin (vitamin B_{12}), shown in Figure 9.8. The presence of a transition metal allows coenzymes and cofactors to bind other ligands or assist with electron transfer.

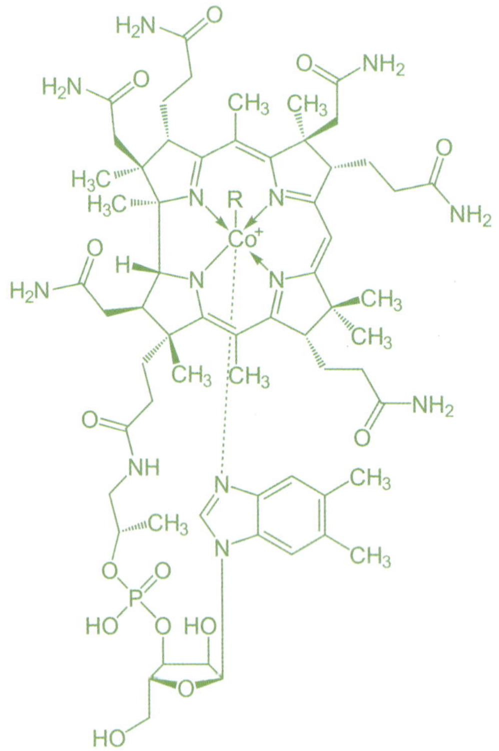

Figure 9.8 Cobalamin (Vitamin B_{12}) Contains a Cobalt Complex

Physical and chemical properties of complex ions are diverse, including a wide range of solubilities and varied chemical reactions. Inorganic complex ions are often fun to characterize because they tend to have vibrant, distinctive colors, as illustrated in Figure 9.9.

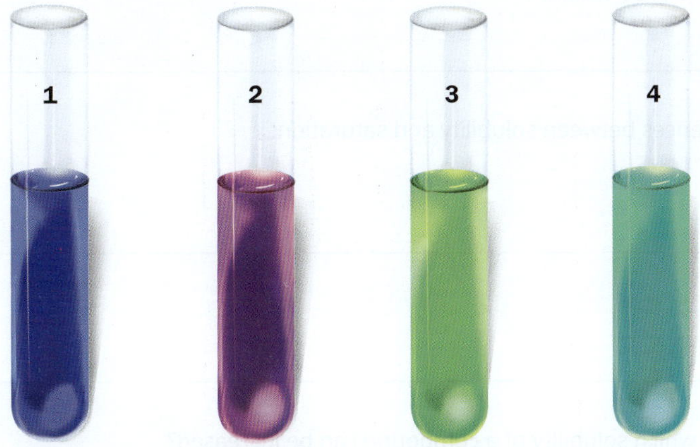

Figure 9.9 Nickel(II) Ion Complexes Display Distinctive Colors
The characteristic colors of Nickel (II) Ion complexes are, from left to right: 1) hexaamminenickel(II), 2) tris(ethylenediamine)nickel(II), 3) tetrachloronickelate(II), and 4) hexaaquanickel(II)

In some complexes, the central cation can be bonded to the same ligand in multiple places. This is called **chelation**, and it generally requires large organic ligands that can double back to form a second (or even third) bond with the central cation. Chelation therapy is often used to sequester toxic metals (lead, arsenic, mercury, and so on). Even biologically necessary metals, such as iron, can be toxic in overload states; an example of iron being chelated is shown in Figure 9.10.

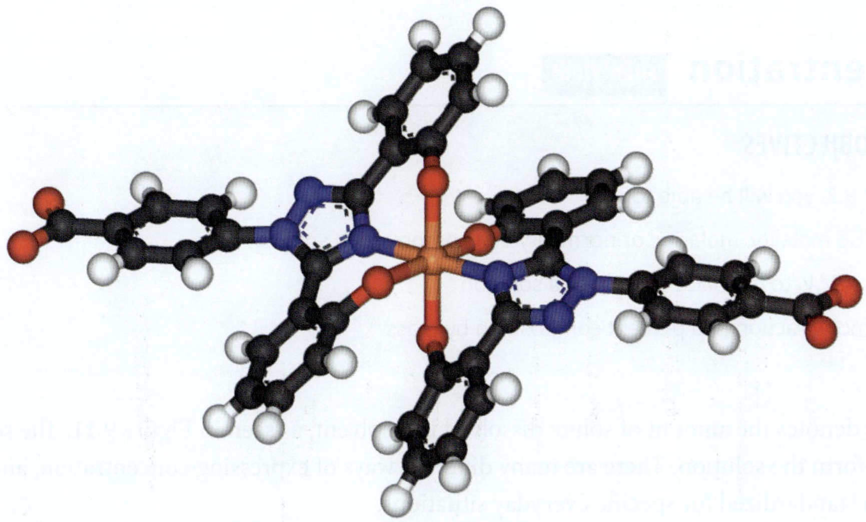

Figure 9.10 Chelation of Iron with Two Molecules of Deferasirox

MCAT CONCEPT CHECK 9.1

Before you move on, assess your understanding of the material with these questions.

1. Describe the process of solvation.

___

2. Describe the differences between solubility and saturation:

 •

___

 •

___

3. What is one way in which solubility of a compound can be increased?

___

4. Name two ions that form salts that are always soluble:

 •

___

 •

___

9.2 Concentration High Yield

LEARNING OBJECTIVES

After Chapter 9.2, you will be able to:

- Calculate the molality, molarity, or normality of a compound in solution
- Apply $M_iV_i = M_fV_f$ to calculate dilution of a solution
- Calculate mole fraction and percent composition by mass

Concentration denotes the amount of solute dissolved in a solvent, as seen in Figure 9.11. The solvent and solute together form the solution. There are many different ways of expressing concentration, and different units have been standardized for specific everyday situations.

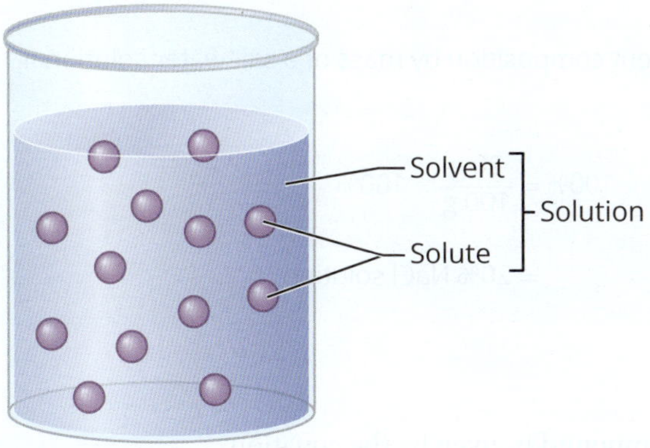

Figure 9.11 A Solution Is Composed of Solute Dissolved in Solvent

For example, alcohol content in liquors like vodka, gin, or rum is expressed in volume percent (volume of solute divided by volume of solution times 100 percent). Alcoholic proof is twice the volume percent. The sugar content of orange juice and other fruit juices is measured in units of degrees Brix (°Bx), which is a mass percent: mass of glucose divided by mass of solution times 100 percent. By convention, placing a substance in brackets, as shown in Figure 9.12, is used to indicate the concentration of that substance.

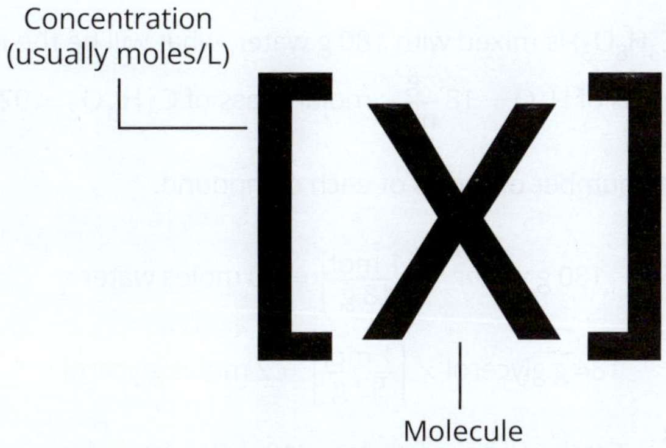

Figure 9.12 Brackets Indicate the Concentration of the Bracketed Substance

Units of Concentration

On the MCAT, concentrations are commonly expressed as percent composition by mass, mole fraction, molarity, molality, and normality.

Percent Composition by Mass

The **percent composition by mass** is given by the equation

$$\frac{\text{mass of solute}}{\text{mass of solution}} \times 100\%$$

Equation 9.1

Percent composition is used not only for aqueous solutions, but also for metal alloys and other solid-in-solid solutions.

MCAT EXPERTISE

It is important to have a good idea of how to work with all of these ways of expressing concentration because more than one may show up on Test Day.

Example: What is the percent composition by mass of a salt water solution if 100 g of the solution contains 20 g of NaCl?

Solution: $\frac{\text{mass of solute}}{\text{mass of solution}} \times 100\% = \frac{20\text{ g}}{100\text{ g}} \times 100\%$

$= 20\%$ NaCl solution

Mole Fraction

The **mole fraction** (*X*) of a compound is given by the equation

$$X_A = \frac{\text{moles of A}}{\text{total moles of all species}}$$

Equation 9.2

The sum of the mole fractions in a system will always equal 1. The mole fraction is used to calculate the vapor pressure depression of a solution, described later in this chapter, as well as the partial pressures of gases in a system, described in Chapter 8 of *MCAT General Chemistry Review.*

Example: If 184 g glycerol ($C_3H_8O_3$) is mixed with 180 g water, what will be the mole fractions of the two components? (Note: Molar mass of $H_2O = 18 \frac{\text{g}}{\text{mol}}$; molar mass of $C_3H_8O_3 = 92 \frac{\text{g}}{\text{mol}}$)

Solution: First, determine the number of moles of each compound:

$$180\text{ g water} \times \left[\frac{1\text{ mol}}{18\text{ g}}\right] = 10\text{ moles water}$$

$$184\text{ g glycerol} \times \left[\frac{1\text{ mol}}{92\text{ g}}\right] = 2\text{ moles glycerol}$$

$$\text{Total number of moles} = 10 + 2 = 12\text{ moles}$$

Then, determine the mole fractions:

$$X_{\text{water}} = \frac{10\text{ mol water}}{12\text{ mol total}} = \frac{5}{6} = 0.83$$

$$X_{\text{glycerol}} = \frac{2\text{ mol glycerol}}{12\text{ mol total}} = \frac{1}{6} = 0.17$$

Molarity

The **molarity** (M) of a solution is defined as

$$\text{M} = \frac{\text{moles of solute}}{\text{liters of solution}}$$

Equation 9.3

Solution concentrations are usually expressed in terms of molarity, and this is the most common unit for concentration on the MCAT. Unless otherwise specified, representations of concentration using brackets—such as $[Na^+]$—indicate molarity. Note that the volume term in the denominator of molarity refers to the solution volume, *not* the volume of solvent used to prepare the solution—although the two values are often close enough to approximate the solution volume using the solvent volume. Molarity is used for rate laws, the law of mass action, osmotic pressure, pH and pOH, and the Nernst equation.

Example: If enough water is added to 11 g of $CaCl_2$ to make 100 mL of solution, what is the molarity of the solution?

Solution: First, calculate the number of moles of $CaCl_2$:

$$11 \text{ g } CaCl_2 \left[\frac{1 \text{ mol}}{111.1 \text{ g}}\right] = 0.1 \text{ mol } CaCl_2$$

Then determine the molarity:

$$M = \frac{\text{moles of solute}}{\text{liters of solution}}$$

$$M = \frac{0.1 \text{ mol}}{100 \text{ mL} \times \frac{1 \text{ L}}{1000 \text{ mL}}} = \frac{0.1}{0.1} = 1 \text{ M}$$

MCAT EXPERTISE

Note that for dilute solutions, the volume of the solution is approximately equal to the volume of solvent used, which simplifies our calculations on Test Day. However, technical questions could ask you to distinguish between these two. For example, when you add two kilograms of sucrose (table sugar) to a liter of water at room temperature (achieving saturation), the volume of solution is certainly larger than 1 L!

Molality

The **molality** (***m***) of a solution is defined as

$$m = \frac{\text{moles of solute}}{\text{kilograms of solvent}}$$

Equation 9.4

For dilute aqueous solutions at 25°C, the molality is approximately equal to molarity because the density of water at this temperature is 1 kilogram per liter. However, note that this is an approximation and true only for dilute aqueous solutions. As aqueous solutions become more concentrated with solute, their densities become significantly different from that of pure water; most water-soluble solutes have molar masses significantly greater than that of water, so the density of the solution increases as the concentration increases. You won't use molality very often, so be mindful of the special situations when it is required: boiling point elevation and freezing point depression.

Example: If 10 g NaOH are dissolved in 500 g of water, what is the molality of the solution?

Solution: First, calculate the number of moles of NaOH:

$$10 \text{ g NaOH} \left[\frac{1 \text{ mol}}{40 \text{ g}}\right] = 0.25 \text{ mol NaOH}$$

Then determine the molality:

$$m = \frac{\text{moles of solute}}{\text{kilograms of solvent}}$$

$$m = \frac{0.25 \text{ mol}}{500 \text{ g} \times \frac{1 \text{ kg}}{1000 \text{ g}}} = \frac{0.25}{0.5} = 0.5\ m$$

Normality

We discussed the related concepts of gram equivalent weight, equivalents, and normality in Chapter 4 of *MCAT General Chemistry Review*. The **normality (N)** of a solution is equal to the number of equivalents of interest per liter of solution. An equivalent is a measure of the reactive capacity of a molecule. Most simply, an equivalent is equal to a mole of the species of interest—protons, hydroxide ions, electrons, or ions.

To calculate the normality of a solution, we need to know what purpose the solution serves because it is the concentration of the reactive species with which we are concerned. For example, in acid–base reactions, we are most concerned with the concentration of hydrogen ions; in oxidation–reduction reactions, we are most concerned with the concentration of electrons. Normality is unique among concentration units in that it is reaction dependent. For example, in acidic solution, 1 mole of the permanganate ion (MnO_4^-) will readily accept 5 moles of electrons, so a 1 M solution would be 5 N. However, in alkaline solution, 1 mole of permanganate will accept only 1 mole of electrons, so in alkaline solution, a 1 M permanganate solution would be 1 N.

MCAT EXPERTISE

Simple ideas on Test Day will make things easier. So, when you come across normality, think of it as *molarity of the stuff of interest* in the reaction.

Dilution

A solution is diluted when solvent is added to a solution of higher concentration to produce a solution of lower concentration. The concentration of a solution after dilution can be determined using the equation

$$M_i V_i = M_f V_f$$

Equation 9.5

where M is the molarity in M, V is volume, and the subscripts i and f refer to the initial and final values, respectively.

MCAT EXPERTISE

This equation is worthy of memorization. Note that a similar equation is used for the equivalence point in acid–base chemistry, as discussed in Chapter 10 of *MCAT General Chemistry Review*.

Example: A chemist wishes to prepare 300 mL of a 1.1 M NaOH solution from a 5.5 M NaOH stock solution. What volume of stock solution should be diluted with pure water to obtain the desired solution?

Solution:

$$M_i V_i = M_f V_f \rightarrow V_i = \frac{M_f V_f}{M_i}$$

$$V_i = \frac{(1.1 \text{ M})(300 \text{ mL})}{(5.5 \text{ M})} = \frac{300}{5} = 60 \text{ mL}$$

Note that one can use mL or L in the equation, as long as the units are consistent.

MCAT CONCEPT CHECK 9.2

Before you move on, assess your understanding of the material with these questions.

1. If you mix 180 g of the following compounds in 250 L of water $\left(\text{density} = 1\,\frac{\text{kg}}{\text{L}}\right)$, what are their concentrations in molality, molarity, and normality (for acid–base chemistry)?

Compound	Molality	Molarity	Normality
Glucose $\left(180\,\frac{\text{g}}{\text{mol}}\right)$			
Carbonate $\left(60\,\frac{\text{g}}{\text{mol}}\right)$			

2. You are working in a sewage treatment facility and are assaying chlorine in a water sample. You need to dilute the water sample from 100 ppm stock to 25 ppm and create 100 mL of solution. Calculate the amount of stock solution needed and determine how you would create your final solution:

____

____

____

3. A stock solution for making typical IV saline bags contains 90.0 g of NaCl per 10 liters of water $\left(\text{density} = 1\,\frac{\text{g}}{\text{mL}}\right)$. What is the mole fraction and the percent composition by mass of NaCl in the saline solutions?
   - Mole fraction:

   ____

   - Percent composition by mass:

   ____

MCAT EXPERTISE

Though not a unique means of measuring concentration or dilution, the term "parts-per" can be used to indicate concentration of a dissolved substance in a solution (most commonly water). Parts-per-million (ppm, 10^{-6}) is the most common usage. If a problem states there is one ppm of substance X in water, that would indicate there is 1 mg/L of water, as there would be 1 millionth of a gram per gram of water, and the density of water is 1 g/mL. On Test Day, prior to converting from ppm, make sure to assess whether conversion to a different unit of measure is actually required, as this conversion can typically be avoided on the MCAT.

9.3 Solution Equilibria **High Yield**

LEARNING OBJECTIVES

After Chapter 9.3, you will be able to:

- Calculate molar solubility for a compound given its K_{sp} and vice versa
- Calculate ion product for a solution
- Given K_{sp}, predict when a solute may dissociate or precipitate in order to reach equilibrium
- Predict the impact of a common ion on the dissolution of a compound

The process of solvation, like other reversible chemical and physical processes, tends toward an equilibrium position, defined as the lowest energy state of a system under a given set of temperature and pressure conditions. Systems move spontaneously toward the equilibrium position, and any movement away from equilibrium is nonspontaneous. In the process of creating a solution, the equilibrium is defined as the **saturation point**, where the solute concentration is at its maximum value for the given temperature and pressure. Immediately after solute has been introduced into a solvent, most of the change taking place is dissociation because no dissolved solute is initially present. However, once solute is dissolved, the reverse process—precipitation of the solute—will begin to occur.

When the solution is dilute (unsaturated), the thermodynamically favored process is dissolution, and initially, the rate of dissolution will be greater than the rate of precipitation. As the solution becomes more concentrated and approaches saturation, the rate of dissolution lessens, while the rate of precipitation increases. Eventually, the saturation point of the solution is reached. The solution now exists in a state of dynamic equilibrium for which the rates of dissolution and precipitation are equal, and the concentration of dissolved solute reaches a steady-state (constant) value. Neither dissolution nor precipitation is more thermodynamically favored at equilibrium because favoring either would necessarily result in the solution no longer being in a state of equilibrium. At this point, the change in free energy is zero, as is the case for all systems at equilibrium.

An ionic solid introduced into a polar solvent dissociates into its component ions, and the dissociation of such a solute in solution may be represented by

$$A_mB_n\ (s) \rightleftharpoons m\ A^{n+}\ (aq) + n\ B^{m-}\ (aq)$$

On Test Day, the first step for any solution stoichiometry or solution equilibrium question is to write out the balanced dissociation reaction for the ionic compound in question. This first step is essential for correctly calculating the solubility product constant, ion product, molar solubility, or for determining the outcome of the common ion effect. In other words, it is the essential first step for nearly every solution chemistry problem on the MCAT.

Solubility Product Constants

Most solubility problems on the MCAT deal with solutions of sparingly soluble salts, which are ionic compounds that have very low solubility in aqueous solutions. You may wonder why any ionic compound would not be highly soluble in water. The degree of solubility is determined by the relative changes in enthalpy and entropy associated with the dissolution of the ionic solute at a given temperature and pressure. One common sparingly soluble salt is silver chloride, AgCl, which dissociates in water according to the following equation:

$$AgCl\ (s) \rightleftharpoons Ag^{+}\ (aq) + Cl^{-}\ (aq)$$

The law of mass action can be applied to a solution at equilibrium; that is to say, when the solution is saturated and the solute concentration is at a maximum and is dynamically stable. For a saturated solution of an ionic compound with the formula A_mB_n, the equilibrium constant for its solubility in aqueous solution, called the **solubility product constant** (**K_{sp}**), can be expressed by:

$$K_{sp} = [A^{n+}]^m[B^{m-}]^n$$

Equation 9.6

where the concentrations of the ionic constituents are equilibrium (saturation) concentrations. For example, we can express the K_{sp} of silver chloride as:

$$K_{sp} = [Ag^{+}][Cl^{-}]$$

MCAT EXPERTISE

On the MCAT, if you remember that K_{sp} is just a specialized form of K_{eq}, then you can simplify a lot of problems by using the same concepts that you do for all equilibria, including Le Châtelier's principle.

You'll notice that, for the law of mass action of solutions, there is no denominator. Remember that pure solids and liquids do not appear in the equilibrium constant. Because the silver chloride solution was formed by adding pure solid silver chloride to pure water, neither the solid silver chloride nor the water is included. Indeed, dissociation reactions—by definition—have a solid salt as a reactant; thus, K_{sp} expressions should never have denominators.

Solubility product constants, like all other equilibrium constants (K_{eq}, K_a, K_b, and K_w) are temperature dependent. When the solution consists of a gas dissolved into a liquid, the value of the equilibrium constant, and hence the position of equilibrium (saturation), will also depend on pressure. Generally speaking, the solubility product constant increases with increasing temperature for non-gas solutes and decreases for gas solutes. Higher pressures favor dissolution of gas solutes, and therefore the K_{sp} will be larger for gases at higher pressures than at lower ones.

As solute dissolves into the solvent, the system approaches saturation, at which point no more solute can be dissolved and any excess will precipitate to the bottom of the container. We may not know whether the solution has reached saturation, and so to determine where the system is with respect to the equilibrium position, we can calculate a value called the **ion product (IP)**, which is analogous to the reaction quotient, *Q*, for other chemical reactions. The ion product equation has the same form as the equation for the solubility product constant:

$$\text{IP} = [\text{A}^{n+}]^m[\text{B}^{m-}]^n$$

Equation 9.7

The difference is that the concentrations used in the ion product equation are the concentrations of the ionic constituents at that given moment in time, which may differ from equilibrium concentrations. As with the reaction quotient *Q*, the utility of the ion product lies in comparing its value to that attained at equilibrium, K_{sp}, as summarized in Figure 9.13.

IP > K_{sp}	Supersaturated
IP = K_{sp}	In equilibrium; saturated
IP < K_{sp}	Unsaturated

Figure 9.13 Saturation States of Solutions

REAL WORLD

Because gases become more soluble in solution as pressure increases, divers who have spent time at significant depths under water will have more nitrogen gas dissolved in their blood because nitrogen gas is the main inert gas in the air we breathe. If divers rise to the surface too quickly, the abrupt decompression will lead to an abrupt decrease in gas solubility in the plasma, resulting in the formation of nitrogen gas bubbles in the bloodstream. The gas bubbles can get lodged in the small vasculature of the peripheral tissue, mostly around the large joints of the body, causing pain and tissue damage (hence the name, the *bends*). The condition is painful and dangerous and can be fatal if not properly treated.

Each salt has its own distinct K_{sp} at a given temperature. If, at a given set of conditions, a salt's IP is less than the salt's K_{sp}, then the solution is not yet at equilibrium and is considered **unsaturated.** As seen in the left-most beaker in Figure 9.14, in an unsaturated solution, more salt is able to go into solution. For unsaturated solutions, dissolution is thermodynamically favored over precipitation. If the IP is greater than the K_{sp}, then the solution is beyond equilibrium, and the solution is considered **supersaturated.** It is possible to create a supersaturated solution by dissolving solute into a hot solvent and then slowly cooling the solution. A supersaturated solution is thermodynamically unstable, and any disturbance to the solution, such as the addition of more solid solute or other solid particles, or further cooling of the solution, will cause spontaneous precipitation of the excess dissolved solute, as seen in the rightmost beaker in Figure 9.14. If the calculated IP is equal to the known K_{sp}, then the solution is at equilibrium—the rates of dissolution and precipitation are equal—and the solution is considered **saturated.** Adding more salt does not cause additional precipitation or dissolution, as seen in the middle beaker in Figure 9.14. The molarity of a solute in a saturated solution is called the **molar solubility** of that substance.

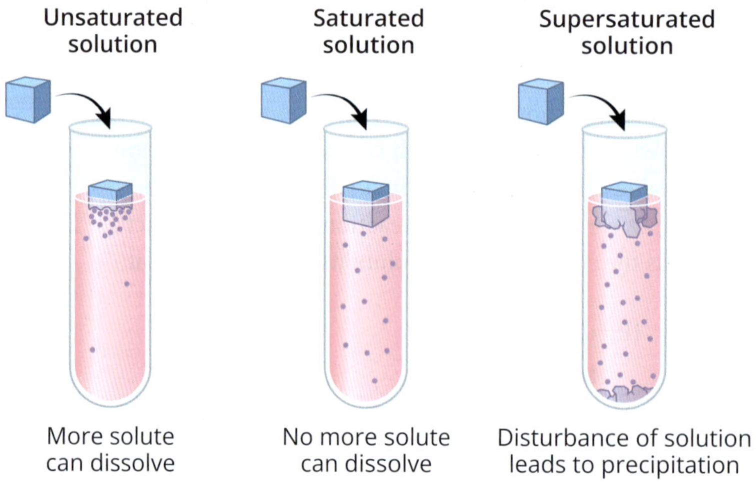

Figure 9.14 Unsaturated, Saturated, and Supersaturated Solutions

Example: The molar solubility of $Fe(OH)_3$ in an aqueous solution was determined to be $4 \times 10^{-10}\ \frac{mol}{L}$. What is the value of the K_{sp} for $Fe(OH)_3$ at the same temperature and pressure?

Solution: The molar solubility is given as 4×10^{-10} M. The equilibrium concentration of each ion can be determined from the molar solubility and the balanced dissociation reaction of $Fe(OH)_3$. The dissociation reaction is:

$$Fe(OH)_3\ (s) \rightleftharpoons Fe^{3+}\ (aq) + 3\ OH^-\ (aq)$$

$$K_{sp} = [Fe^{3+}][OH^-]^3$$

The molar solubility can be expressed as x, the amount of $Fe(OH)_3$ that dissolves to make a saturated solution at equilibrium. As it dissolves, $Fe(OH)_3$ dissociates to create x of Fe^{3+} and $3x$ of OH^-. This can be entered into the K_{sp} equation to give:

$$K_{sp} = [x][3x]^3$$

If the molar solubility x is 4×10^{-10} M, then $x = 4 \times 10^{-10}$ M $Fe(OH)_3$ has dissolved, yielding $x = 4 \times 10^{-10}$ M Fe^{3+} and $3x = 3 \times 4 \times 10^{-10}$ M OH^- (because there are three OH^- ions released per $Fe(OH)_3$ molecule dissolved). Thus,

$$K_{sp} = [Fe^{3+}][OH^-]^3$$

$$K_{sp} = (4 \times 10^{-10}\text{ M})(3 \times 4 \times 10^{-10}\text{ M})^3 = (4 \times 10^{-10}) \times [3^3 \times (4 \times 10^{-10})^3]$$

$$K_{sp} = 3^3 \times (4 \times 10^{-10})^4 = 27(4 \times 10^{-10})^4 = 27 \times 256 \times 10^{-40} \approx 30 \times 250 \times 10^{-40}$$

$$K_{sp} \approx 7500 \times 10^{-40} = 7.5 \times 10^{-37} \text{ (actual} = 6.9 \times 10^{-37})$$

Example: What are the concentrations of each of the ions in a saturated solution of CuBr, given that the K_{sp} of CuBr is 6.27×10^{-9} at 25°C? If 3 g CuBr are dissolved in water to make 1 L of solution at 25°C, would the solution be saturated, unsaturated, or supersaturated?

Solution: The first step is to write out the dissociation reaction:

$$CuBr\ (s) \rightarrow Cu^+\ (aq) + Br^-\ (aq)$$

$$K_{sp} = [Cu^+][Br^-]$$

Let x equal the molar solubility of CuBr, which is the amount of CuBr that dissolves at equilibrium. The concentration of Cu^+ and Br^- will each equal x.

$$K_{sp} = x \cdot x = x^2$$

$$6.27 \times 10^{-9} = x^2$$

$$6.3 \times 10^{-9} \approx x^2$$

$$63 \times 10^{-10} \approx x^2 \approx 64 \times 10^{-10}$$

$$8 \times 10^{-5} \approx x \text{ (actual value} = 7.9 \times 10^{-5})$$

Therefore, $[Cu^+]$ is about 8×10^{-5} M, and $[Br^-]$ is also about 8×10^{-5} M. Note that 8×10^{-5} M also represents the molar solubility of copper(I) bromide.

Next, we convert 3 g of CuBr into moles:

$$3\text{ g} \times \frac{1\text{ mol CuBr}}{143.5\text{ g}} \approx \frac{3}{150} \approx \frac{3}{1.5 \times 10^2} \approx 2 \times 10^{-2}\text{ mol}$$

2×10^{-2} mol CuBr in 1 L of solution represents a molarity of 2×10^{-2} M, which is more than 100 times higher than the molar solubility of CuBr. Therefore, this is a supersaturated solution.

KEY CONCEPT

Every sparingly soluble salt of general formula AB will have $K_{sp} = x^2$, where x is the molar solubility (assuming no common ion effect).

KEY CONCEPT

Every sparingly soluble salt of general formula AB_2 will have $K_{sp} = 4x^3$, where x is the molar solubility (assuming no common ion effect).

KEY CONCEPT

Every sparingly soluble salt of general formula AB_3 will have $K_{sp} = 27x^4$, where x is the molar solubility (assuming no common ion effect).

Finally, let's return to our discussion of complex ions and their solubility factors. Much like the examples we have seen previously, the solubility of complex ion solutions is determined by the K_{sp}. The formation of complex ions increases the solubility of a salt in solution.

For instance, consider free iron(III) (Fe^{3+}) in a solution of water. If a cyanide solution were added, an exceptionally stable iron and cyanide metal complex would form as the water molecules solvating the iron are replaced by excess cyanide ions:

$$Fe^{3+}(aq) + 6\,CN^-(aq) \rightleftharpoons \left[Fe(CN)_6\right]^{3-}(aq) \qquad K_f = 1.0 \times 10^{31}$$

Knowing the intricacies of why complexes are more stable in solution than isolated ions is beyond the scope of the MCAT; however, it should make sense that, if a complex ion contains multiple polar bonds between the ligands and the central metal ion, it should be able to engage in a very large amount of dipole–dipole interactions. This stabilizes the dissolution of the complex ion. The end result is that such complexes tend to have very high K_{sp} values.

When forming a complex ion, one must often use a mixture of solutions. For this reason, a distinction must be made between the K_{sp} of the solution and that of the complex ion itself. The dissolution of the original solution is termed K_{sp}, and the subsequent formation of the complex ion in solution is termed $\mathbf{K_f}$ (the **formation** or **stability constant** of the complex in solution). An example is shown below in which the diamminesilver(I) complex is formed in a silver chloride solution:

$$AgCl(s) \rightleftharpoons Ag^+(aq) + Cl^-(aq) \qquad K_{sp} = 1.8 \times 10^{-10} = \left[Ag^+\right]\left[Cl^-\right]$$

$$Ag^+(aq) + 2\,NH_3(aq) \rightleftharpoons \left[Ag(NH_3)_2\right]^+ \qquad K_f = 1.6 \times 10^7 = \frac{\left[\left[Ag(NH_3)_2\right]^+\right]}{\left[Ag^+\right]\left[NH_3\right]^2}$$

Notice that the formation constant (K_f) of the complex ion is significantly larger than the K_{sp} of the compound providing the metal ion. This is part of the explanation for why the initial dissolution of the metal ion is the rate-limiting step of complex ion formation. However, Le Châtelier's principle is at play in these reactions as well. Ultimately, complex ions form to become more soluble in solution. And as an amount of silver ion is being used up to form the complex ion itself, the dissociation reaction of AgCl shifts to the right, providing more silver for complex ion formation.

Example: A 0.1 mol sample of CuS is added to 1.00 L of 1.00 M NH_3. What is the final concentration of the complex ion, tetraamminecopper(II)?

$$CuS(s) \rightleftharpoons Cu^{2+}(aq) + S^{2-}(aq) \qquad K_{sp} = 8 \times 10^{-37}$$

$$Cu^{2+}(aq) + 4\,NH_3(aq) \rightleftharpoons \left[Cu(NH_3)_4\right]^{2+}(aq) \qquad K_f = 1.1 \times 10^{13}$$

Solution: First determine the amount of copper ion produced from copper sulfide (CuS) in solution. Comparison of the two equilibrium constants shows that the CuS dissociation has a K_{sp} of 8×10^{-37}, indicating that this reaction is unlikely to proceed as the forward reaction is not favorable. However, if the formation of the complex ion occurs simultaneously, the large K_f of 1.1×10^{13} for this process will drive the dissociation of CuS forward as the Cu^{2+} ions are consumed in the second reaction due to Le Châtelier's principle. Note that, even without quantitative analysis, the large value of K_f is a sign that the formation of the product of the second reaction will be highly favorable. In fact, if these two reactions are simultaneous, the CuS will ultimately be completely consumed due to this effect.

Thus, the amount of Cu^{2+} available to react is given by $[Cu^{2+}] = \frac{0.1 \text{ mol}}{1.00 \text{ L}} = 0.1$ M. The reactions given show a 1:1 relationship between the Cu^{2+} available and the $[Cu(NH_3)_4]^{2+}$ that is generated. In other words, almost all of the Cu^{2+} ions will be used up to form the complex. Therefore, the concentration of the $[Cu(NH_3)_4]^{2+}$ complex ion is 0.1 M.

Common Ion Effect

The solubility of a substance varies depending on the temperature of the solution, the solvent, and in the case of a gas-phase solute, the pressure. Solubility is also affected by the addition of other substances to the solution. The effect of a complex ion increasing the solubility of a substance is not typical and is—in fact—opposite to the effect seen in many mixtures of solutions.

One of the more challenging solution chemistry problems on the MCAT is calculation of the equilibrium concentration of a salt in a solution that already contains one of the ions in that salt. The solubility of a salt is considerably reduced when it is dissolved in a solution that already contains one of its constituent ions as compared to its solubility in a pure solvent. This reduction in molar solubility is called the **common ion effect**. As described above, the molar solubility of a compound is its concentration (in moles per liter) at equilibrium at a given temperature. If X moles of A_mB_n (*s*) can be dissolved in one liter of solution to reach saturation, then the molar solubility of A_mB_n (*s*) is X molar.

Pay attention to the effect of the common ion: its presence results in a reduction in the molar solubility of the salt. Note, however, that the presence of the common ion has no effect on the value of the solubility product constant itself. For example, if a salt such as CaF_2 is dissolved into water already containing Ca^{2+} ions (from some other salt, perhaps $CaCl_2$), the solution will dissolve less CaF_2 than would an equal amount of pure water.

The common ion effect is really Le Châtelier's principle in action. Because the solution already contains one of the constituent ions from the products side of the dissociation equilibrium, the system will shift toward the left side, reforming the solid salt. As a result, molar solubility for the solid is reduced, and less of the solid dissolves in the solution—although the K_{sp} remains constant.

One can take advantage of the common ion effect to separate out specific compounds in a solution mixture. For example, in a solution of silver salts, one could add sodium or potassium chloride to preferentially precipitate silver(I) chloride. By adding an appropriate counterion in excess, the dissociation reaction shifts to the left, forming the solid salt.

Example: The K_{sp} of AgI in aqueous solution is 8.5×10^{-17}. If a 1×10^{-5} M solution of $AgNO_3$ is saturated with AgI, what will be the final concentration of the iodide ion?

Solution: The concentration of Ag^+ in the original $AgNO_3$ solution will be 1×10^{-5} M because $AgNO_3$ will fully dissociate (review the solubility rules from earlier in this chapter). Some small amount of AgI will dissociate into the solution, which is the molar solubility x of AgI under these conditions. The net silver concentration from both $AgNO_3$ and AgI will become 1×10^{-5} M + x. Because no iodide was present in solution until the AgI began dissociating, the concentration of iodide will be x. Thus, the K_{sp} expression for the dissociation of AgI can be written as:

$$K_{sp} = [Ag^+][I^-]$$

$$8.5 \times 10^{-17} = (1 \times 10^{-5} \text{ M} + x)(x)$$

Given that the value of K_{sp} for this reaction is 10^{-16}, only a minuscule amount of AgI will be dissociated. Thus, the value of x is sufficiently small to be negligible when added to 10^{-5}. The math simplifies to:

$$8.5 \times 10^{-17} = (1 \times 10^{-5}\ \text{M})(x)$$

$$8.5 \times 10^{-12} = x$$

This question asks for the concentration of iodide, which—based on the equilibrium expression—is represented by x. Thus, $[I^-] = 8.5 \times 10^{-12}$ M.

MCAT CONCEPT CHECK 9.3

Before you move on, assess your understanding of the material with these questions.

1. Calculate the K_{sp} of $Ni(OH)_2$ in water, given that its molar solubility is 5.2×10^{-6} M.

____

____

____

2. The K_{sp} of $Ba(OH)_2$ is 5.0×10^{-3}. Assuming that barium hydroxide is the only salt added to form a solution, calculate the ion product of the following solutions based on the concentration of Ba^{2+}. Then, predict the behavior of the given solutions (dissolution, equilibrium, or precipitation):

$[Ba^{2+}]$	Ion Product	Behavior of Solution
0.5 M		
0.1 M		
0.05 M		

3. What is the molar solubility of $Zn(OH)_2$ ($K_{sp} = 4.1 \times 10^{-17}$) in a 0.1 M solution of NaOH?

____

____

9.4 Colligative Properties

LEARNING OBJECTIVES

After Chapter 9.4, you will be able to:

- Recall the names, equations, and applications of the common colligative properties
- Describe the relationship between molality and molarity for a compound
- Calculate the boiling point, freezing point, vapor pressure, or osmotic pressure of a solution

The **colligative properties** are physical properties of solutions that are dependent on the concentration of dissolved particles but not on the chemical identity of the dissolved particles. These properties—vapor pressure depression, boiling point elevation, freezing point depression, and osmotic pressure—are usually associated with dilute solutions.

Raoult's Law

Raoult's law accounts for **vapor pressure depression** caused by solutes in solution. As solute is added to a solvent, the vapor pressure of the solvent decreases proportionately. For example, consider compound A in Figure 9.15. Compound A in its pure form (mole fraction = 1.0) has a particular vapor pressure, indicated by P_A°. At the same temperature, compound B has a lower vapor pressure, indicated by P_B°. Note that, as the concentration of B increases, the vapor pressure of A decreases. Indeed, as more solute is dissolved into solvent (as more B is dissolved into A), the vapor pressure of the solvent decreases.

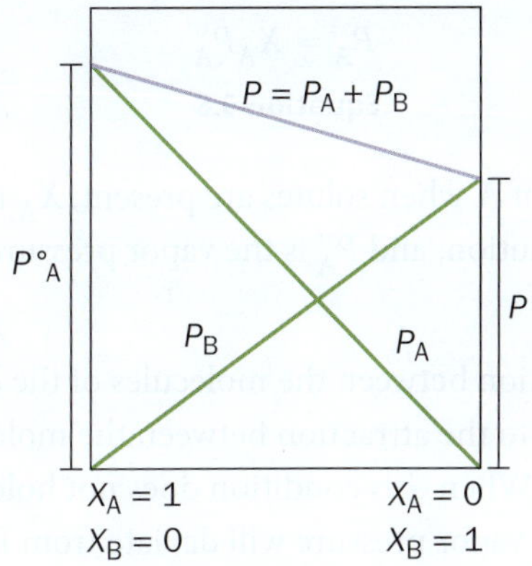

Figure 9.15 Raoult's Law
As more of solute B is dissolved in solvent A, the vapor pressure of solvent A decreases.

On a molecular level, the presence of the solute molecules can block the evaporation of solvent molecules but not their condensation. This reduces the vapor pressure of the solution compared to the pure solvent, as seen in Figure 9.16.

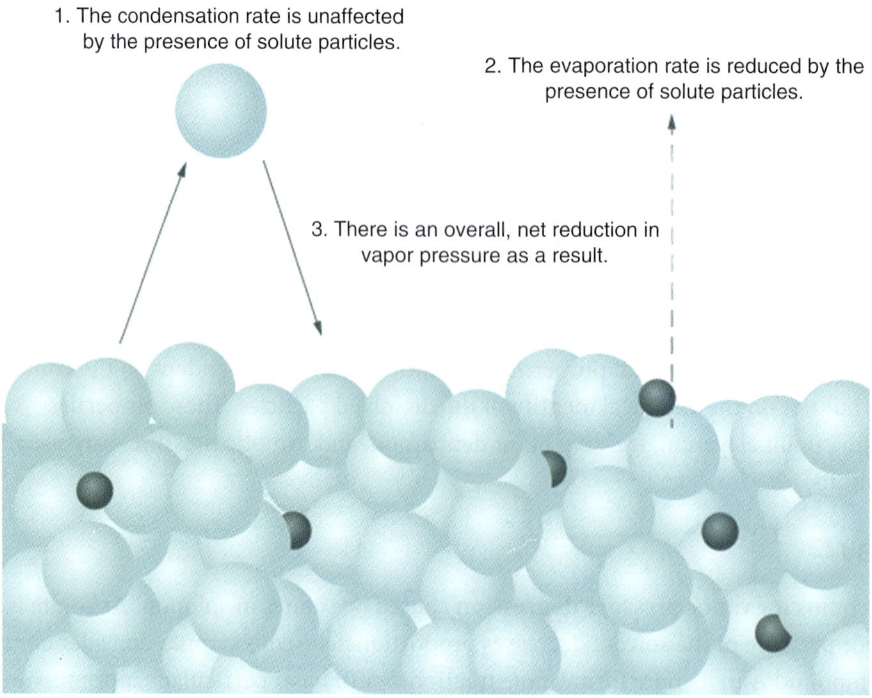

Figure 9.16 Molecular Basis of Raoult's Law

Raoult's law is expressed mathematically as:

$$P_A = X_A P_A^\circ$$

Equation 9.8

where P_A is the vapor pressure of solvent A when solutes are present, X_A is the mole fraction of the solvent A in the solution, and P_A° is the vapor pressure of solvent A in its pure state.

Raoult's law holds only when the attraction between the molecules of the different components of the mixture is equal to the attraction between the molecules of any one component in its pure state. When this condition does not hold, the relationship between mole fraction and vapor pressure will deviate from Raoult's law. Solutions that obey Raoult's law are called ideal solutions.

KEY CONCEPT

Vapor pressure depression goes hand in hand with boiling point elevation. The lowering of a solution's vapor pressure would mean that a higher temperature is required to match atmospheric pressure, thereby raising the boiling point.

Example: What is the change in vapor pressure when 180 grams of glyceraldehyde ($C_3H_6O_3$) are added to 0.18 L of water at 100°C?

Solution: The density of water at 100°C is close to 1 $\frac{\text{g}}{\text{mL}}$, and the vapor pressure of water at the same temperature is 1 atm because this is the boiling point of water.

In order to find the mole fraction of the solvent, first find the molar mass of the solute (glyceraldehyde) and solvent (water). 180 g glyceraldehyde represents 2 moles of glyceraldehyde. 0.18 L of water has a mass around 180 g, which represents 10 moles of water. The mole fraction of water is therefore $\frac{10 \text{ mol water}}{12 \text{ mol total}} = \frac{5}{6} = 0.83$.

To find the vapor pressure change, we want to find the difference in the old pressure and the new pressure. The new pressure can be calculated from Raoult's law:

$$P_A = X_A P_A^\circ = (0.83)(1 \text{ atm}) = 0.83 \text{ atm}.$$

The change in vapor pressure is therefore 1 atm − 0.83 atm = 0.17 atm.

Example: What is the vapor pressure at room temperature of a mixture containing 58 g butane (C_4H_{10}) and 172 g hexane (C_6H_{14})? (Note: The vapor pressures of pure butane and pure hexane are 172 kPa and 17.6 kPa, respectively, at 25°C.)

Solution: First, determine the number of moles of each substance. 58 g butane represents 1 mole of butane. 172 g hexane represents 2 moles of hexane. Then, determine the mole fractions of each component of the mixture.

$$X_{\text{butane}} = \frac{\text{moles of butane}}{\text{total moles}} = \frac{1}{3}$$

$$X_{\text{hexane}} = \frac{\text{moles of hexane}}{\text{total moles}} = \frac{2}{3}$$

Then, calculate the vapor pressure of each component:

$$P^\circ_{\text{butane}} = X_{\text{butane}} P_{\text{butane}} = \frac{1}{3}(172 \text{ kPa}) \approx \frac{1}{3}(180 \text{ kPa}) = 60 \text{ kPa}$$

$$P^\circ_{\text{hexane}} = X_{\text{hexane}} P_{\text{hexane}} = \frac{2}{3}(17.6 \text{ kPa}) \approx \frac{2}{3}(18 \text{ kPa}) = 12 \text{ kPa}$$

The total vapor pressure is the sum of the two vapor pressures. Thus, the total vapor pressure is 60 + 12 = 72 kPa (actual = 69.1 kPa).

Boiling Point Elevation

When a nonvolatile solute is dissolved into a solvent to create a solution, the boiling point of the solution will be greater than that of the pure solvent. The boiling point is the temperature at which the vapor pressure of the liquid equals the ambient (incident) pressure. We've just seen that adding solute to a solvent results in a decrease in the vapor pressure of the solvent in the solution. If the vapor pressure of a solution is lower than that of the pure solvent, then more energy (and consequently a higher temperature) will be required before its vapor pressure equals the ambient pressure. The extent to which the boiling point of a solution is raised relative to that of the pure solvent is given by the formula

$$\Delta T_b = iK_b m$$

Equation 9.9

MCAT EXPERTISE

The boiling point elevation formula calculates the amount that the normal boiling point is raised. The value calculated is not the boiling point itself.

where ΔT_b is the increase in boiling point, i is the van't Hoff factor, K_b is a proportionality constant characteristic of a particular solvent (which will be provided on Test Day), and m is the molality of the solution. The **van't Hoff factor** corresponds to the number of particles into which a compound dissociates in solution. Figure 9.17 shows some examples of solutions with differing van't Hoff factors. For example, $i = 2$ for NaCl because each formula unit of sodium chloride dissociates into two particles—a sodium ion and a chloride ion—when it dissolves. Covalent molecules such as glucose do not readily dissociate in water and thus have i values of 1. Other molecules that only weakly dissociate, such as hydrofluoric acid, have van't Hoff factors that are non-integers.

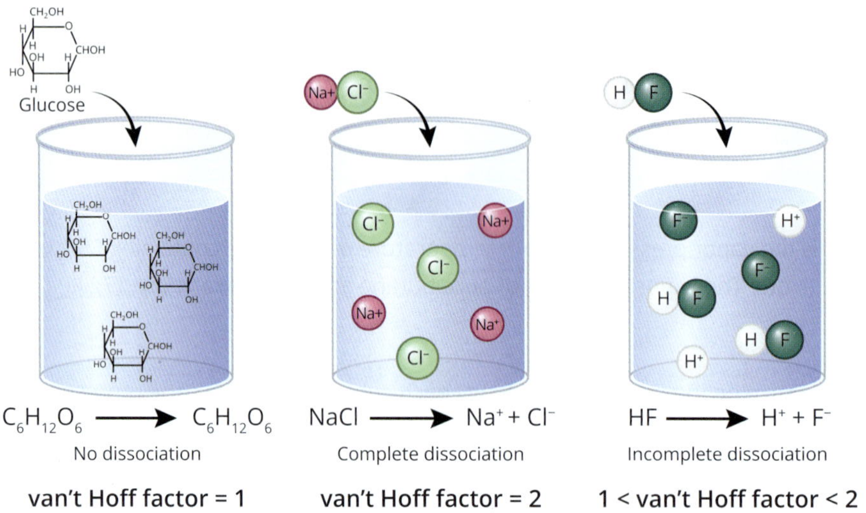

Figure 9.17 van't Hoff Factor of Various Compounds

Example: 400 g $AlCl_3$ is dissolved in 1.5 L of water at room temperature $\left(K_b = 0.512\ \frac{\text{K}\cdot\text{kg}}{\text{mol}}\right)$. How much does the boiling point increase after adding the aluminum chloride?

Solution: Water at room temperature has a density of $1\ \frac{\text{g}}{\text{mL}}$. Therefore, 1.5 L is the same as 1.5 kg. The van't Hoff factor for aluminum chloride is 4 because it breaks down to form 1 aluminum cation and 3 chloride anions. To determine the molality, we will also need to know how many moles 400 g $AlCl_3$ represents.

$$400\text{ g } AlCl_3 \times \frac{1\text{ mol}}{133.5\text{ g}} \approx 3\text{ mol } AlCl_3$$

The molality is therefore $\frac{3\text{ mol } AlCl_3}{1.5\text{ kg}} = 2\ m$.

Then, plug into the boiling point elevation equation.

$$\Delta T_b = iK_b m = (4)\left(0.512\ \frac{\text{K}\cdot\text{kg}}{\text{mol}}\right)(2\ m) \approx 4\text{ K (actual} = 4.1\text{ K)}$$

Freezing Point Depression

The presence of solute particles in a solution interferes with the formation of the lattice arrangement of solvent molecules associated with the solid state. Thus, a greater amount of energy must be removed from the solution (resulting in a lower temperature) in order for the solution to solidify. For example, pure water freezes at 0°C, but for every mole of solute dissolved in 1 kg of water, the freezing point is lowered by 1.86°C. Therefore, the K_f for water is $1.86 \frac{\text{K} \cdot \text{kg}}{\text{mol}}$. As is the case for K_b, the values for K_f are unique to each solvent and will be provided on Test Day. The formula for calculating the freezing point depression for a solution is

$$\Delta T_f = iK_f m$$

Equation 9.10

where ΔT_f is the freezing point depression, i is the van't Hoff factor, K_f is the proportionality constant characteristic of a particular solvent, and m is the molality of the solution. Freezing point depression is a colligative property and depends only on the concentration of particles, not on their identities. Colligative properties of impurities and the van't Hoff factor in boiling point elevation and freezing point depression are illustrated in Figure 9.18.

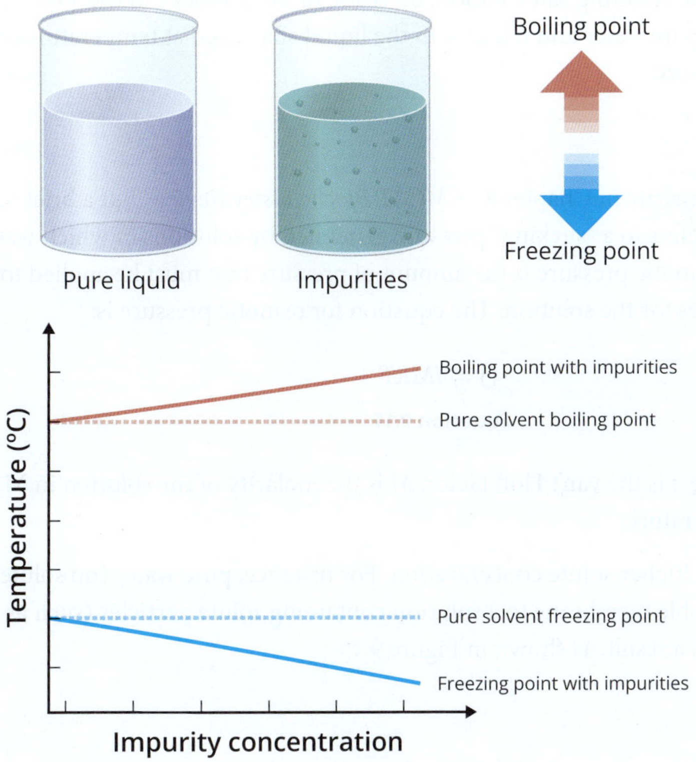

Figure 9.18 Impact of Impurities on Boiling and Freezing Points of a Solvent
The identity of the particles dissolved does not matter, only the amount of particles in solution.

Example: 400 g of $AlCl_3$ is dissolved in 1.5 L of water at room temperature $\left(K_f = 1.86 \frac{\text{K} \cdot \text{kg}}{\text{mol}}\right)$. What is the new freezing point of this solution?

Solution: Using the same variables for i and m from the previous example,

$$\Delta T_f = iK_f m = (4)\left(1.86 \frac{\text{K} \cdot \text{kg}}{\text{mol}}\right)(2\ m) \approx 15\ \text{K}(\text{actual} = 14.9\ \text{K})$$

The normal freezing point of water is 273 K. The freezing point is going to be depressed (or decreased) by 15 K. The new freezing point is therefore 273 − 15 = 258 K = −15°C.

MCAT EXPERTISE

As with boiling point elevation, there is a distinction between the calculated value and a final answer. The freezing point depression calculates the amount that the normal freezing point is lowered. As always, read the question to determine if it is asking for the change in temperature (ΔT) or the new (altered) boiling or freezing point.

This effect is the explanation for why many people in colder climates salt icy roads in the winter. Salt mixes with the snow and ice and initially dissolves into the small amount of liquid water that is in equilibrium with the solid phase (the snow and ice). The solute in solution causes a disturbance to the equilibrium such that the rate of melting is unchanged (because the salt can't interact with the solid water that is stabilized in a rigid lattice arrangement), but the rate of freezing is decreased (the solute displaces some of the water molecules from the solid–liquid interface and prevents liquid water from entering into the solid phase).

This imbalance causes more ice to melt than water to freeze. Melting is an endothermic process, so heat is initially absorbed from the liquid solution, causing the solution temperature to fall below the ambient temperature. Now, there is a temperature gradient, and heat flows from the warmer air to the cooler aqueous solution; this additional heat facilitates more melting—even though the temperature of the solution is actually colder than it was before the solute was added! The more the ice melts into liquid water, the more the solute is dispersed through the liquid. The resulting salt solution, by virtue of the presence of the solute particles, has a lower freezing point than the pure water and remains in the liquid state even at temperatures that would normally cause pure water to freeze.

Osmotic Pressure

Osmotic pressure is covered primarily in Chapter 8 of *MCAT Biochemistry Review*, but a brief recap is provided here. **Osmotic pressure** refers to a "sucking" pressure generated by solutions in which water is drawn into a solution. Formally, the osmotic pressure is the amount of pressure that must be applied to counteract this attraction of water molecules for the solution. The equation for osmotic pressure is:

$$\Pi = iMRT$$

Equation 9.11

where Π is the osmotic pressure, i is the van't Hoff factor, M is the molarity of the solution in M, R is the ideal gas constant, and T is the temperature.

Water moves in the direction of higher solute concentration. For instance, pure water (no solute concentration) will traverse a semipermeable membrane to a solution containing solute particles (such as NaCl) and increase the level of the water as a result, as shown in Figure 9.19.

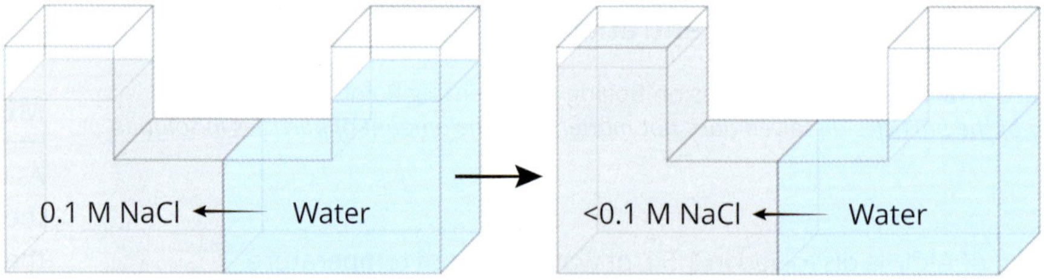

Figure 9.19 Change in Water Level Due to Osmotic Pressure

MCAT CONCEPT CHECK 9.4

Before you move on, assess your understanding of the material with these questions.

1. What is a colligative property?

---

2. How are molality and molarity related for water? How are they related for other solvents?
   - Water:

   - Other solvents:

---

3. Determine the vapor pressure of a solution containing 190 g $MgCl_2$ in 540 g water at room temperature: (Note: The vapor pressure of pure water at 25°C is 3.2 kPa.)

---

4. Determine the new boiling point of a solution containing 190 g $MgCl_2$ in 1500 g water at room temperature: $\left(K_b = 0.512 \ \frac{K \cdot kg}{mol}\right)$

---

5. Determine the freezing point depression of a solution containing 58.5 g of NaCl in 1800 g of water at room temperature: $\left(K_f = 1.86 \ \frac{K \cdot kg}{mol}\right)$

Conclusion

Our review of solution chemistry has provided an opportunity for us to consider the nature of solutions, solutes, and solvents, and the interactions between solutes and solvents in the formation of solutions. We reviewed solubility and the rules that reflect the solubility of common compounds in water. The different ways of expressing the amount of solute in solution were identified, and examples were given for each unit of concentration, including percent composition, mole fraction, molarity, molality, and normality. Next, we reviewed the thermodynamic principles of solution equilibria and defined unsaturated, saturated, and supersaturated solutions with respect to ion product (IP) and solubility product constant (K_{sp}). Subsequently, we discussed the common ion effect from the perspective of Le Châtelier's principle for a solution at equilibrium. And finally, we examined the colligative properties of solutions and the mathematics that govern them. The colligative properties—vapor pressure depression, boiling point elevation, freezing point depression, and osmotic pressure—are physical properties of solutions that depend on the concentration of dissolved particles but not on their chemical identities.

GO ONLINE

You've reviewed the content, now test your knowledge and critical thinking skills by completing a test-like passage set in your online resources!

CONCEPT SUMMARY

Nature of Solutions

- **Solutions** are homogeneous **mixtures** composed of two or more substances.
  - They combine to form a single phase, generally the liquid phase.
  - **Solvent** particles surround **solute** particles via electrostatic interactions in a process called **solvation** or **dissolution**.
  - **Aqueous solutions** are most important for the MCAT; solvation in water can also be called **hydration**.
  - Most dissolutions are endothermic, although the dissolution of gas into liquid is exothermic.
- **Solubility** is the maximum amount of a solute that can be dissolved in a given solvent at a given temperature; it is often expressed as **molar solubility**—the molarity of the solute at saturation.
- **Complex ions** or **coordination compounds** are composed of metallic ions bonded to various neutral compounds and anions, referred to as **ligands**.
  - Formation of **complex ions** increases the solubility of otherwise insoluble ions (the opposite of the common ion effect).
  - The process of forming a complex ion involves electron pair donors and electron pair acceptors such as those seen in **coordinate covalent bonding**.

Concentration

- There are many ways of expressing concentration.
  - **Percent composition by mass** (mass of solute per mass of solution times 100%) is used for aqueous solutions and solid-in-solid solutions.
  - The **mole fraction** (moles of solute per total moles) is used for calculating vapor pressure depression and partial pressures of gases in a system.
  - **Molarity** (moles of solute per liters of solution) is the most common unit for concentration and is used for rate laws, the law of mass action, osmotic pressure, pH and pOH, and the Nernst equation.
  - **Molality** (moles of solute per kilograms of solvent) is used for boiling point elevation and freezing point depression.
  - **Normality** (number of equivalents per liters of solution) is the molarity of the species of interest and is used for acid–base and oxidation–reduction reactions.

Solution Equilibria

- Saturated solutions are in equilibrium at that particular temperature.
- The **solubility product constant** (K_{sp}) is simply the equilibrium constant for a dissociation reaction.
- Comparison of the **ion product (IP)** to K_{sp} determines the level of saturation and behavior of the solution:
  - IP $< K_{sp}$: the solution is unsaturated, and if more solute is added, it will dissolve
  - IP $= K_{sp}$: the solution is saturated (at equilibrium), and there will be no change in concentrations
  - IP $> K_{sp}$: the solution is supersaturated, and a precipitate will form
- Formation of a complex ion in solution greatly increases solubility.
  - The **formation** or **stability constant** (K_f) is the equilibrium constant for complex formation. Its value is usually much greater than K_{sp}.
  - The formation of a complex increases the solubility of other salts containing the same ions because it uses up the products of those dissolution reactions, shifting the equilibrium to the right (the opposite of the common ion effect).
  - The **common ion effect** decreases the solubility of a compound in a solution that already contains one of the ions in the compound. The presence of that ion in solution shifts the dissolution reaction to the left, decreasing its dissociation.

Colligative Properties

- **Colligative properties** are physical properties of solutions that depend on the concentration of dissolved particles but not on their chemical identity.
- **Vapor pressure depression** follows **Raoult's law**.
  - The presence of other solutes decreases the evaporation rate of a solvent without affecting its condensation rate, thus decreasing its vapor pressure.
  - Vapor pressure depression also explains boiling point elevation—as the vapor pressure decreases, the temperature (energy) required to boil the liquid must be raised.
- **Freezing point depression** and **boiling point elevation** are shifts in the phase equilibria dependent on the molality of the solution.
- **Osmotic pressure** is primarily dependent on the molarity of the solution.
- For solutes that dissociate, the **van't Hoff factor** (*i*) is used in freezing point depression, boiling point elevation, and osmotic pressure calculations.

ANSWERS TO CONCEPT CHECKS

9.1

1. Solvation refers to the breaking of intermolecular forces between solute particles and between solvent particles, with formation of intermolecular forces between solute and solvent particles. In an aqueous solution, water is the solvent.
2. Solubility is the amount of solute contained in a solvent. Saturation refers to the maximum solubility of a compound at a given temperature; one cannot dissolve any more of the solute just by adding more at this temperature.
3. Solubility of solids can be increased by increasing temperature. Solubility of gases can be increased by decreasing temperature or increasing the partial pressure of the gas above the solvent (Henry's law).
4. Group I metals, ammonium, nitrate, and acetate salts are always soluble.

9.2

1.

Compound	Molality	Molarity	Normality
Glucose $\left(180\ \frac{\text{g}}{\text{mol}}\right)$	$\frac{1\text{ mol}}{250\text{ kg solvent}} = 0.004\ m$	$\frac{1\text{ mol}}{250\text{ L solution}} = 0.004\text{ M}$	0.004 N (glucose does not dissociate)
Carbonate $\left(60\ \frac{\text{g}}{\text{mol}}\right)$	$\frac{3\text{ mol}}{250\text{ kg solvent}} = 0.012\ m$	$\frac{3\text{ mol}}{250\text{ L solution}} = 0.012\text{ M}$	Approximately 0.024 N (twice the molarity)

Please note that the denominator for molality uses kilograms of *solvent*, whereas the denominator for molarity uses liters of *total solution*. These quantities are not necessarily the same and so you must be careful!

An example will help clarify the difference: Suppose 1 mol of solute were added to 1 L of water. 1 L of water has mass 1 kg, so you would simply use 1 kg solvent in the denominator of the molality computation, because molality's denominator is the mass of the solvent itself. However, when adding 1 mol solute to 1 L water, the volume of the final solution will likely be significantly larger than 1 L, because the solute itself takes up space. Therefore, you could not simply plug 1 L into the molarity equation, because molarity's denominator depends on the total volume of the final, mixed solution. Instead, you would need to remeasure the total, final volume, and use that number when computing molarity.

All that said, in the problem in the concept check, the initial volume of solvent is so large (250 L) that the added solute will not appreciably change the volume of final solution. Therefore, in this case, we were able to add 250 L directly into the molarity computation.

2. $M_\text{i} V_\text{i} = M_\text{f} V_\text{f} \rightarrow V_\text{i} = \frac{M_\text{f} V_\text{f}}{M_\text{i}} = \frac{(25\text{ ppm})(100\text{ mL})}{(100\text{ ppm})} = 25\text{ mL}.$

Thus, start with 25 mL of the stock solution and add 75 mL pure water to get 100 mL of solution with 25 ppm Cl_2.

3. $X_{NaCl} = \dfrac{\text{moles of NaCl}}{\text{total moles}} = \dfrac{90\text{ g}\left[\dfrac{1\text{ mol}}{58.5\text{ g}}\right]}{90\text{ g}\left[\dfrac{1\text{ mol}}{58.5\text{ g}}\right] + 10^4\text{ g}\left[\dfrac{1\text{ mol}}{18\text{ g}}\right]} \approx \dfrac{90\left(\frac{1}{60}\right)}{90\left(\frac{1}{60}\right) + 10^4\left(\frac{1}{20}\right)}$

$\approx \dfrac{1.5}{1.5 + 500} \approx \dfrac{1.5}{500} \approx \dfrac{1.5}{5 \times 10^2} \approx \dfrac{1}{3} \times 10^{-2} \approx 3 \times 10^{-3}$ (actual $= 2.8 \times 10^{-3}$)

Percent composition $= \dfrac{\text{mass of solute}}{\text{mass of solution}} \times 100\% = \dfrac{90\text{ g}}{90\text{ g} + 10^4\text{ g}} \times 100\% \approx$

$\dfrac{90}{10^4} \times 100\% = 0.9\%$ (actual $= 0.89\%$)

9.3

1. First, write out the balanced equation: $Ni(OH)_2 \rightarrow Ni^{2+} + 2OH^-$

   Next, identify that the molar solubility x represents the amount of $Ni(OH)_2$ that dissociates, creating x of Ni^{2+} and $2x$ of OH^-. Write out the K_{sp} equation, and plug in the values of x to solve for K_{sp}:

   $K_{sp} = [Ni^{2+}][OH^-]^2 = x(2x)^2$

   $K_{sp} = (5.2 \times 10^{-6})(2 \times 5.2 \times 10^{-6})^2$

   $K_{sp} = (5 \times 10^{-6})(10 \times 10^{-6})^2 \approx (5 \times 10^{-6})(10^{-5})^2$

   $K_{sp} \approx 5 \times 10^{-6} \times 10^{-10} = 5 \times 10^{-16}$ (actual value $= 5.6 \times 10^{-16}$)

2. Start with the balanced reaction and calculation for K_{sp}, which can also be used to calculate Q. Keep in mind that for every x of $Ba(OH)_2$ that dissolves, x of Ba^{2+} will be produced, and $2x$ of OH^-.

   $Ba(OH)_2 \rightarrow Ba^{2+} + 2OH^-$

   $K_{sp} = [Ba^{2+}][OH^-]^2$

$[Ba^{2+}]$	Ion Product	Behavior of Solution
0.5 M	$(0.5\text{ M})(1\text{ M})^2 = 0.5$	$0.5 > 5.0 \times 10^{-3} \rightarrow$ precipitation
0.1 M	$(0.1\text{ M})(0.2\text{ M})^2 = 4.0 \times 10^{-3}$	$4.0 \times 10^{-3} < 5.0 \times 10^{-3} \rightarrow$ dissolution
0.05 M	$(0.05\text{ M})(0.1\text{ M})^2 = 5.0 \times 10^{-4}$	$5.0 \times 10^{-4} < 5.0 \times 10^{-3} \rightarrow$ dissolution

   Note that the concentration of hydroxide is double that of barium. While there will be a very small contribution of hydroxide from the autoionization of water, this amount is negligible compared to the values given in the question.

3. Start by writing the balanced reaction for the least soluble salt in the problem: $Zn(OH)_2 \rightarrow Zn^{2+} + 2\ OH^-$. Next, write out the K_{sp} equation and enter the variables for the concentrations. The Zn^{2+} concentration will equal x, the molar solubility under these conditions, but the OH^- concentration will come from two contributors: the dissociated $Zn(OH)_2$, and the 0.1 M NaOH solution. This results in the following K_{sp} expression: $K_{sp} = [Zn^{2+}][OH^-]^2 = (x)(0.1 + 2x)^2$. Since the K_{sp} for $Zn(OH)_2$ is 4.1×10^{-17}, x will be negligible compared to the 0.1 M from NaOH. The K_{sp} expression simplifies to: $K_{sp} = (x)(0.1)^2$. Thus, $4.1 \times 10^{-17} = 0.01x$. x = molar solubility of $Zn(OH)_2 = 4.1 \times 10^{-15}$.

9.4

1. Colligative properties are those that depend on the amount of solute present, but not the actual identity of the solute particles. Examples include vapor pressure depression, boiling point elevation, freezing point depression, and osmotic pressure.
2. Molarity (M) and molality (m) are nearly equal at room temperature. This is only because 1 L solution is approximately equal to 1 kg solvent for dilute solutions (the denominators of the molarity and molality equations, respectively). For other solvents, molarity and molality differ significantly because their densities are not 1 $\frac{\text{g}}{\text{mL}}$ like water.
3. $190\ \text{g MgCl}_2 \times \frac{1\ \text{mol}}{95.3\ \text{g}} = 2\ \text{mol MgCl}_2$. $540\ \text{g H}_2\text{O} \times \frac{1\ \text{mol}}{18\ \text{g}} = 30\ \text{mol H}_2\text{O}$

   $$X_{\text{water}} = \frac{30\ \text{moles water}}{32\ \text{total moles}}$$

   $$P_{\text{water}} = X_{\text{water}} P°_{\text{water}} = \frac{30\ \text{moles water}}{32\ \text{total moles}} \times (3.2\ \text{kPa}) = 3.0\ \text{kPa}$$

4. $$T_\text{b} = iK_\text{b}m = (3)\left(0.512\ \frac{\text{K}\cdot\text{kg}}{\text{mol}}\right)\left(\frac{2\ \text{mol MgCl}_2}{1.5\ \text{kg water}}\right) \approx 2\ \text{K (actual} = 2.04\ \text{K)}$$

   The new boiling point will be $373 + 2 = 375$ K.

5. $$\Delta T_\text{f} = iK_\text{f}m = (2)\left(1.86\ \frac{\text{K}\cdot\text{kg}}{\text{mol}}\right)\left(\frac{1\ \text{mol NaCl}}{1.8\ \text{kg water}}\right) \approx 2\ \text{K (actual} = 2.06\ \text{K)}$$

SCIENCE MASTERY ASSESSMENT EXPLANATIONS

1. **A**

The equation $\Delta T_b = iK_bm$ can be used to solve this problem. The change in boiling point is 101.0 – 100 = 1.0°C. Then, plug that into:

$$\Delta T_b = iK_b m \rightarrow m = \frac{\Delta T_b}{iK_b} = \frac{1.0\text{ K}}{(1)\left(0.512\ \frac{\text{K}\cdot\text{kg}}{\text{mol}}\right)} \approx 2\ m$$

The van't Hoff factor for this solute is 1 because the molecule does not dissociate into smaller components. Then, convert to grams of solute using the definition of molality:

$$\text{molality} = \frac{\text{moles of solute}}{\text{kg of solvent}} \rightarrow \text{moles of solute}$$
$$(2\ m)(0.1\text{ kg}) = 0.2\text{ mol.}$$

The mass used in this equation is 0.1 kg because 100 mL of water has a mass of 0.1 kg. Then, determine the molar mass:

$\text{molar mass} = \frac{70\text{ g}}{0.2\text{ mol}} = 350\ \frac{\text{g}}{\text{mol}}$, which is closest to **(A)**.

2. **D**

All three choices can make a solution as long as the two components create a mixture that is of uniform appearance (homogeneous). Hydrogen in platinum is an example of a gas in a solid. Brass and steel are examples of homogeneous mixtures of solids. The air we breathe is an example of a homogeneous mixture of gases; while these are more commonly referred to as mixtures, they still fit the criteria of a solution.

3. **B**

Benzene and toluene are both organic liquids and have very similar properties. They are both nonpolar and are almost exactly the same size. Raoult's law states that ideal solution behavior is observed when solute–solute, solvent–solvent, and solute–solvent interactions are all very similar. Therefore, benzene and toluene in solution will be predicted to behave as a nearly ideal solution.

4. **C**

Melting point depresses upon solute addition, making **(A)** and **(B)** incorrect. Solute particles interfere with lattice formation, the highly organized state in which solid molecules align themselves. Colder-than-normal conditions are necessary to create the solid structure.

5. **D**

The first step will most likely be endothermic because energy is required to break molecules apart. The second step is also endothermic because the intermolecular forces in the solvent must be overcome to allow incorporation of solute particles. The third step will most likely be exothermic because polar water molecules will interact with the dissolved ions, creating a stable solution and releasing energy.

6. **C**

BeF_2 will cause the most negative contribution to $\Delta S°_{soln}$ through the hydration effect because Be^{2+} cation has the highest charge density compared to the other ions. All of the other ions have a charge density of +1 or −1, whereas Be^{2+} has a charge density of magnitude two.

7. **B**

Formation of complex ions between silver ions and ammonia will cause more molecules of solid AgCl to dissociate. The equilibrium is driven toward dissociation because the Ag^+ ions are essentially being removed from solution when they complex with ammonia. This rationale is based upon Le Châtelier's principle, stating that when a chemical equilibrium experiences a change in concentration, the system will shift to counteract that change.

8. **B**

The mass percent of a solute equals the mass of the solute divided by the mass of the total solution times 100%. $\text{mass }\% = \frac{\text{mass of solute}}{\text{total mass of solution}} \times 100\%$. Plug in the values given for sucrose, the volume of water and the density of water to determine the % mass of sucrose:

$$\frac{(100\text{ g sucrose})}{(300\text{ mL }H_2O)(0.975\text{ g/mL}) + 100\text{ g sucrose}} \times 100\%$$
$$\approx \frac{100}{300+100} \times 100\% = \frac{100}{400} \times 100\% = 25\%$$

Keep in mind that in rounding while calculating, the denominator was estimated to be larger than the actual value, thus giving an answer that is slightly lower than the actual value. Thus, the correct answer is **(B)**, 25.5%. **(A)** results if rounding error is not taken into account. While these answers are very close, the mass of the water must be slightly *less* than 300 g, given the density value, so the percent composition of sucrose must be slightly *higher* than 25%. If the solute's mass is not added to the solvent's, the calculated value is 34.2%, which is **(D)**. **(C)** neglects both the addition step and the rounding error.

9. **A**

Mixtures that have a higher vapor pressure than predicted by Raoult's law have stronger solvent–solvent and solute–solute interactions than solvent–solute interactions. Therefore, particles do not want to stay in solution and more readily evaporate, creating a higher vapor pressure than an ideal solution. Two liquids that have different properties, like hexane (hydrophobic) and ethanol (hydrophilic, small) in **(A)**, would not have many interactions with each other and would cause positive deviation (i.e. higher vapor pressure). **(B)** and **(C)** are composed of liquids that are similar to one another and would not show significant deviation from Raoult's law. **(D)** contains two liquids that would interact very well with each other, which would actually cause a negative deviation from Raoult's law—when attracted to one other, solutes and solvents prefer to stay in liquid form and have a lower vapor pressure than predicted by Raoult's law.

10. **A**

Dissolution is governed by enthalpy and entropy, which are related by the equation $\Delta G^\circ_{soln} = \Delta H^\circ_{soln} - T\Delta S^\circ_{soln}$. The cooling of the solution indicates that heat is used up in this bond-breaking reaction. In other words, dissolution is endothermic, and ΔH is positive. The reaction is occurring spontaneously, so ΔG must be negative. The only way that a positive ΔH can result in a negative ΔG is if entropy, ΔS, is a large, positive value as in **(A)**. Conceptually, that means that the only way the solid can dissolve is if the increase in entropy is great enough to overcome the increase in enthalpy. **(B)** is incorrect because it is clearly stated in the question stem that KCl dissolves; further, all salts of Group 1 metals are soluble. **(C)** is incorrect because ΔS°_{soln} must be positive in order for KCl to dissolve. Finally, **(D)** is incorrect because solute dissolution would cause the boiling point to elevate, not depress. It is also not a piece of evidence that could be found simply by observing the beaker's temperature change.

11. **B**

The equation to determine the change in boiling point of a solution is as follows: $\Delta T_b = iK_bm$. m is the molality of the solution, and K_b is the boiling point elevation constant. In this case, the solvent is always water, so K_b will be the same for each solution. What is needed is the number of dissociated particles from each of the original species. This is referred to as the van't Hoff factor (i) and is multiplied by molality to give a normality (the concentration of the species of interest—in this case, all particles). The normality values determine which species causes the greatest change in boiling point.

Species	Number of Moles	Number of Dissolved Particles	$i \times m$ (Normality)
$CaSO_4$	0.4	2	0.8
$Fe(NO_3)_3$	0.5	4	2.0
CH_3COOH	1.0	Between 1 and 2 (acetic acid is a weak acid and a low percentage of the molecules will dissociate into 2 particles)	Between 1.0 and 2.0
$C_{12}H_{22}O_{11}$	1.0	1	1.0

The choice is between iron(III) nitrate and acetic acid. The fact that acetic acid is a weak acid indicates that only a few particles will dissociate into H^+ and acetate. Therefore, the normality of the acetic acid will be much closer to 1.0 than 2.0.

12. **B**

Osmotic pressure is given by the formula $\Pi = iMRT$. Entering the values from the question stem gives:

$$\Pi = (1000 \times 10^{-3}\,\text{mOsm/L})(0.0812\ \text{L}\cdot\text{atm/mol}\cdot\text{K})(298\ \text{K})$$
$$\approx 1 \times 0.08 \times 300 = 24\ \text{atm (actual value} = 24.2\ \text{atm)}$$

Notice that the concentration of seawater is given for all solutes, which represents $i \times M$. It is also given in mOsm/L, which is converted to moles per liter by multiplying by 10^{-3}. Also, the question asks for the minimum pressure required, which means that the correct answer choice must be slightly above the calculated pressure in order for reverse osmosis to proceed.

13. **B**

200 ppb of Pb^{2+} is equivalent to 200 grams of Pb^{2+} in 10^9 grams of solution; given the extremely low concentration of lead, the mass of the water can be assumed to be approximately 10^9 grams, as well. To solve, set up a dimensional analysis question. The units needed at the end are moles per liter (molarity), so convert from grams of lead to moles of lead and grams of water to liters of water:

$$\left[\frac{200\text{ g Pb}^{2+}}{10^9\text{ g H}_2\text{O}}\right]\left[\frac{10^3\text{ g H}_2\text{O}}{1\text{ L}}\right]\left[\frac{1\text{ mol Pb}^{2+}}{207.2\text{ g Pb}^{2+}}\right]\approx\frac{200\times10^3}{200\times10^9}$$

$$= 1\times10^{-6}\text{ M} = 10\times10^{-7}\text{ M}$$

$$(\text{actual value} = 9.67\times10^{-7}\text{ M})$$

Note that the denominator was rounded to a smaller number, meaning the estimated answer is slightly larger than the actual value.

14. **A**

This question is actually more complicated than it seems since hydroxide is involved. In aqueous solution, the concentration of hydroxide from the autoionization of water is 10^{-7} M. This concentration is significantly greater (approximately 10,000× greater) than the amount of hydroxide that would be produced by the dissociation of either salt. Thus, the concentration of hydroxide is set by water, not by the dissociation of cobalt(III) hydroxide and thallium(III) hydroxide. When the two solutions are mixed, the concentration of hydroxide does not change. However, in mixing the two solutions, the concentration of the metal ions decreases as a consequence of dilution. As a result, both solutions would be below saturation, justifying **(A)** as the correct answer.

15. **D**

The solubility of AgBr can be determined using the K_{sp} value given in the equation. Some amount of AgBr will dissolve; this is the molar solubility x for these conditions. When AgBr dissociates, there will be x amount of silver(I) formed and x amount of bromide—which is added to the 0.0010 M Br^- already present from NaBr.

$$\text{AgBr} \rightleftharpoons \text{Ag}^+ + \text{Br}^-$$

$$K_{sp} = [\text{Ag}^+][\text{Br}^-]$$

$$5.35\times10^{-13} = (x)(0.0010\text{ M} + x)$$

Given the K_{sp} of 5.4×10^{-13}, x will be negligible compared to 0.0010 M. Thus, the math can be simplified to:

$$5.35\times10^{-13} = (x)(0.0010)$$

$$x = \frac{5.35\times10^{-13}}{10^{-3}} = 5.35\times10^{-10}$$

Therefore, x, the molar solubility, is 5.35×10^{-10}, which looks like **(C)**. However, the units of the answer choices are grams per liter, not molarity, and the result must be multiplied by the molar mass $\left(187.8\ \frac{\text{g}}{\text{mol}}\right)$:

$$5.35\times10^{-10}\,\frac{\text{mol}}{\text{L}}\times187.8\,\frac{\text{g}}{\text{mol}}\approx5\times10^{-10}\times200$$

$$= 1{,}000\times10^{-10} = 1\times10^{-7}$$

which is close to **(D)**. Note that a very accurate approximation was reached by rounding down the first number and rounding up the second, balancing the error.

GO ONLINE

Consult your online resources for additional practice.

EQUATIONS TO REMEMBER

(9.1) **Percent composition by mass:** $\frac{\text{mass of solute}}{\text{mass of solution}} \times 100\%$

(9.2) **Mole fraction:** $X_A = \frac{\text{moles of A}}{\text{total moles of all species}}$

(9.3) **Molarity:** $\text{M} = \frac{\text{moles of solute}}{\text{liters of solution}}$

(9.4) **Molality:** $m = \frac{\text{moles of solute}}{\text{kilograms of solvent}}$

(9.5) **Dilution formula:** $M_i V_i = M_f V_f$

(9.6) **Solubility product constant:** $K_{sp} = [A^{n+}]^m [B^{m-}]^n$

(9.7) **Ion product:** $\text{IP} = [A^{n+}]^m [B^{m-}]^n$

(9.8) **Raoult's law (vapor pressure depression):** $P_A = X_A P_A^\circ$

(9.9) **Boiling point elevation:** $\Delta T_b = iK_b m$

(9.10) **Freezing point depression:** $\Delta T_f = iK_f m$

(9.11) **Osmotic pressure:** $\Pi = iMRT$

SHARED CONCEPTS

Biology Chapter 10
Homeostasis

General Chemistry Chapter 3
Bonding and Chemical Interactions

General Chemistry Chapter 6
Equilibrium

General Chemistry Chapter 7
Thermochemistry

General Chemistry Chapter 10
Acids and Bases

General Chemistry Chapter 12
Electrochemistry

CHAPTER 10

ACIDS AND BASES

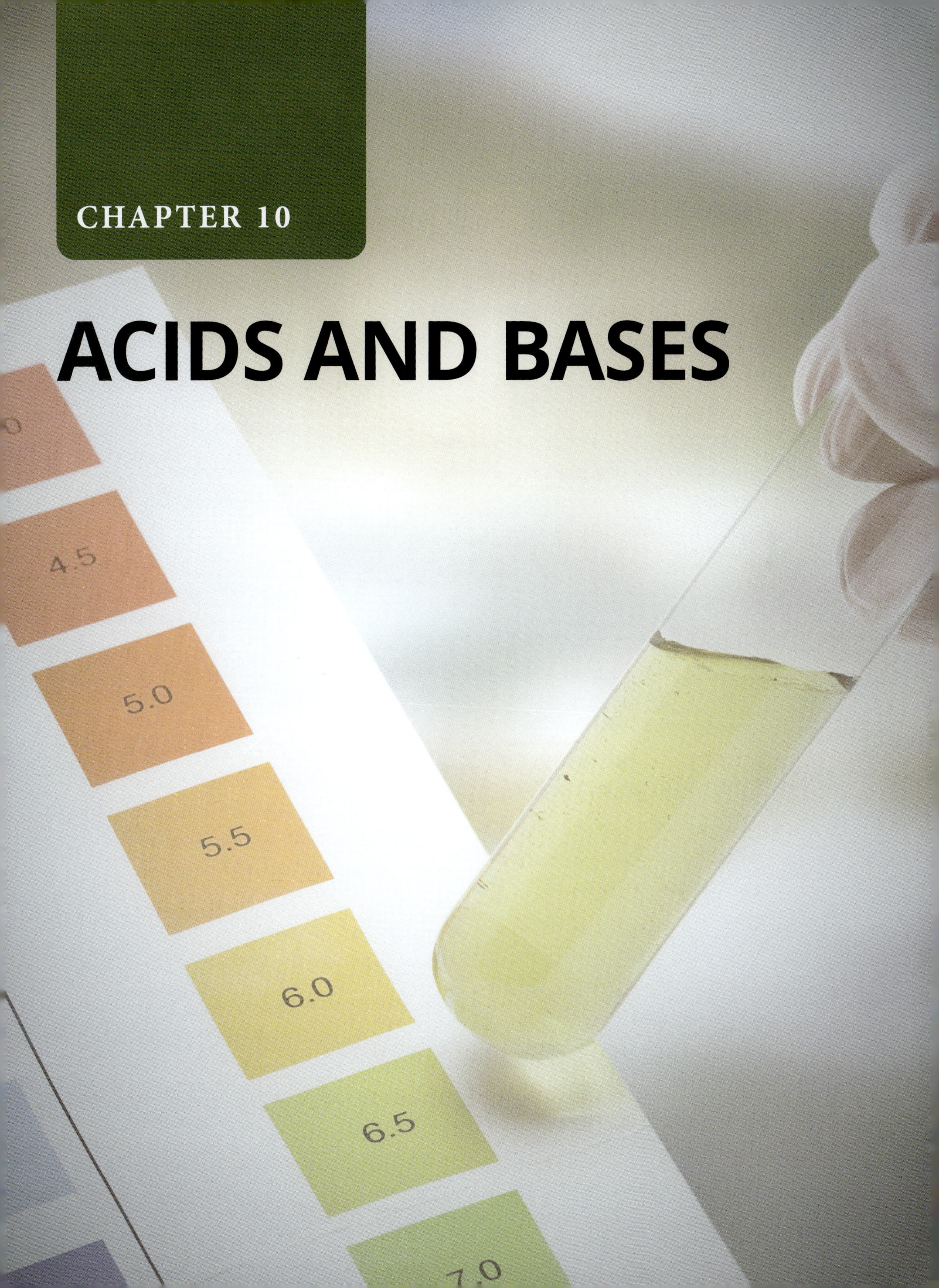

SCIENCE MASTERY ASSESSMENT

Every pre-med knows this feeling: there is so much content I have to know for the MCAT! How do I know what to do first or what's important?

While the high-yield badges throughout this book will help you identify the most important topics, this Science Mastery Assessment is another tool in your MCAT prep arsenal. This quiz (which can also be taken in your online resources) and the guidance below will help ensure that you are spending the appropriate amount of time on this chapter based on your personal strengths and weaknesses. Don't worry though—skipping something now does not mean you'll never study it. Later on in your prep, as you complete full-length tests, you'll uncover specific pieces of content that you need to review and can come back to these chapters as appropriate.

How to Use This Assessment

If you answer 0–7 questions correctly:

Spend about 1 hour to read this chapter in full and take limited notes throughout. Follow up by reviewing **all** quiz questions to ensure that you now understand how to solve each one.

If you answer 8–11 questions correctly:

Spend 20–40 minutes reviewing the quiz questions. Beginning with the questions you missed, read and take notes on the corresponding subchapters. For questions you answered correctly, ensure your thinking matches that of the explanation and you understand why each choice was correct or incorrect.

If you answer 12–15 questions correctly:

Spend less than 20 minutes reviewing all questions from the quiz. If you missed any, then include a quick read-through of the corresponding subchapters, or even just the relevant content within a subchapter, as part of your question review. For questions you answered correctly, ensure your thinking matches that of the explanation and review the Concept Summary at the end of the chapter.

1. Which of the following is not a Brønsted–Lowry base?

   A. 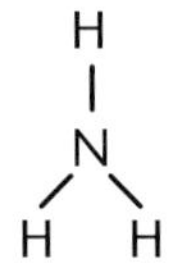

   B. F^-

   C. 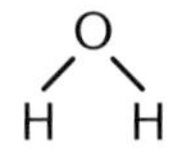

   D. H—O—N=O

2. Which of the following is closest to the pH of a solution containing 5 mM H_2SO_4?

   A. 1

   B. 2

   C. 3

   D. 4

3. Which of the following represents chloric acid?

   A. $HClO_3$

   B. ClO_3^-

   C. $HClO_2$

   D. HClO

4. Which of the following bases is the weakest?

   A. KOH

   B. NH_3

   C. CH_3NH_2

   D. $Ca(OH)_2$

5. The function of a buffer is to:

   A. maintain a neutral pH.

   B. resist changes in pH when small amounts of acid or base are added.

   C. slow down reactions between acids and bases.

   D. speed up reactions between acids and bases.

6. What is the pH of a solution with an ammonium concentration of 70 mM and an ammonia concentration of 712 mM? (Note: The pK_b of ammonia is 3.45.)

   A. 2.45

   B. 4.45

   C. 9.55

   D. 11.55

Questions 7–9 refer to the titration curve of acid X shown below:

Titration Curve of Weak Acid X

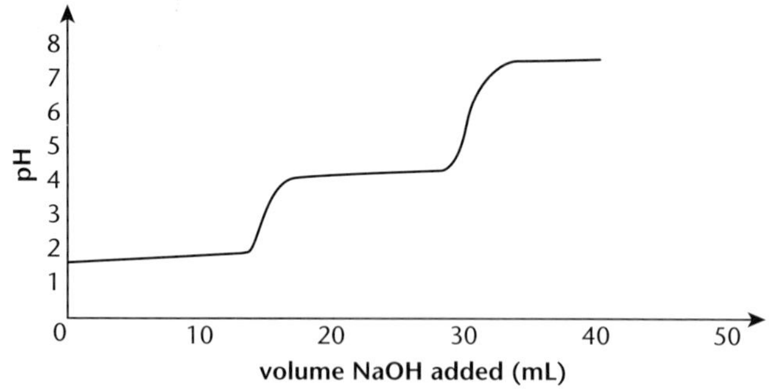

7. What is the approximate value of pK_{a1}?

   A. 1.9

   B. 2.9

   C. 3.8

   D. 4.1

8. At what pH is the second equivalence point?

   A. pH = 3.0

   B. pH = 4.1

   C. pH = 5.9

   D. pH = 7.2

9. What is the approximate value of pK_{a2}?

   A. 3.6

   B. 4.1

   C. 5.5

   D. 7.2

10. What is the gram equivalent weight of phosphoric acid?

    A. 24.5 g

    B. 32.7 g

    C. 49.0 g

    D. 98.0 g

11. What is the $[H_3O^+]$ of a 2 M aqueous solution of a weak acid HXO_2 with $K_a = 3.2 \times 10^{-5}$?

    A. 6.4×10^{-5} M

    B. 1.3×10^{-4} M

    C. 4.0×10^{-3} M

    D. 8.0×10^{-3} M

12. A solution is prepared with an unknown concentration of a theoretical compound with a K_a of exactly 1.0. What is the pH of this solution?

A. Higher than 7
B. Exactly 7
C. Less than 7
D. There is not enough information to answer the question.

13. Which of the following is NOT a characteristic of an amphoteric species?

A. Amphoteric species can act as an acid or a base, depending on its environment.
B. Amphoteric species can act as an oxidizing or reducing agent, depending on its environment.
C. Amphoteric species are sometimes amphiprotic.
D. Amphoteric species are always nonpolar.

14. What is the approximate pH of a 1.2×10^{-5} M aqueous solution of NaOH?

A. 4.92
B. 7.50
C. 9.08
D. 12.45

15. How many liters of 2 M $Ba(OH)_2$ are needed to titrate a 4 L solution of 6 M H_3PO_4?

A. 1.33 L
B. 12 L
C. 18 L
D. 56 L

Answer Key

1. **D** (See section 10.1)
2. **B** (See section 10.2)
3. **A** (See section 10.1)
4. **B** (See section 10.2)
5. **B** (See section 10.4)
6. **D** (See section 10.2)
7. **A** (See section 10.4)
8. **C** (See section 10.4)
9. **B** (See section 10.4)
10. **B** (See section 10.3)
11. **D** (See section 10.2)
12. **C** (See section 10.2)
13. **D** (See section 10.4)
14. **C** (See section 10.2)
15. **C** (See section 10.4)

The relevant section of the chapter to review for each question is given in parentheses after the correct answer. Detailed explanations can be found at the end of the chapter.

CHAPTER 10

ACIDS AND BASES

In This Chapter

CHAPTER PROFILE

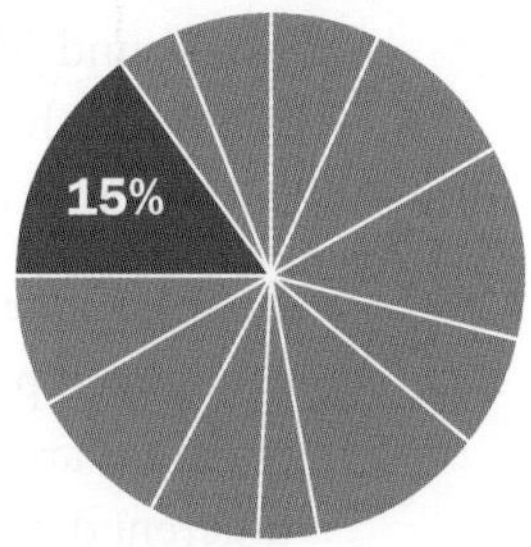

The content in this chapter should be relevant to about 15% of all questions about general chemistry on the MCAT.

This chapter covers material from the following AAMC content categories:

4D: How light and sound interact with matter

5A: Unique nature of water and its solutions

Introduction

Some medications can be applied as drops, salves, or creams to mucous membranes. Others are injected. Some employ a transdermal patch, while others are swallowed or inhaled. The route of administration of a drug compound is related to both the location of its target tissue (local or systemic), as well as the chemical and physical properties of the compound. For example, compounds that are water-soluble can be administered intravenously (an aqueous solution dripped directly into the bloodstream), while those that are lipid-soluble can be administered transcutaneously (via a patch or a cream) or orally (in a pill or liquid suspension). The polarity, size, and charge of the drug compound will determine its solubility in polar or nonpolar environments and will be major contributing factors in determining the most effective and efficient route of administration.

Whether a drug compound has an ionic charge is usually a function of the acidic or basic nature of the compound. For example, a basic organic compound that is insoluble in water when neutral can be reacted with an acid to form a salt; because this salt is ionic, it is water-soluble. Correspondingly, an acidic organic compound that is insoluble in water when neutral can be reacted with a base to form a water-soluble salt. On the other hand, the protonated (acidic cationic) form of an organic compound can be reacted with a base to neutralize the compound and release it from its salt, changing (and usually reversing) its solubility in water.

Medical professionals aren't the only ones concerned about drug solubilities and routes of administration—there's a science to illicit drugs, too. One of the clearest examples of this is the difference between the two major forms of cocaine, a large alkaloid compound derived from the coca plant. Most commonly, the alkaloid compound is reacted with hydrochloric acid (which protonates its tertiary amine functional group), extracted with water, and dried to a water-soluble powder (cocaine hydrochloride); this powder either is snorted (insufflated) into the nasal cavity, where it is absorbed into the capillary beds, or is injected directly into the venous circulation. The second form of cocaine, the salt form, has a very high boiling point, which is close to the temperature at which cocaine degrades, and cannot be smoked. To produce a vaporizable form of cocaine that can be inhaled from a pipe, the cocaine hydrochloride must be reacted with a base, typically either ammonia (to produce pure freebase cocaine) or sodium bicarbonate (to produce crack cocaine, which is less pure). The base reacts with the protonated tertiary amine, removing the hydrogen ion to reform the neutral alkaloid compound. The freebase cocaine is water-insoluble and usually extracted with ether, or it is left in the aqueous solution, which is heated and evaporated. The freebase and crack forms of cocaine have much lower boiling points; consequently, they can be smoked without risk of degradation.

In this chapter, our focus will be on those two classes of compounds—acids and bases—which are involved in so many important reactions. Acid–base reactions are an important topic for the MCAT; in fact, neutralization reactions are some of the most commonly tested reaction types on Test Day. We will begin with a review of the different definitions of acids and bases and their properties, including their characterization as either strong or weak. Focusing on weak acids and bases, we will discuss the significance of the equilibrium constants K_a and K_b for acids and bases, respectively. Finally, we will review acid–base titrations and buffer systems.

10.1 Definitions

LEARNING OBJECTIVES

After Chapter 10.1, you will be able to:

- Compare and contrast the Arrhenius, Brønsted–Lowry, and Lewis definitions for acids and bases
- Predict the acid formula and name for an anion using Arrhenius acid naming trends
- Identify amphoteric species, and determine whether they are amphiprotic as well

Over the last century, chemists have used different definitions to identify compounds as acids or bases. Three definitions emerged, with each more inclusive than the former one.

Arrhenius

The first and most specific definition of an acid or base is the Arrhenius definition, depicted in Figure 10.1. An **Arrhenius acid** will dissociate to form an excess of H^+ in solution, and an **Arrhenius base** will dissociate to form an excess of OH^- in solution. These behaviors are generally limited to aqueous acids and bases. Arrhenius acids and bases are easily identified; acids contain H at the beginning of their formula (HCl, HNO_3, H_2SO_4, and so on) and bases contain OH at the end of their formula (NaOH, $Ca(OH)_2$, $Fe(OH)_3$, and so on).

$$HA \longrightarrow H^+ + A^- \qquad\qquad BOH \longrightarrow B^+ + OH^-$$

Arrhenius acid — Arrhenius base

Figure 10.1 Arrhenius Acid and Base

MCAT EXPERTISE

Any mention of the Arrhenius definition on Test Day will likely be in comparison to other definitions of acids. The Arrhenius definition is by far the most restrictive; the Brønsted–Lowry and Lewis definitions predominate on the MCAT.

Brønsted–Lowry

A more inclusive definition of acids and bases was proposed independently by Johannes Brønsted and Thomas Lowry in 1923 (see Figure 10.2). A **Brønsted–Lowry acid** is a species that donates hydrogen ions (H^+), while a **Brønsted–Lowry base** is a species that accepts them.

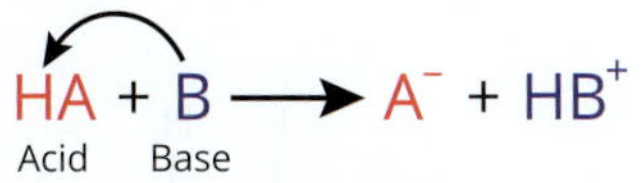

Figure 10.2 Brønsted–Lowry Acid and Base

The advantage of this definition over Arrhenius's is that it is not limited to aqueous solutions. For example, OH^-, NH_3, and F^- are all Brønsted–Lowry bases because each has the ability to accept a hydrogen ion. However, neither NH_3 nor F^- can be classified as Arrhenius bases because they do not dissociate to produce an excess of OH^- ions in aqueous solutions. According to both of these definitions, there is only one way for a species to be an acid: producing hydrogen ions. The only differences between the two definitions for acids are the requirement of an aqueous medium in the Arrhenius definition and the acidity of water. In the Arrhenius definition, water is not considered an acid—it does not produce an excess of H^+ in solution. Water is, on the other hand, a Brønsted–Lowry acid because it is able to donate a proton to other species. Most acid–base chemistry reactions on the MCAT will involve the transfer of hydrogen ions in accordance with the Brønsted–Lowry definitions.

MCAT EXPERTISE

Every Arrhenius acid (or base) can also be classified as a Brønsted–Lowry acid (or base). Every Brønsted–Lowry acid (or base) can also be classified as a Lewis acid (or base). This logic does not always work the other way (for example, NH_3 is a Brønsted–Lowry base, but not an Arrhenius base).

Brønsted–Lowry acids and bases always occur in pairs because the definitions require the transfer of a proton from the acid to the base. These are **conjugate acid–base pairs**, as described in the next section. For example, in the autoionization of water, H_3O^+ is the conjugate acid and OH^- is the conjugate base, as shown in Figure 10.3.

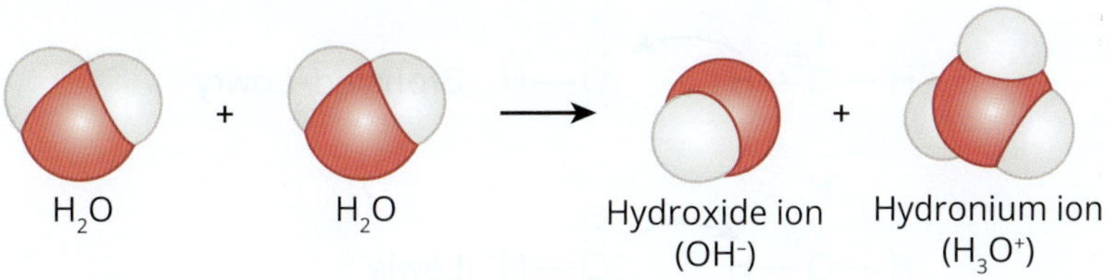

Figure 10.3 Autoionization of Water into Its Conjugate Acid and Conjugate Base
The hydroxide ion is the conjugate base; the oxonium (hydronium) ion is the conjugate acid.
$H_2O\ (l) + H_2O\ (l) \rightleftharpoons H_3O^+\ (aq) + OH^-\ (aq)$

Lewis

At approximately the same time as Brønsted and Lowry's publications, Gilbert Lewis also proposed a definition for acids and bases. A **Lewis acid** is defined as an electron pair acceptor, and a **Lewis base** is defined as an electron pair donor, as shown in Figure 10.4. The electron pair being donated is a lone pair and is not involved in any other bonds.

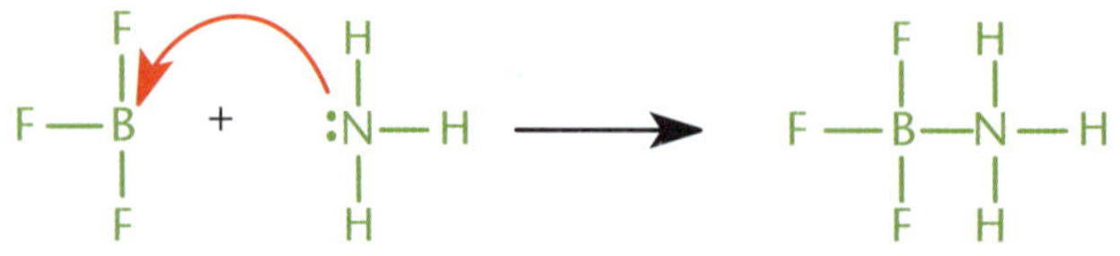

Figure 10.4 Lewis Acid–Base Chemistry
Boron trifluoride serves as the Lewis acid, accepting a lone pair. Ammonia serves as a Lewis base, donating a lone pair.

MNEMONIC

The Br**ø**nsted-L**o**wry definition revolves around pr**o**t**o**ns; the **L**ewis definition around **e**lectrons.

On the MCAT, Lewis acid–base chemistry appears with many names. The underlying idea is that one species pushes a lone pair to form a bond with another. This same chemistry can be called coordinate covalent bond formation (discussed in Chapter 3 of *MCAT General Chemistry Review*), complex ion formation (discussed in Chapter 9 of *MCAT General Chemistry Review*), or nucleophile–electrophile interactions (discussed in Chapter 4 of *MCAT Organic Chemistry Review*).

There is an intuitive approach to understanding the differences in the definitions we have discussed so far. The Lewis definition relies on a behavior that is not vastly different from the Brønsted–Lowry interactions—the only difference is the focus. For Brønsted–Lowry acids and bases, we follow the exchange of the hydrogen ion (H^+), which is essentially a naked proton. In the Lewis definition, the focus of the reaction is no longer on the proton, but instead the electrons forming the coordinate covalent bond. This difference can be seen using curved arrows, as shown in Figure 10.5.

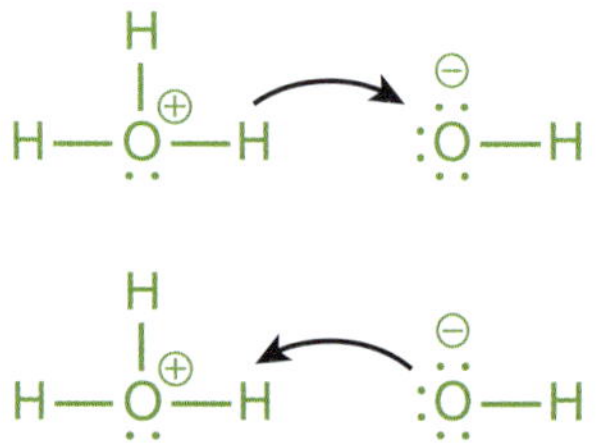

Figure 10.5 Brønsted–Lowry vs. Lewis
In the Brønsted–Lowry definition, the focus is on the transfer of the proton. In the Lewis definition, the focus is on the attack of the Lewis acid (electrophile) by the lone pair of the Lewis base (nucleophile).

Note that the Lewis definition is the most inclusive: every Arrhenius acid is also a Brønsted–Lowry acid, and every Brønsted–Lowry acid is also a Lewis acid (and likewise for bases). However, the converse is not necessarily true. The Lewis definition encompasses some species not included within the Brønsted–Lowry definition; for example, BF_3 and $AlCl_3$ are species that can each accept an electron pair, which qualifies them as Lewis acids, but they lack a hydrogen ion to donate, disqualifying them as both Arrhenius and Brønsted–Lowry acids. It may seem confusing having to memorize the various types and definitions of acids and bases, but they all share similarities. Figure 10.6 helps to visualize the commonalities between the definitions and how they fit with each other.

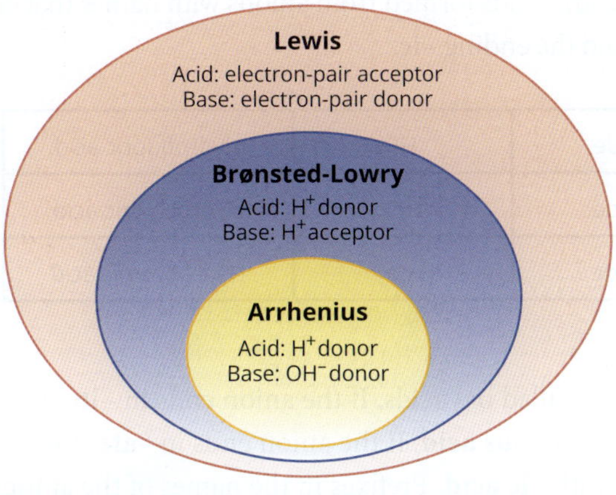

Figure 10.6 Comparison of Acid/Base Definitions

On the MCAT, you may encounter Lewis acids in the context of organic chemistry reactions because Lewis acids are often used as catalysts.

Amphoteric Species

An **amphoteric** species is one that reacts like an acid in a basic environment and like a base in an acidic environment. In the Brønsted–Lowry sense, an amphoteric species can either gain or lose a proton, making it **amphiprotic** as well. On the MCAT, water is the most common example. When water reacts with a base, it behaves as an acid:

$$H_2O + B^- \rightleftharpoons HB + OH^-$$

When water reacts with an acid, it behaves as a base:

$$HA + H_2O \rightleftharpoons H_3O^+ + A^-$$

The partially dissociated conjugate base of a polyvalent acid is usually amphoteric. For example, HSO_4^- can either gain a proton to form H_2SO_4 or lose a proton to form SO_4^{2-}. The hydroxides of certain metals (such as Al, Zn, Pb, and Cr) are also amphoteric. Furthermore, species that can act as both oxidizing and reducing agents are often considered to be amphoteric as well because by accepting or donating electron pairs, they act as Lewis acids or bases, respectively.

KEY CONCEPT

Water, amino acids, and partially deprotonated polyprotic acids such as bicarbonate and bisulfate are common examples of amphoteric and amphiprotic substances. Metal oxides and hydroxides are also considered amphoteric but not necessarily amphiprotic because they do not give off protons.

Complex amphoteric molecules include amino acids that have a *zwitterion* intermediate with both cationic and anionic character, as shown in Figure 10.7. Such species are discussed in great detail in Chapter 1 of *MCAT Biochemistry Review*.

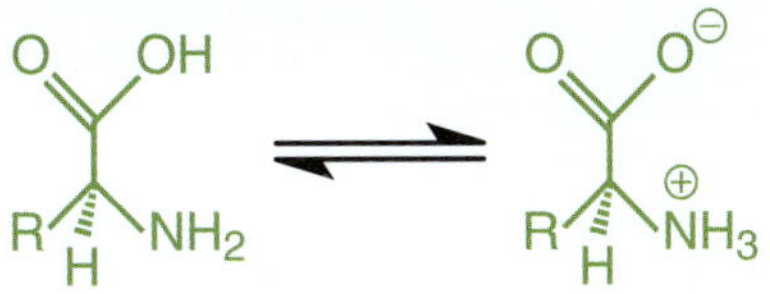

Figure 10.7 Amino Acid Zwitterions Are Complex Amphoteric Species
The amino group can release a proton (acid) and the carboxylate group can accept a proton (base).

Acid–Base Nomenclature

The names of most acids are related to the names of their parent anions (the anion that combines with H^+ to form the acid). Acids formed from anions with names that end in –**ide** have the prefix **hydro**– and the ending –**ic**.

F^-	Fluoride	HF	Hydrofluoric acid
Cl^-	Chloride	HCl	Hydrochloric acid
Br^-	Bromide	HBr	Hydrobromic acid

Acids formed from oxyanions are called oxyacids. If the anion ends in –**ite** (less oxygen), then the acid will end with –**ous acid**. If the anion ends in –**ate** (more oxygen), then the acid will end with –**ic acid**. Prefixes in the names of the anions are retained. Some common examples include the following:

ClO^-	Hypochlorite	HClO	Hypochlorous acid
ClO_2^-	Chlorite	$HClO_2$	Chlorous acid
ClO_3^-	Chlorate	$HClO_3$	Chloric acid
ClO_4^-	Perchlorate	$HClO_4$	Perchloric acid
NO_2^-	Nitrite	HNO_2	Nitrous acid
NO_3^-	Nitrate	HNO_3	Nitric acid
CO_3^{2-}	Carbonate	H_2CO_3	Carbonic acid
SO_4^{2-}	Sulfate	H_2SO_4	Sulfuric acid
PO_4^{3-}	Phosphate	H_3PO_4	Phosphoric acid
BO_3^{3-}	Borate	H_3BO_3	Boric acid
CrO_4^{2-}	Chromate	H_2CrO_4	Chromic acid
CH_3COO^-	Acetate	CH_3COOH	Acetic acid
$HCOO^-$	Formate	HCOOH	Formic Acid
H_2NCOO^-	Carbamate	H_2NCOOH	Carbamic Acid

MCAT EXPERTISE

There are some exceptions to the nomenclature rules. For instance, MnO_4^- is called permanganate even though there are no MnO_3^- or MnO_2^- ions.

MCAT CONCEPT CHECK 10.1

Before you move on, assess your understanding of the material with these questions.

1. Compare and contrast the three definitions for acids and bases:

Definition	Acid	Base
Arrhenius		
Brønsted–Lowry		
Lewis		

2. Utilizing Arrhenius acid naming trends, predict the acid formula and name for the following anions:

Anion	Acid Formula	Acid Name
MnO_4^-		
Titanate (TiO_3^{2-})		
I^-		
IO_4^-		

3. Identify which reactants are amphoteric species in the following reactions. For those species, determine if the compound is also amphiprotic.

Reaction	Amphoteric Reactant	Amphiprotic? (Y or N)
$HCO_3^- + HBr \rightleftharpoons H_2CO_3 + Br^-$		
$3\ HCl + Al(OH)_3 \rightleftharpoons AlCl_3 + 3\ H_2O$		
$2\ HBr + ZnO \rightleftharpoons ZnBr_2 + H_2O$		

10.2 Properties High Yield

LEARNING OBJECTIVES

After Chapter 10.2, you will be able to:

- Predict the behavior of an acid or base in water given its K_a or K_b value, respectively
- Apply the mathematical relationships between pH, pOH, and ion concentration
- Recall the mathematical relationship between K_a, K_b, and K_w
- Determine concentration of hydrogen ions given molarity and K_a or K_b of a solution
- Identify acids, bases, conjugate acids, and conjugate bases in a reaction: $H_2O\ (l) + H_2O\ (l) \rightleftharpoons H_3O^+\ (aq) + OH^-\ (aq)$

Acids and bases are usually characterized according to their relative tendencies to either donate or accept hydrogen ions. Furthermore, aqueous acid and base solutions can be characterized according to their concentrations of hydrogen and hydroxide ions.

Autoionization of Water and Hydrogen Ion Equilibria

Because many acid–base reactions take place in water—especially on the MCAT—it is very important to understand the behavior of acidic and basic compounds in water. Only then can one fully appreciate the meaning and significance of such terms as *strong acid*, *weak base*, or measurements of pH and pOH.

The Acid–Base Behavior of Water

As described above, water is an **amphoteric** species: in the presence of a base it reacts as an acid, and in the presence of an acid, it reacts as a base. As an amphoteric compound, water can react with itself in a process called **autoionization**, seen previously in Figure 10.3. The autoionization of water is represented by the equation:

$$H_2O\ (l) + H_2O\ (l) \rightleftharpoons H_3O^+\ (aq) + OH^-\ (aq)$$

One water molecule donates a hydrogen ion to another water molecule to produce the **hydronium ion** (H_3O^+) and the **hydroxide ion** (OH^-). Many general chemistry courses depict the hydrogen ion simply as H^+, rather than as H_3O^+.

This is acceptable for representing the chemistry, but it is important to remember that the proton is never isolated in the solution; it is always attached to water or some other species that has the ability to accept it. Autoionization of water is a reversible reaction; therefore, the expression above is in equilibrium. For pure water at 298 K, the **water dissociation constant, K_w**, has been experimentally determined:

$$K_w = [H_3O^+][OH^-] = 10^{-14} \text{ at } 25^\circ\text{C (298 K)}$$

Equation 10.1

Each mole of water that autoionizes produces one mole each of hydrogen (or hydronium) ions and hydroxide ions, so the concentrations of the hydrogen ions and hydroxide ions are always equal in pure water at equilibrium. Thus, the concentration of each of the ions in pure water at equilibrium at 298 K is 10^{-7} M.

However, the concentrations of the two ions will not always be equal. In fact, they will only be equal when the solution is neutral. Nevertheless, the product of their respective concentrations will always equal 10^{-14} when the temperature of the solution is 298 K. For example, if a species donates hydrogen ions to pure water, the hydrogen ion concentration will increase, causing the system to shift toward the reactants in the autoionization process. The result is a decrease in the hydroxide ion concentration and a return to the equilibrium state. This is Le Châtelier's principle in action: the addition of product to a system at equilibrium causes the system to shift away from the products and toward the reactants. The shift away from the products necessarily decreases the hydroxide ion concentration such that the product of the concentrations of the dissolved ions equals K_w. The addition of a species that accepts hydrogen ions results in a decrease in the hydrogen ion concentration and causes the system to shift toward the products, thereby replacing hydrogen ions. This shift necessarily increases the hydroxide ion concentration and returns the system to equilibrium.

Before we introduce the scales used in measuring concentrations of hydrogen ions and hydroxide ions in different acid–base solutions, it is worthwhile to emphasize an important thermodynamic principle regarding the water dissociation constant (K_w) expression. K_w is an equilibrium constant; unless the temperature of the water is changed, the value for K_w cannot be changed. Thus, the product of the concentrations of the hydrogen ions and the hydroxide ions in an aqueous solution at 298 K must always equal 10^{-14}. However, at different temperatures, the value for K_w changes. At temperatures above 298 K, K_w will increase; this is a direct result of the endothermic nature of the autoionization reaction.

MCAT EXPERTISE

The MCAT loves to test this concept: the value of K_w, like any other equilibrium constant, is dependent only on temperature. Therefore, isolated changes in concentration, pressure, or volume will not affect K_w.

pH and pOH Scales

The concentrations of hydrogen ions and hydroxide ions in aqueous solutions can vary significantly, making the range of measurements on a linear scale unmanageable. The concentration scales for acidic and basic solutions are condensed into something more manageable through expression in logarithmic terms. These logarithmic scales are the **pH** and the **pOH** scales for the concentrations of hydrogen and hydroxide ions, respectively.

Using a logarithmic scale is not only mathematically convenient, but also useful for calculations. For instance, the reactivity of an acidic solution is not a function of hydrogen ion concentration but instead of the *logarithm* of the hydrogen ion concentration. pH and pOH are prototypical examples of p scales. A **p scale** is defined as the negative logarithm of the number of items.

BRIDGE

Logarithmic scales are used to condense very large absolute differences into small scale differences. Remember that sound level (dB) also uses a logarithmic scale, as discussed in Chapter 7 of *MCAT Physics and Math Review*.

The pH and pOH of a solution are given by:

$$\mathrm{pH} = -\log\,[\mathrm{H^+}] = \log \frac{1}{[\mathrm{H^+}]}$$
$$\mathrm{pOH} = -\log\,[\mathrm{OH^-}] = \log \frac{1}{[\mathrm{OH^-}]}$$

Equation 10.2

For pure water at equilibrium and 298 K, the concentration of hydrogen ions equals the concentration of hydroxide ions (10^{-7} M). Therefore, pure water at 298 K has a pH of 7 and a pOH of 7 ($-\log 10^{-7} = 7$). If we take the negative logarithm of the entire water dissociation constant expression ($[H_3O^+][OH^-] = 10^{-14}$), we find:

$$\mathrm{pH} + \mathrm{pOH} = 14$$

Equation 10.3

Equation 10.3 holds true for all aqueous solutions at 298 K. As pH increases, pOH decreases by the same amount. This relationship can be seen in Figure 10.8 below.

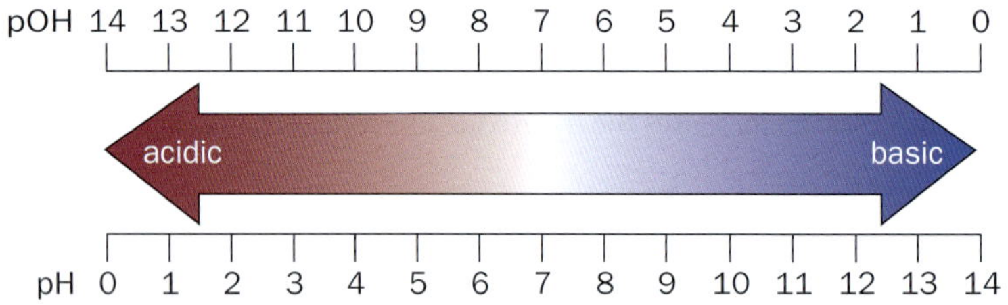

Figure 10.8 pH and pOH Scales
pH + pOH = 14 for aqueous solutions at 298 K.

For an aqueous solution at 298 K, a pH less than 7 (or pOH greater than 7) indicates a relative excess of hydrogen ions, and the solution is acidic; a pH greater than 7 (or pOH less than 7) indicates a relative excess of hydroxide ions, and the solution is basic. A pH (and pOH) equal to 7 indicates equal concentrations of hydrogen and hydroxide ions, resulting in a neutral solution.

MCAT EXPERTISE

The K_w (like all equilibrium constants) will change if the temperature changes and, in turn, will change the significance of the pH scale. Be careful and read the system conditions given on the MCAT: pH = 7 = neutral is only valid at 25°C.

Estimating Scale Values

An essential skill to hone for Test Day is the ability to quickly convert pH, pOH, pK_a, and pK_b values into nonlogarithmic form and vice-versa.

When the original value is a power of ten, the operation is relatively straightforward: changing the sign on the exponent gives the corresponding p scale value directly. For example, if $[H^+] = 0.001$ or 10^{-3}, then the pH = 3 and pOH = 11. Or, if $K_b = 1.0 \times 10^{-12}$, then $pK_b = 12$.

More difficulty arises when the value is not an exact power of ten. Rest assured that the MCAT is not a math test and is not interested in determining your ability to perform complex logarithmic calculations; an exact logarithmic calculation of a number that is not an integer power of ten is unnecessary on the MCAT. The testmakers are interested, however, in testing the ability to apply mathematical concepts appropriately in solving certain problems.

One can obtain a relatively close approximation of a p scale value using the following shortcut: if the nonlogarithmic value is written in proper scientific notation, it will be in the form $n \times 10^{-m}$, where n is a number between 1 and 10. Taking the negative logarithm and simplifying, the p value will be:

$$-\log(n \times 10^{-m}) = -\log(n) - \log(10^{-m})$$
$$= m - \log(n)$$

BRIDGE

In general, math using logarithms frequently appears on the MCAT; make sure to review how these mathematical concepts work in Chapter 10 of *MCAT Physics and Math Review*. Specifically, the equation pH + pOH = 14 comes from the fact that the log of a product is equal to the sum of logs; that is, $\log(xy) = \log x + \log y$.

Because n is a number between 1 and 10, its logarithm will be a decimal between 0 and 1 (log 1 = 0 and log 10 = 1). The closer n is to 1, the closer log n will be to 0; the closer n is to 10, the closer log n will be to 1. As a reasonable approximation, one can say that:

$$\text{p value} \approx m - 0.n$$

Equation 10.4

where $0.n$ represents sliding the decimal point of n one position to the left (dividing n by ten).

Example: If the K_a of an acid is 1.8×10^{-5}, then what is its pK_a?

Solution: $pK_a = -\log(1.8 \times 10^{-5}) = 5 - \log 1.8 \approx 5 - 0.18$

$= 4.82$ (actual $= 4.74$)

MCAT EXPERTISE

Learning how to estimate when using logarithms is an important skill that can save a lot of time on Test Day.

Strong Acids and Bases

Strong acids and bases completely dissociate into their component ions in aqueous solutions. For example, when sodium hydroxide is added to water, the ionic compound dissociates according to the net ionic equation:

$$NaOH\ (s) \rightarrow Na^+\ (aq) + OH^-\ (aq)$$

Hence, in a 1 M NaOH solution, complete dissociation yields 1 M Na^+ and 1 M OH^-. The pH and pOH for this solution can be calculated as follows:

$$pH = 14 - pOH = 14 - (-\log[OH^-]) = 14 + \log(1\ M) = 14 + 0 = 14$$

Virtually no undissociated strong acid or base, such as NaOH, will remain in solution. This is why the dissociation of strong acids and bases is said to go to completion. In the NaOH example above, we assume that the concentration of OH^- from the autoionization of water is negligible due to addition of a strong base. The contribution of OH^- and H^+ ions from the autoionization of water is negligible if the concentration of the acid or base is significantly greater than 10^{-7} M. On the other hand, if the concentration of acid or base is close to 10^{-7} M, then the contribution from the autoionization of water is important.

MCAT EXPERTISE

Acid–base reactions that consist of a single-headed arrow generally indicate strong acids or bases (complete dissociation with no reversibility).

Example: Calculate the pH of a 1×10^{-8} M solution of HCl.

Solution: At first, one may calculate the pH as $-\log[H^+] = -\log 10^{-8}\ M = 8$. However, this answer is not feasible: a pH of 8 cannot describe an acidic solution at 298 K because the presence of the acid will increase the hydrogen ion concentration to above 10^{-7} M, resulting in an acidic pH below 7.

Recognize that the acid concentration in this question is actually ten times less than the equilibrium concentration of hydrogen ions in pure water generated by the autoionization of water. Consequently, the hydrogen ion concentration from the water itself is significant and cannot be ignored. This can be represented in the equilibrium expression in which x represents the concentration of H_3O^+ and OH^- resulting from the autoionization of water:

$$K_w = [H_3O^+][OH^-] = [x + 10^{-8}][x] = 10^{-14}$$

Solving for x (which would require a quadratic equation—math that is beyond the scope of the MCAT) gives $x = 9.5 \times 10^{-8}$ M. The total concentration of hydrogen ions is $[H^+]_{total} = (9.5 \times 10^{-8}) + (1.0 \times 10^{-8}) = 1.05 \times 10^{-7}$ M. Notice that this is extremely close to the concentration of H^+ in pure water. The pH of this acidic solution can now be calculated as $pH = -\log(1.05 \times 10^{-7}) \approx 7$ (actual = 6.98). This pH is slightly lower than 7, as expected for a very dilute acidic solution. The point of all of this is: *stay alert and keep thinking critically, no matter how familiar the problem setups might seem to you!*

Strong acids commonly encountered on the MCAT include HCl (hydrochloric acid), HBr (hydrobromic acid), HI (hydroiodic acid), H_2SO_4 (sulfuric acid), HNO_3 (nitric acid), and $HClO_4$ (perchloric acid). Strong bases commonly encountered include NaOH (sodium hydroxide), KOH (potassium hydroxide), and other soluble hydroxides of Group IA metals. Calculation of the pH and pOH of strong acids and bases assumes complete dissociation of the acid or base in solution.

Example: What is the pH of a solution with $[HClO_4] = 10$ M?

Solution: Because perchloric acid is a strong acid, it will fully dissociate in solution. Therefore, $[H^+] = 10$ M (note that the contribution from the autoionization of water is negligible). $pH = -\log [H^+] = -\log 10 \text{ M} = -1$.

This question points out that the pH scale does not "end" at 0 and 14. There can be negative pH values and pH values greater than 14—but this implies a very high concentration of a strong acid or base.

Weak Acids and Bases

Before going any further in our discussion of acids and bases as *strong* or *weak*, verify that you are making the distinction between the chemical behavior of an acid or base with respect to its tendency to dissociate (that is, strong bases completely dissociate in aqueous solutions) and the concentrations of acid and base solutions. Although we may casually describe a solution's concentration as *strong* or *weak*, it is preferable to use the terms *concentrated* and *dilute*, respectively, because they are unambiguously associated with concentrations, rather than chemical behavior.

Continuing our focus on the chemical behavior of acids and bases, we will now consider those acids and bases that only partially dissociate in aqueous solutions. These are called **weak acids and bases**. A weak monoprotic acid, HA, will dissociate partially in water to achieve an equilibrium state:

$$HA\ (aq) + H_2O\ (l) \rightleftharpoons H_3O^+\ (aq) + A^-\ (aq)$$

Because the system exists in an equilibrium state, we can write the dissociation equation to determine the **acid dissociation constant** (K_a) as:

$$K_a = \frac{[H_3O^+][A^-]}{[HA]}$$

Equation 10.5

The smaller the K_a, the weaker the acid, and consequently, the less it will dissociate. Note that water, as a pure liquid, is not incorporated into the equilibrium expression.

A weak monovalent Arrhenius base, BOH, undergoes dissociation to yield B^+ and OH^- in solution:

$$BOH\ (aq) \rightleftharpoons B^+\ (aq) + OH^-\ (aq)$$

The **base dissociation constant** (K_b) can be calculated as:

$$K_b = \frac{[B^+][OH^-]}{[BOH]}$$

Equation 10.6

The smaller the K_b, the weaker the base, and consequently, the less it will dissociate. As with the acid dissociation expression, water is not included because it is a pure liquid.

Generally speaking, we can characterize a species as a weak acid if its K_a is less than 1.0 and as a weak base if its K_b is less than 1.0. On the MCAT, molecular (nonionic) weak bases are almost exclusively amines.

Conjugate Acid–Base Pairs

Because the Brønsted–Lowry definition of an acid–base reaction is one in which a hydrogen ion (proton) is transferred from an acid to a base, the two always occur in pairs called conjugates. A **conjugate acid** is the acid formed when a base gains a proton, and a **conjugate base** is the base formed when an acid loses a proton. Consider the example in Figure 10.9.

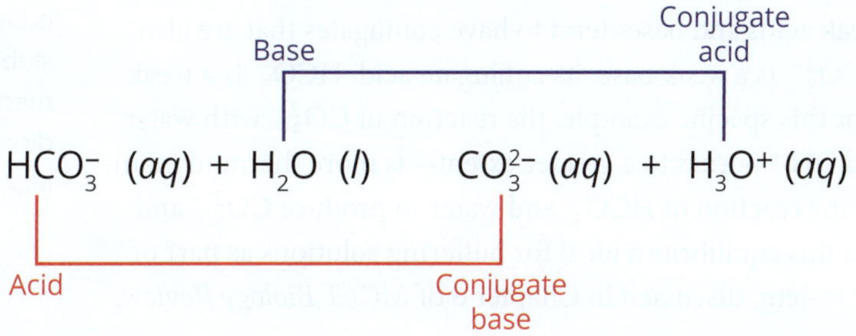

Figure 10.9 Conjugate Acid-Base Pair of Bicarbonate Ion (HCO_3^-)

CO_3^{2-} is the conjugate base of HCO_3^-, a weak acid, and H_3O^+ is the conjugate acid of H_2O, a weak base. To find the K_a, we consider the equilibrium concentrations of the dissolved species:

$$K_a = \frac{[CO_3^{2-}][H_3O^+]}{[HCO_3^-]}$$

The reaction between bicarbonate and water is reversible. The reverse reaction would be:

$$CO_3^{2-}\ (aq) + H_2O\ (l) \rightleftharpoons HCO_3^-\ (aq) + OH^-\ (aq)$$

We can write the K_b for CO_3^{2-} as:

$$K_b = \frac{[HCO_3^-][OH^-]}{[CO_3^{2-}]}$$

If one adds the previous two reversible reactions, the net reaction is simply the dissociation of water:

$$\begin{array}{l} \cancel{HCO_3^-} + H_2O \rightleftharpoons \cancel{CO_3^{2-}} + H_3O^+ \\ \underline{\cancel{CO_3^{2-}} + H_2O \rightleftharpoons \cancel{HCO_3^-} + OH^-} \\ 2\ H_2O \rightleftharpoons H_3O^+ + OH^- \end{array}$$

Because the net reaction is the autoionization of water, the equilibrium constant for the reaction is $K_w = [H_3O^+][OH^-] = 10^{-14}$, which is the product of K_a and K_b. Remember: the product of the concentrations of the hydrogen ion and the hydroxide ion must always equal 10^{-14} for acidic or basic aqueous solutions. Because water is an amphoteric species (both a weak acid and a weak base), all acid–base reactivity in water ultimately reduces to the acid–base behavior of water, and all acidic or basic aqueous solutions are governed by the dissociation constant for water. Thus, if the dissociation constant for one species or its conjugate is known, then the dissociation constant for the other can be determined using the following equations:

$$K_{a,\text{acid}} \times K_{b,\text{conjugate base}} = K_w = 10^{-14}$$

$$K_{b,\text{base}} \times K_{a,\text{conjugate acid}} = K_w = 10^{-14}$$

Equation 10.7

KEY CONCEPT

Be aware of the relationship between conjugate acids and bases because you will need to recognize these entities on the MCAT. Removing a proton from a molecule produces the conjugate base, and adding a proton produces the conjugate acid.

As is evident from these equations, K_a and K_b are inversely related. In other words, if K_a is large, then K_b is small, and vice-versa. By this logic, a strong acid (K_a approaching ∞) will produce a very weak conjugate base (for example, HCl is a strong acid and Cl^- is a very weak base), and a strong base will produce a very weak conjugate acid (for example, NaOH is a strong base and H_2O is a very weak acid). The conjugate of a strong acid or base is sometimes termed **inert** because it is almost completely unreactive.

On the other hand, weak acids and bases tend to have conjugates that are also weak. As seen above, CO_3^{2-} is a weak base; its conjugate acid, HCO_3^- is a weak acid. As it turns out, for this specific example, the reaction of CO_3^{2-} with water to produce HCO_3^- and OH^- occurs to a greater extent—is more thermodynamically favorable—than the reaction of HCO_3^- and water to produce CO_3^{2-} and H_3O^+. This fact makes this equilibrium ideal for buffering solutions as part of the bicarbonate buffer system, discussed in Chapter 6 of *MCAT Biology Review*.

BRIDGE

This thermodynamic preference for the bicarbonate ion intermediate is a major reason why the bicarbonate buffer system in the body is ideal for maintaining a stable pH. The homeostatic mechanisms involved are discussed in Chapter 6 of *MCAT Biology Review*.

One important theme for acid strength is the effect of induction. Electronegative elements positioned near an acidic proton increase acid strength by pulling electron density out of the bond holding the acidic proton. This weakens proton bonding and facilitates dissociation. Thus, acids that have electronegative elements nearer to acidic hydrogens are stronger than those that do not, as shown in Figure 10.10.

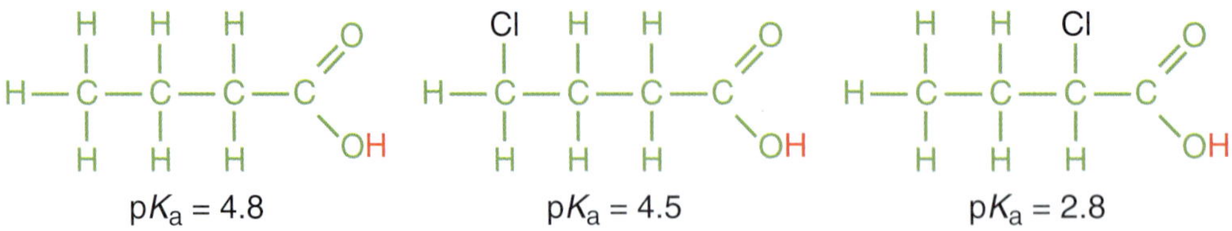

Figure 10.10 Inductive Effects from Electronegative Elements Increase Acidity

Applications of K_a and K_b

The most common use of acid and base dissociation constants is to determine the concentration of one of the species in solution at equilibrium. On Test Day, you may be asked to calculate the concentration of the hydrogen ion (or pH), the concentration of the hydroxide ion (or pOH), or the concentration of either the original acid or base.

Example: Calculate the concentration of H_3O^+ in a 2.0 M aqueous solution of acetic acid, CH_3COOH. (Note: $K_a = 1.8 \times 10^{-5}$)

Solution: First, write the equilibrium reaction:

$$CH_3COOH\ (aq) + H_2O\ (l) \rightleftharpoons H_3O^+\ (aq) + CH_3COO^-\ (aq)$$

Next, write the expression for the acid dissociation constant:

$$K_a = \frac{[H_3O^+][CH_3COO^-]}{[CH_3COOH]} = 1.8 \times 10^{-5}$$

Then, recognize that acetic acid is a weak acid, so the concentration of CH_3COOH at equilibrium is equal to its initial concentration, 2.0 M, minus the amount dissociated, *x*. Likewise, $[H_3O^+] = [CH_3COO^-] = x$ because each molecule of CH_3COOH dissociates into one H^+ ion and one CH_3COO^- ion. Note that the contribution of H_3O^+ from water is negligible. Thus, the equation can be rewritten as follows:

$$K_a = \frac{[X][X]}{[2.0\ M - x]} = 1.8 \times 10^{-5}$$

Remember that the value of *x* is generally very small. Therefore, we can approximate that $2.0\ M - x \approx 2.0\ M$. This is further supported because acetic acid is a weak acid and only slightly dissociates in water. This simplifies the calculations:

$$K_a = \frac{[X][X]}{2.0\ M} = 1.8 \times 10^{-5}$$

$$x^2 = 3.6 \times 10^{-5} = 36 \times 10^{-6}$$

$$x = 6 \times 10^{-3}\ M$$

x represents the concentration of H_3O^+; therefore, $[H_3O^+] = 6 \times 10^{-3}$ M. Note: When required to take the square root, adjust the coefficient as needed to make the power of 10 an even number. This way the square root only requires cutting the power of 10 in half.

In this example, note that *x* is significantly lower than the initial concentration of acetic acid (2.0 M), which validates the approximation; otherwise, it would have been necessary to solve for *x* using the quadratic formula. Fortunately, the value of *x* on Test Day is almost always sufficiently small to make this approximation. A rule of thumb is that the approximation is valid as long as *x* is less than 5 percent of the initial concentration. This typically occurs when K_a is at least 100 times smaller than the concentration of the starting solution. For example, if K_a is 10^{-4} and the concentration of the starting solution is 0.01 M (10^{-2} M), then the ratio between the values is 10^2 or 100. The error in this calculation should be no more than $\frac{1}{100} = 1\%$. On the other hand, if the K_a is 10^{-3} and the concentration is still 0.01 M, then the ratio between the values becomes 10, which could lead to $\frac{1}{10} = 10\%$ error. This degree of error may not be useful when identifying an answer choice on the MCAT.

Students often feel nervous making the assumption that x is negligible because they want to see precise answer choices. However, keep in mind that the MCAT quite deliberately tests students' ability to make reasonable assumptions under timed conditions to arrive at a feasible answer choice. Part of the skill of taking the MCAT is rounding appropriately to simplify math.

Salt Formation

Acids and bases may react with each other to form a salt and often (but not always) water, in what is termed a **neutralization reaction**. For example,

$$HA\ (aq) + BOH\ (aq) \rightarrow BA\ (s) + H_2O\ (l)$$

The salt may precipitate out or remain ionized in solution, depending on its solubility and the amount produced. In general, neutralization reactions go to completion. The reverse reaction, in which the salt ions react with water to give back the acid or base, is known as **hydrolysis**.

BRIDGE

Remember the reaction types discussed in Chapter 4 of *MCAT General Chemistry Review*? Go back and review the section on neutralization reactions if this equation doesn't look familiar to you.

Four combinations of strong and weak acids and bases are possible:

- Strong acid + strong base: $HCl + NaOH \rightarrow NaCl + H_2O$
- Strong acid + weak base: $HCl + NH_3 \rightarrow NH_4Cl$
- Weak acid + strong base: $HClO + NaOH \rightarrow NaClO + H_2O$
- Weak acid + weak base: $HClO + NH_3 \rightarrow NH_4ClO$

The products of a reaction between equal concentrations of a strong acid and a strong base are equimolar amounts of salt and water. The acid and base neutralize each other, so the resulting solution is neutral ($pH = 7$), and the ions formed in the reaction will not react with water because they are inert conjugates.

The product of a reaction between a strong acid and a weak base is also a salt, but often no water will be formed because weak bases are often not hydroxides. In this case, the cation of the salt is a weak acid and will react with the water solvent, re-forming some of the weak base through hydrolysis. For example:

- Reaction I: $HCl\ (aq) + NH_3\ (aq) \rightarrow NH_4^+\ (aq) + Cl^-\ (aq)$
- Reaction II: $NH_4^+\ (aq) + H_2O\ (l) \rightarrow NH_3\ (aq) + H_3O^+\ (aq)$

NH_4^+ is the conjugate acid of a weak base (NH_3) and is stronger than the conjugate base (Cl^-) of the strong acid, HCl. NH_4^+ will then transfer a proton to H_2O to form the hydronium ion. The increase in the concentration of the hydronium ion causes the system to shift away from autoionization, thereby reducing the concentration of hydroxide ion. Consequently, the concentration of the hydronium ion will be greater than that of the hydroxide ion at equilibrium, and as a result, the pH of the solution will fall below 7. This should make sense: a strong acid and a weak base produce a slightly acidic solution.

On the other hand, when a weak acid reacts with a strong base, the pH of the solution at equilibrium will be within the basic range because the salt hydrolyzes, with concurrent formation of hydroxide ions. The increase in hydroxide ion concentration will cause the system to shift away from autoionization, thereby reducing the concentration of the hydronium ion. Consequently, the concentration of the hydroxide ion will be greater than that of the hydronium ion at equilibrium, and as a result, the pH of the solution will rise above 7. Consider the reaction of acetic acid, CH_3COOH (weak acid) with sodium hydroxide, NaOH (strong base):

- Reaction I: $CH_3COOH\ (aq) + NaOH\ (aq) \rightarrow Na^+\ (aq) + CH_3COO^-\ (aq) + H_2O\ (l)$
- Reaction II: $CH_3COO^-\ (aq) + H_2O\ (l) \rightarrow CH_3COOH\ (aq) + OH^-\ (aq)$

The pH of a solution containing a weak acid and a weak base depends on the relative strengths of the reactants. For example, the weak acid HClO has a K_a of 3.2×10^{-8}, and the weak base NH_3 has a $K_b = 1.8 \times 10^{-5}$. Thus, an aqueous solution of HClO and NH_3 is basic because the K_a for HClO is less than the K_b for NH_3. That is, HClO is weaker as an acid than NH_3 is as a base. At equilibrium, therefore, the concentration of hydroxide ions will be greater than the concentration of hydronium ions in the aqueous solution.

In biology and biochemistry, neutralization reactions are often condensation reactions because they form bonds with a small molecule as a byproduct (usually water). The peptide bonds in proteins, for example, are created from the reaction of a carboxyl group (acid) and an amino group (base), while forming a water molecule, as shown in Figure 10.11. The salt in this reaction is the polypeptide itself; breaking it apart requires hydrolysis.

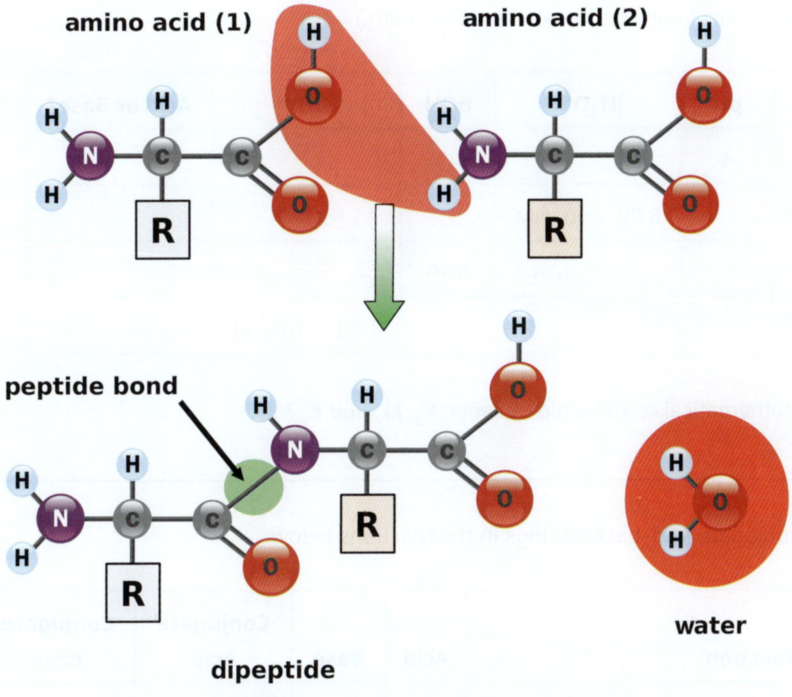

Figure 10.11 Peptide Bond Formation
An acidic carboxyl group reacts with a basic amino group.

MCAT CONCEPT CHECK 10.2

Before you move on, assess your understanding of the material with these questions.

1. What is an amphoteric species?

---

2. If a compound has a K_a value $\gg$ water, what does it mean about its behavior in solution? How does this compare with a solution that has only a slightly higher K_a than water?

---

3. If a compound has a K_b value $\gg$ water, what does it mean about its behavior in solution? How does this compare with a solution that has only a slightly higher K_b than water?

---

4. Complete the blank cells in the table by utilizing the mathematical relationships between pH, pOH, and ion concentrations. (Note: Round the numbers given and use logarithmic approximations to determine p values, without a calculator, to simulate Test Day math.)

pH	$[H_3O^+]$	pOH	$[OH^-]$	Acid or Base?
4				
	8.89×10^{-4} M			
		5.19		
			1.88×10^{-6} M	

5. What is the mathematical relationship between K_a, K_b, and K_w?

---

6. Identify the conjugate acid–base pairings in the reactions below:

Reaction	Acid	Base	Conjugate Acid	Conjugate Base
$H_2CO_3 + H_2O \rightleftharpoons HCO_3^- + H_3O^+$				
$H_2PO_4^- + H_2O \rightleftharpoons H_3PO_4 + OH^-$				

7. Determine the concentration of hydrogen ions and pH of a solution of 0.2 M acetic acid ($K_a = 1.8 \times 10^{-5}$).

10.3 Polyvalence and Normality

LEARNING OBJECTIVES

After Chapter 10.3, you will be able to:

- Describe how equivalents of acid or base are calculated
- Calculate the normality of a solution given its formula and molarity

The relative acidity or basicity of an aqueous solution is determined by the relative concentrations of acid and base equivalents. An **acid equivalent** is equal to one mole of H^+ (or, more properly, H_3O^+) ions; a **base equivalent** is equal to one mole of OH^- ions. Some acids and bases are **polyvalent**; that is, each mole of the acid or base liberates more than one acid or base equivalent. Under the Brønsted–Lowry definition, such acids or bases could also be termed **polyprotic**. For example, the divalent diprotic acid H_2SO_4 undergoes the following dissociation in water:

$$H_2SO_4\ (aq) + H_2O\ (l) \rightarrow H_3O^+\ (aq) + HSO_4^-\ (aq)$$
$$HSO_4^-\ (aq) + H_2O\ (l) \rightleftharpoons H_3O^+\ (aq) + SO_4^{2-}\ (aq)$$

One mole of H_2SO_4 produces two acid equivalents (2 moles of H_3O^+). Notice that the first dissociation goes to completion, but the second dissociation reaches an equilibrium state. The acidity or basicity of a solution depends on the concentration of acidic or basic equivalents that can be liberated. The quantity of acidic or basic capacity is directly indicated by the solution's **normality**, described in Chapter 9 of *MCAT General Chemistry Review*. For example, each mole of H_3PO_4 yields three moles (equivalents) of H_3O^+. Therefore, a 2 M H_3PO_4 solution would be 6 N.

Another measurement useful for acid–base chemistry is **gram equivalent weight**. Chapter 4 of *MCAT General Chemistry Review* defined and discussed this term extensively. The gram equivalent weight is the mass of a compound that produces one equivalent (one mole of charge). For example, H_2SO_4 (molar mass: 98 $\frac{\text{g}}{\text{mol}}$) is a divalent acid, so each mole of the acid compound yields two acid equivalents. The gram equivalent weight is $98 \div 2 = 49$ grams. That is, the complete dissociation of 49 grams of H_2SO_4 will yield one acid equivalent (one mole of H_3O^+). Common polyvalent acids include H_2SO_4, H_3PO_4, and H_2CO_3. Common polyvalent bases include $Al(OH)_3$, $Ca(OH)_2$, and $Mg(OH)_2$.

BRIDGE

To review normality in more detail, revisit the calculations performed in Chapter 4 of *MCAT General Chemistry Review*. These are critical calculations for polyvalent acids and bases.

MCAT CONCEPT CHECK 10.3

Before you move on, assess your understanding of the material with these questions.

1. What species are considered the equivalents for acids and bases, respectively?
   - Acids:

   - Bases:

   ---

2. Calculate the normality of the following solutions:
   - 2 M $Al(OH)_3$:

   - 16 M H_2SO_4:

10.4 Titration and Buffers High Yield

LEARNING OBJECTIVES

After Chapter 10.4, you will be able to:

- Select an appropriate indicator for a given acid–base reaction
- Explain the purpose of a buffer solution
- Identify the pH range of the equivalence point for different combinations of acids and bases, for example, weak acid + weak base
- Calculate the pH or pOH of a known solution
- Identify the buffering region, half-equivalence point, equivalence point, and endpoint of a titration reaction:

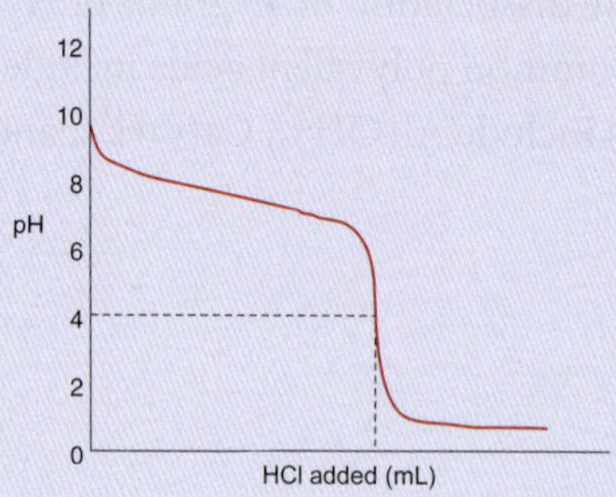

Titration is a procedure used to determine the concentration of a known reactant in a solution. There are different types of titrations, including acid–base, oxidation–reduction, and complexometric (metal ion). The MCAT frequently tests the first two types. Complexometric (metal ion) titrations are outside the scope of the MCAT but focus on formation of complex ions, as described in Chapter 9 of *MCAT General Chemistry Review*.

General Principles

Titrations are performed by adding small volumes of a solution of known concentration (the **titrant**) to a known volume of a solution of unknown concentration (the **titrand**), both represented in Figure 10.12, until completion of the reaction is achieved at the **equivalence point**.

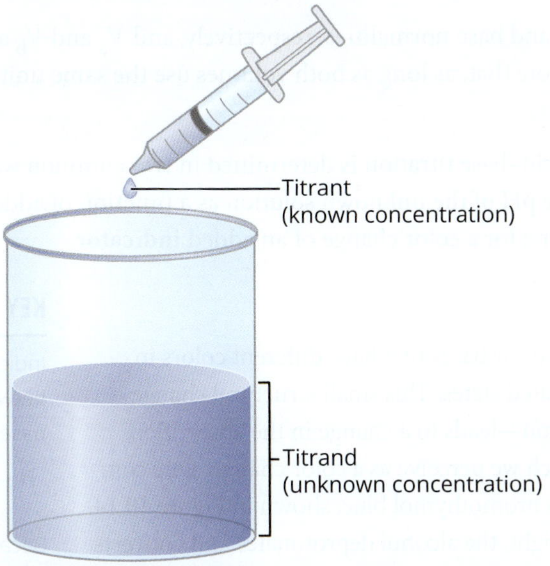

Figure 10.12 Titrant and Titrand in Acid-Base Titration

Acid–Base Equivalence Points

In acid–base titrations, the equivalence point is reached when the number of acid equivalents present in the original solution equals the number of base equivalents added, or vice-versa. It is important to emphasize that, while a strong acid/strong base titration will have its equivalence point at a pH of 7, the equivalence point does *not* always occur at pH 7. When titrating polyprotic acids or bases (discussed later in this chapter), there are multiple equivalence points, as each acidic or basic conjugate species is titrated separately. This is shown in the speciation plot in Figure 10.13.

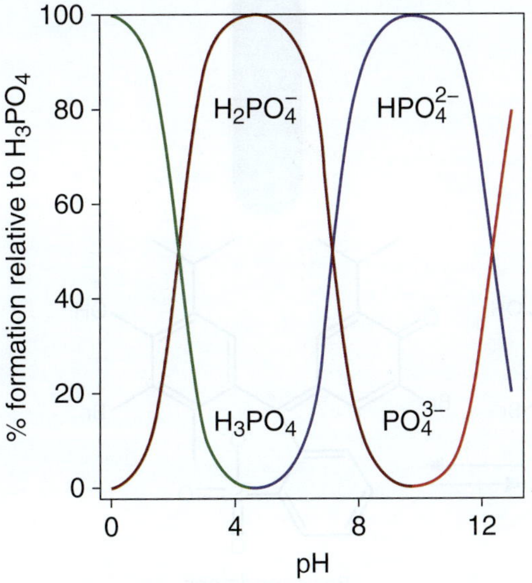

Figure 10.13 Speciation Plot of Phosphoric Acid
At any given pH, only two forms of the acid exist in solution; thus, each conjugate is titrated separately.

At the equivalence point, the number of equivalents of acid and base are equal. This fact allows us to calculate the unknown concentration of the titrand through the equation:

$$N_a V_a = N_b V_b$$

Equation 10.8

where N_a and N_b are the acid and base normalities, respectively, and V_a and V_b are the volumes of acid and base solutions, respectively. Note that, as long as both volumes use the same units, the units used do not have to be liters.

The equivalence point in an acid–base titration is determined in two common ways: evaluated by using a graphical method, plotting the pH of the unknown solution as a function of added titrant by using a **pH meter**, or estimated by watching for a color change of an added **indicator**.

Indicators

Indicators are weak organic acids or bases that have different colors in their protonated and deprotonated states. This small structural change—the binding or release of a proton—leads to a change in the absorption spectrum of the molecule, which we perceive as a color change. One common example of an indicator is bromothymol blue, shown in Figure 10.14. In basic conditions, as on the right, the alcohol deprotonates and converts into a ketone, and the resulting structure has more extensive conjugation, leading to the blue color. Indicators are generally vibrant and can be used in low concentrations without significantly altering the equivalence point.

KEY CONCEPT

Indicators change color as they shift between their conjugate acid and base forms:

$$\underset{\text{(color 1)}}{\text{H} - \text{Indicator}} \rightleftharpoons \text{H}^+ + \underset{\text{(color 2)}}{\text{Indicator}^-}$$

Because this is an equilibrium process, we can apply Le Châtelier's principle. Adding H^+ shifts the equilibrium to the left. Adding OH^- removes H^+ and therefore shifts the equilibrium to the right.

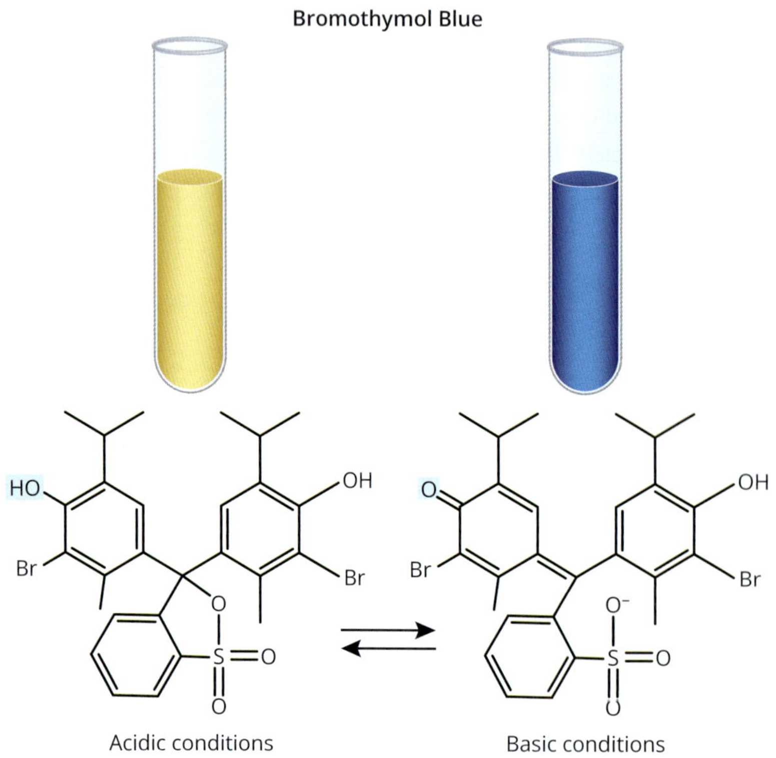

Figure 10.14 Color Change of an Indicator under Acidic/Basic Conditions

MCAT EXPERTISE

Any question involving the selection of an ideal indicator will require you to know what the pH of the reaction at the equivalence point will be, whether graphically or mathematically. Once you have determined where the equivalence point is, select the indicator that has the closest pK_a value to it.

The indicator must always be a weaker acid or base than the acid or base being titrated; otherwise, the indicator would be titrated first! The point at which the indicator changes to its final color is not the equivalence point but rather the **endpoint**. If the indicator is chosen correctly and the titration is performed well, the volume difference between the endpoint and the equivalence point is negligible and may be corrected for or simply ignored.

Acid–base titrations can be performed for different combinations of strong and weak acids and bases. The most useful combinations involve at least one strong species. Weak acid/weak base titrations can be done but are not very accurate and therefore are rarely performed. The pH curve for the titration of a weak acid and weak base lacks the sharp change that normally indicates the equivalence point. Furthermore, indicators are less useful because the pH change is far more gradual.

Strong Acid and Strong Base

Let's consider the titration of 10 mL of a 0.1 N solution of HCl with a 0.1 N solution of NaOH. Plotting the pH of the solution vs. the quantity of NaOH added gives the curve shown in Figure 10.15.

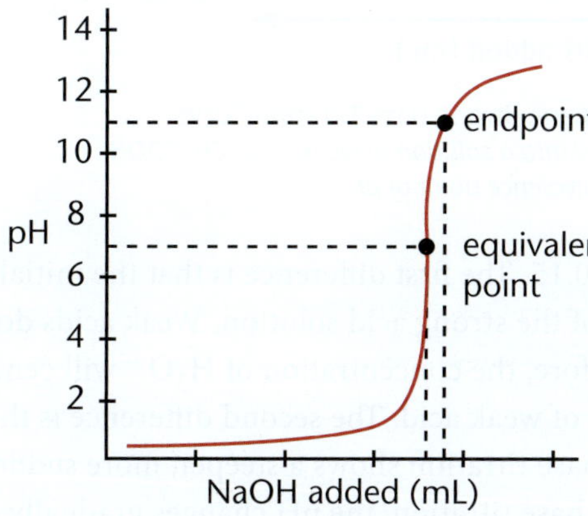

Figure 10.15 Monoprotic Strong Acid and Strong Base Titration Curve
A strong base, NaOH, is titrated into a solution of strong acid, HCl, to yield an equivalence point of pH = 7.

KEY CONCEPT

Compare the relative strength of the two solutions in a titration to determine if the pH of the equivalence point is less than, equal to, or greater than 7:

- Strong acid + weak base: equivalence point pH < 7
- Strong acid + strong base: equivalence point pH $= 7$
- Weak acid + strong base: equivalence point pH > 7

Because HCl is a strong acid and NaOH is a strong base, the equivalence point of the titration will be at pH 7, and the solution will be neutral. Note that the endpoint shown is close to, but not exactly equal to, the equivalence point; selection of a better indicator, one that changes colors at, say, pH 8, would have given a better approximation. Still, the amount of error introduced by the use of an indicator that changes color around pH 11 rather than pH 8 is not especially significant; it represents a mere fraction of a milliliter of excess NaOH solution.

In the early part of the curve when little base has been added, the acidic species predominates, so the addition of small amounts of base will not appreciably change either the $[OH^-]$ or the pH. Similarly, in the last part of the titration curve when an excess of base has been added, the addition of small amounts of base will not change the $[OH^-]$ significantly, and the pH will remain relatively constant. The addition of base will alter the concentrations of H^+ and OH^- near the equivalence point, and will elicit the most substantial changes in pH in that region. Remember: the equivalence point for strong acid/strong base titrations is always at pH 7 (for monovalent species).

If one uses a pH meter to chart the change in pH as a function of volume of titrant added, a good approximation can be made of the equivalence point by locating the midpoint of the region of the curve with the steepest slope.

Weak Acid and Strong Base

Titration of a weak acid, such as CH_3COOH, with a strong base, such as NaOH, produces the titration curve shown in Figure 10.16.

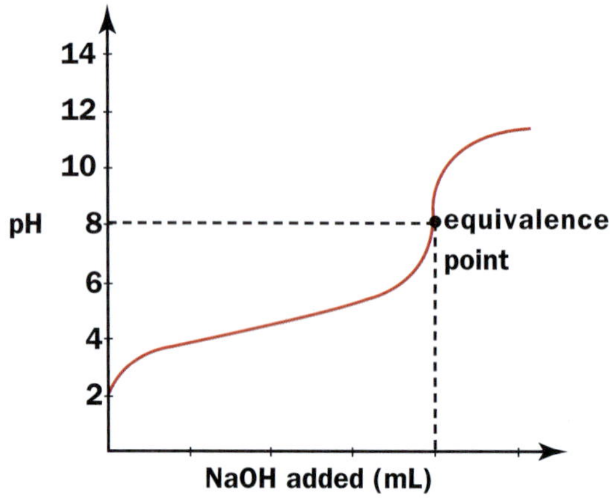

Figure 10.16 Weak Acid and Strong Base Titration Curve
A strong base, NaOH, is titrated into a solution of weak acid, CH_3COOH, to yield an equivalence point of pH > 7.

Compare Figure 10.16 with the curve in Figure 10.15. The first difference is that the initial pH of the weak acid solution is greater than the initial pH of the strong acid solution. Weak acids do not dissociate to the same degree that strong acids do; therefore, the concentration of H_3O^+ will generally be lower (and pH will be higher) in an equimolar solution of weak acid. The second difference is the shapes of the curves. The pH curve for the strong acid/strong base titration shows a steeper, more sudden rise in pH at the equivalence point. In the weak acid/strong base titration, the pH changes gradually early on in the titration and has a less sudden rise at the equivalence point. The third difference is the position of the equivalence point. While the equivalence point for a strong acid/strong base titration is pH 7, the equivalence point for a weak acid/strong base titration is above 7. This is because the reaction between the weak acid (HA) and strong base (OH^-) produces a weak conjugate base (A^-) and even weaker conjugate acid (H_2O). This produces a greater concentration of hydroxide ions than hydrogen ions at equilibrium (due to the common ion effect on the autoionization of water). Therefore, the equivalence point for weak acid/strong base titration is always in the basic range of the pH scale.

Strong Acid and Weak Base

The appearance of the titration curve for a weak base titrand and strong acid titrant will look like an inversion of the curve for a weak acid titrand and strong base titrant. The initial pH will be in the basic range (typical range: pH 10–12) and will demonstrate a gradual drop in pH with the addition of strong acid. The equivalence point will be in the acidic pH range because the reaction between the weak base and strong acid will produce a weak conjugate acid and even weaker conjugate base, as shown in Figure 10.17. The stronger conjugate acid will result in an equilibrium state with a concentration of hydrogen ions greater than that of the hydroxide ions. Therefore, the equivalence point for a weak base/strong acid titration is always in the acidic range of the pH scale.

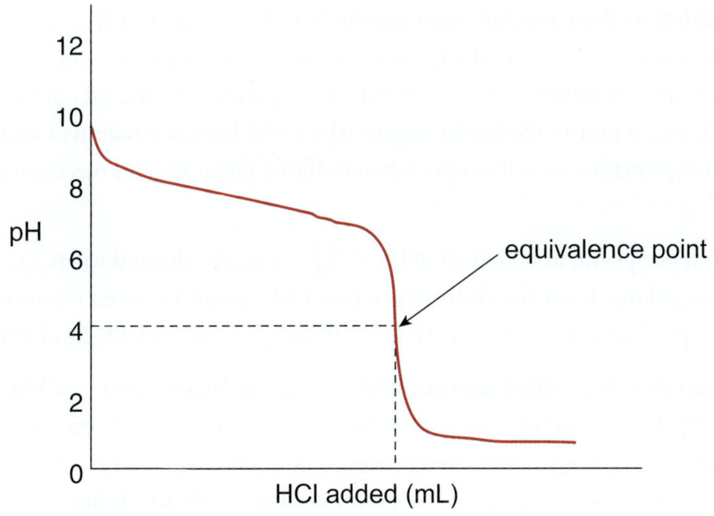

Figure 10.17 Strong Acid and Weak Base Titration Curve
A strong acid, HCl, is titrated into a solution of weak base, NH_3, to yield an equivalence point of pH < 7.

Weak Acid and Weak Base

The appearance of the titration curve for a weak base titrand and weak acid titrant will look like an intermediate of the previous types discussed. Because both the titrant and the titrand are weak, the initial pH is generally in the 3–11 range and will demonstrate a very shallow drop at the equivalence point. The equivalence point will be near neutral pH because the reaction is partially dissociative for both species.

MCAT EXPERTISE

To identify which type of titration is being shown in a graph, identify the starting position in the graph ($pH \gg 7$ = titrand is a strong base, > 7 (slightly) = weak base, < 7 (slightly) = weak acid, and $\ll 7$ pH = strong acid), and determine where the equivalence point is. Think of titrations like tug-of-war: the stronger the acid or base, the more it pulls the equivalence point into its pH territory.

Polyvalent Acids and Bases

The titration curve for a polyvalent acid or base looks different from that for a monovalent acid or base. Figure 10.18 shows the titration of Na_2CO_3 with HCl, in which the divalent (diprotic) acid H_2CO_3 is the ultimate product.

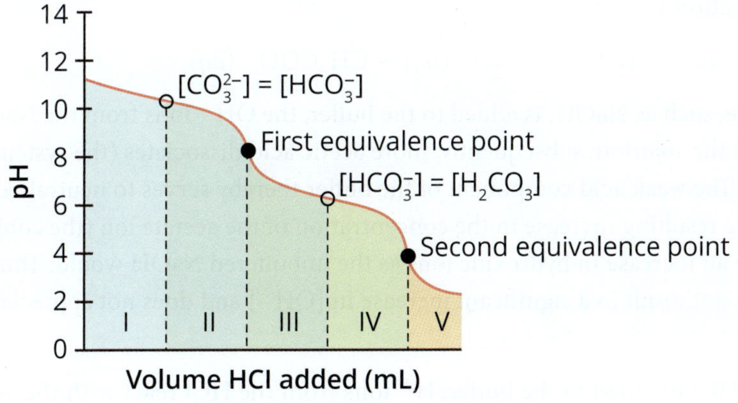

Figure 10.18 Polyvalent Titration
The multiple equivalence points indicate that this is a polyvalent titration.

In region I, little acid has been added, and the predominant species is CO_3^{2-}. In region II, more acid has been added, and the predominant species are CO_3^{2-} and HCO_3^-, in relatively equal concentrations. The flat part of the curve is the first buffer region (discussed in the next section), corresponding to the pK_a of HCO_3^- ($K_a = 5.6 \times 10^{-11}$; p$K_a = 10.25$). The center of the buffer region (the point between regions I and II) is sometimes termed the **half-equivalence point** because it occurs when half of a given species has been protonated (or deprotonated).

Region III begins with the equivalence point, at which all of the CO_3^{2-} is finally titrated to HCO_3^-. As the curve illustrates, a rapid change in pH occurs at the equivalence point (the point between regions II and III). In the latter part of region III, the predominant species is HCO_3^-, although some H_2CO_3 has formed as well.

At the beginning of region IV, the acid has neutralized approximately half of the HCO_3^-, and now H_2CO_3 and HCO_3^- are in roughly equal concentrations. This flat region is the second buffer region (and second half-equivalence point, between regions III and IV) of the titration curve, corresponding to the pK_a of H_2CO_3 ($K_a = 4.3 \times 10^{-7}$; p$K_a = 6.37$). Region V starts with the second equivalence point, as all of the HCO_3^- is finally converted to H_2CO_3. Again, a rapid change in pH is observed near the equivalence point (the point between regions IV and V) as acid is added.

The titrations of the acidic and basic amino acids (which have acidic or basic side chains, respectively) will show curves similar to the one shown in Figure 10.18. But rather than two equivalence points, there will in fact be three: one corresponding to the titration of the carboxyl group and a second corresponding to the titration of the amino group, both of which are attached to the central carbon, as well as a third corresponding to either the acidic or basic side chain.

Buffers

A **buffer solution** consists of a mixture of a weak acid and its salt (which is composed of its conjugate base and a cation) or a mixture of a weak base and its salt (which is composed of its conjugate acid and an anion). Two examples of buffers that are common in the laboratory—and commonly tested on the MCAT—are a solution of acetic acid (CH_3COOH) and its salt, sodium acetate ($CH_3COO^-Na^+$), and a solution of ammonia (NH_3) and its salt, ammonium chloride ($NH_4^+Cl^-$). The acetic acid/sodium acetate solution is considered an acid buffer, and the ammonium chloride/ammonia solution is a base buffer. Buffer solutions have the useful property of resisting changes in pH when small amounts of acid or base are added. Consider a buffer solution of acetic acid and sodium acetate: (Note: The sodium ion has not been included because it is not involved in the acid–base reaction.)

$$CH_3COOH\ (aq) + H_2O\ (l) \rightleftharpoons H_3O^+\ (aq) + CH_3COO^-\ (aq)$$

When a small amount of strong base, such as NaOH, is added to the buffer, the OH^- ions from the NaOH react with the H_3O^+ ions present in the solution; subsequently, more acetic acid dissociates (the system shifts to the right), restoring the $[H_3O^+]$. The weak acid component of the buffer thereby serves to neutralize the strong base that has been added. The resulting increase in the concentration of the acetate ion (the conjugate base) does not create nearly as large an increase in hydroxide ions as the unbuffered NaOH would. Thus, the addition of the strong base does not result in a significant increase in $[OH^-]$ and does not appreciably change the pH.

Likewise, when a small amount of HCl is added to the buffer, H^+ ions from the HCl react with the acetate ions to form acetic acid. Acetic acid is weaker than the added hydrochloric acid (which has been neutralized by the acetate ions), so the increased concentration of acetic acid does not significantly contribute to the hydrogen ion concentration in the solution. Because the buffer maintains $[H^+]$ at approximately constant values, the pH of the solution is relatively unchanged.

The Bicarbonate Buffer System

In the human body, one of the most important buffers is the H_2CO_3/HCO_3^- conjugate pair in the plasma component of the blood, called the **bicarbonate buffer system**. Specifically, carbonic acid (H_2CO_3) and its conjugate base, bicarbonate (HCO_3^-), form a weak acid buffer for maintaining the pH of the blood within a fairly narrow physiological range. CO_2 (*g*), one of the waste products of cellular respiration, also has low solubility in aqueous solutions. The majority of the CO_2 transported from peripheral tissues to the lungs (where it will be exhaled out) is dissolved in the plasma in a "disguised" form through the bicarbonate buffer system. CO_2 (*g*) and water react in the following manner:

$$CO_2\,(g) + H_2O\,(l) \rightleftharpoons H_2CO_3\,(aq) \rightleftharpoons H^+\,(aq) + HCO_3^-\,(aq)$$

The bicarbonate buffer system is tied to the respiratory system. In conditions of metabolic acidosis (production of excess plasma H^+ not caused by the respiratory system itself), the breathing rate will increase to compensate and blow off a greater amount of carbon dioxide gas; this causes the system to shift to the left, thereby reducing $[H^+]$ and buffering against dramatic and dangerous changes to the blood pH. It is interesting to note that the bicarbonate buffer system ($pK_a = 6.37$) maintains a pH around 7.4, which is actually slightly outside the optimal buffering capacity of the system. Buffers have a narrow range of optimal activity ($pK_a \pm 1$). This actually makes sense—it is far more common for acidemia (too much acid in the blood) to occur than alkalemia (too much base in the blood). As acidemia becomes more severe, the buffer system actually becomes more effective and more resistant to further lowering of the pH.

REAL WORLD

A number of conditions can affect the delicate pH balance of tissues in the body, including chronic obstructive pulmonary disease (COPD), renal tubular acidosis (RTA), diabetic ketoacidosis (DKA), lactic acidosis, metabolic diseases, poisonings and ingestions, and hyperventilation. The buffer system must be well maintained to mitigate these changes.

The Henderson–Hasselbalch Equation

The **Henderson–Hasselbalch equation** is used to estimate the pH or pOH of a buffer solution. For a weak acid buffer solution:

$$pH = pK_a + \log \frac{[A^-]}{[HA]}$$

Equation 10.9

where $[A^-]$ is the concentration of the conjugate base and [HA] is the concentration of the weak acid. Note that when [conjugate base] = [weak acid], the pH = pK_a because log (1) = 0. This occurs at the half-equivalence points in a titration, and buffering capacity is optimal at this pH.

Likewise, for a weak base buffer solution:

$$pOH = pK_b + \log \frac{[B^+]}{[BOH]}$$

Equation 10.10

where $[B^+]$ is the concentration of conjugate acid and [BOH] is the concentration of the weak base. Similar to acid buffers, $pOH = pK_b$ when [conjugate acid] = [weak base]. Buffering capacity is optimal at this pOH.

The Henderson–Hasselbalch equation is, in reality, just a rearrangement of the acid (or base) dissociation constant:

$$\begin{aligned} K_a &= \frac{[H_3O^+][A^-]}{[HA]} \\ -\log K_a &= -\log \frac{[H_3O^+][A^-]}{[HA]} \\ -\log K_a &= -\log [H_3O^+] - \log \frac{[A^-]}{[HA]} \\ pK_a &= pH - \log \frac{[A^-]}{[HA]} \\ pH &= pK_a + \log \frac{[A^-]}{[HA]} \end{aligned}$$

One subtlety of buffer systems and Henderson–Hasselbalch calculations that usually goes unnoticed or is misunderstood by students is the effect of changing the concentrations of the conjugate pair but not changing the ratio of their concentrations. Clearly, changing the ratio of the conjugate base to the acid will lead to a change in the pH of the buffer solution. But what about changing the concentrations while maintaining a constant ratio? What would happen if the concentrations of both the acid and its conjugate base were doubled? While the pH would not change, the **buffering capacity**—the ability to which the system can resist changes in pH—has doubled. In other words, addition of a small amount of acid or base to this system will now cause even less deviation in the pH. As mentioned earlier, the buffering capacity is generally maintained within 1 pH unit of the pK_a value.

Example: What is the pH of a solution made from 1 L of 0.05 M acetic acid (CH_3COOH, $K_a = 1.8 \times 10^{-5}$) mixed with 500 mL of 1 M acetate (CH_3COO^-)?

Solution: First, determine the concentrations of acetic acid and acetate in the final solution. Because two solutions were mixed, there will be some dilution of both the acetic acid and acetate.

$$N_{i,CH_3COOH}V_{i,CH_3COOH} = N_{f,CH_3COOH}V_{f,CH_3COOH} \rightarrow N_{f,CH_3COOH} = \frac{N_{i,CH_3COOH}V_{i,CH_3COOH}}{V_{f,CH_3COOH}}$$

$$N_{f,CH_3COOH} = \frac{(0.05\text{ N})(1\text{ L})}{(1.5\text{ L})} = 0.033\text{ N}$$

$$N_{i,CH_3COO^-}V_{i,CH_3COO^-} = N_{f,CH_3COO^-}V_{f,CH_3COO^-} \rightarrow N_{f,CH_3COO^-} = \frac{N_{i,CH_3COO^-}V_{i,CH_3COO^-}}{V_{f,CH_3COO^-}}$$

$$N_{f,CH_3COO^-} = \frac{(1\text{ N})(0.5\text{ L})}{(1.5\text{ L})} = 0.33\text{ N}$$

Then, use the Henderson–Hasselbalch equation.

$$pH = pK_a + \log \frac{[A^-]}{[HA]} = -\log(1.8 \times 10^{-5}) + \log \frac{0.33\text{ N}}{0.033\text{ N}}$$

$$pH \approx 4.82 + 1 = 5.82\ (\text{actual} = 5.74)$$

MCAT CONCEPT CHECK 10.4

Before you move on, assess your understanding of the material with these questions.

1. Describe each of the following parts of a titration curve:
   - Buffering region:

   - Half-equivalence point:

   - Equivalence point:

   - Endpoint:

   ---

2. For a reaction involving a strong base and a weak acid, which of the following indicators would be best to indicate the endpoint of the titration? (Circle the correct answer.)
   - Phenolphthalein ($pK_a = 9.7$)
   - Bromothymol blue ($pK_a = 7.1$)
   - Bromocresol green ($pK_a = 4.7$)
   - Methyl yellow ($pK_a = 3.3$)

3. In which part of the pH range (acidic, basic, or neutral) will the equivalence points fall for each of the following titrations?
   - Strong acid + weak base:

   - Strong base + weak acid:

   - Strong acid + strong base:

   - Weak acid + weak base:

   ---

4. What is the purpose of a buffer solution?

   ---

5. What are the pH and pOH of a solution containing 5 mL of 5 M benzoic acid ($K_a = 6.3 \times 10^{-5}$) and 100 mL of 0.005 M benzoate solution?

Conclusion

In this chapter, we have reviewed the important principles of acid–base chemistry. We clarified the differences among the three definitions of acids and bases, including the nomenclature of some common Arrhenius acids. We investigated important properties of acids and bases, including the important acid–base behavior of water (autoionization) and hydrogen ion equilibria. We explained the mathematics of the pH and pOH logarithmic scales and demonstrated a useful Test Day shortcut for approximating the logarithmic value of hydrogen ion or hydroxide ion concentrations. Strong acids and bases are defined as compounds that completely dissociate in aqueous solutions, and weak acids and bases are compounds that only partially dissociate (to an equilibrium state). We discussed neutralization and salt formation upon reaction of acids and bases, and finally, we applied our fundamental understanding of acid–base reactivity to titrations and buffer systems. Titrations are useful for determining the concentration of a known acid or base solution. Weak acid and weak base buffers are useful for minimizing changes in pH upon addition of a strong acid or base.

You've just accomplished a major task in the overall effort to earn points on Test Day. It's okay if you didn't understand everything on this first pass. Go back and review the concepts that were challenging for you and then complete the questions at the end of the chapter and MCAT practice passages to test your knowledge. Don't be alarmed if you find yourself reviewing parts or all of a chapter a second or third time—repetition is the key to success.

You are now two chapters away from completing this review of general chemistry. While we don't want to offer our congratulations prematurely, we want to acknowledge all the hard work you've invested in this process. Keep it up: success on Test Day is within your reach!

GO ONLINE

You've reviewed the content, now test your knowledge and critical thinking skills by completing a test-like passage set in your online resources!

CONCEPT SUMMARY

Definitions

- **Arrhenius acids** dissociate to produce an excess of hydrogen ions in solution. **Arrhenius bases** dissociate to produce an excess of hydroxide ions in solution.
- **Brønsted–Lowry acids** are species that can donate hydrogen ions. **Brønsted–Lowry bases** are species that can accept hydrogen ions.
- **Lewis acids** are electron-pair acceptors. **Lewis bases** are electron-pair donors.
- All Arrhenius acids and bases are Brønsted–Lowry acids and bases, and all Brønsted–Lowry acids and bases are Lewis acids and bases; however, the converse of these statements is not necessarily true (that is, not all Lewis acids and bases are Brønsted–Lowry acids and bases, and not all Brønsted–Lowry acids and bases are Arrhenius acids and bases).
- **Amphoteric** species are those that can behave as an acid or base. **Amphiprotic** species are amphoteric species that specifically can behave as a Brønsted–Lowry acid or Brønsted–Lowry base.
    - Water is a classic example of an amphoteric, amphiprotic species—it can accept a hydrogen ion to become a hydronium ion, or it can donate a hydrogen ion to become a hydroxide ion.
    - Conjugate species of polyvalent acids and bases can also behave as amphoteric and amphiprotic species.

Properties

- The **water dissociation constant,** K_w, is 10^{-14} at 298 K. Like other equilibrium constants, K_w is only affected by changes in temperature.
- **pH** and **pOH** can be calculated given the concentrations of H_3O^+ and OH^- ions, respectively. In aqueous solutions, pH + pOH = 14 at 298 K.
- **Strong acids and bases** completely dissociate in solution.
- **Weak acids and bases** do not completely dissociate in solution and have corresponding **dissociation constants** (**K_a** and **K_b**, respectively).
- In the Brønsted–Lowry definition, acids have conjugate bases that are formed when the acid is deprotonated. Bases have conjugate acids that are formed when the base is protonated.
    - Strong acids and bases have very weak (**inert**) conjugates.
    - Weak acids and bases have weak conjugates.
- **Neutralization reactions** form salts and (sometimes) water.

Polyvalence and Normality

- An **equivalent** is defined as one mole of the species of interest.
- In acid–base chemistry, **normality** is the concentration of acid or base equivalents in solution.
- **Polyvalent** acids and bases are those that can donate or accept multiple electrons. The normality of a solution containing a polyvalent species is the molarity of the acid or base times the number of protons it can donate or accept.

Titration and Buffers

- **Titrations** are used to determine the concentration of a known reactant in a solution.
  - The **titrant** has a known concentration and is added slowly to the titrand to reach the equivalence point.
  - The **titrand** has an unknown concentration but a known volume.
- The **half-equivalence point** is the midpoint of the **buffering region**, in which half of the titrant has been protonated (or deprotonated); thus, $[HA] = [A^-]$ and a buffer is formed.
- The **equivalence point** is indicated by the steepest slope in a titration curve; it is reached when the number of acid equivalents in the original solution equals the number of base equivalents added, or vice-versa.
  - Strong acid and strong base titrations have equivalence points at $pH = 7$.
  - Weak acid and strong base titrations have equivalence points at $pH > 7$.
  - Weak base and strong acid titrations have equivalence points at $pH < 7$.
  - Weak acid and weak base titrations can have equivalence points above or below 7, depending on the relative strength of the acid and base.
- **Indicators** are weak acids or bases that display different colors in their protonated and deprotonated forms.
  - The indicator chosen for a titration should have a pK_a close to the pH of the expected equivalence point.
  - The **endpoint** of a titration is when the indicator reaches its final color.
- Multiple buffering regions and equivalence points are observed in polyvalent acid and base titrations.
- **Buffer solutions** consist of a mixture of a weak acid and its conjugate salt or a weak base and its conjugate salt; they resist large fluctuations in pH.
- **Buffering capacity** refers to the ability of a buffer to resist changes in pH; maximal buffering capacity is seen within 1 pH point of the pK_a of the acid in the buffer solution.
- The **Henderson–Hasselbalch equation** quantifies the relationship between pH and pK_a for weak acids and between pOH and pK_b for weak bases; when a solution is optimally buffered, $pH = pK_a$ and $pOH = pK_b$.

ANSWERS TO CONCEPT CHECKS

10.1

1.

Definition	Acid	Base
Arrhenius	Dissociates to form excess H^+ in solution	Dissociates to form excess OH^- in solution
Brønsted–Lowry	H^+ donor	H^+ acceptor
Lewis	Electron pair acceptor	Electron pair donor

2.

Anion	Acid Formula	Acid Name
MnO_4^-	$HMnO_4$	Permanganic acid
Titanate (TiO_2^{2-})	H_2TiO_3	Titanic acid
I^-	HI	Hydroiodic acid
IO_4^-	HIO_4	Periodic acid

3.

Reaction	Amphoteric Reactant	Amphiprotic? (Y or N)
$HCO_3^- + HBr \rightarrow H_2CO_3 + Br^-$	HCO_3^-	Yes
$3\ HCl + Al(OH)_3 \rightarrow AlCl_3 + 3\ H_2O$	$Al(OH)_3$	No
$2\ HBr + ZnO \rightarrow ZnBr_2 + H_2O$	ZnO	No

10.2

1. An amphoteric species can act as an acid or a base.
2. High K_a indicates a strong acid, which will dissociate completely in solution. Having a K_a slightly greater than water means the acid is a weak acid with minimal dissociation.
3. High K_b indicates a strong base, which will dissociate completely in solution. Having a K_b slightly greater than water means the base is a weak base with minimal dissociation.

4.

pH	$[H_3O^+]$	pOH	$[OH^-]$	Acid or Base?
4	10^{-4} M	10	10^{-10} M	Acid
3.05	8.89×10^{-4} M	10.95	1.12×10^{-11} M	Acid
8.81	1.55×10^{-9} M	5.19	6.46×10^{-6} M	Base
8.27	5.32×10^{-9} M	5.73	1.88×10^{-6} M	Base

(Note: Exact answers are provided; your rounded answers should be relatively close to those listed here.)

5. $K_a \times K_b = K_w$

6.

Reaction	Acid	Base	Conjugate Acid	Conjugate Base
$H_2CO_3 + H_2O \rightleftharpoons HCO_3^- + H_3O^+$	H_2CO_3	H_2O	H_3O^+	HCO_3^-
$H_2PO_4^- + H_2O \rightleftharpoons H_3PO_4 + OH^-$	H_2O	$H_2PO_4^-$	H_3PO_4	OH^-

7. $K_a = \frac{[CH_3COO^-][H_3O^+]}{[CH_3COOH]} = \frac{[x][x]}{[0.2\text{ M} - x]} \approx \frac{x^2}{0.2}$. Therefore, $x^2 = 3.6 \times 10^{-6}$ $\rightarrow x \approx 2 \times 10^{-3}$ M (actual $= 1.9 \times 10^{-3}$ M). Then, pH $= -\log H_3O^+ \approx$ $3 - 0.2 = 2.8$ (actual $= 2.72$)

10.3

1. Acids use moles of H^+ (H_3O^+) as an equivalent. Bases use moles of OH^- as an equivalent.
2. 6 N $Al(OH)_3$; 32 N H_2SO_4

10.4

1. The buffering region occurs when $[HA] \approx [A^-]$ and is the flattest portion of the titration curve (resistant to changes in pH). The half-equivalence point is the center of the buffering region, where $[HA] = [A^-]$. The equivalence point is the steepest point of the titration curve, and occurs when the equivalents of acid present equal the equivalents of base added (or vice-versa). The endpoint is the pH at which an indicator turns its final color.
2. Phenolphthalein would be the preferred indicator for this titration.
3. A strong acid and weak base have an equivalence point in the acidic range. A strong base and weak acid have an equivalence point in the basic range. A strong acid and strong base have an equivalence point at pH = 7 (neutral). A weak acid and weak base can have an equivalence point in the acidic, neutral, or basic range, depending on the relative strengths of the acid and base.
4. A buffer solution is designed to resist changes in pH and has optimal buffering capacity within 1 pH point from its pK_a.

5. Recall from section 10.2 on Properties that the concentrations of the conjugate acid and conjugate base in the final solution must first be calculated due to the dilution from mixing the two solutions together. The calculation below follows that step, but leaves the values unsolved for so that some of their components can be cancelled and simplified:

$$\text{pH} = \text{p}K_\text{a} + \log\frac{[\text{A}^-]}{[\text{HA}]} = -\log(6.3\times10^{-5}) + \log\frac{\left[\dfrac{(0.005\text{ N})(100\text{ mL})}{(105\text{ mL})}\right]}{\left[\dfrac{(5\text{ N})(5\text{ mL})}{(105\text{ mL})}\right]}$$

$$\text{pH} \approx 4.37 + \log\frac{(0.005\text{ N})(100\text{ mL})}{(5\text{ N})(5\text{ mL})} = 4.37 + \log\frac{0.5}{25} = 4.37 + \log(2\times10^{-2})$$

$$\approx 4.37 - 1.8 = 2.57\ (\text{actual} = 2.50)$$

$$\text{pOH} \approx 14 - 2.57 = 11.43\ (\text{actual} = 11.5)$$

SCIENCE MASTERY ASSESSMENT EXPLANATIONS

1. **D**

A Brønsted–Lowry base is defined as a proton acceptor. Ammonia, fluoride, and water—**(A)**, **(B)**, and **(C)**, respectively—each accept a proton. **(D)**, HNO_2, is a far better Brønsted–Lowry acid, donating a proton to a solution.

2. **B**

First, convert the concentration to 5×10^{-3} M. Next, because sulfuric acid is a strong acid, we can assume that, for the majority of sulfuric acid molecules (although not all), both protons will dissociate. The concentration of hydrogen ions is therefore $2 \times 5 \times 10^{-3}$, or 10^{-2}. The equation for pH is $pH = -\log [H^+]$. If $[H^+] = 10^{-2}$ M, then pH = 2.

3. **A**

Answering this question is simply a matter of knowing nomenclature. Acids ending in **–ic** are derivatives of anions ending in **–ate**, while acids ending in **–ous** are derivatives of anions ending in **–ite**. ClO_3^-, **(B)**, is chlorate because it has more oxygen than the other commonly occurring ion, ClO_2^-, which is named chlorite. Therefore, $HClO_3$ is chloric acid. $HClO_2$, **(C)**, represents chlorous acid. HClO, **(D)**, represents hypochlorous acid.

4. **B**

Soluble hydroxides of Group IA and IIA metals are strong bases, eliminating **(A)** and **(D)**. **(B)** and **(C)** are both weak bases; however, methylamine contains an alkyl group, which is electron-donating. This increases the electron density on the nitrogen in methylamine, making it a stronger (Lewis) base. Therefore, ammonia is the weakest base.

5. **B**

The purpose of a buffer is to resist changes in the pH of a reaction. Buffers are not generally used to affect the kinetics of a reaction, so **(C)** and **(D)** are incorrect. **(A)** is true only in specific circumstances where the pH of the buffer solution itself is neutral. Many natural buffer systems maintain pH in the acidic or basic ranges.

6. **D**

The question is asking for pH, but because of the information given, we must first find the pOH and then subtract it from 14 to get the pH. Use the Henderson–Hasselbalch equation:

$$\begin{aligned} \text{pOH} &= \text{p}K_b + \log \frac{[\text{conjugate acid}]}{[\text{base}]} \\ &= 3.45 + \log \frac{70 \text{ mM}}{712 \text{ mM}} \\ &\approx 3.45 + \log \frac{1}{10} \\ &= 3.45 - 1 = 2.45 \end{aligned}$$

If the pOH = 2.45, the pH = 14 − 2.45 = 11.55.

7. **A**

The first pK_a in this curve can be estimated by eye. It is located halfway between the starting point (when no base had yet been added) and the first equivalence point (the first steep portion of the graph, around 15 mL). This point is at approximately 7–8 mL on the *x*-axis, which corresponds to a pH of approximately 1.9. Notice that this region experiences very little change in pH, which is the defining characteristic of a buffer region.

8. **C**

The second equivalence point is the midpoint of the second steep increase in slope. This corresponds to approximately pH = 5.9.

9. **B**

The value of the second pK_a is found at the midpoint between the first and second equivalence points. In this curve, that corresponds to $pH = 4.1$. Just like the first pK_a, it is in the center of a flat buffering region.

10. **B**

Gram equivalent weight is the weight (in grams) that releases 1 acid or base equivalent from a compound. Because H_3PO_4 contains 3 protons, we find the gram equivalent weight by dividing the mass of one mole of the species by 3. The molar mass of phosphoric acid is $98\ \frac{\text{g}}{\text{mol}}$, so the gram equivalent weight is 32.7 g.

11. **D**

This question requires the application of the acid dissociation constant. Weak acids do not dissociate completely; therefore, all three species that appear in the balanced equation will be present in solution. Hydrogen ions and conjugate base anions dissociate in equal amounts, so $[H^+] = [XO_2^-]$. If the initial concentration of HXO_2 was 2 M and some amount x dissociates, we will have x amount of H_3O^+ and XO_2^- at equilibrium, with $2\ \text{M} - x$ amount of HXO_2 at equilibrium.

$$K_a = \frac{[H_3O^+][XO_2^-]}{[HXO_2]} = \frac{(x)(x)}{2\ \text{M} - x} \approx \frac{x^2}{2}$$

Note that x was considered negligible when added or subtracted, per usual. Solving for x, we get:

$$\frac{x^2}{2} = 3.2 \times 10^{-5} \rightarrow x^2 = 6.4 \times 10^{-5} = 64 \times 10^{-6}$$

$$\rightarrow x = 8 \times 10^{-3}\ \text{M}$$

12. **C**

A higher K_a implies a stronger acid. Weak acids usually have a K_a that is several orders of magnitude below 1. The pK_a of a compound is the pH at which there are equal concentrations of acid and conjugate base; the pK_a of this compound would be $-\log 1 = 0$. With such a low pK_a, this compound must be an acid. Therefore, the pH of any concentration of this compound must be below 7.

13. **D**

An amphoteric species is one that can act either as an acid or a base, depending on its environment. Proton transfers are classic oxidation–reduction reactions, so **(A)** and **(B)** are true. **(C)** is true because many amphoteric species, such as water and bicarbonate, can either donate or accept a proton. **(D)** is false, and thus the correct answer because amphoteric species can be either polar or nonpolar in nature.

14. **C**

NaOH is a strong base; as such, there will be 1.2×10^{-5} M OH^- in solution. Based on this information alone, the pOH must be between 4 and 5, and the pH must be between 9 and 10. Using the shortcut, $pOH \approx 5 - 0.12 = 4.88$. $pH = 14 - pOH = 9.12$ (actual $= 9.08$).

15. **C**

Use the equivalence point equation: $N_aV_a = N_bV_b$. $Ba(OH)_2$ can dissociate to give two hydroxide ions, so its normality is $2\ \text{M} \times 2 = 4\ \text{N}$. H_3PO_4 can dissociate to give three hydronium ions, so its normality is $6\ \text{M} \times 3 = 18\ \text{N}$. Plugging into the equation, we get $(18\ \text{N})(4\ \text{L}) = (4\ \text{N})(V_b)$. Therefore, V_b is 18 L.

GO ONLINE

Consult your online resources for additional practice.

EQUATIONS TO REMEMBER

(10.1) **Autoionization constant for water:** $K_w = [H_3O^+][OH^-] = 10^{-14}$ at 25°C (298 K)

(10.2) **Definitions of pH and pOH:** $\text{pH} = -\log[H^+] = \log \frac{1}{[H^+]}$

$$\text{pOH} = -\log[OH^-] = \log \frac{1}{[OH^-]}$$

(10.3) **Relationship of pH and pOH at 298 K:** $\text{pH} + \text{pOH} = 14$

(10.4) **p scale value approximation:** p value $\approx m - 0.n$

(10.5) **Acid dissociation constant:** $K_a = \frac{[H_3O^+][A^-]}{[HA]}$

(10.6) **Base dissociation constant:** $K_b = \frac{[B^+][OH^-]}{[BOH]}$

(10.7) **Relationship of K_a and K_b at 298 K:** $K_{a,\text{acid}} \times K_{b,\text{conjugate base}} = K_w = 10^{-14}$;

$$K_{b,\text{base}} \times K_{a,\text{conjugate acid}} = K_w = 10^{-14}$$

(10.8) **Equivalence point:** $N_a V_a = N_b V_b$

(10.9) **Henderson–Hasselbalch equation (acid buffer):** $\text{pH} = \text{p}K_a + \log \frac{[A^-]}{[HA]}$

(10.10) **Henderson–Hasselbalch equation (base buffer):** $\text{pOH} = \text{p}K_b + \log \frac{[B^+]}{[BOH]}$

SHARED CONCEPTS

Biology Chapter 6
The Respiratory System

Biology Chapter 10
Homeostasis

General Chemistry Chapter 3
Bonding and Chemical Interactions

General Chemistry Chapter 9
Solutions

Organic Chemistry Chapter 4
Analyzing Organic Reactions

Physics and Math Chapter 10
Mathematics

CHAPTER 11

OXIDATION–REDUCTION REACTIONS

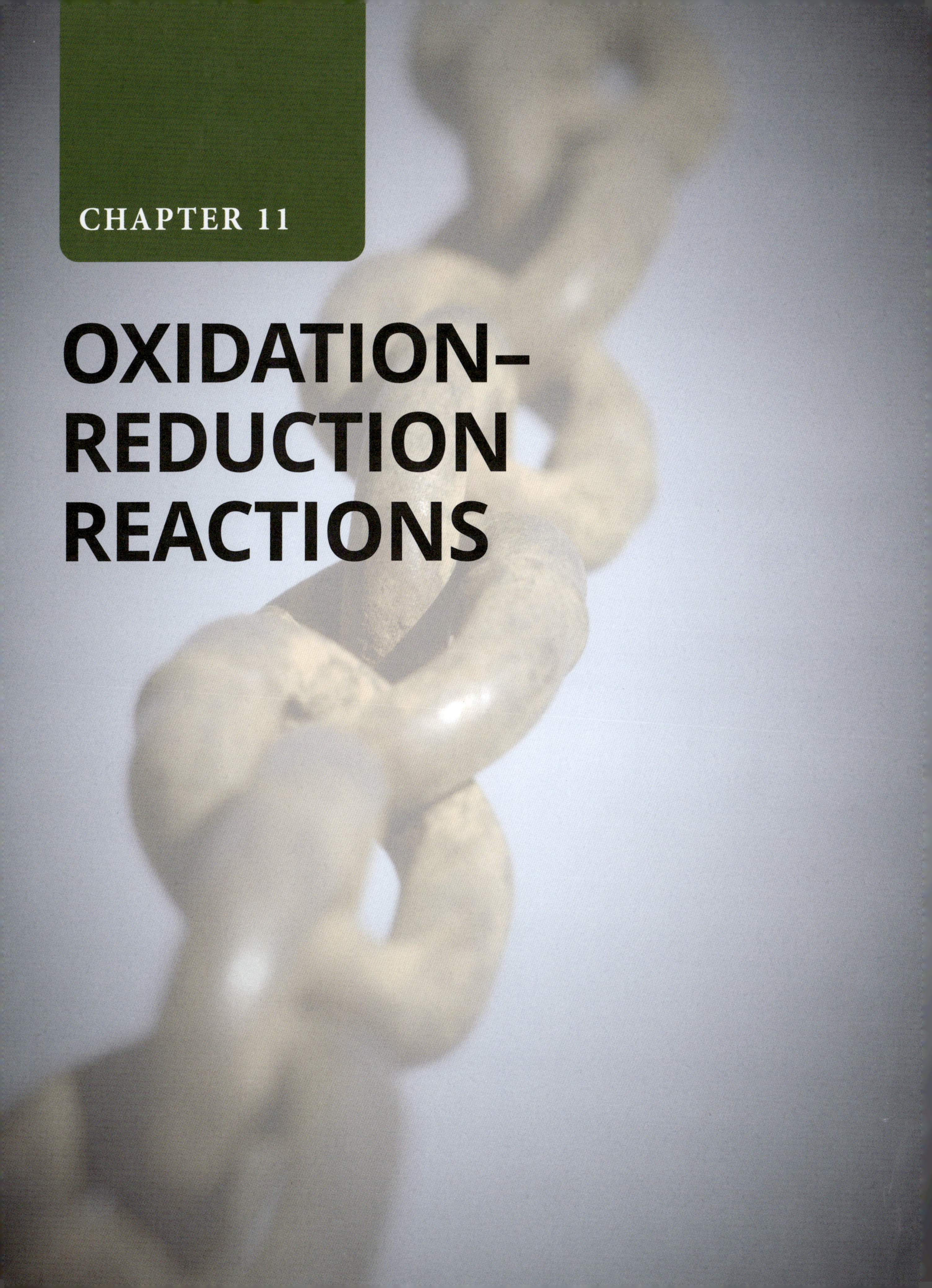

SCIENCE MASTERY ASSESSMENT

Every pre-med knows this feeling: there is so much content I have to know for the MCAT! How do I know what to do first or what's important?

While the high-yield badges throughout this book will help you identify the most important topics, this Science Mastery Assessment is another tool in your MCAT prep arsenal. This quiz (which can also be taken in your online resources) and the guidance below will help ensure that you are spending the appropriate amount of time on this chapter based on your personal strengths and weaknesses. Don't worry though—skipping something now does not mean you'll never study it. Later on in your prep, as you complete full-length tests, you'll uncover specific pieces of content that you need to review and can come back to these chapters as appropriate.

How to Use This Assessment

If you answer 0–7 questions correctly:

Spend about 1 hour to read this chapter in full and take limited notes throughout. Follow up by reviewing **all** quiz questions to ensure that you now understand how to solve each one.

If you answer 8–11 questions correctly:

Spend 20–40 minutes reviewing the quiz questions. Beginning with the questions you missed, read and take notes on the corresponding subchapters. For questions you answered correctly, ensure your thinking matches that of the explanation and you understand why each choice was correct or incorrect.

If you answer 12–15 questions correctly:

Spend less than 20 minutes reviewing all questions from the quiz. If you missed any, then include a quick read-through of the corresponding subchapters, or even just the relevant content within a subchapter, as part of your question review. For questions you answered correctly, ensure your thinking matches that of the explanation and review the Concept Summary at the end of the chapter.

OXIDATION–REDUCTION REACTIONS

1. Consider the following equation:

$$6\ Na\ (s) + 2\ NH_3\ (aq) \rightarrow 2\ Na_3N\ (s) + 3\ H_2\ (g)$$

Which species acts as an oxidizing agent?

A. Na
B. N in NH_3
C. H in NH_3
D. H_2

2. How many electrons are involved in the following half-reaction after it is balanced?

$$Cr_2O_7^{2-} + H^+ + e^- \rightarrow Cr^{2+} + H_2O$$

A. 2
B. 8
C. 12
D. 16

3. Lithium aluminum hydride ($LiAlH_4$) is often used in laboratories because of its tendency to donate a hydride ion. Which of the following roles would lithium aluminum hydride likely play in a reaction?

A. Strong reducing agent only
B. Strong oxidizing agent only
C. Both a strong reducing agent and strong oxidizing agent
D. Neither a strong reducing agent nor a strong oxidizing agent

4. What is the oxidation number of chlorine in NaClO?

A. −1
B. 0
C. +1
D. +2

5. The following electronic configurations represent elements in their neutral form. Which element is the strongest oxidizing agent?

A. $1s^22s^22p^63s^23p^64s^2$
B. $1s^22s^22p^63s^23p^64s^23d^5$
C. $1s^22s^22p^63s^23p^64s^23d^{10}4p^1$
D. $1s^22s^22p^63s^23p^64s^23d^{10}4p^5$

6. Which of the following is the correct net ionic reaction for the reaction of copper with silver(I) nitrate?

A. $Cu + AgNO_3 \rightarrow Cu(NO_3)_2 + Ag$
B. $Cu + 2\ Ag^+ + 2\ NO_3^- \rightarrow Cu^{2+} + 2\ NO_3^- + 2\ Ag$
C. $2\ Ag^+ + 2\ NO_3^- \rightarrow 2\ NO_3^- + 2\ Ag^+$
D. $Cu + 2\ Ag^+ \rightarrow Cu^{2+} + 2\ Ag$

7. One way to test for the presence of iron in solution is by adding potassium thiocyanate to the solution. The product when this reagent reacts with iron is $FeSCN^{2+}$, which creates a dark red color in solution via the following net ionic equation:

$$Fe^{3+} + SCN^- \rightarrow FeSCN^{2+}$$

How many grams of iron sulfate would be needed to produce 2 moles of $FeSCN^{2+}$?

A. 110 g
B. 220 g
C. 400 g
D. 500 g

8. During the assigning of oxidation numbers, which of the following elements would most likely be determined last?
   - A. Ar
   - B. F
   - C. Sr
   - D. Ir

9. As methanol is converted to methanal, and then methanoic acid, the oxidation number of the carbon:
   - A. increases.
   - B. decreases.
   - C. increases, then decreases.
   - D. decreases, then increases.

10. In the compound KH_2PO_4, which element has the highest oxidation number?
   - A. K
   - B. H
   - C. P
   - D. O

11. If a certain metal has multiple oxidation states, its acidity as an oxide generally increases as the oxidation state increases. Therefore, which of the following tungsten compounds is likely to be the strongest acid?
   - A. WO_2
   - B. WO_3
   - C. W_2O_3
   - D. W_2O_5

12. Consider the following steps in the reaction between oxalic acid and chlorine:
   - I. $Cl_2 + H_2O \rightarrow HOCl + Cl^- + H^+$
   - II. $H_2C_2O_4 \rightarrow H^+ + HC_2O_4^-$
   - III. $HOCl + HC_2O_4^- \rightarrow H_2O + Cl^- + 2\ CO_2$

   Which of these steps, occurring in aqueous solution, is an example of a disproportionation reaction?
   - A. I only
   - B. III only
   - C. I and III only
   - D. I, II, and III

13. Potentiometry in an oxidation–reduction titration is analogous to performing an acid–base titration with a(n):
   - A. acidic indicator.
   - B. basic indicator.
   - C. pH meter.
   - D. oxidizing agent.

14. After balancing the following oxidation–reduction reaction, what is the sum of the stoichiometric coefficients of all of the reactants and products?

$$S_8\ (s) + NO_3^-\ (aq) \rightarrow SO_3^{2-}\ (aq) + NO\ (g)$$

   - A. 4
   - B. 50
   - C. 91
   - D. 115

15. An assay is performed to determine the gold content in a supply of crushed ore. One method for pulling gold out of ore is to react it in a concentrated cyanide (CN^-) solution. The equation is provided below:

$$Au + NaCN + O_2 + H_2O \rightarrow Na[Au(CN)_2] + NaOH$$

   An indicator is used during this reaction, and approximately 100 mL of a 2 M NaCN solution is used to reach the endpoint. How many moles of Au are present in the crushed ore?
   - A. 0.01 mol
   - B. 0.02 mol
   - C. 0.10 mol
   - D. 0.20 mol

Answer Key

1. **C** (See section 11.1)
2. **B** (See section 11.1)
3. **A** (See section 11.1)
4. **C** (See section 11.1)
5. **D** (See section 11.1)
6. **D** (See section 11.2)
7. **C** (See section 11.2)
8. **D** (See section 11.1)
9. **A** (See section 11.1)
10. **C** (See section 11.1)
11. **B** (See section 11.1)
12. **A** (See section 11.2)
13. **C** (See section 11.2)
14. **D** (See section 11.1)
15. **C** (See section 11.2)

The relevant section of the chapter to review for each question is given in parentheses after the correct answer. Detailed explanations can be found at the end of the chapter.

CHAPTER 11

OXIDATION–REDUCTION REACTIONS

In This Chapter

CHAPTER PROFILE

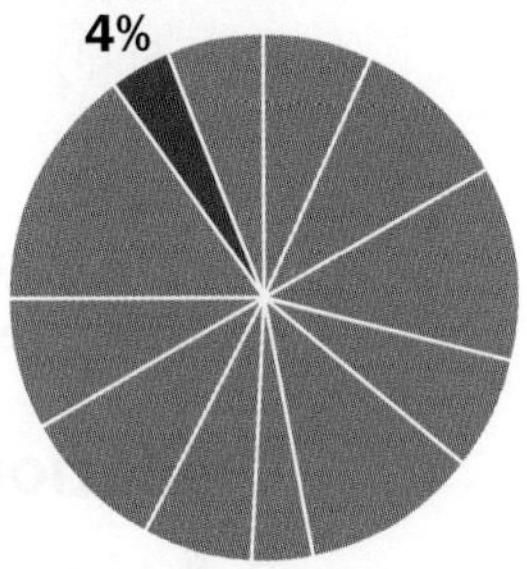

The content in this chapter should be relevant to about 4% of all questions about general chemistry on the MCAT.

This chapter covers material from the following AAMC content categories:

4E: Atoms, nuclear decay, electronic structure, and atomic chemical behavior

5A: Unique nature of water and its solutions

Introduction

You're on a night call in the emergency department (ED) when a 5-month-old infant patient's chart appears on your screen. You click through the triage notes and read what the caregiver reports: *poor sucking ability and loss of head control and motor skills.* You're puzzled by the findings and the previous ED admissions of lactic acidosis. You suspect diabetic ketoacidosis (DKA), liver, or kidney diseases—and possibly even poisoning—but nothing seems to fit. Minutes later, the child is brought into the examination room and does not stop crying. Over the course of an hour, another episode of lactic acidosis develops. The child is eventually admitted to the neonatal intensive care unit for long-term care.

Later, you ask the neonatologist about the patient. They point you to the charts and a genetic test performed shortly after birth. The child was diagnosed with Leigh disease, an extremely rare mitochondrial disorder. In Leigh disease, a number of key mitochondrial enzymes are disrupted and the process of oxidative phosphorylation is never achieved. Specifically, some of the most important enzymes that catalyze oxidation–reduction reactions, such as the *pyruvate dehydrogenase complex* and *succinate dehydrogenase complex,* are affected. When pyruvate cannot be oxidized to acetyl-CoA, it is instead fermented to lactic acid.

In biological systems, oxidation is coincident with the loss of electrons, sometimes in the form of hydrogen (dehydrogenation). The enzymes that catalyze these oxidations are called *dehydrogenases.* Many other macromolecules besides enzymes, such as vitamins, also carry out their functions by oxidizing or reducing other compounds. Iron in hemoglobin likewise undergoes rounds of oxidation and reduction as it carries oxygen from the lungs to tissues.

In this chapter, we focus our attention on the movement of electrons in chemical reactions. Such reactions are called oxidation–reduction (redox) reactions because they always occur in pairs. Oxidation–reduction reactions are particularly important because they tie into a number of topics in organic chemistry and biochemistry. In fact, Chapters 5 through 10 of *MCAT Organic Chemistry Review* and Chapters 9 through 11 of *MCAT Biochemistry Review* all touch on oxidation–reduction reactions in different sets of molecules.

11.1 Oxidation–Reduction Reactions

LEARNING OBJECTIVES

After Chapter 11.1, you will be able to:

- Separate a redox reaction into oxidation and reduction half-reactions
- Balance a redox reaction
- Identify the oxidizing agent, reducing agent, and relevant oxidation states for a given reaction: $SnCl_2 + PbCl_4 \rightarrow SnCl_4 + PbCl_2$

Reactions that involve the transfer of electrons from one chemical species to another can be classified as **oxidation–reduction (redox) reactions.**

Oxidation and Reduction

The law of conservation of charge states that electrical charge can be neither created nor destroyed. Thus, an isolated loss or gain of electrons cannot occur; **oxidation** (loss of electrons) and **reduction** (gain of electrons) must occur simultaneously, resulting in an electron transfer called a **redox reaction**. An **oxidizing agent** causes another atom in a redox reaction to undergo oxidation and is itself reduced. A **reducing agent** causes the other atom to be reduced and is itself oxidized. A visual illustration of oxidizing and reducing agents can be seen in Figure 11.1. There are various mnemonics to remember these terms, as highlighted in the sidebar.

MNEMONIC

Redox reactions: choose one of the mnemonics and stick with it!

- **OIL RIG**: **O**xidation **I**s **L**oss of electrons, **R**eduction **I**s **G**ain of electrons.
- **LEO** the lion says **GER**: **L**oss of **E**lectrons is **O**xidation, **G**ain of **E**lectrons is **R**eduction.
- **LEORA** says **GEROA**: **L**oss of **E**lectrons is **O**xidation (**R**educing **A**gent), **G**ain of **E**lectrons is **R**eduction (**O**xidizing **A**gent).

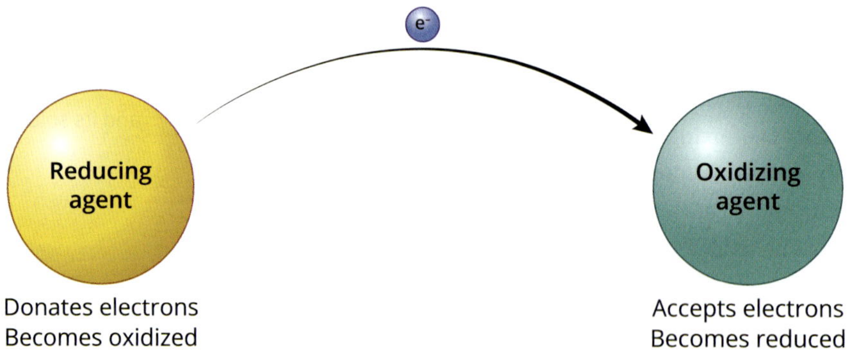

Figure 11.1 Oxidizing and Reducing Agents

Being familiar with some common oxidizing and reducing agents can save significant time on Test Day, especially in organic chemistry reactions. Some of the commonly used agents on the MCAT are listed in Table 11.1. Note that almost all oxidizing agents contain oxygen or another strongly electronegative element (such as a halogen). Reducing agents often contain metal ions or hydrides (H^-).

Oxidizing Agents	Reducing Agents
O_2	CO
H_2O_2	C
F_2, Cl_2, Br_2, I_2 (halogens)	B_2H_6
H_2SO_4	Sn^{2+} and other pure metals
HNO_3	Hydrazine*
NaClO	Zn(Hg)*
$KMnO_4$*	Lindlar's catalyst*
CrO_3, $Na_2Cr_2O_7$*	$NaBH_4$*
Pyridinium chlorochromate (PCC)*	$LiAlH_4$*
NAD^+, FADH**	NADH, $FADH_2$**

* These oxidizing agents and reducing agents are commonly seen in organic chemistry reactions.

** These and other biochemical redox reagents often act as energy carriers in biochemistry reactions.

Table 11.1 Common Oxidizing and Reducing Agents

Note that biochemical redox reagents such as NAD^+ tend to act as both oxidizing and reducing agents at different times during metabolic pathways. As such, they act as mediators of energy transfer during many metabolic processes, as shown in Figure 11.2.

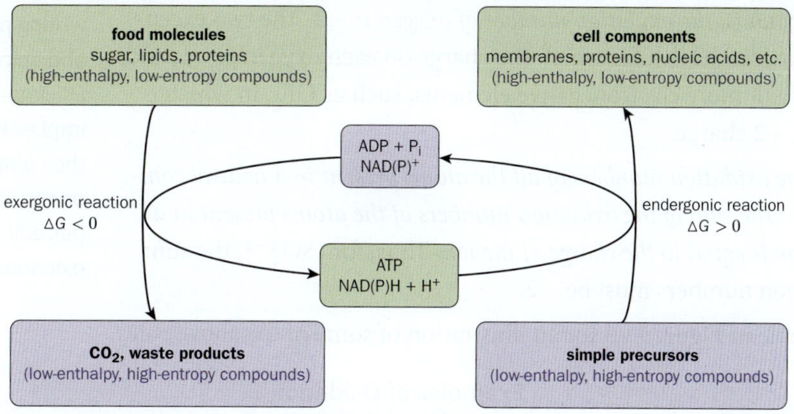

Figure 11.2 Oxidation and Reduction of Biochemical Compounds Serves as a Method of Energy Transfer

On a technical level, the term oxidizing agent or reducing agent is applied specifically to the atom that gains or loses electrons, respectively. However, many science texts will describe the compound as a whole (CrO_3, rather than Cr^{6+}) as the oxidizing or reducing agent.

Assigning Oxidation Numbers

It is important, of course, to know which atom is oxidized and which is reduced. **Oxidation numbers** are assigned to atoms in order to keep track of the redistribution of electrons during chemical reactions. Based on the oxidation numbers of the reactants and products, it is possible to determine how many electrons are gained or lost by each atom.

The oxidation number of an atom in a compound is assigned according to the following rules:

1. *The oxidation number of a free element is zero.* For example, the atoms in N_2, P_4, S_8, and He all have oxidation numbers of zero.
2. *The oxidation number for a monatomic ion is equal to the charge of the ion.* For example, the oxidation numbers for Na^+, Cu^{2+}, Fe^{3+}, Cl^-, and N^{3-} are +1, +2, +3, −1, and −3, respectively.
3. *The oxidation number of each Group IA element in a compound is +1.*
4. *The oxidation number of each Group IIA element in a compound is +2.*
5. *The oxidation number of each Group VIIA element in a compound is −1, except when combined with an element of higher electronegativity.* For example, in HCl, the oxidation number of Cl is −1; in HOCl, however, the oxidation number of Cl is +1.
6. *The oxidation number of hydrogen is usually +1; however, its oxidation number is −1 in compounds with less electronegative elements (Groups IA and IIA).* Hydrogen is +1 in HCl, but −1 in NaH.
7. *In most compounds, the oxidation number of oxygen is −2.* The two exceptions are peroxides (O_2^{2-}), for which the charge on each oxygen is −1, and compounds with more electronegative elements, such as OF_2, in which oxygen has a +2 charge.
8. *The sum of the oxidation numbers of all the atoms present in a neutral compound is zero. The sum of the oxidation numbers of the atoms present in a polyatomic ion is equal to the charge of the ion.* Thus, for (SO_4^{2-}), the sum of the oxidation numbers must be −2.

Consider the example in Figure 11.3 for an illustration of some of the above rules.

Examples of Oxidation Numbers

C (0) O_2 (0) H_2 (0) Zn (0)

Na^+ (+1) Ca^{2+} (+2) Cl^- (−1)

$KMnO_4$ (+1)(+7)(−2) ZnO (+2)(−2) HCl (+1)(−1) HCO_3^- (+1)(−2)

Figure 11.3 Examples of Oxidation Numbers Assigned to Atoms
The bottom row of molecules is color coded with assigned oxidation numbers.

BRIDGE

In Chapter 3 of *MCAT General Chemistry Review,* we illustrated that metals form cations and nonmetals form anions. To form a cation, a metal must lose electrons. Therefore, metals like to get oxidized (lose electrons) and act as good reducing agents. Nonmetals, on the other hand, like to get reduced (gain electrons) and act as good oxidizing agents.

MCAT EXPERTISE

Think of the oxidation number as the typical charge of an element based on its group number, metallicity, and general location in the periodic table.

KEY CONCEPT

The conventions of formula writing put cation first and anion second. Thus HCl implies H^+, and NaH implies H^-. Use the way the compound is written on the MCAT along with the periodic table to determine oxidation states.

Oxidation number is often confused with **formal charge**, discussed in Chapter 3 of *MCAT General Chemistry Review*. Both account for the perceived charge on an element, but do so in different ways. Oxidation number assumes unequal division of electrons in bonds, "awarding" the electrons to the more electronegative element. Formal charge, on the other hand, assumes equal division of electrons in bonds, "awarding" one electron to each atom in the bond. In reality, the distribution of electron density lies somewhere between these two extremes. The assigning of oxidation numbers can be seen in Figure 11.4.

MCAT EXPERTISE

Don't forget that you can click on "Periodic table" to pull it up on Test Day. Note the trends for assigning oxidation numbers; these general rules will help reduce the need to memorize individual oxidation numbers. Be aware that the transition metals can take on multiple oxidation states and therefore multiple oxidation numbers.

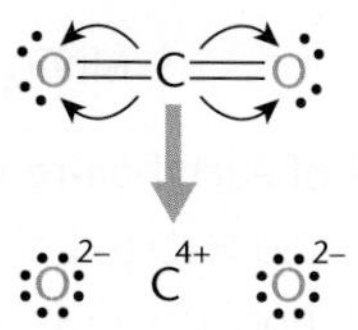

Figure 11.4 Assigning Oxidation Numbers to Carbon Dioxide

When assigning oxidation numbers, start with the known atoms (usually Groups I and II, halides, and oxygen) and use this information to determine the oxidation states of the other atoms. Keep in mind that most transition metals can take on multiple oxidation states. When transition metals are oxidized or reduced, the absorption and emission of light from a metal is altered such that different frequencies are absorbed. For this reason, changes of oxidation state in transition metals usually correspond to a color change.

Example: Assign oxidation numbers to the atoms in the following reaction to determine the oxidizing and reducing agents.

$$SnCl_2 + PbCl_4 \rightarrow SnCl_4 + PbCl_2$$

Solution: All of these species are neutral, so the oxidation numbers of each compound must add up to zero. In $SnCl_2$, tin must have an oxidation number of +2 because there are two chlorines present and each chlorine has an oxidation number of −1. Similarly, the oxidation number of Sn in $SnCl_4$ is +4; the oxidation number of Pb is +4 in $PbCl_4$ and +2 in $PbCl_2$.

The oxidation number of Sn goes from +2 to +4; it loses electrons and thus is oxidized, making it the reducing agent. Because the oxidation number of Pb has decreased from +4 to +2, it gains electrons and is reduced, making it the oxidizing agent. The sum of the charges on both sides of the reaction is equal to zero, so charge has been conserved. Keep in mind that oxidation state also plays a role in nomenclature; the reactants in this reaction would be called tin(II) chloride and lead(IV) chloride.

Balancing Oxidation–Reduction Reactions

By assigning oxidation numbers to the reactants and products, one can determine how many moles of each species are required for conservation of charge and mass, which is necessary to balance the equation. To balance a redox reaction, both the net charge and the number of atoms must be equal on both sides of the equation. The most common method for balancing redox equations is the **half-reaction method**, also known as the **ion–electron method**, in which the equation is separated into two half-reactions—the oxidation part and the reduction part. Each half-reaction is balanced separately, and they are then added to give a balanced overall reaction. While it is important to understand this process, it is unlikely that the MCAT will require you to perform a full balancing of a redox reaction.

KEY CONCEPT

Oxidizing agents oxidize *other* molecules, but are themselves *reduced*. Reducing agents reduce *other* molecules, but are themselves *oxidized*. If you determine one ion to be an oxidizing agent then the other must be a reducing agent.

MCAT EXPERTISE

Methodical, step-by-step approaches like the half-reaction method are great for the MCAT. Usually, you will not have to go through *all* of these steps before you can narrow down your answer choices and may be able to find the correct answer partway through the problem with a little critical thinking.

Example: Balance this redox reaction using the half-reaction method:

$$MnO_4^- + I^- \rightarrow I_2 + Mn^{2+}$$

Step 1: Separate the two half-reactions.

$$I^- \rightarrow I_2$$

$$MnO_4^- \rightarrow Mn^{2+}$$

Step 2: Balance the atoms of each half-reaction. First, balance all atoms except H and O. Next, in an acidic solution, add H_2O to balance the O atoms and then add H^+ to balance the H atoms. In a basic solution, use OH^- and H_2O to balance the O and H atoms.

$$2\ I^- \rightarrow I_2$$

$$MnO_4^- + 8\ H^+ \rightarrow Mn^{2+} + 4\ H_2O$$

Step 3: Balance the charges of each half-reaction. Add electrons as necessary to one side of the reaction so that the charges are equal on both sides.

$$2\ I^- \rightarrow I_2 + 2\ e^-$$

$$MnO_4^- + 8\ H^+ + 5\ e^- \rightarrow Mn^{2+} + 4\ H_2O$$

Step 4: Both half-reactions must have the same number of electrons so that they cancel each other out in the next step. In this example, you need to multiply the oxidation half-reaction by 5 and the reduction half-reaction by 2.

$$10\ I^- \rightarrow 5\ I_2 + 10\ e^-$$

$$2\ MnO_4^- + 16\ H^+ + 10\ e^- \rightarrow 2\ Mn^{2+} + 8\ H_2O$$

Step 5: Add the half-reactions, canceling out terms that appear on both sides of the reaction arrow.

$$2\ MnO_4^- + 16\ H^+ + 10\ I^- \rightarrow 2\ Mn^{2+} + 5\ I_2 + 8\ H_2O$$

Step 6: Confirm that mass and charge are balanced. There is a +4 net charge on each side of the reaction equation, and the atoms are stoichiometrically balanced.

MCAT CONCEPT CHECK 11.1

Before you move on, assess your understanding of the material with these questions.

1. For each of the reactions below, identify the oxidation states of the relevant atoms, the oxidizing agent, and the reducing agent:

Reaction	Oxidation Numbers	Oxidizing Agent	Reducing Agent
$2\ KI + H_2 \rightarrow 2\ K + 2\ HI$			
$Al + BPO_4 \rightarrow B + AlPO_4$			

2. Identify the oxidation and reduction half-reactions in the following redox reaction:

$$Zn + Cu^{2+} \rightarrow Zn^{2+} + Cu$$

- Oxidation:

- Reduction:

---

3. Balance the following redox reaction using the half-reaction method:

$$Mg\ (s) + HNO_3\ (aq) \rightarrow Mg^{2+}\ (aq) + NO\ (g)$$

11.2 Net Ionic Equations

LEARNING OBJECTIVES

After Chapter 11.2, you will be able to:

- Identify the element undergoing disproportionation and the oxidation state of the products for a given reaction
- Apply redox reaction principles to balance and solve application-style problems, such as ones that involve redox titrations
- Determine the net ionic equation for a reaction:

$$Zn\ (s) + CuSO_4\ (aq) \rightarrow Cu\ (s) + ZnSO_4\ (aq)$$

When we discussed reaction types in Chapter 4 of *MCAT General Chemistry Review*, we left out the rationale for why certain elements come together and others do not. Now that we have discussed oxidation–reduction reactions, it should be clearer that the gain and loss of electrons drives the formation of many compounds, especially ionic ones. Below, we will revisit many important reaction types and understand their basis in oxidation–reduction reactions.

Overview

In our discussion of acids and bases, we focused only on the presence of protons and hydroxide ions, with little concern for which species actually provided those ions. Similarly, in redox reactions, our focus is on the shifting of electrons more so than the identities of the ions themselves. Consider the following single-displacement reaction:

$$\text{Zn}\ (s) + \text{CuSO}_4\ (aq) \rightarrow \text{Cu}\ (s) + \text{ZnSO}_4\ (aq)$$

If we split the various species into all of the ions present, we get the **complete ionic equation**:

$$\text{Zn}\ (s) + \text{Cu}^{2+}\ (aq) + \text{SO}_4^{2-}\ (aq) \rightarrow \text{Cu}\ (s) + \text{Zn}^{2+}\ (aq) + \text{SO}_4^{2-}\ (aq)$$

Note that the sulfate ion is present on both sides of the equation in the same form; this ion is chemically inert during this reaction. In other words, the sulfate is not taking part in the overall reaction but simply remaining in the solution unchanged. We call such species **spectator ions**. Because the sulfate ion is not involved in the oxidation–reduction reaction, we can simplify the reaction to its **net ionic equation**, showing only the species that actually participate in the reaction:

$$\text{Zn}\ (s) + \text{Cu}^{2+}\ (aq) \rightarrow \text{Cu}\ (s) + \text{Zn}^{2+}\ (aq)$$

When writing net ionic equations, all aqueous compounds should be split into their constituent ions. Solid salts, on the other hand, should be kept together as a single entity. Let's return to some of the other reactions we have seen previously, including combination, decomposition, combustion, and double-displacement (metathesis) reactions.

MCAT EXPERTISE

Look for compounds such as polyatomic anions that retain their charge before and after reactions; these are usually spectator ions and will *not* be found in the net ionic equation.

Combination Reactions

In **combination reactions**, two or more species come together to form a product. Consider the example in Figure 11.5.

Reaction	(0) (0) (+1)(−1) $H_2(g) + F_2(g) \rightarrow 2HF(aq)$ oxidation reduction
Half-reactions	$H_2 \rightarrow 2H^+ + 2e^-$ $F_2 + 2e^- \rightarrow 2F^-$
Net ionic equation	$H_2 + F_2 \rightarrow 2H^+ + 2F^-$

Figure 11.5 Formation of Hydrogen Fluoride as an Example of Redox in a Combination Reaction

In this reaction, molecular hydrogen acts as a reducing agent as it reduces fluorine, turning hydrogen's oxidation state from 0 to +1. Molecular fluorine is the oxidizing agent as it oxidizes hydrogen, turning fluorine's oxidation state from 0 to −1. The half-reactions in the second row show that two electrons are transferred from hydrogen to fluorine. In this reaction, there is no spectator ion.

Decomposition Reactions

In **decomposition reactions**, one product breaks down into two or more species. See Figure 11.6 for an example.

Reaction	(−3)(+1) (+6) (−2) → (0) (+3) (−2) (+1)(−2) $(NH_4)_2Cr_2O_7(aq) \longrightarrow N_2(g) + Cr_2O_3(s) + 4\,H_2O(g)$ oxidation; reduction
Half-reactions	$2\,NH_4^+ \longrightarrow N_2 + 8\,H^+ + 6\,e^-$ $Cr_2O_7^{2-} + 8\,H^+ + 6\,e^- \longrightarrow Cr_2O_3 + 4\,H_2O$
Net ionic equation	$2\,NH_4^+ + Cr_2O_7^{2-} \longrightarrow N_2 + Cr_2O_3 + 4\,H_2O$

Figure 11.6 Redox of the Decomposition of Ammonium Chromate

In this reaction, the nitrogen atom in the ammonium cation acts as a reducing agent to reduce chromium, turning nitrogen's oxidation state from −3 to 0. The chromium in the dichromate anion acts as the oxidizing agent to oxidize ammonium, turning chromium's oxidation state from +6 to +3. In this reaction, there is no spectator ion. The half-reactions show that six electrons are transferred from ammonium to chromium. Note that the net ionic equation is not significantly different from the original balanced equation.

Combustion Reactions

In **combustion reactions**, a fuel (usually a hydrocarbon) is mixed with an oxidant (usually oxygen), forming carbon dioxide and water, as illustrated in Figure 11.7.

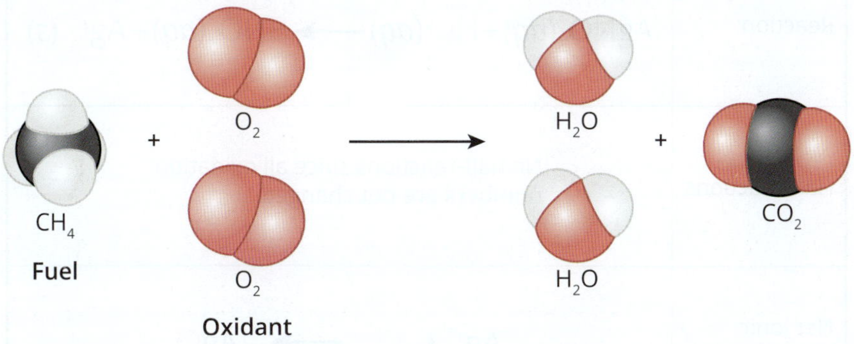

Figure 11.7 Combustion of Methane

The redox of a combustion reaction can be seen in Figure 11.8.

Reaction	(−4)(+1) (0) (+4)(−2) (+1)(−2) $CH_4(g) + 2O_2(g) \longrightarrow CO_2(g) + 2H_2O(g)$ oxidation reduction
Half-reactions	$CH_4 + 2H_2O \longrightarrow CO_2 + 8H^+ + 8e^-$ $2O_2 + 8H^+ + 8e^- \longrightarrow 4H_2O$
Net ionic equation	$CH_4 + 2O_2 \longrightarrow CO_2 + H_2O$

Figure 11.8 Redox of the Complete Combustion of Methane

The net ionic equation is identical to the overall balanced equation because there are no spectator ions and no aqueous species.

Combustion reactions can have complex half-reactions, depending on the type of fuel used. In this instance, carbon in methane is the reducing agent to reduce oxygen, turning carbon's oxidation state from −4 to +4. Molecular oxygen is the oxidizing agent as it oxidizes methane, turning oxygen's oxidation state from 0 to −2. The half-reactions show that eight electrons are transferred from methane to oxygen.

Double-Displacement (Metathesis) Reactions

Double-displacement, metathesis, or **ping-pong reactions** involve the switching of counterions. Because all ions generally retain their oxidation state, these are not usually oxidation–reduction reactions. An example of a double-displacement reaction is seen in Figure 11.9.

Reaction	(+1) (−1) (+1)(−1) (+1)(−1) (+1)(−1) $AgNO_3(aq) + HCl(aq) \longrightarrow HNO_3(aq) + AgCl(s)$
Half-reactions	No half-reactions since all oxidation numbers are not changed
Net ionic equation	$Ag^+ + Cl^- \longrightarrow AgCl$

Figure 11.9 Double-Displacement of Sliver Nitrate and Hydrochloric Acid

Because all species retain the same oxidation numbers, this is not considered oxidation–reduction. The nitrate anion and hydrogen cation both act as spectator ions in this reaction, so they are not present in the net ionic equation.

In double-displacement reactions where both reactants and both products are aqueous, there is no net ionic reaction. For example:

$$\overset{+1}{\text{Na}}\overbrace{\text{NO}_3}^{-1}\,(aq) + \overset{+1}{\text{H}}\,\overset{-1}{\text{Cl}}\,(aq) \rightarrow \overset{+1}{\text{H}}\overbrace{\text{NO}_3}^{-1}\,(aq) + \overset{+1}{\text{Na}}\,\overset{-1}{\text{Cl}}\,(aq)$$

This reaction is not an oxidation–reduction reaction because no species change their oxidation states. Further, because all species are aqueous, the complete ionic reaction is:

$$\text{Na}^+ + \text{NO}_3^- + \text{H}^+ + \text{Cl}^- \rightarrow \text{H}^+ + \text{NO}_3^- + \text{Na}^+ + \text{Cl}^-$$

Because all of the ions appear on both sides of the reaction, there is no net ionic reaction.

Disproportionation Reactions

Disproportionation (or **dismutation**) is a specific type of redox reaction in which an element undergoes both oxidation and reduction in producing its products. Many biological enzymes utilize a disproportionation mechanism. An example of such a reaction is the catalysis of peroxides by *catalase*, an enzyme found in peroxisomes. Catalase is a critical biological enzyme used to protect cells from excessive oxidation by free radicals or reactive oxygen species. The activity of catalase can be seen when disinfecting a wound with hydrogen peroxide. The disproportionation of hydrogen peroxide is seen in Figure 11.10.

Reaction	$2\,\overset{(+1)(-1)}{\text{H}_2\text{O}_2}(aq) \xrightarrow{\text{catalase}} 2\,\overset{(+1)(-2)}{\text{H}_2\text{O}}(l) + \overset{(0)}{\text{O}_2}(g)$ (reduction; oxidation)
Half-reactions	$\text{H}_2\text{O}_2 + 2\text{H}^+ + 2e^- \longrightarrow 2\,\text{H}_2\text{O}$ $\text{H}_2\text{O}_2 \longrightarrow \text{O}_2 + 2\text{H}^+ + 2e^-$
Net ionic equation	$2\,\text{H}_2\text{O}_2 \longrightarrow 2\,\text{H}_2\text{O} + \text{O}_2$

Figure 11.10 Redox of Disproportionation of Hydrogen Peroxide

As can be seen from this reaction, oxygen is disproportioned between water and molecular oxygen. In hydrogen peroxide, each oxygen has an oxidation state of -1 (the peroxide ion has a charge of -2 overall). In water, oxygen has an oxidation state of -2, and in molecular oxygen, it has an oxidation state of 0. Therefore, the oxygen is both reduced and oxidized in this reaction. The half-reactions show that two electrons are transferred from hydrogen peroxide to form molecular oxygen and water.

Another related biological disproportionation mechanism is that of the enzyme *superoxide dismutase*. As the name implies, a *dismutase* catalyzes dismutation. This enzyme disproportions oxygen free radicals in the reaction shown in Figure 11.11.

Reaction	Oxidation states: $O_2^{\bullet-}$ (−½), H^+ (+1), H_2O_2 (+1)(−1), O_2 (0) $2\,O_2^{\bullet-}(aq) + 2\,H^+(aq) \xrightarrow{\text{dismutase}} H_2O_2(aq) + O_2(g)$ reduction: $O_2^{\bullet-} \rightarrow H_2O_2$; oxidation: $O_2^{\bullet-} \rightarrow O_2$
Half-reactions	$O_2^{\bullet-} \longrightarrow O_2 + e^-$ $O_2^{\bullet-} + 2\,H^+ + e^- \longrightarrow H_2O_2$
Net ionic equation	$2\,O_2^{\bullet-} + 2\,H^+ \longrightarrow H_2O_2 + O_2$

Figure 11.11 Redox of Disproportionation of Oxygen Free Radical

Hydrogen peroxide and oxygen are the disproportioned products. The oxidation state of oxygen in the free radical is $-\frac{1}{2}$ (a negative charge divided over two oxygen atoms), and it is reduced to -1 in the peroxide and oxidized to 0 in molecular oxygen. The half-reactions show that one electron is transferred from the oxygen free radical to form hydrogen peroxide and molecular oxygen.

Biochemical disproportionation reactions—and oxidation–reduction reactions in biological systems in general—are usually accomplished by enzymes. Structurally, these enzymes often have metals such as Cu (copper) and Zn (zinc) in their active sites that act as reducing agents, as shown in Figure 11.12.

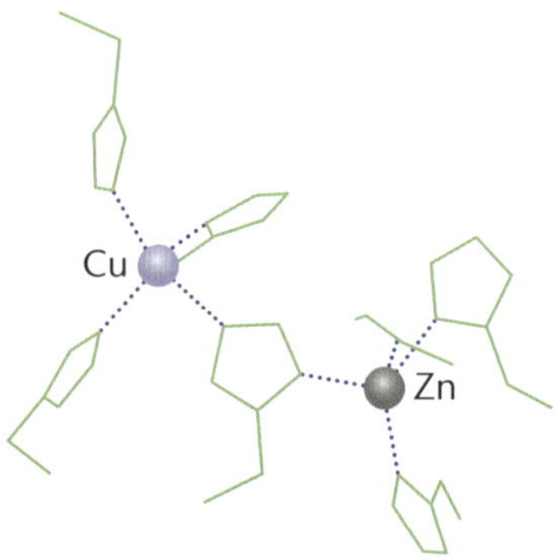

Figure 11.12 Active Site of Superoxide Dismutase
Cu and Zn atoms act as reducing agents, losing electrons during catalysis. The atoms are stabilized in position by histidine residues.

Oxidation–Reduction Titrations

Oxidation–reduction titrations are similar in setup to acid–base titrations, but the focus is different. Whereas acid–base titrations follow the movement of protons, as discussed in Chapter 10 of *MCAT General Chemistry Review*, redox titrations follow the transfer of charge (as electrons) to reach the equivalence point. Redox titrations can utilize indicators that change color at a particular voltage (emf) value. Some common indicators are listed in Table 11.2. As for acid–base titrations, it is not necessary to memorize these indicators, but rather to understand their utility.

Indicator	Voltage of Color Change	Oxidized Form	Reduced Form
Bipyridine metal complexes	About +1 V	Colorless (Ru), Cyan (Fe)	Yellow (Ru), Red (Fe)
Diphenylamine	+0.76 V	Violet	Colorless
Safranin	+0.24/−0.29 V*	Red-Violet	Colorless

* Safranin is unique in that its color change is not only voltage dependent, but also pH dependent.

Table 11.2 Common Indicators for Oxidation–Reduction (Redox) Titrations

One prototypical redox titration involves the use of starch indicators to identify iodine complexes. This specific redox titration is called an iodimetric titration because it relies on the titration of free iodine radicals. The presence of iodine is initially determined by a dark solution in the presence of starch, and at the endpoint of the titration, a colorless solution develops. A common general chemistry laboratory experiment involves the standardization of a thiosulfate solution using iodimetry, as described in the example below.

Example: A group of students prepares to standardize a $Na_2S_2O_3$ solution. 32 mL of the $Na_2S_2O_3$ solution is titrated into 50 mL of a 0.01 M KIO_3 solution to reach the equivalence point. They first titrate the KIO_3 solution until it loses color, then add a starch indicator until the reaction is complete. The reaction proceeds in these two steps:

$$IO_3^- + I^- + H^+ \rightarrow I_3^- + H_2O$$

$$I_3^- + S_2O_3^{2-} \rightarrow I^- + S_4O_6^{2-}$$

Determine the concentration of the sodium thiosulfate solution at the beginning of the experiment.

Solution: The titration is performed in two steps. In the first step, the iodate is converted into triiodide anions. The initial titration creates a colorless I_3^- solution in water, which then requires a starch indicator for the remainder of the titration.

In the second step, the triiodide ions are then reduced in the presence of thiosulfate to determine its concentration. Note that the reactions are unbalanced. It would be tempting to balance the first equation as:

$$IO_3^- + 2\,I^- + 6\,H^+ \rightarrow I_3^- + 3\,H_2O$$

However, this reaction has a charge of +3 on the reactants side and −1 on the products side. In oxidation-reduction chemistry, we must balance not only for stoichiometry but also for charge. The correct balanced equations are:

$$IO_3^- + 8\,I^- + 6\,H^+ \rightarrow 3\,I_3^- + 3\,H_2O$$

$$I_3^- + 2\,S_2O_3^{2-} \rightarrow 3\,I^- + S_4O_6^{2-}$$

Keeping in mind that each iodate is used to make three triiodide anions, and each triiodide anion interacts with two thiosulfate anions, the mole ratio of thiosulfate to iodate is six to one:

$$IO_3^- + 8\,I^- + 6\,H^+ \rightarrow 3\,I_3^- + 3\,H_2O$$

$$3\,I_3^- + 6\,S_2O_3^{2-} \rightarrow 9\,I^- + 3\,S_4O_6^{2-}$$

Then, use stoichiometry to determine the molarity of the thiosulfate solution from the 50 mL potassium iodate solution.

$$0.01\text{ M } IO_3^-[0.05\text{ L}]\left[\frac{6\text{ mol } S_2O_3^{2-}}{1\text{ mol } IO_3^-}\right] = 3\times10^{-3}\text{ mol}$$

Now, we can use the volume to find the molarity.

$$M_{S_2O_3^{2-}} = \frac{3\times10^{-3}\text{ mol}}{32\text{ mL}\left[\frac{1\text{ L}}{1000\text{ mL}}\right]} = \frac{3\times10^{-3}}{32\times10^{-3}} \approx \frac{3}{30} = 0.1\text{ M (actual} = 0.094\text{ M)}$$

Potentiometric titration is a form of redox titration where no indicator is used. Instead, the electrical potential difference (voltage) is measured using a voltmeter. As a redox titration progresses, its voltage changes; this is analogous to following an acid–base titration with a pH meter instead of a color indicator.

MCAT CONCEPT CHECK 11.2

Before you move on, assess your understanding of the material with these questions.

1. Write the net ionic equations for the reactions below:
   - $CuNO_3\ (aq) + NaCl\ (aq) \rightarrow CuCl\ (s) + NaNO_3\ (aq)$

   ____

   - $Mg\ (s) + AlCl_3\ (aq) \rightarrow Al\ (s) + MgCl_2\ (aq)$

   ____

2. In each of the reactions below, which element undergoes disproportionation? What are that element's oxidation states in the products?

$$3\,Cl_2\ (g) + 6\,NaOH\ (aq) \rightarrow 5\,NaCl\ (aq) + NaClO_3\ (aq) + 3\,H_2O\ (l)$$

$$S_2O_3^{2-}\ (aq) + 2\,H^+\ (aq) \rightarrow S\ (s) + SO_2\ (g) + H_2O\ (l)$$

   - Element undergoing disproportionation:

   ____

   - Oxidation states in products:

   ____

- Element undergoing disproportionation:

- Oxidation states in products:

---

3. A sample is assayed for lead by a redox titration with I_3^- (*aq*). A 10.00 g sample is crushed, dissolved in sulfuric acid, and passed over a reducing agent so that all the lead is in the form Pb^{2+}. The Pb^{2+} (*aq*) is completely oxidized to Pb^{4+} by 32.60 mL of a 0.7 M solution of NaI_3. The balanced equation for the reaction is:

$$I_3^- + (aq) + Pb^{2+}\ (aq) \rightarrow Pb^{4+}\ (aq) + 3\ I^-\ (aq)$$

Calculate the mass of lead in the sample.

Conclusion

In this chapter, we covered the essential MCAT topic of oxidation–reduction reactions. We reviewed the rules for assigning oxidation numbers to help us keep track of the movement of electrons from the species that are oxidized (reducing agents) to the species that are reduced (oxidizing agents). We also covered the sequence of steps involved in balancing half-reactions, redox titrations, and disproportionation reactions.

In addition to understanding the fundamental chemical principles behind these reactions, you will begin to see these concepts resurface in *MCAT Organic Chemistry Review* and *MCAT Biochemistry Review*. Oxidation–reduction reactions are often used for energy transfer in biological systems, and any deficiencies in such systems are profoundly deleterious (such as metabolic, mitochondrial, and immunologic diseases). Our next chapter—the last of *MCAT General Chemistry Review*—brings the principles of oxidation–reduction reactions to their application in electrochemical cells. By the end of the next chapter, you will have reviewed all of the general chemistry knowledge required for Test Day!

GO ONLINE

You've reviewed the content, now test your knowledge and critical thinking skills by completing a test-like passage set in your online resources!

CONCEPT SUMMARY

Oxidation–Reduction Reactions

- **Oxidation** is a loss of electrons, and **reduction** is a gain of electrons; the two are paired together in what is known as an **oxidation–reduction** (**redox**) reaction.
- An **oxidizing agent** facilitates the oxidation of another compound and is reduced itself in the process; a **reducing agent** facilitates the reduction of another compound and is itself oxidized in the process.
  - Common oxidizing agents almost all contain oxygen or a similarly electronegative element.
  - Common reducing agents often contain metal ions or hydrides (H^-).
- To assign oxidation numbers, one must know the common oxidation states of the representative elements.
  - Any free element or diatomic species has an oxidation number of zero.
  - The oxidation number of a monatomic ion is equal to the charge of the ion.
  - When in compounds, Group IA metals have an oxidation number of $+1$; Group IIA metals have an oxidation number of $+2$.
  - When in compounds, Group VIIA elements have an oxidation number of -1 (unless combined with an element with higher electronegativity).
  - The oxidation state of hydrogen is $+1$ unless it is paired with a less electronegative element, in which case it is -1.
  - The oxidation state of oxygen is usually -2, except in peroxides (when its charge is -1) or in compounds with more electronegative elements.
  - The sum of the oxidation numbers of all the atoms present in a compound is equal to the overall charge of that compound.
- When balancing redox reactions, the **half-reaction method**, also called the **ion–electron method**, is the most common.
  - Separate the two half-reactions.
  - Balance the atoms of each half-reaction. Start with all the elements besides H and O. In acidic solution, balance H and O using water and H^+. In basic solution, balance H and O using water and OH^-.
  - Balance the charges of each half-reaction by adding electrons as necessary to one side of the reaction.
  - Multiply the half-reactions as necessary to obtain the same number of electrons in both half-reactions.
  - Add the half-reactions, canceling out terms on both sides of the reaction arrow.
  - Confirm that the mass and charge are balanced.

Net Ionic Equations

- A **complete ionic equation** accounts for all of the ions present in a reaction. To write a complete ionic reaction, split all aqueous compounds into their relevant ions. Keep solid salts intact.
- **Net ionic equations** ignore spectator ions to focus only on the species that actually participate in the reaction. To obtain a net ionic reaction, subtract the ions appearing on both sides of the reaction, which are called **spectator ions**.

- For reactions that contain no aqueous salts, the net ionic equation is generally the same as the overall balanced reaction.
- For double displacement (metathesis) reactions that do not form a solid salt, there is no net ionic reaction because all ions remain in solution and do not change oxidation number.

- **Disproportionation (dismutation) reactions** are a type of redox reaction in which one element is both oxidized and reduced, forming at least two molecules containing the element with different oxidation states.
- **Oxidation–reduction titrations** are similar in methodology to acid–base titrations. These titrations follow transfer of charge.
    - Indicators used in such titrations change color when certain voltages of solutions are achieved.
    - **Potentiometric titration** is a form of redox titration in which a voltmeter or external cell measures the electromotive force (emf) of a solution. No indicator is used, and the equivalence point is determined by a sharp change in voltage.

ANSWERS TO CONCEPT CHECKS

11.1

1.

Reaction	Oxidation Numbers	Oxidizing Agent	Reducing Agent
$2\,KI + H_2 \rightarrow 2\,K + 2\,HI$	$2\,\overset{+1}{K}\overset{-1}{I} + \overset{0}{H_2} \rightarrow 2\,\overset{0}{K} + 2\,\overset{+1}{H}\overset{-1}{I}$	K^+ (charge goes from +1 to 0)	H_2 (charge goes from 0 to +1)
$Al + BPO_4 \rightarrow B + AlPO^4$	$\overset{0}{Al} + \overset{+3}{B}\overset{-3}{PO_4} \rightarrow \overset{0}{B} + \overset{+3}{Al}\overset{-3}{PO_4}$	B^{3+} (charge goes from +3 to 0)	Al (charge goes from 0 to +3)

2. Oxidation: $Zn \rightarrow Zn^{2+} + 2\,e^-$

   Reduction: $Cu^{2+} + 2\,e^- \rightarrow Cu$

3. 1. $\begin{cases} Mg \rightarrow Mg^{2+} \\ HNO_3 \rightarrow NO \end{cases}$

   2. $\begin{cases} Mg \rightarrow Mg^{2+} \\ HNO_3 + 3\,H^+ \rightarrow NO + 2\,H_2O \end{cases}$

   3. $\begin{cases} Mg \rightarrow Mg^{2+} + 2\,e^- \\ HNO_3 + 3\,H^+ + 3\,e^- \rightarrow NO + 2\,H_2O \end{cases}$

   4. $\begin{cases} 3\,Mg \rightarrow 3\,Mg^{2+} + 6\,e^- \\ 2\,HNO_3 + 6\,H^+ + 6\,e^- \rightarrow 2\,NO + 4\,H_2O \end{cases}$

   5. $2\,HNO_3 + 3\,Mg + 6\,H^+ \rightarrow 2\,NO + 3\,Mg^{2+} + 4\,H_2O$

11.2

1. $Cu^+ + Cl^- \rightarrow CuCl$
   $3\,Mg + 2\,Al^{3+} \rightarrow 3\,Mg^{2+} + 2\,Al$ (don't forget to balance the reaction!)
2. In the first reaction, chlorine undergoes disproportionation to have a −1 oxidation state in NaCl and a +5 oxidation state in $NaClO_3$.

   In the second reaction, sulfur undergoes disproportionation to have a 0 oxidation state in elemental sulfur and +4 oxidation state in SO_2.

3. $0.7\text{ M } I_3^-[32.60 \times 10^{-3}\text{ L}]\left[\frac{1\text{ mol }Pb^{2+}}{1\text{ mol }I_3^-}\right]\left[\frac{207.2\text{ g }Pb^{2+}}{1\text{ mol }Pb^{2+}}\right] \approx 0.7 \times 3 \times 2 = 4.2\text{ g}$

   (actual = 4.73 g)

   Note that question 3 also included the extraneous value 10.0 g, which is not needed to calculate the mass of lead produced.

SCIENCE MASTERY ASSESSMENT EXPLANATIONS

1. **C**

The oxidizing agent is the species that is reduced in any given equation. In this problem, six hydrogen atoms with +1 oxidation states in NH_3 are reduced to three neutral H_2 molecules.

2. **B**

First, balance the atoms in the equation:

$$Cr_2O_7^{2-} + 14\ H^+ \rightarrow 2\ Cr^{2+} + 7\ H_2O$$

Now, adjust the number of electrons to balance the charge. Currently, the left side has a charge of +12 (−2 from dichromate and +14 from protons). The right side has a charge of +4 (+2 from each chromium cation). To decrease the charge on the left side from +12 to +4, we should add 8 electrons:

$$Cr_2O_7^{2-} + 14\ H^+ + 8\ e^- \rightarrow 2\ Cr^{2+} + 7\ H_2O$$

3. **A**

Hydride ions are composed of a hydrogen nucleus with two electrons, thereby giving it a negative charge and a considerable tendency to donate electrons. $LiAlH_4$ is therefore a strong reducing agent. Strong reducing agents tend to have metals or hydrides; strong oxidizing agents tend to have oxygen or a similarly electronegative element.

4. **C**

In NaClO (sodium hypochlorite), sodium carries its typical +1 charge, and oxygen carries its typical −2 charge. This means that the chlorine atom must carry a +1 charge in order to balance the overall charge of zero.

5. **D**

A strong oxidizing agent will be easily reduced, meaning that it will have a tendency to gain electrons. Atoms usually gain electrons if they are one or two electrons away from filling up their valence shell. **(A)** has a full 4*s*-orbital, meaning that it can only gain an electron if it gains an entire subshell. **(B)** has a stable, half-full 3*d*-orbital, so it is unlikely to pick up electrons unless it can gain five. **(C)** has only a single electron in the outer shell, which is more likely lost upon ionization. **(D)** would fill up its 4*p*-orbital by gaining one electron, so it is easily reduced.

6. **D**

A net ionic equation represents each of the aqueous ions comprising the reactants and products as individual ions, instead of combining them as formula units. Thus, **(A)** is not a net ionic reaction. The term *net* means that the correct answer does not include any spectator ions (ions that do not participate in the reaction). In this reaction, nitrate (NO_3^-) remains unchanged. Therefore, **(B)** and **(C)** are eliminated.

7. **C**

What you are shown is a net ionic equation. If two moles of FeSCN are created, two moles of Fe^{3+} must be used because the mole ratio is 1:1. Iron sulfate has the formula $Fe_2(SO_4)_3$ because sulfate has a charge of −2 and iron has a charge of +3 (based on the net ionic equation). Therefore, one mole of iron sulfate is needed to make two moles of iron for the reaction. The molar mass of iron sulfate is

$$2 \times 55.8\frac{g}{mol} + 3 \times 32.1\frac{g}{mol} + 12 \times 16.0\frac{g}{mol} = 399.9\frac{g}{mol}$$

This most closely matches answer **(C)**. The most common error would be to calculate the amount of iron, which would be 111.6 g, **(A)**.

8. **D**

When assigning oxidation numbers, one starts with elements of known oxidation state first, and determines the oxidation state of the other elements by deduction. As a noble gas, argon, **(A)**, will always have an oxidation state of 0. As a Group VIIA element, fluorine, **(B)**, will have an oxidation state of 0 (by itself) or −1 (in a compound). As a Group IIA element, strontium, **(C)**, will have an oxidation state of 0 (by itself) or +2 (in a compound). Like most transition metals, iridium, **(D)**, can have various oxidation states, ranging from −3 to +8. Therefore, one would have to determine the oxidation states of other atoms in an iridium-containing compound to determine iridium's oxidation number.

9. **A**

The formula for methanol is H_3COH, for methanal is HCHO, and for methanoic acid is HCOOH. If we assign oxidation numbers to carbon in each molecule, it starts at -2, then becomes 0, then becomes $+2$:

$$\overset{+1}{H_3}\overset{-2}{C}\overset{-2}{O}\overset{+1}{H} \rightarrow \overset{+1}{H}\overset{0}{C}\overset{+1}{H}\overset{-2}{O} \rightarrow \overset{+1}{H}\overset{+2}{C}\overset{-2}{O}\overset{-2}{O}\overset{+1}{H}$$

In general, it is often easier to think of oxidation as a gain of bonds to oxygen (or a similarly electronegative element) or loss of bonds to hydrogen for organic compounds. Therefore, because the carbon is oxidized as one converts from an alcohol to an aldehyde to a carboxylic acid, the oxidation number must increase.

10. **C**

Start with the atoms that have oxidation states of which you are certain. Potassium is a Group IA metal, and therefore must have an oxidation state of $+1$. Hydrogen is almost always $+1$, unless it is paired with a less electronegative element (which is not the case here). Oxygen is generally -2. Because there are four oxygens, they create a total negative charge of -8 which is partially balanced by two hydrogens ($+2$) and potassium ($+1$). Therefore, phosphorus has a $+5$ charge, making it the highest oxidation state.

11. **B**

Recall that oxygen has an oxidation state of -2. Therefore, in tungsten(IV) oxide, **(A)**, tungsten has an oxidation state of $+4$. In tungsten(VI) oxide, **(B)**, it has an oxidation state of $+6$. In tungsten(III) oxide, **(C)**, it is $+3$. In tungsten pentoxide, **(D)**, it is $+5$.

12. **A**

Step I is a disproportionation reaction because chlorine starts with an oxidation state of 0 in the reactants and ends up with an oxidation state of $+1$ in HOCl and -1 as Cl^-. In the other reactions, no element appears with different oxidation states in two different products. Therefore, only step I is a disproportionation reaction.

13. **C**

Potentiometry refers to carrying out an oxidation–reduction titration with a voltmeter present to get precise readings of the reaction's electromotive force (emf) to determine the endpoint. This is analogous to using a pH meter in an acid–base titration because it uses technology to get precise readings for plotting a titration curve. Indicators, as in **(A)** and **(B),** can be used in both acid–base and redox titrations, but provide a qualitative (rather than quantitative) analysis of the titration. Oxidizing and reducing agents are used in redox titrations, not acid–base titrations, eliminating **(D)**.

14. **D**

Utilize the method described earlier to balance this redox reaction. The balanced half-reactions are:

$$S_8 + 24\,H_2O \rightarrow 8\,SO_3^{2-} + 48\,H^+ + 32\,e^-$$

$$NO_3^- + 4\,H^+ + 3\,e^- \rightarrow NO + 2\,H_2O$$

To get equal numbers of electrons in each half-reaction, the oxidation half-reaction will have to be multiplied by 3, and the reduction half-reaction will have to be multiplied by 32:

$$3\,S_8 + 72\,H_2O \rightarrow 24\,SO_3^{2-} + 144\,H^+ + 96\,e^-$$

$$32\,NO_3^- + 128\,H^+ + 96\,e^- \rightarrow 32\,NO + 64\,H_2O$$

This makes the overall reaction:

$$3\,S_8 + 32\,NO_3^- + 8\,H_2O \rightarrow 24\,SO_3^{2-} + 32\,NO + 16\,H^+$$

The sum of the stoichiometric coefficients is therefore: $3 + 32 + 8 + 24 + 32 + 16 = 115$.

15. **C**

First, balance the chemical equation:

$$4\,Au + 8\,NaCN + O_2 + 2\,H_2O \rightarrow 4\,Na[Au(CN)_2] + 4\,NaOH$$

Now, determine the number of moles of NaCN used in the reaction:

$$0.1\ L \times 2\,\frac{mol}{L} = 0.2\ mol\ NaCN$$

If 0.2 mol NaCN are used in the reaction, then 0.2 mol NaCN $\times \dfrac{4\ mol\ Au}{8\ mol\ NaCN} = 0.1$ mol Au is oxidized.

GO ONLINE

Consult your online resources for additional practice.

SHARED CONCEPTS

Biochemistry Chapter 2
Enzymes

Biochemistry Chapter 10
Carbohydrate Metabolism II

Biology Chapter 7
The Cardiovascular System

General Chemistry Chapter 10
Acids and Bases

General Chemistry Chapter 12
Electrochemistry

Organic Chemistry Chapter 4
Analyzing Organic Reactions

CHAPTER 12

ELECTROCHEMISTRY

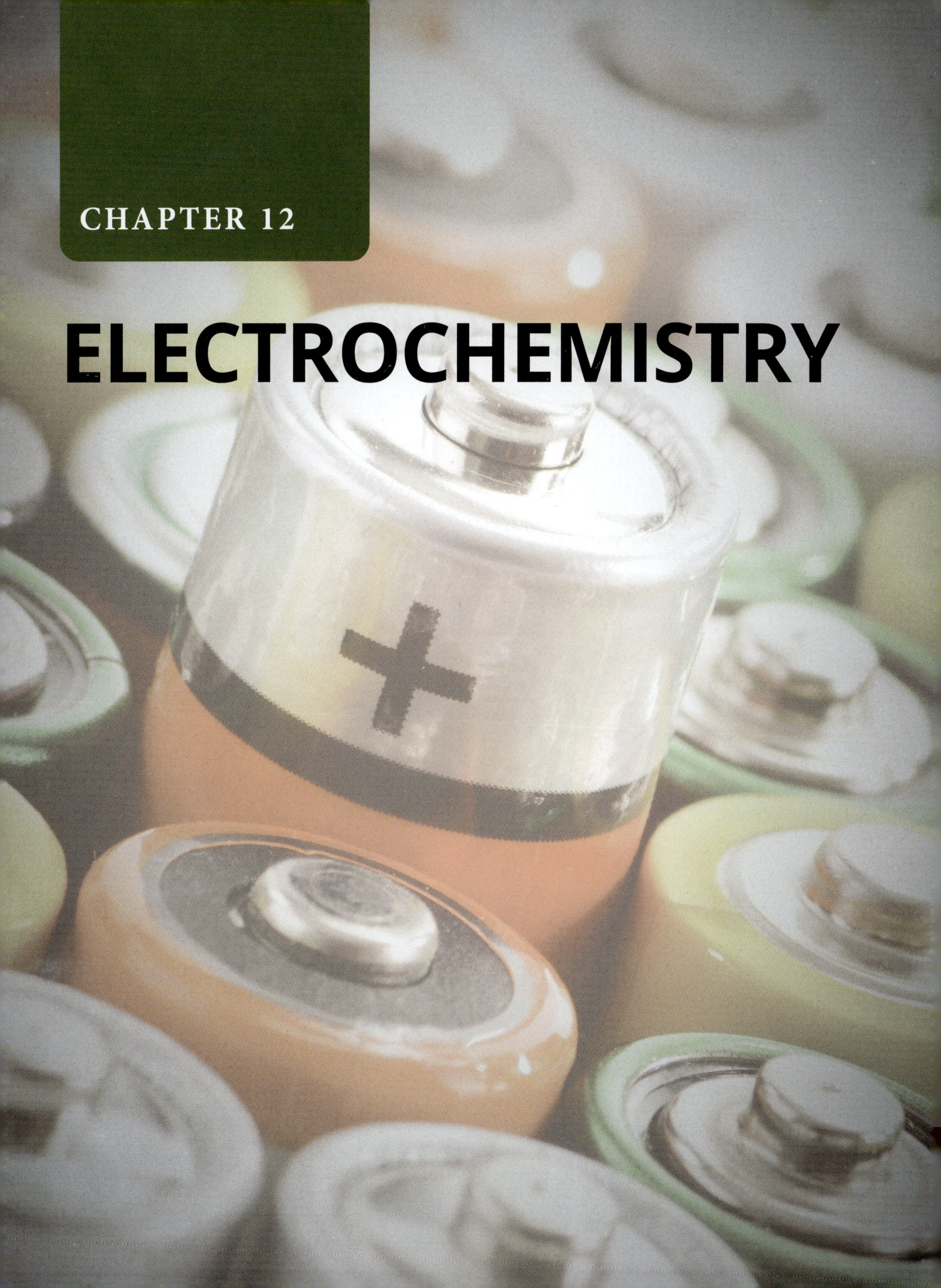

SCIENCE MASTERY ASSESSMENT

Every pre-med knows this feeling: there is so much content I have to know for the MCAT! How do I know what to do first or what's important?

While the high-yield badges throughout this book will help you identify the most important topics, this Science Mastery Assessment is another tool in your MCAT prep arsenal. This quiz (which can also be taken in your online resources) and the guidance below will help ensure that you are spending the appropriate amount of time on this chapter based on your personal strengths and weaknesses. Don't worry though—skipping something now does not mean you'll never study it. Later on in your prep, as you complete full-length tests, you'll uncover specific pieces of content that you need to review and can come back to these chapters as appropriate.

How to Use This Assessment

If you answer 0–7 questions correctly:

Spend about 1 hour to read this chapter in full and take limited notes throughout. Follow up by reviewing **all** quiz questions to ensure that you now understand how to solve each one.

If you answer 8–11 questions correctly:

Spend 20–40 minutes reviewing the quiz questions. Beginning with the questions you missed, read and take notes on the corresponding subchapters. For questions you answered correctly, ensure your thinking matches that of the explanation and you understand why each choice was correct or incorrect.

If you answer 12–15 questions correctly:

Spend less than 20 minutes reviewing all questions from the quiz. If you missed any, then include a quick read-through of the corresponding subchapters, or even just the relevant content within a subchapter, as part of your question review. For questions you answered correctly, ensure your thinking matches that of the explanation and review the Concept Summary at the end of the chapter.

1. Rusting occurs due to the oxidation–reduction reaction of iron with environmental oxygen:

$$4\ Fe\ (s) + 3\ O_2\ (g) \rightarrow 2\ Fe_2O_3\ (s)$$

Some metals cannot react with oxygen in this fashion.

Which of the following best explains why iron can?

A. Iron has a more positive reduction potential than those metals, making it more likely to donate electrons to oxygen.
B. Iron has a more positive reduction potential than those metals, making it more likely to accept electrons from oxygen.
C. Iron has a less positive reduction potential than those metals, making it more likely to donate electrons to oxygen.
D. Iron has a less positive reduction potential than those metals, making it more likely to accept electrons from oxygen.

2. Given the following standard reduction potentials:

$Zn^{2+} + 2\ e^- \rightarrow Zn$ $\quad E^\circ_{red} = -0.763\ V$

$Ag^+ + e^- \rightarrow Ag$ $\quad E^\circ_{red} = +0.337\ V$

What is the standard electromotive force of the following reaction?

$$Zn^{2+} + 2\ Ag \rightarrow 2\ Ag^+ + Zn$$

A. -2.2 V
B. -1.1 V
C. $+1.1$ V
D. $+2.2$ V

3. Consider the following data:

$Hg^{2+} + 2\ e^- \rightarrow Hg$ $\quad E^\circ_{red} = +0.85\ V$

$Cu^+ + e^- \rightarrow Cu$ $\quad E^\circ_{red} = +0.52\ V$

$Zn^{2+} + 2\ e^- \rightarrow Zn$ $\quad E^\circ_{red} = -0.76\ V$

$Al^{3+} + 3\ e^- \rightarrow Al$ $\quad E^\circ_{red} = -1.66\ V$

The anode of a certain galvanic cell is composed of copper. Which of the metals from the data table can be used at the cathode, assuming equal concentrations of the two electrolyte solutions?

A. Hg
B. Cu
C. Zn
D. Al

4. An electrolytic cell is filled with water. Which of the following will move toward the cathode of such a cell?

I. H^+ ions
II. O^{2-} ions
III. Electrons

A. I only
B. II only
C. I and III only
D. II and III only

5. If the value of E°_{cell} is known, what other data is needed to calculate ΔG°?

A. Equilibrium constant
B. Reaction quotient
C. Temperature of the system
D. Half-reactions of the cells

6. Which of the following compounds is LEAST likely to be found in the salt bridge of a galvanic cell?
   A. NaCl
   B. SO_3
   C. $MgSO_3$
   D. NH_4NO_3

7. If the surface area of electrode material in an electrochemical cell is tripled, what else is necessarily tripled?
   I. E°_{cell}
   II. Current
   III. K_{eq}

   A. I only
   B. II only
   C. I and II only
   D. II and III only

8. Which of the following can alter the emf of an electrochemical cell?
   A. The mass of the electrodes
   B. The length of the wire connecting the half-cells
   C. The overall size of the battery
   D. The temperature of the solutions in the half-cells

9. Which of the following statements could be true about a Na–Cd cell, based on the information below?

$$Na^+ + e^- \rightarrow Na \qquad E^\circ_{red} = -2.71 \text{ V}$$

$$Cd^{2+} + 2e^- \rightarrow Cd \qquad E^\circ_{red} = -0.40 \text{ V}$$

   A. It is a galvanic cell, and sodium is the cathode.
   B. It is an electrolytic cell, and cadmium is the anode.
   C. It is a galvanic cell, with $E^\circ_{cell} = 3.11$ V.
   D. It is an electrolytic cell, with $E^\circ_{cell} = -3.11$ V.

10. Which of the following expressions correctly describes the relationship between standard electromotive force and standard change in free energy?
   A. $\Delta G^\circ = -nF(E^\circ_{red,anode} - E^\circ_{red,cathode})$
   B. $E^\circ_{cell} = \frac{nF}{RT} \ln K_{eq}$
   C. $E^\circ_{cell} = -\frac{RT}{nF} \ln K_{eq}$
   D. $\Delta G^\circ = nF(E^\circ_{red,anode} - E^\circ_{red,cathode})$

11. Which of the following choices is indicative of a spontaneous reaction, assuming standard conditions?
   A. E°_{cell} is negative.
   B. $Q = K_{eq}$
   C. The cell is a concentration cell.
   D. $K_{eq} > 1$

12. For a cell with the following half-reactions:

Anode: $SO_2 + 2\ H_2O \rightarrow SO_4^{2-} + 4\ H^+ + 2\ e^-$

Cathode: $Pd^{2+} + 2\ e^- \rightarrow Pd$

How would decreasing the pH of the solution inside the cell affect the electromotive force (emf)?
   A. The emf would decrease.
   B. The emf would remain the same.
   C. The emf would increase.
   D. The emf would become zero.

13. An electrolytic cell necessarily has:
   A. $\Delta S^\circ > 0$
   B. $\Delta G^\circ < 0$
   C. $K_{eq} < 1$
   D. $E^\circ_{cell} > 0$

14. Which of the following is the best explanation for the fact that a larger mass of electrodes are required for lead–acid batteries, as compared to other batteries, to produce a certain current?

A. The lead–acid electrolyte, sulfuric acid, is diprotic and incompletely dissociates in solution.

B. The energy density of lead–acid electrodes is higher than that of other batteries.

C. The electrolytes in other batteries less readily dissociate than those of lead–acid batteries.

D. The energy density of lead–acid electrodes is lower than that of other batteries.

15. Which of the following best describes why overcharging a Ni–Cd battery is not detrimental?

A. The energy density of a Ni–Cd battery is high, so it can store more charge than other batteries per its mass.

B. The electrodes of a Ni–Cd battery can discharge through the circuit when they are fully charged.

C. The Ni–Cd battery will stop accepting electrons from an outside source when its electrodes are recharged.

D. Ni–Cd batteries have a high surge current and can dissipate the overcharge before damage can occur to electrodes.

Answer Key follows on next page.

Answer Key

1. **C** (See section 12.1)
2. **B** (See section 12.2)
3. **A** (See section 12.2)
4. **C** (See section 12.1)
5. **D** (See section 12.3)
6. **B** (See section 12.1)
7. **B** (See section 12.1)
8. **D** (See section 12.2)
9. **B** (See section 12.2)
10. **D** (See section 12.3)
11. **D** (See section 12.3)
12. **A** (See section 12.2)
13. **C** (See section 12.3)
14. **D** (See section 12.1)
15. **C** (See section 12.1)

The relevant section of the chapter to review for each question is given in parentheses after the correct answer. Detailed explanations can be found at the end of the chapter.

CHAPTER 12

ELECTROCHEMISTRY

In This Chapter

CHAPTER PROFILE

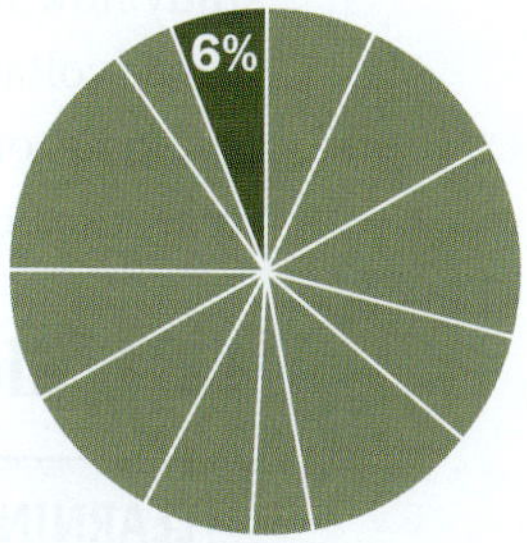

The content in this chapter should be relevant to about 6% of all questions about general chemistry on the MCAT.

This chapter covers material from the following AAMC content categories:

1D: Principles of bioenergetics and fuel molecule metabolism

3A: Structure and functions of the nervous and endocrine systems and ways in which these systems coordinate the organ systems

4C: Electrochemistry and electrical circuits and their elements

5E: Principles of chemical thermodynamics and kinetics

Introduction

The mitochondria are powerhouses of energy. Their primary purpose is to manufacture a deliverable and usable form of energy. By now, you are well aware of the complex processes by which the potential energy in the chemical bonds of carbohydrates, amino acids, and lipids is converted into the potential energy of the phosphate bond in adenosine triphosphate (ATP). ATP is then delivered to different parts of the cell, where it is used to energize most of the processes essential to the maintenance of life.

The mitochondria generate tremendous amounts of ATP—in humans, the average daily turnover of ATP is more than 50 kilograms! Without a continuous supply and replenishment of ATP, we wouldn't survive. ATP powers the contraction of our heart muscle and maintains the membrane potential essential for neurological function, among thousands of other essential roles. How do the mitochondria manufacture these packets of life-sustaining energy? Remember that mitochondria rely on their double-membrane structure to carry out the electron transport chain and oxidative phosphorylation. As such, mitochondria truly act as batteries of the cell. In fact, note the similarity between the proton-motive force of the mitochondria and the electromotive force of electrochemistry. Are these two terms the same thing or—at the very least—similar in nature?

Indeed, mitochondria and batteries do function in similar ways. Specifically, mitochondria function most similarly to concentration cells. In both concentration cells and mitochondria, a concentration gradient of ions between two separated compartments—connected to each other by some means of charge conduction—establishes an electrical potential difference (voltage).

This voltage, called electromotive force in concentration cells and proton-motive force in the mitochondria, provides the drive to move charge from one compartment to the other, creating current. In the concentration cell, an oxidation–reduction reaction takes place, and electrons move in the direction that causes the concentration gradient to be dissipated. In the mitochondria, the charge buildup is in the form of a hydrogen ion (proton) gradient between the intermembrane space and the matrix. Embedded in the inner membrane is *ATP synthase*, which serves a dual role as a proton channel and a catalyst for the formation of the high-energy phosphate bond in ATP. As the hydrogen ions flow down their electrochemical gradient, energy is dissipated, and this energy is harnessed by ATP synthase to form ATP.

In this final chapter of *MCAT General Chemistry Review*, we will focus our attention on the study of various electrochemical cells. Utilizing our knowledge of oxidation–reduction reactions from Chapter 11, we will study how these principles can be applied to create different types of electrochemical cells, including galvanic (voltaic), electrolytic, and concentration cells. Regarding the thermodynamics of electrochemistry, we will focus on the significance of reduction potentials and examine the relationship between electromotive force, the equilibrium constant, and Gibbs free energy.

12.1 Electrochemical Cells High Yield

LEARNING OBJECTIVES

After Chapter 12.1, you will be able to:

- Distinguish between electrolytic and galvanic cells
- Describe electrolytic and galvanic cells
- Predict which electrode will act as the cathode or anode in an electrolytic or a galvanic cell
- Calculate ΔG and emf values for a given galvanic or electrolytic cell
- Apply the Nernst equation to electrochemical cell questions

Electrochemical cells are contained systems in which oxidation–reduction reactions occur. There are three fundamental types of electrochemical cells: galvanic cells (also known as voltaic cells), electrolytic cells, and concentration cells. In addition, there are specific commercial cells such as Ni–Cd batteries through which we can understand these fundamental models.

Galvanic cells and concentration cells house spontaneous reactions, whereas electrolytic cells contain nonspontaneous reactions. Remember that spontaneity is indicated by the change in Gibbs free energy, ΔG. All three types contain **electrodes** where oxidation and reduction take place. For all electrochemical cells, the electrode where oxidation occurs is called the **anode**, and the electrode where reduction occurs is called the **cathode**. Other descriptors of electrochemical cells include the **electromotive force** (**emf**), which corresponds to the voltage or electrical potential difference of the cell. If the emf is positive, the cell is able to release energy ($\Delta G < 0$), which means it is spontaneous. If the emf is negative, the cell must absorb energy ($\Delta G > 0$), which means it is nonspontaneous.

MNEMONIC

Electrodes in an electrochemical cell: **AN OX** and a **RED CAT**

The **an**ode is the site of **ox**idation; **red**uction occurs at the **cat**hode.

Furthermore, we can also state that, for all electrochemical cells, the movement of electrons is from anode to cathode, and the current (I) runs from cathode to anode. This point can be a point of confusion among students. In physics, it is typical to state that current is the direction of flow of a positive charge through a circuit; this model was first proposed by Ben Franklin and continues to be used among physicists. Modern chemists are interested in the flow of electrons, but may discuss the current (a theoretical flow of positive charge) as a proxy for the flow of electrons; the current and the flow of electrons are always of equal magnitude but in opposite directions.

KEY CONCEPT

Electrons move through an electrochemical cell opposite to the flow of current (I).

Last, it is important to note that all batteries are influenced by temperature changes. For instance, lead–acid batteries in cars, like most galvanic cells, tend to fail most in cold weather. The thermodynamic reasons behind this will be discussed later in this chapter.

Galvanic (Voltaic) Cells

All of the nonrechargeable batteries you own are **galvanic cells**, also called **voltaic cells**. Accordingly, because household batteries are used to supply energy to a flashlight or remote control, the reactions in these cells must be spontaneous. This means that the reaction's free energy is decreasing ($\Delta G < 0$) as the cell releases energy to the environment. By extension, if the free energy change is negative for these cells, their electromotive force (E_{cell}) must be positive; the free energy change and electromotive force always have opposite signs.

REAL WORLD

Galvanic cells are commonly used as batteries; to be worthwhile (that is, producing energy to power some device or appliance), these batteries must be spontaneous!

Let's examine the inner workings of a galvanic (voltaic) cell. Two electrodes of distinct chemical identity are placed in separate compartments, which are called **half-cells**. The two electrodes are connected to each other by a conductive material, such as a copper wire. Along the wire, there may be other various components of a circuit, such as resistors or capacitors, but for now, we'll focus on the battery itself.

Surrounding each of the electrodes is an aqueous **electrolyte** solution composed of cations and anions. As shown in the **Daniell cell** illustrated in Figure 12.1, the cations in the two half-cell solutions can be of the same element as the respective metal electrode. Connecting the two solutions is a structure called a **salt bridge**, which consists of an inert salt. When the electrodes are connected to each other by a conductive material, charge will begin to flow as the result of an oxidation–reduction reaction that is taking place between the two half-cells. The redox reaction in a galvanic cell is spontaneous, and therefore the change in Gibbs free energy for the reaction is negative ($\Delta G < 0$). As the spontaneous reaction proceeds toward equilibrium, the movement of electrons results in a conversion of electrical potential energy into kinetic energy. By separating the reduction and oxidation half-reactions into two compartments, we are able to harness this energy and use it to do work by connecting various electrical devices into the circuit between the two electrodes.

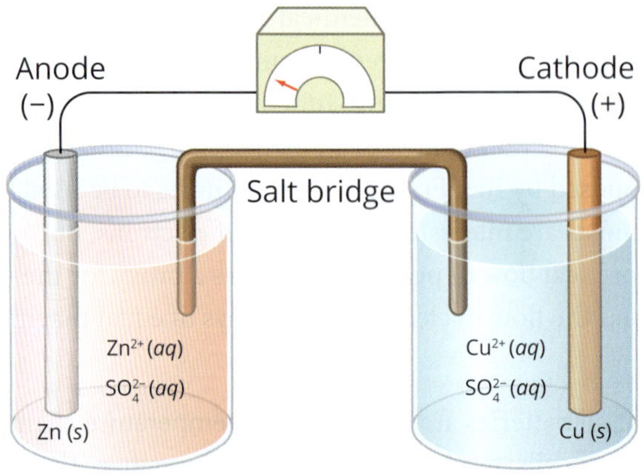

Figure 12.1 Daniell Cell
In this galvanic cell, zinc is the anode and copper is the cathode; each electrode is bathed in an electrolyte solution containing its cation and sulfate.

In the Daniell cell, a zinc electrode is placed in an aqueous $ZnSO_4$ solution, and a copper electrode is placed in an aqueous $CuSO_4$ solution. The anode of this cell is the zinc bar where Zn (*s*) is oxidized to Zn^{2+} (*aq*). The cathode is the copper bar, and it is the site of the reduction of Cu^{2+} (*aq*) to Cu (*s*). The half-cell reactions are written as follows:

$$\text{Zn}\ (s) \rightarrow \text{Zn}^{2+}\ (aq) + 2\ \text{e}^- \qquad E_{\text{red}} = -0.762\ \text{V (anode)}$$

$$\text{Cu}^{2+}\ (aq) + 2\ \text{e}^- \rightarrow \text{Cu}\ (s) \qquad E_{\text{red}} = +0.340\ \text{V (cathode)}$$

The net reaction is

$$\text{Zn}\ (s) + \text{Cu}^{2+}\ (aq) \rightarrow \text{Zn}^{2+}\ (aq) + \text{Cu}\ (s) \qquad E_{\text{cell}} = +1.102\ \text{V}$$

We will discuss the calculation of cell potential in the next section. For now, appreciate that the calculation can be accomplished by knowing each half-reaction. If the two half-cells were not separated, the Cu^{2+} ions would react directly with the zinc bar, and no useful electrical work would be done. Because the solutions and electrodes are physically separated, they must be connected by a conductive material to complete the circuit.

However, if only a wire were provided for this electron flow, the reaction would soon stop because an excess positive charge would build up on the anode, and an excess negative charge would build up on the cathode. Eventually, the excessive charge accumulation would provide a countervoltage large enough to prevent the oxidation–reduction reaction from taking place, and the current would cease. This charge gradient is dissipated by the presence of a **salt bridge**, which permits the exchange of cations and anions, as seen in Figure 12.2.

KEY CONCEPT

The purpose of the salt bridge is to exchange anions and cations to balance, or dissipate, newly generated charges.

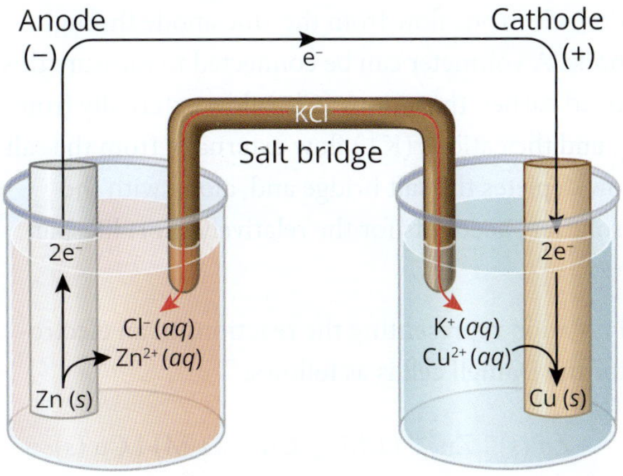

Figure 12.2 Salt Bridge in an Electrochemical Cell
The cations of the salt bridge (K^+) balance the charge on the cathode side, while the anions of the salt bridge (Cl^-) balance the charge on the anode side.

The salt bridge contains an inert electrolyte, usually KCl or NH_4NO_3, which contains ions that will not react with the electrodes or with the ions in solution. While the anions from the salt bridge (Cl^-) diffuse into the solution on the anode side ($ZnSO_4$) to balance out the charge of the newly created Zn^{2+} ions, the cations of the salt bridge (K^+) flow into the solution on the cathode side ($CuSO_4$) to balance out the charge of the sulfate ions left in solution when the Cu^{2+} ions are reduced to Cu and precipitate onto the electrode. This precipitation process onto the cathode itself can also be called **plating** or **galvanization**, as seen in Figure 12.3. This is often used to provide a coating to steel and iron to prevent rusting.

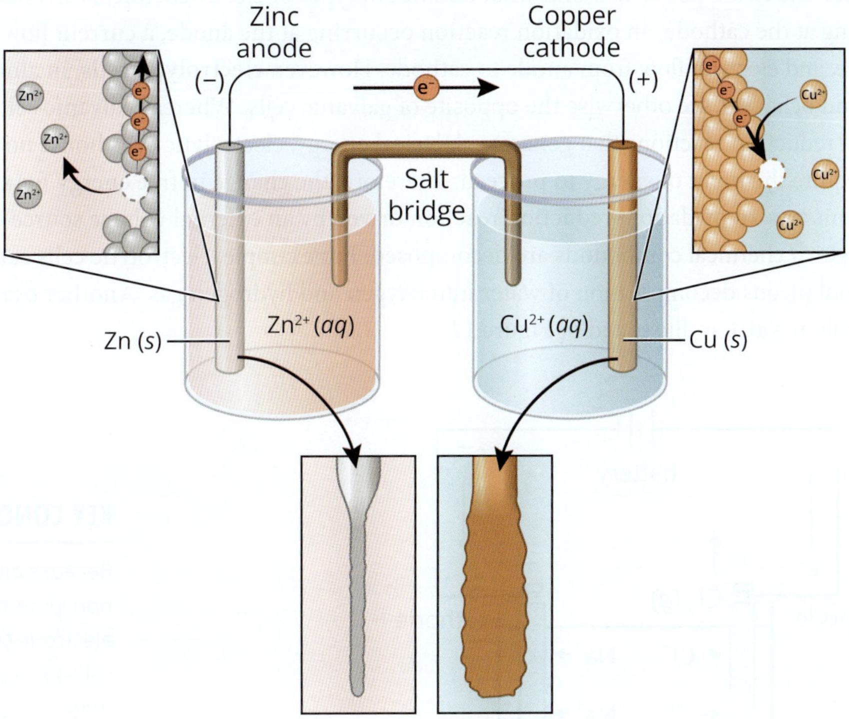

Figure 12.3 Plating in Electrochemical Cells
Precipitation of cations from solution builds up on the cathode.

During the course of the reaction, electrons flow from the zinc anode through the wire and to the copper cathode. A voltmeter can be connected to measure this electromotive force. As mentioned earlier, the anions (Cl^-) flow externally from the salt bridge into the $ZnSO_4$, and the cations (K^+) flow externally from the salt bridge into the $CuSO_4$. This flow depletes the salt bridge and, along with the finite quantity of Cu^{2+} in the solution, accounts for the relatively short lifespan of the cell.

A **cell diagram** is a shorthand notation representing the reactions in an electrochemical cell. A cell diagram for the Daniell cell is as follows:

$$Zn\ (s)\ |\ Zn^{2+}\ (1\ M)\ ||\ Cu^{2+}\ (1\ M)\ |\ Cu\ (s)$$

The following rules are used in constructing a cell diagram:

1. The reactants and products are always listed from left to right in this form: anode | anode solution (concentration) || cathode solution (concentration) | cathode
2. A single vertical line indicates a phase boundary.
3. A double vertical line indicates the presence of a salt bridge or some other type of barrier.

MNEMONIC

Electron flow in an electrochemical cell: **A** → **C** (order in the alphabet)

Electrons flow from **a**node to **c**athode in all types of electrochemical cells.

MCAT EXPERTISE

Recognize and understand the shorthand cell notation for electrochemical cells on Test Day. Passages frequently use this format rather than spelling out which reactions take place at the anode and cathode.

Electrolytic Cells

When comparing and contrasting galvanic and electrolytic cells, it is important to keep straight what remains consistent between the two types of cells and what differs. All types of electrochemical cells have a reduction reaction occurring at the cathode, an oxidation reaction occurring at the anode, a current flowing from cathode to anode, and electron flow from anode to cathode. However, **electrolytic cells**, in almost all of their characteristics and behavior, are otherwise the opposite of galvanic cells. Whereas galvanic cells house spontaneous oxidation–reduction reactions that generate electrical energy, electrolytic cells house nonspontaneous reactions that require the input of energy to proceed. Therefore, the change in free energy for an electrolytic cell is positive. This type of oxidation–reduction reaction driven by an external voltage source is called **electrolysis**, in which chemical compounds are decomposed. For example, electrolytic cells can be used to drive the nonspontaneous decomposition of water into oxygen and hydrogen gas. Another example, the electrolysis of molten NaCl, is illustrated in Figure 12.4.

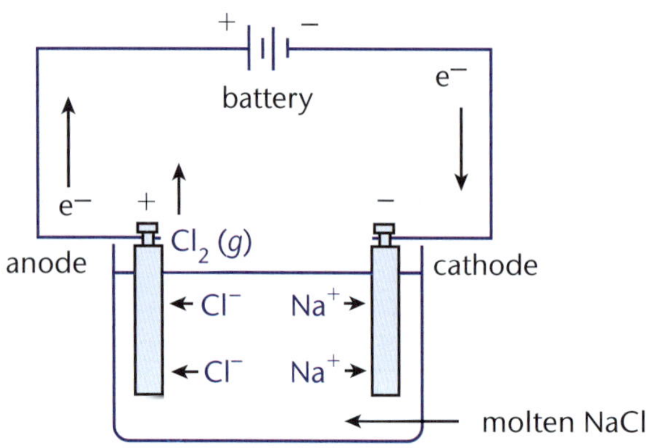

Figure 12.4 Electrolysis of Molten NaCl

KEY CONCEPT

Because electrolysis is nonspontaneous, the electrode (anode or cathode) can consist of any material so long as it can resist the high temperatures and corrosion of the process.

In this electrolytic cell, molten NaCl is decomposed into Cl_2 (*g*) and Na (*l*). The external voltage source—a battery—supplies energy sufficient to drive the oxidation–reduction reaction in the direction that is thermodynamically unfavorable (nonspontaneous).

In this example, Na^+ ions migrate toward the cathode, where they are reduced to Na (*l*). At the same time, Cl^- ions migrate toward the anode, where they are oxidized to Cl_2 (*g*). Notice that the half-reactions do not need to be separated into different compartments; this is because the desired reaction is nonspontaneous. Note that sodium is a liquid at the temperature of molten NaCl; it is also less dense than the molten salt and, thus, is easily removed as it floats to the top of the reaction vessel.

This cell is used in industry as the major means of sodium and chlorine production. You may wonder why one would do so much work to obtain pure sodium and chlorine. Remember that these elements are never found naturally in their elemental form because they are so reactive. Thus, to use elemental sodium or chlorine gas in a reaction, it must be manufactured through processes such as these.

Michael Faraday was the first to define certain quantitative principles governing the behavior of electrolytic cells. He theorized that the amount of chemical change induced in an electrolytic cell is directly proportional to the number of moles of electrons that are exchanged during the oxidation–reduction reaction. The number of moles exchanged can be determined from the balanced half-reaction. In general, for a reaction that involves the transfer of *n* electrons per atom M:

$$M^{n+} + n\,e^- \rightarrow M\,(s)$$

Equation 12.1

According to this equation, one mole of metal M (*s*) will logically be produced if *n* moles of electrons are supplied to one mole of M^{n+}. Additionally, the number of moles of electrons needed to produce a certain amount of M (*s*) can now be related to the measurable electrical property of charge. One electron carries a charge of 1.6×10^{-19} coulombs (C). The charge carried by one mole of electrons can be calculated by multiplying this number by Avogadro's number, as follows:

$$\left[\frac{1.6 \times 10^{-19}\ \text{C}}{\text{electron}}\right]\left[\frac{6.02 \times 10^{23}\,\text{electrons}}{1\ \text{mol e}^-}\right] = 96{,}485\ \frac{\text{C}}{\text{mol e}^-}$$

This number is called the **Faraday constant** (*F*), and one **faraday** (**F**) is equivalent to the amount of charge contained in one mole of electrons (1 F = 96,485 C) or one equivalent. On the MCAT, you should round up this number to $10^5\ \frac{\text{C}}{\text{mol e}^-}$ to make calculations more manageable.

The **electrodeposition equation** summarizes this process and helps determine the number of moles of element being deposited on a plate:

$$\text{mol Me} = \frac{It}{nF}$$

Equation 12.2

where mol Me is the amount of metal ion being deposited at a specific electrode, *I* is current, *t* is time, *n* is the number of electron equivalents for a specific metal ion, and *F* is the Faraday constant. This equation can also be used to determine the amount of gas liberated during electrolysis.

KEY CONCEPT

Faraday's laws state that the liberation of gas and deposition of elements on electrodes is directly proportional to the number of electrons being transferred during the oxidation–reduction reaction. Here, normality or gram equivalent weight is used. These observations are proxy measurements of the amount of current flowing in a circuit.

KEY CONCEPT

One faraday (F) is equivalent to the amount of charge contained in one mole of electrons (1 F = 96,485 C).

MNEMONIC

Electrodeposition equation: Calculating **Moles of Me**tal, **It** is **N**ot **F**un.

mol Me $= \frac{It}{nF}$

Example: What mass of copper will be deposited in a Daniell cell if a current of 2 A flows through the cell for 3 hours?

Solution: We will use the equation mol Me $= \frac{It}{nF}$

A Daniell cell uses a copper electrode in copper sulfate ($CuSO_4$) solution. Because the oxidation state of copper in solution is +2, $n = 2$. Now we can plug into the equation.

$$\text{mol Me} = \frac{It}{nF} = \frac{(2\text{ A})(3\text{ hr})\left(3600\ \frac{\text{s}}{\text{hr}}\right)}{(2\text{ mol e}^-)\left(96{,}485\ \frac{\text{C}}{\text{mol e}^-}\right)} \approx \frac{3 \times 3600}{10^5}$$
$$= 0.1\text{ mol Cu (actual} = 0.11\text{ mol Cu)}$$

Then, we must determine the actual mass of copper being deposited.
0.1 mol Cu should have a mass of 6.35 g because the molar mass of copper is $63.5\ \frac{\text{g}}{\text{mol}}$ (actual = 7.11 g).

Concentration Cells

A **concentration cell** is a special type of galvanic cell. Like all galvanic cells, it contains two half-cells connected by a conductive material, allowing a spontaneous oxidation–reduction reaction to proceed, which generates a current and delivers energy. The distinguishing characteristic of a concentration cell is in its design: the electrodes are chemically identical. For example, if both electrodes are copper metal, they have the same reduction potential. Therefore, current is generated as a function of a concentration gradient established between the two solutions surrounding the electrodes. The concentration gradient results in a potential difference between the two compartments and drives the movement of electrons in the direction that results in equilibration of the ion gradient. The current will stop when the concentrations of ionic species in the half-cells are equal. This implies that the voltage (V) or electromotive force of a concentration cell is zero when the concentrations are equal; the voltage, as a function of concentrations, can be calculated using the **Nernst equation**.

In a biological system, a concentration cell is best represented by the cell membrane of a neuron, as shown in Figure 12.5. Sodium and potassium cations, and chlorine anions, are exchanged as needed to produce an electrical potential. The actual value depends on both the concentrations and charges of the ions. In this way, a **resting membrane potential** (**V_m**) can be maintained. Disturbances of the resting membrane potential, if sufficiently large, may stimulate the firing of an action potential.

BRIDGE

The maintenance of a resting membrane potential is discussed in Chapter 8 of *MCAT Biochemistry Review.* The conduction of an action potential is discussed in Chapter 4 of *MCAT Biology Review.* The transfer of ions and electrons during an action potential produces biochemical work.

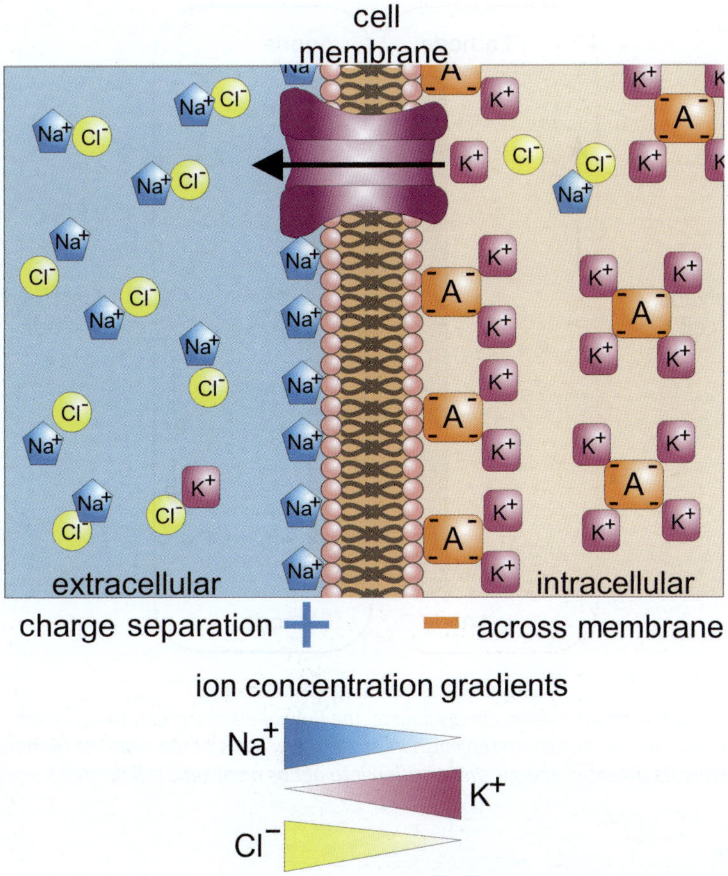

Figure 12.5 The Cell Membrane as an Example of a Concentration Cell
The electrochemical gradient created by separation of ions across the cell membrane is analogous to a cell with two electrodes composed of the same material.

Rechargeable Cells

A **rechargeable cell** or **rechargeable battery** (Figure 12.6) is one that can function as both a galvanic and electrolytic cell. During discharge, the battery functions as a galvanic (voltaic) cell, in which a spontaneous redox reaction produces an electric current that powers an external device. During recharge, an external voltage is applied, causing the cell to operate as an electrolytic cell. This external energy source drives the nonspontaneous reverse reaction, regenerating the original reactants and restoring the cell's chemical potential. The reversibility of this electrochemical process is what enables the battery to be rechargeable.

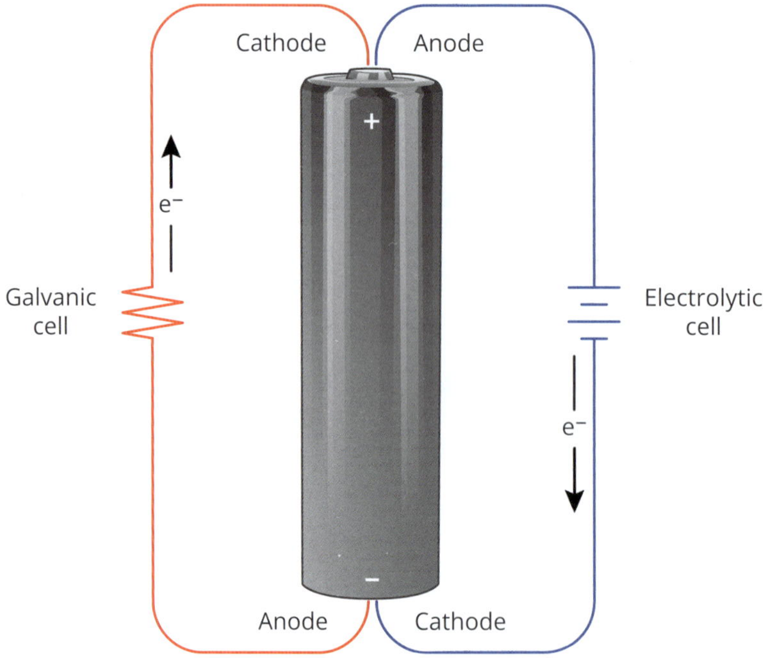

Figure 12.6 Rechargeable Battery
By applying an outside energy source, the flow of electrons can be reversed, allowing for the battery to replenish its store of electrons at the negative terminal, restore its potential energy, and position it to act as a galvanic cell (battery) again.

Lead–Acid Batteries

A **lead–acid battery**, also known as a **lead storage battery**, is a specific type of rechargeable battery. As a voltaic cell, when fully charged, it consists of two half-cells—a Pb anode and a porous PbO_2 cathode, connected by a conductive material (concentrated 4 M H_2SO_4). When fully discharged, it consists of two $PbSO_4$ electroplated lead electrodes with a dilute concentration of H_2SO_4, as shown in Figure 12.7.

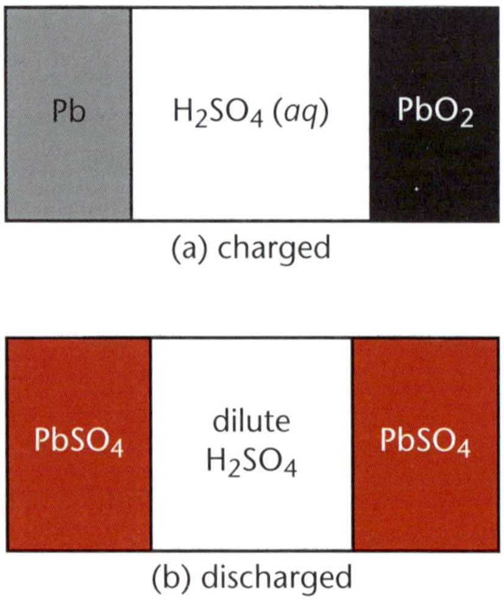

Figure 12.7 Lead–Acid Battery
When charged (a), the cell contains a Pb anode and PbO2 cathode; when discharged (b), both electrodes are coated with lead sulfate.

The oxidation half-reaction at the lead (negative) anode is:

$$Pb\ (s) + HSO_4^-\ (aq) \rightarrow PbSO_4\ (s) + H^+\ (aq) + 2\ e^- \qquad E^\circ_{red} = -0.356\ V$$

The reduction half-reaction at the lead(IV) oxide (positive) cathode is:

$$PbO_2\ (s) + SO_4^{2-}\ (aq) + 4H^+ + 2\ e^- \rightarrow PbSO_4\ (s) + 2\ H_2O \qquad E^\circ_{red} = 1.685\ V$$

Both half-reactions cause the electrodes to plate with lead sulfate ($PbSO_4$) and dilute the acid electrolyte when **discharging**. The lead anode is negatively charged and attracts the anionic bisulfate. The lead(IV) oxide cathode is a bit more complicated. This electrode is porous, which allows the electrolyte (sulfuric acid) to solvate the cathode into lead and oxide ions. Then, the hydrogen ions in solution react with the oxide ions to produce water, and the remaining sulfate ions react with the lead to produce the electroplated lead sulfate.

Overall, the net equation for a discharging lead–acid battery is:

$$Pb\ (s) + PbO_2\ (s) + 2\ H_2SO_4\ (aq) \rightarrow 2\ PbSO_4\ (s) + 2\ H_2O$$

$$E^o_{cell} = 1.685 - (-0.356) = 2.041\ V$$

When **charging**, the lead–acid cell is part of an electrolytic circuit. These equations and electrode charge designations are the opposite because an external source reverses the electroplating process and concentrates the acid solution—this external source is very evident when one uses jumper cables to restart a car.

Lead–acid batteries, as compared to other cells, have some of the lowest energy-to-weight ratios (otherwise known as energy density). **Energy density** is a measure of a battery's ability to produce power as a function of its weight. Lead–acid batteries, therefore, require a heavier amount of battery material to produce a certain output as compared to other batteries.

Nickel–Cadmium Batteries

Nickel–cadmium batteries are also rechargeable cells. They consist of two half-cells made of solid cadmium (the anode) and nickel(III) oxide-hydroxide (the cathode) connected by a conductive material, typically potassium hydroxide (KOH). Most of us are familiar with AA and AAA cells made of Ni–Cd materials, inside of which the electrodes are layered and wrapped around in a cylinder, as shown in Figure 12.8.

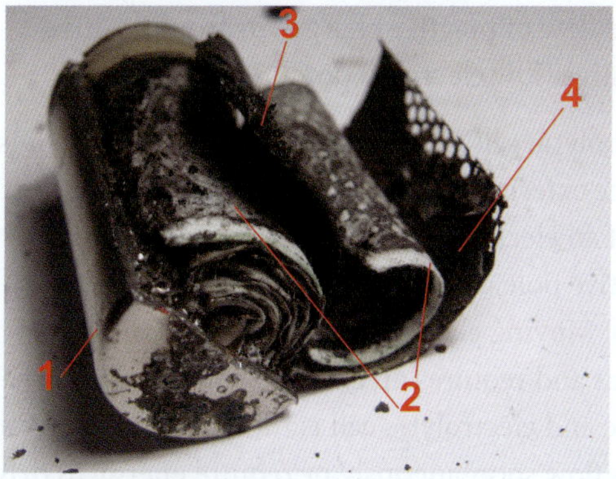

Figure 12.8 A Nickel–Cadmium Battery
(1) Metal casing, (2) salt bridge, (3) NiO(OH) cathode, (4) Cd anode

The oxidation half-reaction at the cadmium (negative) anode is:

$$Cd\ (s) + 2\ OH^-(aq) \rightarrow Cd(OH)_2(s) + 2\ e^- \qquad E^\circ_{red} = -0.86\ V$$

The reduction half-reaction at the nickel oxide–hydroxide (positive) cathode is:

$$2\ NiO(OH)\ (s) + 2\ H_2O + 2\ e^- \rightarrow 2\ Ni(OH)_2(s) + 2\ OH^- \qquad E^\circ_{red} = 0.49\ V$$

Both half-reactions cause the electrodes to plate with their respective products. Overall, the net equation for a Ni–Cd battery is:

$$2\ NiO(OH)\ (s) + Cd + 2\ H_2O \rightarrow 2\ Ni(OH)_2(s) + Cd(OH)_2(s)$$

$$E^o_{cell} = 0.49 - (-0.86) = 1.35\ V$$

As in our previous example, charging reverses the electrolytic cell potentials. Some Ni–Cd designs are vented for this reason to allow for the release of built-up hydrogen and oxygen gas during electrolysis.

Ni–Cd batteries have a higher energy density than lead–acid batteries. The electrochemistry of the Ni–Cd half-reactions also tends to provide higher surge current. **Surge currents** are periods of large current (amperage) early in the discharge cycle. This is preferable in appliances such as remote controls that demand rapid responses. It is important to note that modern Ni–Cd batteries have largely been replaced by more efficient **nickel–metal hydride** (**NiMH**) **batteries**. These newer batteries have more energy density, are more cost effective, and are significantly less toxic. As the name suggests, in lieu of a pure metal anode, a metal hydride is used instead.

Electrode Charge Designations

In a galvanic cell, current is spontaneously generated as electrons are released by the oxidized species, which has a lower reduction potential, at the anode and travel through the conductive material to the cathode, where reduction takes place since the reduced species has a higher reduction potential. By convention, the lower reduction potential is assigned the negative designation; the higher reduction potential is assigned the positive designation. Electrons, therefore, move from negative (low electrical potential) to positive (high electrical potential), while the current—the flow of positive charge—is from positive (high electrical potential) to negative (low electrical potential).

Conversely, the anode of an electrolytic cell is considered positive because it is attached to the positive pole of the external voltage source and attracts anions from the solution. The cathode of an electrolytic cell is considered negative because it is attached to the negative pole of the external voltage source and attracts cations from the solution. Moving electrons from higher potential to lower potential is nonspontaneous and requires an external source of energy. The real difference between a galvanic and electrolytic cell is the direction of electron flow and whether those electrons flow spontaneously or require energy to drive them in that direction. Figure 12.9 demonstrates this difference.

MNEMONIC

In a galva**N**ic cell, the a**N**ode is **N**egative.

KEY CONCEPT

In a galvanic cell, the anode is negative and the cathode is positive. In an electrolytic cell, the anode is positive and the cathode is negative. This is because an external source is used to reverse the charge of an electrolytic cell. However, in both types of cells, reduction occurs at the cathode, and oxidation occurs at the anode; cations are attracted to the cathode, and anions are attracted to the anode.

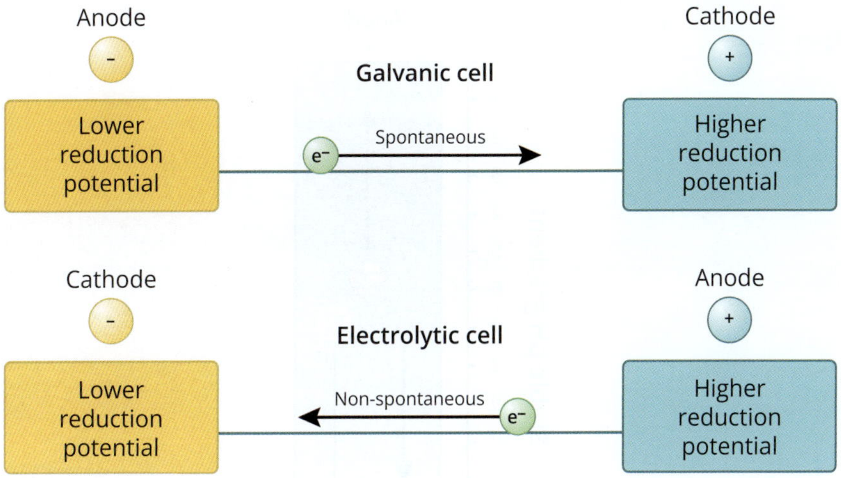

Figure 12.9 Galvanic vs. Electrolytic Cells
Spontaneity and direction of electron flow are the key differences.

Note that the positive and negative terminals do not change sides as reduction potential is an intrinsic property, but the label of anode and cathode does. Also note that in both types of cells, the electron always moves towards the cathode. This can help you remember the sign convention. Electrons are negatively charged, and are spontaneously attracted to a positive cathode in galvanic cells. Electrolytic cells are nonspontaneous, meaning energy must be applied to drive the negative electrons towards the negative cathode.

In spite of this difference in designating charge (sign), oxidation always takes place at the anode and reduction always takes place at the cathode *in both types of cells*; electrons always flow through the wire *from the anode to the cathode* and current flows from cathode to anode. Finally, note that—regardless of its charge designation—the cathode always attracts cations and the anode always attracts anions. In the Daniell cell, for example, the electrons created at the anode by the oxidation of elemental zinc travel through the wire to the copper half-cell. There, they attract copper(II) cations to the cathode, resulting in the reduction of the copper ions to elemental copper, and drawing cations out of the salt bridge into the compartment. The anode, having lost electrons, attracts anions from the salt bridge at the same time that zinc(II) ions formed by the oxidation process dissolve away from the anode.

This is an important rule to understand not only for electrochemistry in the *Chemical and Physical Foundations of Biological Systems* section on Test Day, but also for electrophoresis in both this section and *Biological and Biochemical Foundations of Living Systems*. **Isoelectric focusing** is a technique used to separate amino acids or polypeptides based on their **isoelectric points** (**pI**). The positively charged amino acids (protonated at the solution's pH) will migrate toward the cathode; negatively charged amino acids (deprotonated at the solution's pH) will migrate toward the anode, as demonstrated in Figure 12.10. The technique of isoelectric focusing is discussed in detail in Chapter 3 of *MCAT Biochemistry Review*.

REAL WORLD

Recognize that in any system in which batteries are placed, it is important to line up cathodes and anodes. Electronics tend to have (+) and (−) designations to line up the electrodes—think jumper cables, television remotes, and button batteries in watches.

MNEMONIC

Anions are attracted to the **an**ode. **Cat**ions are attracted to the **ca**thode. This is true regardless of the type of cell (galvanic, electrolytic, or concentration cells).

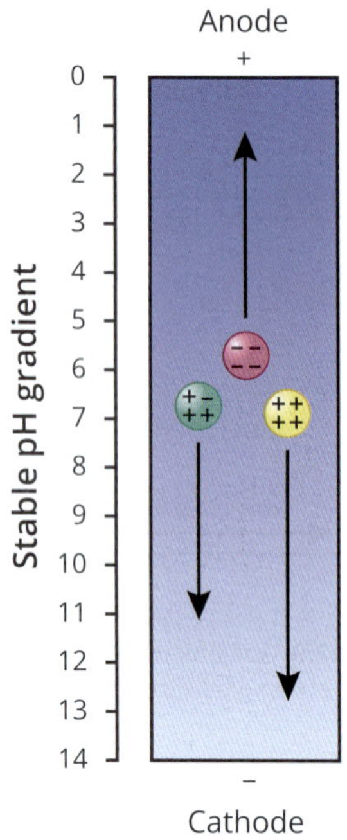

Figure 12.10 Isoelectric Focusing Gel as an Electrolytic Cell
Cations are attracted to the cathode; anions are attracted to the anode.

MCAT CONCEPT CHECK 12.1

Before you move on, assess your understanding of the material with these questions.

1. Circle which electrode each of the following statements describes in a galvanic (voltaic) cell:

• Site of oxidation:	Anode	Cathode
• Electrons flow toward it:	Anode	Cathode
• Current flows toward it:	Anode	Cathode
• Has (−) designation:	Anode	Cathode
• Attracts cations:	Anode	Cathode

2. Circle which electrode each of the following statements describes in an electrolytic cell:

• Site of oxidation:	Anode	Cathode
• Electrons flow toward it:	Anode	Cathode
• Current flows toward it:	Anode	Cathode
• Has (−) designation:	Anode	Cathode
• Attracts cations:	Anode	Cathode

3. Write the cell diagram for the discharging state of a lead–acid battery:

____

4. Which type of cell has a positive ΔG? A positive E_{cell}?

   • Positive ΔG:

____

   • Positive E_{cell}:

____

5. How much current is required to produce 0.23 kg Na from a molten NaCl electrolytic cell that runs for 30 hours? Assume the cell is 100% efficient.

____

6. Fill in the following chart to summarize electrode charge designations of batteries we have analyzed:

Battery	State of Use	Galvanic or Electrolytic	Anode Material	Anode Charge	Cathode Material	Cathode Charge
Ni—Cd	Discharging					
Ni—Cd	Charging					
Molten NaCl	Discharging					
Daniell cell	Discharging					
Lead–acid	Charging					
Lead–acid	Discharging					

12.2 Cell Potentials

LEARNING OBJECTIVES

After Chapter 12.2, you will be able to:

- Describe how standard reduction potentials are measured
- Explain the importance of the sign for electromotive force
- Determine whether a cell using a given reaction is galvanic or electrolytic
- Calculate the net E value for a redox reaction between two species:

$$Ag^{+} + e^{-} \rightarrow Ag\ (s) \qquad E^{\circ}_{red} = +0.80\ V$$

$$Tl^{+} + e^{-} \rightarrow Tl\ (s) \qquad E^{\circ}_{red} = -0.34\ V$$

For galvanic cells, the direction of spontaneous movement of charge is from the anode, the site of oxidation, to the cathode, the site of reduction. This is simple enough to remember, but it begs the question: how do we determine which electrode species will be oxidized and which will be reduced? The relative tendencies of different chemical species to be reduced have been determined experimentally, using the tendency of the hydrogen ion (H^+) to be reduced as an arbitrary zero reference point.

Reduction Potentials

A reduction potential is measured in volts (V) and defined relative to the **standard hydrogen electrode** (SHE), which is given a potential of 0 V by convention. The species in a reaction that will be oxidized or reduced can be determined from the **reduction potential** of each species, defined as the tendency of a species to gain electrons and to be reduced. Each species has its own intrinsic reduction potential; the more positive the potential, the greater the tendency to be reduced.

Standard reduction potential (E°_{red}) is measured under **standard conditions**: 25°C (298 K), 1 atm pressure, and 1 *M* concentrations. The relative reactivities of different half-cells can be compared to predict the direction of electron flow. A more positive E°_{red} means a greater relative tendency for reduction to occur, while a less positive E°_{red} means a greater relative tendency for oxidation to occur. A list of common half-reactions and their standard reduction potentials is provided in Table 12.1. Note that reduction potential values do not need to be memorized for Test Day, but be prepared to know how to use the values given in a passage or question if asked.

KEY CONCEPT

A reduction potential is exactly what it sounds like. It tells us how likely a compound is to be reduced. The more positive the value, the more likely it is to be reduced—the more it *wants* to be reduced.

Half-Reaction	E°_{red} (V)
$F_2\ (g) + 2\ e^- \rightarrow 2\ F^-\ (aq)$	+2.87
$O_2\ (g) + 4\ H^+\ (aq) + 4\ e^- \rightarrow 2\ H_2O\ (l)$	+1.23
$Cu^{2+}\ (aq) + 2\ e^- \rightarrow Cu\ (s)$	+0.34
$2\ H^+\ (aq) + 2\ e^- \rightarrow H_2\ (g)$	0.00
$Zn^{2+}\ (aq) + 2\ e^- \rightarrow Zn\ (s)$	−0.76
$Li^+\ (aq) + e^- \rightarrow Li\ (s)$	−3.05

Table 12.1 Standard Reduction Potentials at 25°C

For galvanic cells, the electrode with the more positive reduction potential is the cathode, and the electrode with the less positive reduction potential is the anode. Because the species with a stronger tendency to gain electrons (that *wants* to gain electrons more) is actually doing so, the reaction is spontaneous and ΔG is negative. For electrolytic cells, the electrode with the more positive reduction potential is forced by the external voltage source to be oxidized and is, therefore, the anode. The electrode with the less positive reduction potential is forced to be reduced and is, therefore, the cathode. Because the movement of electrons is in the direction against the tendency or desires of the respective electrochemical species, the reaction is nonspontaneous and ΔG is positive.

Example: Given the following half-reactions and E°_{red} values, determine which species would be oxidized and which would be reduced in a galvanic cell.

$$Ag^+ + e^- \rightarrow Ag\ (s) \quad E^\circ_{red} = +0.80\text{ V}$$

$$Tl^+ + e^- \rightarrow Tl\ (s) \quad E^\circ_{red} = -0.34\text{ V}$$

Solution: E°_{red} indicates the reduction potential, or the likelihood of a compound to be reduced via a given reaction. A positive E°_{red} value indicates a spontaneous reduction, and a negative value indicates a non-spontaneous reduction. In a galvanic cell, Ag^+ will be spontaneously reduced to Ag (*s*) and Tl (*s*) will be spontaneously oxidized to Tl^+ because Ag^+ has the more positive E°_{red} and thus the more favorable reduction reaction. Therefore, the net ionic equation would be:

$$Ag^+ + Tl\ (s) \rightarrow Tl^+ + Ag\ (s)$$

which is the sum of the two spontaneous half-reactions.

It should be noted that reduction and oxidation are opposite processes. Therefore, to obtain the oxidation potential of a given half-reaction, both the reduction half-reaction and the sign of the reduction potential are reversed. For instance, from the example above, the oxidation half-reaction and oxidation potential of Tl (*s*) are:

$$Tl\ (s) \rightarrow Tl^+ + e^- \qquad E^\circ_{ox} = +0.34\text{ V}$$

Note that, in the examples of batteries given above (lead–acid storage batteries and nickel–cadmium batteries), the oxidation half-reaction was given with the reduction potential of the reverse reaction. These two quantities have equal magnitudes but opposite signs. On the MCAT, reduction potentials are generally given rather than oxidation potentials. Therefore, all references in this book (with exception of the thallium example immediately above) are given using reduction potentials—not oxidation potentials.

The Electromotive Force

Standard reduction potentials are also used to calculate the **standard electromotive force** (**emf** or E°_{cell}) of a reaction, which is the difference in potential (voltage) between two half-cells under standard conditions. The emf of a reaction is determined by calculating the difference in reduction potentials between the two half-cells:

$$E^\circ_{cell} = E^\circ_{red,cathode} - E^\circ_{red,anode}$$

Equation 12.3

When subtracting standard potentials, do not multiply them by the number of moles oxidized or reduced. This is because the potential of each electrode does not depend on the size of the electrode (the amount of material), but rather the identity of the material. The standard reduction potential of an electrode will not change unless the chemical identity of that electrode is changed.

KEY CONCEPT

If you need to multiply each half-reaction by a common denominator to cancel out electrons when coming up with the net ionic equation, do *not* multiply the reduction potential, E°_{red}, by that number. That would indicate a change in the chemical identity of the electrode, which is not occurring.

Example: Given that the standard reduction potentials for Sm^{3+} and $[RhCl_6]^{3-}$ are −2.41 V and +0.44 V, respectively, calculate the electromotive force of the following reaction:

$$Sm^{3+} + Rh + 6\ Cl^- \rightarrow [RhCl_6]^{3-} + Sm$$

Solution: First, determine the oxidation and reduction half-reactions. As written, the Rh is oxidized, and the Sm^{3+} is reduced:

$$Sm^{3+} + 3\ e^- \rightarrow Sm$$

$$Rh + 6\ Cl^- \rightarrow [RhCl_6]^{3-} + 3\ e^-$$

Now, we simply take the difference between the samarium(III) reduction potential and the hexachlororhodate(III) reduction potential. We need not change the sign on the hexachlororhodate(III) reduction potential because we are *subtracting* it from that of samarium(III).

Using the equation provided, the emf can be calculated as:
−2.41 V − (+0.44 V) = −2.85 V. The cell is thus electrolytic. If this were instead a galvanic cell the reaction would proceed spontaneously to the left, toward reactants, in which case the Sm would be oxidized while $[RhCl_6]^{3-}$ would be reduced with an emf of +2.85 V.

MCAT CONCEPT CHECK 12.2

Before you move on, assess your understanding of the material with these questions.

1. How are standard reduction potentials measured?

___

2. If a cell's electromotive force (emf) is denoted as a positive value, what does that mean? What if it is negative?

   - Positive emf:

   ___

   - Negative emf:

   ___

3. Given the following reactions, determine whether the cell is galvanic or electrolytic:

   - $2\ Fe^{3+}\ (aq) + 2\ Cl^-\ (aq) \rightarrow 2\ Fe^{2+}\ (aq) + Cl_2\ (g)$ ($E^\circ_{cell} = -0.59$ V):

   ___

   - $2\ Fe^{3+}\ (aq) + 2\ I^-\ (aq) \rightarrow 2\ Fe^{2+}\ (aq) + I_2\ (aq)$ ($E^\circ_{cell} = +0.25$ V):

   ___

4. Given the two half-reactions below, what would be the spontaneous oxidation–reduction reaction between these two species?

$$Fe^{3+} + 3\,e^- \rightarrow Fe \qquad E^\circ_{red} = -0.036\text{ V}$$

$$I_3^- + 2\,e^- \rightarrow 3\,I^- \qquad E^\circ_{red} = +0.534\text{ V}$$

12.3 Electromotive Force and Thermodynamics

LEARNING OBJECTIVES

After Chapter 12.3, you will be able to:

- Apply the formula $\Delta G^\circ = -RT \ln K_{eq}$ to calculations of Gibbs free energy or electromotive force
- Predict E_{cell} given reaction quotients and equilibrium constants

Throughout our discussion of electrochemistry and the different types of electrochemical cells, we have been making references to the spontaneity or nonspontaneity of the redox reactions housed in each of the different cell types. Let's now look more formally at this topic by relating free energy to electromotive force (emf) and the concentrations of the oxidation–reduction reactants and products to the voltage of a cell at a given point in time.

Gibbs Free Energy

By now, you should be familiar with the thermodynamic criterion for determining the spontaneity of a reaction: the change in Gibbs free energy, ΔG. This is the change in the amount of energy available in a chemical system to do work. In an electrochemical cell, the work done is dependent on the number of coulombs of charge transferred and the energy available. Thus, ΔG° and emf are related as follows:

$$\Delta G^\circ = -nFE^\circ_{cell}$$

Equation 12.4

where ΔG° is the standard change in free energy, n is the number of moles of electrons exchanged, F is the Faraday constant, and E°_{cell} is the standard emf of the cell. Keep in mind that, if the Faraday constant is expressed in coulombs $\left(\frac{\text{J}}{\text{V}}\right)$, then ΔG° must be expressed in J, not kJ. Notice the similarity of this relationship to that expressed in the physics formula $W = q\Delta V$ for the amount of work available or needed in the transport of a charge q across a potential difference ΔV: $n \times F$ is a charge, and E°_{cell} is a voltage. This application in electrostatics is discussed in Chapter 5 of *MCAT Physics and Math Review.*

BRIDGE

Recall from Chapter 6 of *MCAT General Chemistry Review* that, if ΔG is positive, the reaction is nonspontaneous; if ΔG is negative, the reaction is spontaneous.

Note the significance of the negative sign on the right side of the equation. ΔG° and E°_{cell} will always have opposite signs. Therefore, galvanic cells have negative ΔG° and positive E°_{cell} values; electrolytic cells have positive ΔG° and negative E°_{cell} values.

Example: Determine the standard change in free energy of a cell with the following net reaction. (Note: The standard reduction potential of iron(III) is +0.77 V; the standard reduction potential of molecular chlorine is +1.36 V.)

$$2\ Fe^{3+}\ (aq) + 2\ Cl^-\ (aq) \rightarrow 2\ Fe^{2+}\ (aq) + Cl_2\ (g)$$

Solution: First, separate the reaction into the half-reactions:

$$2\ Fe^{3+} + 2\ e^- \rightarrow 2\ Fe^{2+}$$

$$2\ Cl^- \rightarrow Cl_2 + 2\ e^-$$

In this reaction, iron(III) is reduced and is the cathode, whereas Cl^- is oxidized and is the anode. The reduction potential of chlorine is actually higher than that of iron(III); this means that the electrodes are serving the *opposite* role from their natural tendency, and the reaction is nonspontaneous. This is an electrolytic cell, and should have a negative emf value.

Now, determine the emf:

$$E^\circ_{cell} = E^\circ_{red,cathode} - E^\circ_{red,anode} = 0.77\ V - 1.36\ V = -0.59\ V$$

Use the emf to determine the free energy change (note that as 2 electrons are transferred, $n = 2$):

$$\Delta G^\circ = -nFE^\circ_{cell} = -\ (2\ mol\ e^-)\left(96{,}485 \frac{C}{mol\ e^-}\right)(-0.59\ V)$$

$$\approx 2 \times 10^5 \times (0.6) = 1.2 \times 10^5\ J\ (actual = 1.14 \times 10^5\ J)$$

The free energy change is about +120 kJ, which represents a non-spontaneous reaction.

Reaction Quotients

So far, we have considered the calculation of a cell's emf only under standard conditions. However, electrochemical cells may have ionic concentrations that deviate from 1 M. Also, for the concentration cell, the concentrations of the ions in the two compartments *must* be different for there to be a measurable voltage and current. Concentration and the emf of a cell are related: emf varies with the changing concentrations of the species in the cell. When conditions deviate from standard conditions, one can use the **Nernst equation**:

$$E_{cell} = E^\circ_{cell} - \frac{RT}{nF} \ln Q$$

Equation 12.5

where E_{cell} is the emf of the cell under nonstandard conditions, E°_{cell} is the emf of the cell under standard conditions, R is the ideal gas constant, T is the temperature in kelvin, n is the number of moles of electrons, F is the Faraday constant, and Q is the reaction quotient for the reaction at a given point in time. The following simplified version of the equation can be used, assuming $T = 298$ K:

$$E_{cell} = E^\circ_{cell} - \frac{0.0592}{n} \log Q$$

Equation 12.6

This simplified version of the equation brings together R, T (298 K), and F, and converts the natural logarithm to the base-ten logarithm to make calculations easier.

MCAT EXPERTISE

If the Nernst equation is needed on Test Day, stick with the $\log_{10}$ version because natural logarithm calculations get very tedious.

Remember that the reaction quotient, Q, for a general reaction $aA + bB \rightarrow cC + dD$ has the form:

$$Q = \frac{[C]^c[D]^d}{[A]^a[B]^b}$$

Equation 12.7

Although the expression for the reaction quotient Q has two terms for the concentrations of reactants and two terms for the concentrations of products, remember that only the species in solution are included. When considering the case of the Daniell cell, for example, only the concentrations of zinc and copper ions are considered:

$$Zn\,(s) + Cu^{2+}(aq) \rightarrow Zn^{2+}(aq) + Cu\,(s)$$

$$Q = \frac{[Zn^{2+}]}{[Cu^{2+}]}$$

The emf of a cell can be measured with a **voltmeter**. A **potentiometer** is a kind of voltmeter that draws no current and gives a more accurate reading of the difference in potential between two electrodes. Figure 12.11 shows where a voltmeter should be placed to obtain an accurate reading.

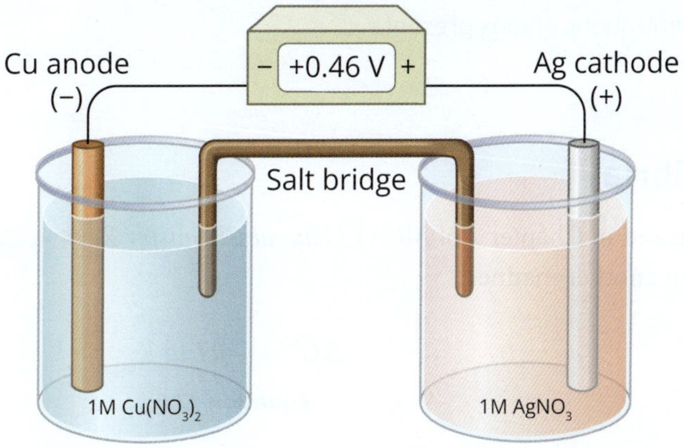

Figure 12.11 Placement of Voltmeter in Electrochemical Cell

Example: Find the emf of a galvanic cell at 25°C based on the following standard reduction potentials:

$Fe^{2+} + 2\,e^- \rightarrow Fe \qquad E^\circ_{red} = -0.44\ V$

$Cl_2 + 2\,e^- \rightarrow 2\,Cl^- \qquad E^\circ_{red} = +1.36\ V$

In this cell, $[Fe^{2+}] = 0.01$ M and $[Cl^-] = 0.1$ M.

BRIDGE

While a mathematically rigorous equation, the Nernst equation has a powerful use in biochemistry for calculating resting and depolarized membrane potentials based on concentrations of ions. Its more extended version, the Goldman–Hodgkin–Katz equation, is discussed in Chapter 8 of *MCAT Biochemistry Review.* Equation 8.2 in that chapter looks slightly different than Equation 12.6 here. This is because the temperature is different (310 K rather than 298 K) and the units are different (mV instead of V).

Solution: First, determine the standard cell potential. Because the chlorine half-reaction has a higher reduction potential, it will be the cathode. Iron will act as the anode. The standard cell potential is:

$$E^\circ_{\text{cell}} = E^\circ_{\text{red,cathode}} - E^\circ_{\text{red,anode}} = 1.36\text{ V} - (-0.44\text{ V}) = +1.80\text{ V}$$

Now, determine the net ionic equation. Remember that iron is being oxidized, so its reduction half-reaction in the question stem will have to be reversed. The net ionic equation is:

$$\text{Fe} + \text{Cl}_2 \rightarrow \text{Fe}^{2+} + 2\text{ Cl}^-$$

From this equation, we can determine the value of the reaction quotient:

$$Q = [\text{Fe}^{2+}][\text{Cl}^-]^2 = (0.01\text{ M})(0.1\text{ M})^2 = 10^{-4}$$

Now, plug into the Nernst equation, keeping in mind that two electrons are transferred ($n = 2$):

$$E_{\text{cell}} = E^\circ_{\text{cell}} - \frac{0.0592}{n}\log Q = 1.8 - \frac{0.0592}{2}\log 10^{-4}$$

$$= 1.8 + \frac{4 \times 0.0592}{2} \approx 1.8 + (2 \times 0.06) = 1.92\text{ V}$$

In this case, the cell actually has a higher voltage than it normally would due to the concentrations of ions present.

Equilibria

As discussed in Chapter 7 of *MCAT General Chemistry Review*, ΔG° can also be determined in another manner:

$$\Delta G^\circ = -RT \ln K_{\text{eq}}$$

Equation 12.8

where R is the ideal gas constant, T is the absolute temperature, and K_{eq} is the equilibrium constant for the reaction.

MCAT EXPERTISE

Whether it is log or ln, remember that a logarithm will be positive when equilibrium constants are greater than 1, negative when equilibrium constants are less than 1, and 0 when equilibrium constants are equal to 1.

Combining the two expressions that solve for standard free energy change, we see that

$$\Delta G^\circ = -nFE^\circ_{\text{cell}} = -RT \ln K_{\text{eq}}$$

or

$$nFE^\circ_{\text{cell}} = RT \ln K_{\text{eq}}$$

By extension, if the values for n, T, and K_{eq} are known, then E°_{cell} for the reaction is easily calculated. On the MCAT, you will not be expected to calculate natural logarithm values in your head. That being said, these equations can still be tested but in a conceptual way.

Analysis of the equations shows us that, for redox reactions with equilibrium constants less than 1 (equilibrium state favors the reactants), the E°_{cell} will be negative because the natural logarithm of any number between 0 and 1 is negative. These properties are characteristic of electrolytic cells, which house nonspontaneous oxidation–reduction reactions. Instead, if the equilibrium constant for the reaction is greater than 1 (equilibrium state favors the products), the E°_{cell} will be positive because the natural logarithm of any number greater than 1 is positive. These properties are characteristic of galvanic cells, which house spontaneous oxidation–reduction reactions. If the equilibrium constant is equal to 1 (concentrations of the reactants and products are equal at equilibrium), the E°_{cell} will be equal to zero. An easy way to remember this is that $E^\circ_{cell} = 0$ V for any concentration cell with equimolar concentrations in both half-cells because there is no net ionic equation (both half-cells contain the same ions).

KEY CONCEPT

If E°_{cell} is positive, ln K_{eq} is positive. This means that K_{eq} must be greater than one and that the equilibrium lies to the right (products are favored).

Knowing the effects of concentration on equilibria, we can now derive the change in Gibbs free energy of an electrochemical cell with varying concentrations using the equation:

$$\Delta G = \Delta G^\circ + RT \ln Q$$

Equation 12.9

where ΔG is the free energy change under nonstandard conditions, ΔG° is the free energy change under standard conditions (which can be determined from Equation 12.4 or Equation 12.8 above), R is the ideal gas constant, T is the temperature, and Q is the reaction quotient.

MCAT CONCEPT CHECK 12.3

Before you move on, assess your understanding of the material with these questions.

1. Fill in the table to show the relationships between the equilibrium constant, Gibbs free energy, and electromotive force (emf), assuming standard conditions:

K_{eq}	ΔG°: (+) or (−)?	Reaction: Spontaneous or Nonspontaneous?	E°_{cell}: (+) or (−)?
1.2×10^{-2}			
2×10^2			
1			

2. Given the following reaction quotients and equilibrium constants, determine the direction of the reaction and the sign of E_{cell}:

Q	K_{eq}	Reaction Direction (Forward, Backward, or Equilibrium)	Sign of E_{cell}
10^{-3}	10^{-2}		
10^2	1.1		
1	1		

Conclusion

In this chapter, we covered the essential MCAT topic of electrochemistry. We reviewed the behavior of many different types of electrochemical cells. Galvanic cells rely on spontaneous oxidation–reduction reactions to produce current and supply energy. The concentration cell is a special type of galvanic cell for which the current is dependent on an ion concentration gradient rather than a difference in reduction potential between two chemically distinct electrodes. Electrolytic cells rely on external voltage sources to drive a nonspontaneous oxidation–reduction reaction called electrolysis. Finally, we considered the thermodynamics of the different cell types. Galvanic and concentration cells have positive electromotive forces (emf) and negative free energy changes, whereas electrolytic cells have negative electromotive forces and positive free energy changes.

In retrospect, the content you have learned in *MCAT General Chemistry Review* has numerous organic (biological) and inorganic applications. And as you prepare to be a physician, you must begin to understand and treat the individual as a sum of many intertwining systems and parts. Many body systems and parts rely on electrochemical cells: the heart is a self-paced electrochemical cell, the neurons of the brain and spinal cord are rechargeable concentration cells, and every cell that contains mitochondria (all cells except erythrocytes) rely on the proton-motive force across the inner mitochondrial membrane to function. Our discussion here of inorganic systems has value through analogy to many biological systems.

Without further delay, we want to offer you our heartiest congratulations for completing this final chapter of *MCAT General Chemistry Review*. The hard work, time, and energy you have invested in a careful and thorough review of the topics covered within the pages of this book will pay off on Test Day. We hope that we have been successful in meeting our goals in writing this *Kaplan MCAT Review* series: to assess the general concepts and principles essential to correctly and efficiently answer the general chemistry questions on the MCAT; to guide you in the development of critical thinking skills necessary for analyzing passages, question stems, and answer choices; and to provide holistic preparation for your Test Day experience. In addition to all of these, we aimed to relate the science to everyday life experiences and future experiences as a physician, demystify the concepts, and have some fun in the process. We are grateful for the opportunity to have been a part of your journey to success on the MCAT, and—beyond that—success in your medical education and future practice as the great physician you deserve to be!

GO ONLINE

You've reviewed the content, now test your knowledge and critical thinking skills by completing a test-like passage set in your online resources!

CONCEPT SUMMARY

Electrochemical Cells

- An **electrochemical cell** describes any cell in which oxidation–reduction reactions take place. Certain characteristics are shared between all types of electrochemical cells.
  - **Electrodes** are strips of metal or other conductive materials placed in an **electrolyte** solution.
  - The **anode** is always the site of oxidation. It attracts anions.
  - The **cathode** is always the site of reduction. It attracts cations.
  - Electrons flow from the anode to the cathode.
  - Current flows from the cathode to the anode.
- **Cell diagrams** are shorthand notation that represent the reactions taking place in an electrochemical cell.
  - Cell diagrams are written from anode to cathode with electrolytes (the solution) in between.
  - A vertical line represents a phase boundary, and a double vertical line represents a salt bridge or other physical boundary.
- **Galvanic (voltaic) cells** house spontaneous reactions ($\Delta G < 0$) with a positive electromotive force.
- **Electrolytic cells** house nonspontaneous reactions ($\Delta G > 0$) with a negative electromotive force. These nonspontaneous cells can be used to create useful products through electrolysis.
- **Concentration cells** are a specialized form of a galvanic cell in which both electrodes are made of the same material. Rather than a potential difference causing the movement of charge, it is the concentration gradient between the two solutions.
- The charge on an electrode is dependent on the type of electrochemical cell one is studying.
  - For galvanic cells, the anode is negatively charged and the cathode is positively charged.
  - For electrolytic cells, the anode is positively charged and the cathode is negatively charged.
- **Rechargeable batteries** are electrochemical cells that can experience **charging** (electrolytic) and **discharging** (galvanic) states. Rechargeable batteries are often ranked by **energy density**—the amount of energy a cell can produce relative to the mass of battery material.
  - **Lead–acid batteries**, when discharging, consist of a Pb anode and a PbO_2 cathode in a concentrated sulfuric acid solution. When charging, the $PbSO_4$-plated electrodes are dissociated to restore the original Pb and PbO_2 electrodes and concentrate the electrolyte. These cells have a low energy density.
  - **Nickel–cadmium batteries (Ni–Cd)**, when discharging, consist of a Cd anode and a NiO(OH) cathode in a concentrated KOH solution. When charging, the $Ni(OH)_2$ and $Cd(OH)_2$ plated electrodes are dissociated to restore the original Cd and NiO(OH) electrodes and concentrate the electrolyte. These cells have a higher energy density than lead–acid batteries.
  - **Nickel–metal hydride (NiMH)** batteries have more or less replaced Ni–Cd batteries because they have higher energy density, are more cost effective, and are significantly less toxic.
- **Surge current** is an above-average current transiently released at the beginning of the discharge phase; it wanes rapidly until a stable current is achieved.

Cell Potentials

- A **reduction potential** quantifies the tendency for a species to gain electrons and be reduced. The higher the reduction potential, the more a given species wants to be reduced.
    - **Standard reduction potentials (E°_{red})** are calculated by comparison to the **standard hydrogen electrode (SHE)** under the standard conditions of 298 K, 1 atm pressure, and 1 M concentrations.
    - The standard hydrogen electrode has a standard reduction potential of 0 V.
- **Standard electromotive force (E°_{cell})** is the difference in standard reduction potential between the two half-cells.
- For galvanic cells, the difference of the reduction potentials of the two half-reactions is positive; for electrolytic cells, the difference of the reduction potentials of the two half-reactions is negative.

Electromotive Force and Thermodynamics

- Electromotive force and change in free energy always have opposite signs.
    - When E°_{cell} is positive, ΔG° is negative. This is the case in galvanic cells.
    - When E°_{cell} is negative, ΔG° is positive. This is the case in electrolytic cells.
    - When E°_{cell} is 0, ΔG° is 0. This is the case in concentration cells.
- The **Nernst equation** describes the relationship between the concentration of species in a solution under nonstandard conditions and the electromotive force.
- There exists a relationship between the equilibrium constant (K_{eq}) and E°_{cell}.
    - When K_{eq} (the ratio of products' concentrations at equilibrium over reactants', raised to their stoichiometric coefficients) is greater than 1, E°_{cell} is positive.
    - When K_{eq} is less than 1, E°_{cell} is negative.
    - When K_{eq} is equal to 1, E°_{cell} is 0.

ANSWERS TO CONCEPT CHECKS

12.1

1. In a galvanic cell, the anode is the site of oxidation, has current flowing toward it, and has a (−) designation. The cathode has electrons flowing toward it and attracts cations.
2. In an electrolytic cell, the anode is the site of oxidation and has current flowing toward it. The cathode has electrons flowing toward it, has a (−) designation, and attracts cations.
3. Pb (s) | H_2SO_4 (4 M) || H_2SO_4 (4 M) | PbO_2 (s)
4. Electrolytic cells are nonspontaneous and have a positive ΔG. Galvanic cells are spontaneous and have a negative ΔG; therefore, they have a positive E_{cell}.
5. $$\text{mol Me} = \frac{It}{nF} \rightarrow I = \frac{(\text{mol Me})nF}{t} = \frac{\left[\dfrac{230\ \text{g}}{23\ \dfrac{\text{g}}{\text{mol}}}\right](1\ \text{mol e}^-)\left[96{,}485\ \dfrac{\text{C}}{\text{mol e}^-}\right]}{30\ \text{hr}\left[\dfrac{3600\ \text{s}}{1\ \text{hr}}\right]} \approx \frac{10 \times 10^5}{10^5}$$
   $= 10$ A (actual $= 8.93$ A)
6.

Battery	State of Use	Galvanic or Electrolytic	Anode Material	Anode Charge	Cathode Material	Cathode Charge
Ni—Cd	Discharging	Galvanic	Cd	Negative	NiO(OH)	Positive
Ni—Cd	Charging	Electrolytic	$Cd(OH)_2$	Positive	$Ni(OH)_2$	Negative
Molten NaCl	Discharging	Electrolytic	Any	Positive	Any	Negative
Daniell cell	Discharging	Galvanic	Zn	Negative	Cu	Positive
Lead–acid	Charging	Electrolytic	$PbSO_4$	Positive	$PbSO_4$	Negative
Lead–acid	Discharging	Galvanic	Pb	Negative	PbO_2	Positive

12.2

1. A sample is measured by setting up a cell relative to a standard hydrogen electrode, which is given a reduction potential of 0 V by convention.
2. A positive emf means the cell is spontaneous (galvanic); a negative emf means the cell is nonspontaneous (electrolytic).
3. The first cell is electrolytic because it has a negative emf. The second cell is galvanic because it has a positive emf.
4. The reduction potential of triiodide is higher than iron(III), so triiodide will be reduced and iron will be oxidized: $2\ Fe + 3\ I_3^- \rightarrow 2\ Fe^{3+} + 9\ I^-$ ($E^\circ_{cell} = +0.57$ V).

12.3

1.

K_{eq}	ΔG°: (+) or (−)?	Reaction: Spontaneous or Nonspontaneous?	E°_{cell}: (+) or (−)?
1.2×10^{-2}	+	Nonspontaneous	−
2×10^2	−	Spontaneous	+
1	0	Not applicable—applies to any cell at equilibrium	0

Remember that $\Delta G^\circ = -RT \ln K_{eq}$; if $K_{eq} < 1$, $\ln K_{eq} < 0$, and $\Delta G^\circ > 0$. If $K_{eq} > 1$, $\ln K_{eq} > 0$, and $\Delta G^\circ < 0$. If $K_{eq} = 1$, $\ln K_{eq} = 0$, and $\Delta G^\circ = 0$.

2.

Q	K_{eq}	Reaction Direction (Forward, Backward, or Equilibrium)	Sign of E_{cell}
10^{-3}	10^{-2}	Forward	+
10^2	1.1	Backward	−
1	1	Equilibrium	0

Note that these calculations do not assume standard conditions, unlike question 1.

SCIENCE MASTERY ASSESSMENT EXPLANATIONS

1. **C**

In the oxidation–reduction reaction of a metal with oxygen, the metal will be oxidized (donate electrons) and oxygen will be reduced (accept electrons). This fact allows us to immediately eliminate **(B)** and **(D)**. A species with a higher reduction potential is more likely to be reduced, and a species with a lower reduction potential is more likely to be oxidized. Based on the information in the question, iron is oxidized more readily than those metals; this means that iron has a lower reduction potential.

2. **B**

To determine the standard electromotive force of a cell, simply subtract the standard reduction potentials of the two electrodes. In this case, the cathode is zinc because it is being reduced; the anode is silver because it is being oxidized. Thus,

$$E^{\circ}_{\text{cell}} = E^{\circ}_{\text{red,cathode}} - E^{\circ}_{\text{red,anode}} = -\ 0.763 - 0.337 = -\ 1.10\ \text{V}$$

While we must multiply the silver half-reaction by two to balance electrons, the actual value for the reduction potential does not change. Remember that the standard reduction potential is determined by the identity of the electrode, not the amount of it present.

3. **A**

Oxidation occurs at the anode, and reduction occurs at the cathode. Because Cu is the anode, it must be oxidized. The reduction potential of the cathode cannot be less than that of the anode for a galvanic cell. Therefore, mercury, **(A)**, must be the cathode. In a concentration cell, the same material is used as both the cathode and anode; however, this question assumes equal concentrations. If both electrolyte solutions have the same concentration, there will be no oxidation–reduction reaction and, therefore, no anode or cathode. This eliminates **(B)**.

4. **C**

In an electrolytic cell, ionic compounds are broken up into their constituents; the cations (positively charged ions) migrate toward the cathode, and the anions (negatively charged ions) migrate toward the anode. In this case, the cations are H^+ ions (protons), so option I is correct. Electrons flow from anode to cathode in all types of cells, meaning that option III is also correct. Option II is incorrect for two reasons. First, it is unlikely that the anions in any cell would be O^{2-} rather than OH^-. Second, and more significantly, these anions would flow to the anode, not the cathode.

5. **D**

This answer comes directly from the equation relating Gibbs free energy and E°_{cell}. $\Delta G^{\circ} = -nFE^{\circ}_{\text{cell}}$, where n is the number of moles of electrons transferred and F is the Faraday constant, $96{,}485\ \frac{\text{C}}{\text{mol e}^-}$. To determine n, one must look at the balanced half-reactions occurring in the oxidation–reduction reaction.

6. **B**

Salt bridges contain inert electrolytes. Ionic compounds, such as **(A)**, **(C)**, and **(D)**, are known to be strong electrolytes because they completely dissociate in solution. **(B)** cannot be considered an electrolyte because its atoms are covalently bonded and will not dissociate in aqueous solution. **(B)** and **(C)** may appear similar, but there is an important distinction to be made. **(C)** implies that Mg^{2+} and SO_3^{2-} are the final, dissociated ionic constituents, while **(B)** implies that neutral SO_3 would have to be dissolved in solution.

7. **B**

Potential, as measured by E°_{cell}, is dependent only on the identity of the electrodes and not the amount present. Similarly, the equilibrium constant depends only on the identity of the electrolyte solutions and the temperature. However, as the electrode material is increased, the surface area participating in oxidation–reduction reactions is increased and more electrons are released, making statement II correct.

8. **D**

E°_{cell} is dependent upon the change in free energy of the system through the equation $RT \ln K_{eq} = nFE^\circ_{cell}$. The temperature, T, appears in this equation; thus, a change in temperature will impact the E°_{cell}.

9. **B**

If this were a galvanic cell, the species with the more positive reduction potential (cadmium) would be reduced. The cathode is always reduced in an electrochemical cell, so sodium could not be the cathode in such a galvanic cell, eliminating **(A)**. Sodium would be the cathode in an electrolytic cell, however, which would make cadmium the anode. Thus, the answer is **(B)**. Note that we do not have to determine E°_{cell} because we already know the answer. However, the E°_{cell} would be $-2.71 - (-0.40) = -2.31$ V for an electrolytic cell, and $+2.31$ V for a galvanic cell, eliminating **(C)** and **(D)**.

10. **D**

There are only two equations involving standard change in free energy in electrochemical cells: $\Delta G^\circ = -nFE^\circ_{cell}$ and $\Delta G^\circ = -RT \ln K_{eq}$. Substituting $E^\circ_{cell} = E^\circ_{red,cathode} - E^\circ_{red,anode}$ into the first equation and distributing the negative sign gives **(D)**. **(A)** would be the opposite of ΔG°. Setting the two equations equal to each other, we get $RT \ln K_{eq} = nFE^\circ_{cell}$. Solving for E°_{cell}, we get $E^\circ_{cell} = \frac{RT}{nF} \ln K_{eq}$, which is the opposite of **(B)**. **(C)** incorrectly solves the algebra.

11. **D**

A spontaneous electrochemical reaction has a negative ΔG. Using the equation $\Delta G^\circ = -RT \ln K_{eq}$, $K_{eq} > 1$ would result in $\ln K_{eq} > 0$, which means $\Delta G^\circ < 0$. A negative electromotive force, **(A)**, or equilibrium state, **(B)**, would not correspond to a spontaneous reaction. Concentration cells can be spontaneous; however, if the concentration cell had reached equilibrium, it would cease to be a spontaneous reaction, eliminating **(C)**. When an answer choice *may* be true, but does not *have to* be—it is the wrong answer on Test Day.

12. **A**

A change in pH has a direct correlation to the hydrogen ion (H^+) concentration. Decreasing the pH increases the H^+ concentration, which means the concentration of products has increased in the oxidation of sulfur dioxide. This means it would be harder to liberate electrons, thus decreasing the emf. One could also view this decrease in oxidation potential as an increase in reduction potential. If $E^\circ_{red,anode}$ increases, then E°_{cell} must decrease according to $E^\circ_{cell} = E^\circ_{red,cathode} - E^\circ_{red,anode}$.

13. **C**

An electrolytic cell is nonspontaneous. Therefore, the ΔG° must be positive and E°_{cell} must be negative, eliminating **(B)** and **(D)**. The change in entropy may be positive or negative, depending on the species involved, eliminating **(A)**. According to the equation $\Delta G^\circ = -RT \ln K_{eq}$, $K_{eq} < 1$ would result in $\ln K_{eq} < 0$, which means $\Delta G^\circ > 0$.

14. **D**

Compared to other cell types, lead–acid batteries have a characteristically low energy density, **(D)**. While **(A)** is a true statement, the incomplete dissociation of sulfuric acid does not fully explain the low energy density of lead–acid batteries. **(C)** is likely to be an opposite; the more easily the electrodes dissociate, the easier it is to carry out oxidation–reduction reactions with them.

15. **C**

During the recharge cycle, Ni–Cd cells will accept current from an outside source until the Cd and NiO(OH) electrodes are pure; at this point, the reaction will stop because $Cd(OH)_2$ runs out and no more electrons can be accepted. **(A)** and **(B)** are both true statements, but they fail to explain why overcharging the battery (continuing to try to run current into the battery even when the electrodes are reverted to their original state) is not a problem with Ni–Cd batteries. Finally, surge current refers to the initial burst of current seen in some batteries; once charged, the surge current will not increase even if the power source continues to be run because no additional charge will be stored on the electrodes, eliminating **(D)**.

GO ONLINE

Consult your online resources for additional practice.

EQUATIONS TO REMEMBER

(12.1) **Moles of electrons transferred during reduction:** $M^{n+} + n\,e^- \rightarrow M\,(s)$

(12.2) **Electrodeposition equation:** $\text{mol Me} = \frac{It}{nF}$

(12.3) **Standard electromotive force of a cell:** $E^\circ_{\text{cell}} = E^\circ_{\text{red,cathode}} - E^\circ_{\text{red,anode}}$

(12.4) **Standard change in free energy from standard emf:** $\Delta G^\circ = -nFE^\circ_{\text{cell}}$

(12.5) **Nernst equation (full):** $E_{\text{cell}} = E^\circ_{\text{cell}} - \frac{RT}{nF} \ln Q$

(12.6) **Nernst equation (simplified):** $E_{\text{cell}} = E^\circ_{\text{cell}} - \frac{0.0592}{n} \log Q$

(12.7) **Reaction quotient:** $Q = \frac{[C]^c[D]^d}{[A]^a[B]^b}$

(12.8) **Standard change in free energy from equilibrium constant:**
$\Delta G^\circ = -RT \ln K_{\text{eq}}$

(12.9) **Free energy change (nonstandard conditions):** $\Delta G = \Delta G^\circ + RT \ln Q$

SHARED CONCEPTS

Biochemistry Chapter 3
Nonenzymatic Protein Function and Protein Analysis

Biochemistry Chapter 8
Biological Membranes

General Chemistry Chapter 7
Thermochemistry

General Chemistry Chapter 11
Oxidation–Reduction Reactions

Physics and Math Chapter 5
Electrostatics and Magnetism

Physics and Math Chapter 6
Circuits

GLOSSARY

Absolute zero–The temperature at which all substances have no thermal energy; 0 K or −273.15°C.

Absorption spectrum–The series of discrete lines at characteristic frequencies representing the energy required to excite an electron from the ground state.

Acid–A species that donates hydrogen ions or accepts electrons.

Acid dissociation constant (K_a)–The equilibrium constant that measures the degree of dissociation of an acid under specific conditions.

Acidic solution–An aqueous solution that contains more H^+ ions than OH^- ions; pH <7 under standard conditions.

Actinide series–The series of chemical elements atomic numbered 89–103 and falling between the *s* and *d* blocks on the periodic table.

Activation energy (E_a)–The minimum amount of energy required for a reaction to reach the transition state; also called energy barrier.

Actual yield–The experimental quantity of a substance obtained at the end of a reaction.

Adiabatic process–A process that occurs without the transfer of heat into or out of the system.

Alkali metals–Elements found in Group IA of the periodic table; highly reactive, readily losing one valence electron to form ionic compounds with nonmetals.

Alkaline earth metals–Elements found in Group IIA of the periodic table; chemistry is similar to that of the alkali metals, except that they have two valence electrons and, thus, form +2 cations.

Amphiprotic species–A species that may either gain or lose a proton.

Amphoteric species–A species capable of reacting as either an acid or base, depending on the nature of the reactants.

Angular momentum–The rotational analog of linear momentum.

Anion–An ionic species with a negative charge.

Anode–The electrode at which oxidation occurs.

Antibonding orbital–A molecular orbital formed by the overlap of two or more atomic orbitals; energy is greater than the energy of the combining atomic orbitals.

Aqueous solution–A solution in which water is the solvent.

Arrhenius acid–A species that donates protons (H^+) in aqueous solution.

Arrhenius base–A species that donates hydroxide ions (OH^-) in aqueous solution.

Arrhenius equation–A chemical kinetics equation that relates the rate constant (k) of a reaction with the frequency factor (A), the activation energy (E_a), the ideal gas constant (R), and temperature (T) in kelvin.

Atom–The smallest unit of an element that retains the properties of the element; it cannot be further broken down by chemical means.

Atomic mass–The mass of a given isotope of an element; closely related to the mass number.

Atomic mass unit (amu)–A unit of mass defined as $\frac{1}{12}$ the mass of a carbon-12 atom; approximately equal to the mass of one proton or one neutron.

Atomic number–The number of protons in a given element.

Atomic orbital–Describes the region of space where there is a high probability of finding an electron.

Atomic radius–The average distance between a nucleus and its outermost electron; usually measured as one-half the distance between two nuclei of an element in its elemental form.

Atomic weight–The weighted average mass of the atoms of an element, taking into account the relative abundance of all naturally occurring isotopes.

Aufbau principle–The concept that electrons fill energy levels in order of increasing energy, completely filling one sublevel before beginning to fill the next.

Autoionization–The process by which a molecule (usually water) spontaneously dissociates into cations and anions.

Avogadro's number–The number of atoms or molecules in one mole of a substance: $6.02 \times 10^{23}\ mol^{-1}$.

Avogadro's principle–The law stating that under the same conditions of temperature and pressure, equal volumes of different gases will have the same number of molecules.

Azimuthal quantum number (l)–The quantum number denoting the sublevel or subshell in which an electron can be found; reveals the shape of the orbital.

Balanced equation–An equation for a chemical reaction in which the number of atoms for each element in the reaction and the total charge are the same for the reactants and the products.

Balmer series–Part of the emission spectrum for hydrogen, representing transitions of an electron from energy levels $n > 2$ to $n = 2$.

Barometer–A tool for measuring pressure.

Base–A species that donates hydroxide ions or electron pairs or that accepts protons.

Base dissociation constant (K_b)–The equilibrium constant that measures the degree of dissociation for a base under specific conditions.

Basic solution–An aqueous solution that contains more OH^- ions than H^+ ion; pH > 7 under standard conditions.

Bohr model–The model of the hydrogen atom in which electrons assume certain circular orbits around a positive nucleus.

Boiling point–The temperature at which the vapor pressure of a liquid is equal to the incident pressure; the normal boiling point of any liquid is defined as its boiling point at a pressure of 1 atmosphere.

Boiling point elevation–The amount by which a given quantity of solute raises the boiling point of a liquid; a colligative property.

Bond energy–The energy (enthalpy change) required to break a particular bond under given conditions.

Bond enthalpy–The average energy that is required to break a particular type of bond between atoms in the gas phase.

Bonding electrons–Electrons located in the valence shell of an atom and involved in a covalent bond.

Bonding orbital–A molecular orbital formed by the overlap of two or more atomic orbitals; energy is less than that of the combining orbitals.

Bond length–The average distance between two nuclei in a bond; as the number of shared electron pairs increases, the bond length decreases.

Bond order–The number of shared electron pairs between two atoms; a single bond has a bond order of 1, a double bond has a bond order of 2, a triple bond has a bond order of 3.

Boyle's law–The law stating that at constant temperature, the volume of a gaseous sample is inversely proportional to its pressure.

Broken-order reaction–A reaction with noninteger orders in its rate law.

Brønsted–Lowry acid–A proton donor.

Brønsted–Lowry base–A proton acceptor.

Buffer–A solution containing a weak acid and its salt (or a weak base and its salt) that tends to resist changes in pH.

Buffer region–The portion of a titration curve in which the concentration of an acid is approximately equal to that of its conjugate base; pH remains relatively constant through this region.

Buffering capacity–The degree to which a system can resist changes in pH.

Calorie (cal)–A unit of thermal energy.

Calorimeter–An apparatus used to measure the heat absorbed or released by a reaction.

Catalyst–A substance that increases the rates of the forward and reverse directions of a specific reaction by lowering activation energy, but is itself left unchanged.

Cathode–The electrode at which reduction takes place.

Cation–An ionic species with a positive charge.

Celsius (°C)–A temperature scale defined by having 0°C equal to the freezing point of water and 100°C equal to the boiling point of water; otherwise known as the centigrade temperature scale.

Chalcogens–Elements found in Group VIA of the periodic table with diverse chemistry; the group contains metals, nonmetals (like oxygen), and metalloids; typically form –2 anions.

Charging–A state of an electrochemical cell in which an external electromotive force is being used to return a cell to its original state; during this process, electrons are transferred nonspontaneously from cathode to anode.

Charles's law–The law stating that the volume of a gas at constant pressure is directly proportional to its absolute (kelvin) temperature.

Chelation–The process of binding metal ions to the same ligand at multiple points.

Chemical bond–The interaction between two atoms resulting from the sharing or transfer of electrons.

Chemical equation–An expression used to describe the quantity and identity of the reactants and products of a reaction.

Chemical properties–Those properties of a substance related to the chemical changes that it undergoes, such as ionization energy and electronegativity.

Closed system–A system that can exchange energy but not matter with its surroundings.

Colligative properties–Those properties of solutions that depend only on the number of solute particles present but not on the nature of those particles.

Collision theory of chemical kinetics–A theory that states that the rate of a reaction is proportional to the number of collisions per second between reacting molecules that have sufficient energy to overcome the activation energy barrier; implies that only a fraction of collisions are sufficient.

Combination reaction–A reaction in which two or more reactants form a single product.

Combined gas law–A gas law that combines Boyle's law, Charles's law, and Gay-Lussac's law to state that pressure and volume are inversely proportional to each other, and each is directly proportional to temperature.

Combustion reaction–A reaction in which an oxidant (typically oxygen) reacts with a fuel (typically a hydrocarbon) to yield water and an oxide (such as carbon dioxide if between a hydrocarbon and oxygen).

Common ion effect–A shift in the equilibrium of a solution due to the addition of ions of a species already present in the reaction mixture.

Complexation reaction–A reaction in which a central cation is bound to one or more ligands.

Complex ion–A polyatomic molecule in which a central cation is bonded to electron pair donors called ligands.

Compound–A pure substance that can be decomposed to produce elements, other compounds, or both.

Compression–Reduction in the volume of a gas.

Concentrated solution–A solution with a high concentration value; the cutoff for the term "concentrated" depends on the purpose and identity of the solution.

Concentration–The amount of solute per unit of solvent or the relative amount of one component in a mixture.

Concentration cell–A cell that creates an electromotive force (emf or voltage) using a single chemical species in half-cells of varying concentration.

Condensation–The process in which a gas transitions to the liquid state.

Conductor–A material in which electrons are able to transfer energy in the form of heat or electricity.

Conjugate acid–base pair–The relationship between a Brønsted–Lowry acid and its deprotonated form, or a Brønsted–Lowry base and its protonated form.

Coordinate covalent bond–A covalent bond in which both electrons of the bonding pair are donated by one of the bonded atoms.

Coordination number–The number of atoms that are bound to a central atom.

Covalent bond–A chemical bond formed by the sharing of an electron pair between two atoms; can be in the form of single bonds, double bonds, or triple bonds.

Critical point–The point in a phase diagram beyond which the phase boundary between liquid and gas no longer exists.

Critical pressure–The vapor pressure at the critical temperature of a given substance.

Critical temperature–Also known as the critical point. The highest temperature at which the liquid and gas phases of a substance can coexist; above this temperature, the liquid and gas phases are indistinguishable.

Crystal–A solid in which atoms, ions, or molecules are arranged in a regular, three-dimensional lattice structure.

***d* subshell**–Subshell corresponding to the angular momentum quantum number $l = 2$; contains five orbitals and is found in the third and higher principal energy levels.

Dalton's law of partial pressures–The law stating that the sum of the partial pressures of the components of a gaseous mixture must equal the total pressure of the sample.

Daniell cell–An electrochemical cell in which the anode is the site of Zn metal oxidation and the cathode is the site of Cu^{2+} ion reduction.

Decomposition reaction–A reaction in which a single compound breaks down into two or more products.

Delocalized orbitals–Molecular orbitals in which electron density is spread over an entire molecule, or a portion thereof, rather than being localized between two atoms.

Density (ρ)–A physical property of a substance, defined as the mass contained in a unit of volume.

Deposition–In most chemical processes, the direct transition of a substance from the gaseous state to the solid state; in electrochemical reactions, the build-up of a solid precipitate onto an electrode.

Diamagnetism–A condition that arises when a substance has no unpaired electrons and is slightly repelled by a magnetic field.

Diffusion–The random motion of gas or solute particles across a concentration gradient, leading to uniform distribution of the gas or solute throughout the container.

Dilute solution–A solution with a low concentration of a given solute.

Dipole–A species containing bonds between elements of different electronegativities, resulting in an unequal distribution of charge.

Dipole–dipole interactions–The attractive forces between two dipoles; magnitude is dependent on both the dipole moments and the distance between the two species.

Dipole moment–A vector quantity with a magnitude that is dependent on the product of the charges and the distance between them; oriented from the positive to the negative pole.

Discharging–The state of a rechargeable electrochemical cell that is providing an electromotive force by allowing electrons to flow spontaneously from anode to cathode.

Disproportionation–An oxidation–reduction reaction in which the same species acts as the oxidizing agent and as the reducing agent; also called dismutation.

Dissociation–The separation of a single species into two separate species; usually used in reference to salts or weak acids or bases.

Double-displacement reaction–A reaction in which ions from two different compounds swap their associated counterions; typically, one of the products of this type of reaction is insoluble in solution and will precipitate; also called metathesis or ping-pong reaction.

Ductility–The property of metals that allows a material to be drawn into thinly stretched wires.

Effective nuclear charge (Z_{eff})–The charge perceived by an electron from the nucleus; applies most often to valence electrons and influences periodic trends such as atomic radius and ionization energy.

Effusion–The movement of gas from one compartment to another under pressure through a small opening; follows Graham's law.

Electrochemical cell–A cell within which an oxidation–reduction reaction takes place, containing two electrodes between which there is an electrical potential difference.

Electrode–An electrical conductor through which an electrical current enters or leaves a medium.

Electrolysis–The process in which an electrical current is used to power an otherwise nonspontaneous decomposition reaction.

Electrolyte–A compound that ionizes in water and increases the conductance of the solution.

Electrolytic cell–An electrochemical cell that uses an external voltage source to drive a nonspontaneous oxidation–reduction reaction.

Electromagnetic radiation–A wave composed of electric and magnetic fields oscillating perpendicular to each other and to the direction of propagation.

Electromagnetic spectrum–The range of all possible frequencies or wavelengths of electromagnetic radiation.

Electromotive force (emf)–The potential difference developed between the cathode and the anode of an electrochemical cell; also called voltage.

Electron (e^-)–A subatomic particle that remains outside the nucleus and carries a single negative charge; in most cases, its mass is considered to be negligible.

Electron affinity–The energy dissipated by a gaseous species when it gains an electron.

Electron configuration–The symbolic representation used to describe the electron arrangement within the energy sublevels in a given atom.

Electron spin–The intrinsic angular momentum of an electron, represented by *ms*; has arbitrary values of $+\frac{1}{2}$and $-\frac{1}{2}$.

Electronegativity–A measure of the ability of an atom to attract the electrons in a bond; commonly measured with the Pauling scale.

Electronic geometry–The spatial arrangement of all pairs of electrons around a central atom, including both the bonding and lone pairs.

Electron shell–The space occupied by/path followed by an electron around an atom's nucleus. Electron shell (also called principal energy level) for a given electron is indicated by its principal quantum number.

Element–A substance that cannot be further broken down by chemical means; defined by its number of protons (atomic number).

Emission spectrum–A series of discrete lines at characteristic frequencies, each representing the energy emitted when electrons in an atom return from an excited state to their ground state.

Empirical formula–The simplest whole-number ratio of the different elements in a compound.

Endothermic reaction–A reaction that absorbs heat from the surroundings as the reaction proceeds (positive ΔH).

Endpoint–The point in a titration at which the indicator changes to its final color.

Energy density–An equivalence unit regarding the amount of electrochemical energy capable of being stored per unit weight; a battery with a large energy density can produce a large amount of energy with a small amount of material.

Enthalpy (*H*)–The heat content of a system at constant pressure; the change in enthalpy (ΔH) in the course of a reaction is the difference between the enthalpies of the products and the reactants.

Entropy (*S*)–A property related to dispersion of energy through a system or the degree of disorder in that system; the change in entropy (ΔS) in the course of a reaction is the difference between the entropies of the products and the reactants.

Equilibrium–The state of balance in which the forward and reverse reaction rates of a reversible reaction are equal; the concentrations of all species will remain constant over time unless there is a change in the reaction conditions.

Equilibrium constant (K_{eq})–The ratio of the concentrations of the products to the concentrations of the reactants for a certain reaction at equilibrium, all raised to their stoichiometric coefficients.

Equivalence point–The point in a titration at which the moles of acid present equal the moles of base added, or vice-versa.

Equivalent–A mole of charge in the form of electrons, protons, ions, or other measurable quantities that are produced by a substance.

Evaporation–The transition from a liquid to a gaseous state.

Excess reagent–In a chemical reaction, any reagent that does not limit the amount of product that can be formed.

Excitation–The promotion of an electron to a higher energy level by absorption of an energy quantum.

Excited state–An electronic state having a higher energy than the ground state; typically attained by the absorption of a photon of a certain energy.

Exothermic reaction–A reaction that gives off heat to the surroundings (negative ΔH) as the reaction proceeds.

***f* subshell**–The subshell corresponding to the angular momentum quantum number $l = 3$; contains seven orbitals and is found in the fourth and higher principal energy levels.

Faraday constant (*F*)–The total charge on 1 mole of electrons $\left(F = 96,485\ \frac{\text{C}}{\text{mol e}^-}\right)$; not to be confused with the farad (denoted F), a unit of capacitance.

First law of thermodynamics–The law stating that the total energy of a system and its surroundings remains constant.

First-order reaction–A reaction in which the rate is directly proportional to the concentration of only one reactant.

Fluid–A substance that flows due to weak intermolecular attractions between molecules and that takes the shape of its container; liquids and gases are considered fluids.

Formal charge–The conventional assignment of charges to individual atoms of a Lewis structure for a molecule; the total number of valence electrons in the free atom minus the total number of electrons when the atom is bonded (assuming equal splitting of the electrons in bonds).

Formula weight–The sum of the atomic weights of constituent ions according to an ionic compound's empirical formula.

Freezing–The process in which a liquid transitions to the solid state; also known as solidification or crystallization.

Freezing point–At a given pressure, the temperature at which the solid and liquid phases of a substance coexist in equilibrium; identical to the melting point.

Freezing point depression–Amount by which a given quantity of solute lowers the freezing point of a liquid; a colligative property.

Galvanic cell–An electrochemical cell that uses a spontaneous oxidation–reduction reaction to generate an electromotive force; also called a voltaic cell.

Galvanization–In electrochemical cells, the precipitation process onto the cathode itself; also called plating.

Gas–The physical state of matter possessing the most disorder, in which molecules interact through very weak attractions; found at relatively low pressure and high temperatures.

Gas constant (*R*)–A proportionality constant that appears in the ideal gas law equation, $PV = nRT$. Its value depends on the units of pressure, temperature, and volume used in a given situation.

Gay-Lussac's law–The law stating that the pressure of a gaseous sample at constant volume is directly proportional to its absolute temperature.

Gibbs free energy (*G*)–The energy of a system available to do work. The change in Gibbs free energy, ΔG, can be determined for a given reaction equation from the enthalpy change, temperature, and entropy change; a negative ΔG denotes a spontaneous reaction, while a positive ΔG denotes a nonspontaneous reaction.

Graham's law–The law stating that the rate of effusion or diffusion for a gas is inversely proportional to the square root of the gas's molar mass.

Gram equivalent weight (GEW)–The amount of a compound that contains 1 mole of reacting capacity when fully dissociated; one GEW equals the molar mass divided by the reactive capacity (how many of the species of interest is obtained) per formula unit.

Ground state–The unexcited state of an electron.

Group–A vertical column of the periodic table containing elements that are similar in their chemical properties; also called a family.

Half-cell–The separated compartments housing the electrodes and solutions in an electrochemical reaction.

Half-equivalence point–The point at which half a given species within a titration has been protonated or deprotonated.

Half-reaction–Either the reduction half or oxidation half of an oxidation–reduction reaction; in an electrochemical cell, each half-reaction occurs at one of the electrodes.

Halogens–The active nonmetals in Group VIIA of the periodic table, which have high electronegativities and high electron affinities.

Heat–The energy transferred spontaneously from a warmer sample to a cooler sample.

Heat of formation (ΔH_f)–The heat absorbed or released during the formation of a pure substance from its elements at a constant pressure.

Heat of fusion (ΔH_{fus})–The enthalpy change for the conversion of 1 gram or 1 mole of a solid to a liquid at constant temperature and pressure.

Heat of sublimation (ΔH_{sub})–The enthalpy change for the conversion of 1 gram or 1 mole of a solid to a gas at constant temperature and pressure.

Heat of vaporization (ΔH_{vap})–The enthalpy change for the conversion of 1 gram or 1 mole of a liquid to a gas at constant temperature and pressure.

Heisenberg uncertainty principle–The concept that states that it is impossible to determine both the momentum and position of an electron simultaneously with perfect accuracy.

Henderson–Hasselbalch equation–Equation showing the relationship of the pH or pOH of a solution to the pK_a or pK_b and the ratio of the concentrations of the dissociated species.

Henry's law–The law stating that the mass of a gas that dissolves in a solution is directly proportional to the partial pressure of the gas above the solution.

Hess's law–The law stating that the energy change in an overall reaction is equal to the sum of the energy changes in the individual reactions that comprise it.

Heterogeneous–Nonuniform in composition.

Heterogeneous catalyst–A catalyst that is not in the same phase of matter as the reactants (for example, a solid platinum catalyst reacting with hydrogen gas).

Homogeneous–Uniform in composition.

Homogeneous catalyst–A catalyst that is in the same phase of matter as the reactants (for example, an aqueous enzyme in the cytoplasm of a cell).

Hund's rule–The rule that electrons will fill into separate orbitals with parallel spins before pairing within an orbital.

Hybridization–The combination of two or more atomic orbitals to form new orbitals with properties that are intermediate between those of the original orbitals.

Hydration–The process in which a substance combines with water, either through molecules surrounding an ion in a solution or by incorporating water directly into a solid crystal structure.

Hydration shell–The sphere of water molecules that surrounds an ion when it is dissolved in an aqueous solution.

Hydrogen bonding–The strong attraction between a hydrogen atom bonded to a highly electronegative atom (such as nitrogen, oxygen, or fluorine) in one molecule and a highly electronegative atom in another molecule.

Hydrolysis–A reaction in which water is consumed during the breakdown of another molecule.

Hydronium ion–The H_3O^+ ion.

Hydroxide ion–The OH^- ion.

Ideal bond angle–An angle between nonbonding or bonding electron pairs that minimizes the repulsion between them.

Ideal gas–A hypothetical gas with behavior that is described by the ideal gas law under all conditions; assumes that its particles have zero volume and do not exhibit interactive forces.

Ideal gas law–The equation stating $PV = nRT$, where R is the gas constant; can be used to describe the behavior of many real gases at moderate pressures and temperatures significantly above absolute zero.

Ideal solution–A solution with an enthalpy of dissolution that is equal to zero.

Indicator–A substance used in low concentrations during a titration that changes color over a certain pH range (acid–base titrations) or at a particular electromotive force (oxidation–reduction titrations); the final color change of an indicator occurs at the endpoint of a titration.

Inert–Unreactive.

Inert gases–The elements in Group VIIIA, which contain a full octet of valence electrons in their outermost shells and are therefore very unreactive; also called noble gases.

Intermediate–A molecule that transiently exists in a multistep reaction; does not appear in the overall balanced equation.

Intermolecular forces–The attractive and repulsive forces between molecules.

Intramolecular forces–The attractive forces between atoms within a single molecule (ionic and covalent bonds).

Ion–A charged atom or molecule that results from the loss or gain of electrons.

Ion product (IP)–The general term for the reaction quotient of a dissolving ionic compound; compared to K_{sp} to determine the saturation status of a solution.

Ionic bond–A chemical bond formed through electrostatic interaction between positive and negative ions.

Ionic radius–The average distance from the center of the nucleus to the edge of its electron cloud; cationic radii are generally smaller than their parent metal, whereas anionic radii are generally larger than their parent nonmetal.

Ionic solid–A solid consisting of positive and negative ions arranged into crystals that are made up of regularly repeated units held together by ionic bonds.

Ionization energy–The energy required to remove an electron from the valence shell of a gaseous atom.

Irreversible reaction–A reaction that proceeds in one direction only and goes to completion.

Isobaric process–A process that occurs at constant pressure.

Isoelectric focusing–A technique used to separate amino acids or polypeptides based on their isoelectric points.

Isolated system–A system that can exchange neither matter nor energy with its surroundings.

Isothermal process–A process that occurs at constant temperature.

Isotopes–Atoms containing the same number of protons but different numbers of neutrons.

Isovolumetric process–A process that occurs at constant volume in which the system performs no work; also called an isochoric process.

Joule (J)–The unit of energy;1 $J = 1\ \frac{Kg \cdot m^2}{s^2}$.

Kelvin (K)–A temperature scale with units equal to the units of the Celsius scale and absolute zero defined as 0 K; also called the absolute temperature scale.

Kinetic molecular theory–The theory proposed to account for the observed behavior of gases; considers gas molecules to be pointlike, volumeless particles exhibiting no intermolecular forces that are in constant random motion and undergo only completely elastic collisions with the container or other gas particles.

Kinetic product–The product of a reaction that is formed favorably at a lower temperature because thermal energy is not available to form the transition state required to create a more stable thermodynamic product; has a smaller overall difference in free energy between the products and reactants than the thermodynamic product.

Lanthanide series–The series of chemical elements atomic numbered 57–71 and falling between the S and D blocks on the periodic table.

Latent heat–The enthalpy of an isothermal process.

Law of conservation of charge–The law stating that, in a given reaction, the charge of ions in the products is equal to the charge of ions in the reactants.

Law of conservation of mass–The law stating that, in a given reaction, the mass of the products is equal to the mass of the reactants.

Law of constant composition–The law stating that the elements in a pure compound are found in specific mass ratios.

Law of mass action–The form of the equilibrium constant; has the concentrations of products over concentrations of reactants, each raised to their stoichiometric coefficients.

Le Châtelier's principle–The observation that when a system at equilibrium is disturbed or stressed, the system will react in such a way as to relieve the stress and restore equilibrium.

Lead–acid battery–An electrochemical cell in which the anode is the site of Pb metal oxidation and the cathode is the site of Pb^{4+} ion reduction. The electrolyte is a strong acid, usually sulfuric acid.

Lewis acid–A species capable of accepting an electron pair.

Lewis base–A species capable of donating an electron pair.

Lewis structure–A method of representing the shared and unshared electrons of an atom, molecule, or ion; also called a Lewis dot diagram.

Ligand–A molecule bonded to a metal ion in a coordination compound; ligands are Lewis bases that form coordinate covalent bonds with the central metal ion.

Limiting reagent–In a chemical reaction, the reactant present in such quantity as to limit the amount of product that can be formed.

Liquid–The state of matter in which intermolecular attractions are intermediate between those in gases and in solids, distinguished from the gas phase by having a definite volume and from the solid phase because molecules may mix freely.

London dispersion forces–Intermolecular forces arising from interactions between temporary dipoles in molecules.

Lyman series–A portion of the emission spectrum for hydrogen representing electronic transitions from energy levels $n > 1$ to $n = 1$.

Magnetic quantum number (m_l)–The third quantum number, defining the particular orbital of a subshell in which an electron resides; conveys information about the orientation of the orbital in space.

Malleability–A physical property of metals that defines how well an element can be shaped using a hammer.

Mass–A physical property representing the amount of matter in a given sample.

Mass number–The sum of protons and neutrons in an atom's nucleus. Can also be called atomic mass number.

Maxwell–Boltzmann distribution curve–The distribution of the molecular speeds of gas particles at a given temperature; as temperature increases, average speed increases and the distribution becomes wider and flatter.

Mechanism–The series of steps involved in a given reaction.

Melting point–The temperature at which the solid and liquid phases of a substance coexist in equilibrium; identical to the freezing point.

Metal–One of a class of elements on the left side of the periodic table possessing low ionization energies and electronegativities; readily give up electrons to form cations and possess relatively high electrical conductivity.

Metalloid–An element possessing properties intermediate between those of a metal and those of a nonmetal; also called a semimetal.

Microstate–In thermodynamics, a specific way in which energy of a system is organized.

Millimeters of mercury (mmHg)–A unit of pressure defined as the number of millimeters that mercury in a barometer is raised above its surface in a capillary tube by an external pressure; 1 torr is equal to 1 mmHg by definition, and 1 atmosphere is equal to 760 mmHg.

Mixed-order reaction–A reaction in which the reaction order changes over time in the rate law.

Mixture–A system containing multiple substances (2+) that have been physically combined but are not chemically combined.

Molality (m)–A concentration unit equal to the number of moles of solute per kilogram of solvent.

Molarity (M)–A concentration unit equal to the number of moles of solute per liter of solution.

Molar mass (M)–The mass in grams of one mole of an element or compound.

Molar solubility–The molarity of a solute in a saturated solution.

Mole (mol)–An amount of substance equal to Avogadro's number of molecules or atoms; the mass of 1 mole of substance in grams is the same as the mass of one molecule or atom in atomic mass units.

Mole fraction (X)–A unit of concentration equal to the ratio of the number of moles of a particular component to the total number of moles for all species in the system.

Molecular formula–A formula showing the actual number and identity of all atoms in each molecule of a compound; always a whole-number multiple of the empirical formula.

Molecular geometry–The spatial arrangement of only the bonding pairs of electrons around a central atom.

Molecular orbital–The region of electron density in chemical bonding that results from the overlap of two or more atomic orbitals.

Molecular weight–The sum of the atomic weights of all the atoms in a molecule.

Molecule–The smallest polyatomic unit of an element or compound that exists with distinct chemical and physical properties.

Nernst equation–An equation that relates the voltage of an electrochemical cell to the concentrations of the reactants and products within that cell.

Net ionic equation–A reaction equation showing only the species actually participating in the reaction.

Neutral solution–An aqueous solution in which the concentration of H^+ and OH^- ions are equal (pH = 7 at 298 K).

Neutralization reaction–A reaction between an acid and base in which a salt is formed (and sometimes water).

Neutron (n^0)–A subatomic particle contained within the nucleus of an atom; carries no charge and has a mass slightly larger than that of a proton.

Nickel-cadmium battery–A rechargeable electrochemical cell in which the anode is the site of Cd metal oxidation and the cathode is the site of Ni^{2+} ion reduction.

Nickel-metal hydride battery–A rechargeable electrochemical cell in which the anode is the site of metal hydride oxidation and the cathode is the site of nickel ion reduction; the nickel may be in one of many oxidation states.

Nonbonding electrons–Electrons located in the valence shell of an atom but not involved in covalent bonds.

Nonelectrolyte–A compound that does not ionize in water.

Nonmetal–One of a class of elements with high ionization energies and electron affinities that generally gain electrons to form anions; located in the upper right corner of the periodic table.

Nonpolar covalent bond–A covalent bond between elements of similar electronegativity; contains no charge separation.

Nonpolar molecule–A molecule that exhibits no net separation of charge and, therefore, no net dipole moment.

Nonrepresentative element–Elements with an expanded valence shell that includes *d*- and *f*-block electrons; also called Group B or transition elements.

Nonspontaneous process–A process that will not occur on its own without energy input from the surroundings; has a positive change in free energy.

Normality (N)–A concentration unit equal to the number of equivalents per liter of solution.

Nucleus–The small central region of an atom; a dense, positively charged area containing protons and neutrons.

Octet–Eight valence electrons in a subshell around a nucleus; imparts great stability to an atom.

Octet rule–A rule stating that bonded atoms tend to undergo reactions that will produce a complete octet of valence electrons; applies without exception only to C, N, O, and F.

Open system–A system that can exchange both energy and matter with its surroundings.

Orbital–A region of electron density around an atom or molecule containing no more than two electrons of opposite spin.

Osmosis–The movement of water through a semipermeable membrane down its concentration gradient, from low solute concentration to high solute concentration.

Osmotic pressure–The pressure that must be applied to a solution to prevent the passage of water through a semipermeable membrane down its concentration gradient; best thought of as a "sucking" pressure drawing water into solution.

Oxidation–A reaction involving the net loss of electrons, increasing oxidation number.

Oxidation number–Also called oxidation state, the number assigned to an atom in an ion or molecule that denotes its real or hypothetical charge, assuming that the most electronegative element in a bond is awarded all of the electrons in that bond.

Oxidation potential–The ability of a substance to be spontaneously oxidized; a more positive oxidation potential (measured in volts) is indicative of a substance that is easier to oxidize and will therefore more likely act as an anode in an electrochemical cell.

Oxidation-reduction (redox) reaction–A reaction that involves the transfer of electrons from one chemical species to another.

Oxidizing agent–In an oxidation–reduction reaction, the atom that facilitates the oxidation of another species; the oxidizing agent gains electrons and is thereby reduced.

***p* subshell**–The subshell corresponding to the angular momentum quantum number $l = 1$; contains three dumbbell-shaped orbitals oriented perpendicular to each other (p_x, p_y, and p_z) and is found in the second and higher principal energy levels.

Paired electrons–Two electrons in the same orbital with assigned spins of $+\frac{1}{2}$ and $-\frac{1}{2}$.

Parallel spin–In quantum mechanics, electrons in different orbitals of an atom with the same m_s values.

Paramagnetism–A condition that arises when a substance has unpaired electrons and is slightly attracted to a magnetic field.

Partial pressure–The pressure that one component of a gaseous mixture would exert if it were alone in the container.

Pascal (Pa)–The SI unit for pressure, equivalent to $\frac{N}{m^2}$; 1 atm = 101,325 Pa.

Paschen series–Part of the emission spectrum for hydrogen, representing transitions of an electron from energy levels $n \geq 4$ to $n = 3$.

Pauli exclusion principle–The principle stating that no two electrons within an atom may have an identical set of quantum numbers.

Pauling electronegativity scale–The most common scale used to express electronegativity of the elements.

Percent composition–The percentage of the total formula weight of a compound attributable to a given element.

Percent yield–The percentage of the theoretical product yield that is actually recovered when a chemical reaction occurs; obtained by dividing the actual yield by the theoretical yield and multiplying by 100%.

Period–A horizontal row of the periodic table containing elements with the same number of electron shells.

Periodic law–The law stating that the chemical properties of elements depend on the atomic number of the elements and change in a periodic fashion.

Periodic table–The visual display of all known chemical elements arranged in rows (periods) and columns (groups) according to their atomic number and electron structure.

pH–A measure of the hydrogen ion content of an aqueous solution,
defined as the negative log of the
H^+ (H_3O^+) concentration.

pH meter–A device used to measure the concentration of hydrogen ions in solution and report it as a pH value.

Phase–One of the three forms of matter: solid, liquid, or gas; also called state.

Phase change–Reversible transition between solid, liquid, and/or gas phase caused by shifts in temperature or pressure.

Phase diagram–A plot, usually of pressure vs. temperature, showing which phases of a compound will exist under any set of conditions.

Photon–The form of light which displays particulate and quantal behavior.

Physical property–A property of a substance unrelated to its chemical behavior, such as melting point, boiling point, density, or odor.

Pi (π) bond–A bond with two parallel electron cloud densities formed between two *p*-orbitals that limits the possibility of free rotation; π bonds are the second bond in a double bond and both the second and third bonds in a triple bond.

pOH–A measure of the hydroxide (OH^-) ion content of an aqueous solution, defined as the negative log of the OH^- concentration.

Polar covalent bond–A covalent bond between atoms with different electronegativities in which electron density is unevenly distributed, giving the bond positive and negative ends.

Polar molecule–A molecule possessing one or more polar covalent bonds and a geometry that allows the bond dipole moments to sum to a net dipole moment.

Polyprotic–A molecule capable of donating more than one proton.

Polyvalent acid–An acid capable of donating more than one acid equivalent.

Polyvalent base–A base capable of donating more than one hydroxide or accepting more than one proton.

Potential energy diagram–A graph that shows the potential energies of the reactants and products of a reaction during the course of the reaction; by convention, the *x*-axis shows the progress of the reaction and the *y*-axis shows potential energy.

Potentiometer–A device used to measure electromotive force (voltage). Potentiometers can be used in potentiometric titrations: redox titrations with no indicator.

Precipitate–An insoluble solid that separates from a solution; generally the result of mixing two or more solutions or of a temperature change.

Pressure–Average force per unit area measured in atmospheres (atm), torr or mmHg, or pascals (Pa); 1 atm $=$ 760 torr $\equiv$ 760 mmHg $=$ 101.325 kPa.

Principal quantum number (*n*)–The first quantum number, which defines the energy level or shell occupied by an electron.

Process–In a system, when a change in one or more of the properties of the system occurs.

Proton (p^+)–A subatomic particle that carries a single positive charge and has a mass slightly less than 1 amu.

Quanta–In Planck's theory, discrete bundles of energy that are emitted as electromagnetic radiation from matter.

Quantum number–A number used to describe the energy levels in which electrons reside; all electrons in an element are described by a unique set of four quantum numbers.

Radioactivity–A phenomenon exhibited by certain unstable isotopes in which they undergo spontaneous nuclear transformation via emission of one or more particles.

Raoult's law–A law stating that the partial pressure of a component in a solution is proportional to the mole fraction of that component in the solution; provides an explanation for vapor pressure depression seen in solutions.

Rate constant–The proportionality constant in the rate law of a reaction; specific to a particular reaction at a given temperature.

Rate-determining step–The slowest step of a reaction mechanism; this step serves as a bottleneck on the progress of the reaction.

Rate law–A mathematical expression giving the rate of a reaction as a function of the concentrations of the reactants; must be determined experimentally.

Rate order–The exponential effect of a change in concentration of a reactant on the change of rate in a reaction; the overall rate order is the sum of all the individual reactant rate orders.

Reaction mechanism–The series of steps that occurs in the course of a chemical reaction, often including the formation and destruction of reaction intermediates.

Reaction order–In a calculation of the rate law for a reaction, the sum of the exponents to which the concentrations of reactants must be raised.

Reaction quotient (*Q*)–Has the same form as the equilibrium constant, but the concentrations of products and reactants may not be at equilibrium; when compared to K_{eq}, it dictates the direction a reaction will proceed spontaneously.

Reaction rate–The speed at which a substance is produced or consumed by a reaction.

Real gas–A gas that exhibits deviations from the ideal gas law due to molecular attractions and the actual volume of the gas molecules themselves.

Rechargeable battery–An electrochemical cell that can undergo a reversible oxidation–reduction process; when discharging, it functions as a galvanic (voltaic) cell, and when charging, it functions as an electrolytic cell.

Redox titration–A specific method used to determine the concentration of an unknown solution using reducible titrants or titrands, typically by measuring voltage changes.

Reducing agent–In an oxidation–reduction reaction, the atom that facilitates the reduction of another species; the reducing agent loses electrons and is thereby oxidized.

Reduction–A reaction involving the net gain of electrons, decreasing the oxidation number.

Reduction potential–The ability of a substance to be spontaneously reduced; a more positive reduction potential (measured in volts) is indicative of a substance that is easier to reduce and will therefore more likely act as a cathode in an electrochemical cell.

Representative elements–Elements in Groups 1, 2, and 13 through 18 in the modern IUPAC table (the *s*- and *p*-blocks of the table, also called A group elements); these elements tend to have valence shells that follow the octet rule.

Resonance–A difference in the arrangement of electron pairs but not the bond connectivity or overall charge within a Lewis structure.

Resonance hybrid–A Lewis structure that represents the weighted average (by stability) of all possible resonance structures.

Reversible reaction–A reaction that can proceed in either the forward or reverse direction, and typically does not go to completion.

Root-mean-square speed (u_{rms})–The average speed of a gas molecule at a given temperature; as a scalar, it does not take direction into account.

***s* subshell**–Subshell corresponding to the angular momentum quantum number $l = 0$ and containing one spherical orbital; found in all energy levels.

Salt–An ionic substance consisting of cations and anions.

Salt bridge–A component of an electrochemical cell composed of an inert electrolyte that allows the charge gradient that builds up in the half-cells to be dissipated as a reaction occurs; contains ions that will not react with electrodes or ions in solution and that can move to balance charge.

Saturated solution–A solution containing the maximum amount of solute that can be dissolved in a particular solvent at a given temperature.

Second law of thermodynamics–The law stating that all spontaneous processes lead to an increase in the entropy of the universe.

Second-order reaction–A reaction in which the rate is directly proportional to the concentration of two reactants, or to the square of one single reactant.

Semipermeable–A quality of a membrane allowing only some components of a solution to pass through, usually including the solvent, while limiting the passage of other species.

Sigma (σ) bond–A head-to-head bond between two orbitals of different atoms that allows free rotation about its axis.

Single-displacement reaction–A reaction in which an ion of one compound is replaced with another ion; also known as a single-replacement reaction.

Solid–The phase of matter possessing the greatest order; molecules are fixed in a rigid structure.

Solubility–A measure of the amount of solute that can be dissolved in a solvent at a certain temperature.

Solubility product (K_{sp})–The equilibrium constant for the ionization reaction of a sparingly soluble salt.

Solute–The component of a solution that is present in a lesser concentration than the solvent.

Solution–A homogeneous mixture of two or more substances. It may be solid (brass), liquid (HCl (*aq*)), or gas (air).

Solvation–The electrostatic interaction between solute and solvent molecules; also called dissolution. The term hydration can be used when water is the solvent.

Solvation layer–The shell of solvent molecules that arranges itself in an ordered fashion around a dissolved solute particle.

Solvent–The component of a solution present in the greatest amount; the substance in which the solute is dissolved.

Sparingly soluble salt–An ionic compound that has a low solubility at a given temperature.

Specific heat–The amount of heat required to raise the temperature of one gram of a substance by 1°C.

Spectator ions–Ions involved in a reaction that do not change formula, charge, or phase; normally omitted from the net ionic equation.

Spectrum–The characteristic wavelengths of electromagnetic radiation emitted or absorbed by an object, atom, or molecule.

Spectroscopic notation–The shorthand representation of the principal and azimuthal quantum numbers, in which the azimuthal number is designated by a letter rather than a number.

Sphygmomanometer–A tool for measuring blood pressure.

Spin quantum number (m_s)–The fourth quantum number, which indicates the orientation of the intrinsic spin of an electron in an atom; can only assume values of $+\frac{1}{2}$ and $-\frac{1}{2}$.

Spontaneous process–A process that will occur on its own without energy input from the surroundings; defined by a negative change in free energy.

Standard conditions–Conditions defined as 25°C, 1 atm pressure, and 1 M concentrations; used for measuring the standard Gibbs free energy, enthalpy, entropy, and cell electromotive force.

Standard free energy ($G°$)–The Gibbs free energy for a reaction under standard conditions.

Standard heat of combustion (ΔH°_{comb})–The enthalpy change associated with the combustion of a fuel.

Standard hydrogen electrode (SHE)–The electrode defined as having a potential of zero under standard conditions; all oxidation and reduction potentials are measured relative to the standard hydrogen electrode at 25°C and with 1 M concentrations of each ion in solution.

Standard potential–The voltage associated with a half-reaction of a specific oxidation–reduction reaction; generally tabulated as reduction potentials, compared to the standard hydrogen electrode.

Standard state–The phase of matter for a certain element under standard conditions.

Standard temperature and pressure (STP)–Defined as 0°C (273 K) and 1 atm; used for measuring characteristics of an ideal gas.

State function–A function that depends on the state of a system but not on the path used to arrive at that state; includes pressure, density, temperature, volume, enthalpy, internal energy, Gibbs free energy, and entropy.

Stoichiometric coefficient–In a reaction, the number placed in front of each compound to indicate relative number of moles of that species involved in the reaction.

Stoichiometry–A form of dimensional analysis focusing on the relationships between amounts of reactants and products in a reaction.

Strong acid–An acid that undergoes complete dissociation in an aqueous solution.

Strong base–A base that undergoes complete dissociation in an aqueous solution.

Structural formula–The graphic representation of a molecule depicting how its atoms are arranged.

Sublimation–A change of phase from solid to gas without passing through the liquid phase.

Subshell–The division of electron shells or energy levels into different values of the azimuthal quantum number (*s*, *p*, *d*, and *f*); composed of orbitals.

Supercritical fluid–A substance whose current state is simultaneously a liquid and a gas—there is no distinction between the two phases.

Supersaturated–A solution which is beyond equilibrium, where ion product is greater than the solubility product constant. Supersaturated solutions are thermodynamically unstable.

Surge current–An above-average current transiently released at the beginning of the discharge phase of a battery.

Surroundings–All matter and energy in the universe not included in the particular system under consideration.

System–The matter and energy under consideration.

Temperature–A measure of the average kinetic energy of the particles in a system.

Theoretical yield–The maximal amount of product that can be obtained in a reaction; determined by stoichiometric analysis of the limiting reagent.

Thermodynamic product–The product of a reaction that is formed favorably at a higher temperature because thermal energy is available to form the transition state of the more stable product; has a larger overall difference in free energy between the products and reactants than the kinetic product.

Titrand–A solution of unknown concentration to which a solution of known concentration is added to determine its concentration.

Titrant–A solution of known concentration that is slowly added to a solution of unknown concentration to determine its concentration.

Titration–A method used to determine the concentration of an unknown solution by gradual reaction with a solution of known concentration.

Titration curve–A plot of the pH of a solution vs. the volume of acid or base added in an acid–base titration, or a plot of the electromotive force of a solution vs. the volume of oxidizing or reducing agent added in an oxidation–reduction titration.

Transition metal–Any of the elements in the B groups of the periodic table, all of which have partially filled *d* subshells.

Transition state–The point during a reaction in which old bonds are partially broken and new bonds are partially formed; has a higher energy than the reactants or products of the reaction and is also called the activated complex.

Triple point–The pressure and temperature at which the solid, liquid, and gas phases of a particular substance coexist in equilibrium.

Unsaturated solution–A solution into which more solute may be dissolved before reaching saturation.

Valence electron–An electron in the highest occupied energy level of an atom; the tendency of a given valence electron to be retained or lost determines the chemical properties of an element.

Valence shell–The outermost shell of an atom.

Valence shell electron pair repulsion (VSEPR) theory–A system that reflects the geometric arrangement of a molecule based on its Lewis dot structure; the three-dimensional structure is determined by the repulsions between bonding and nonbonding electron pairs in the valence shells of atoms.

van der Waals equation of state–One of several real gas laws, which corrects for attractive forces and the volumes of gas particles, which are assumed to be negligible in the ideal gas law.

van der Waals forces–Attractive or repulsive forces between molecules that don't arise from covalent or ionic bonds.

van't Hoff factor–The number of particles into which a compound dissociates in solution.

Vapor pressure–The partial pressure of a gaseous substance in the atmosphere above the liquid or solid with which it is in equilibrium.

Vapor pressure depression–The decrease in the vapor pressure of a liquid caused by the presence of dissolved solute; a colligative property.

Vaporization–The transformation of a liquid into a gas.

Water dissociation constant (K_w)–The equilibrium constant of the water dissociation reaction at a given temperature; equal to 10^{-14} at 25°C (298 K).

Weak acid–An acid that undergoes partial dissociation in an aqueous solution.

Weak base–A base that undergoes partial dissociation in an aqueous solution.

Yield–The amount of product obtained from a reaction.

Zero-order reaction–A reaction in which the concentrations of reactants have no effect on the overall rate.

INDEX

Note: Material in figures or tables is indicated by italic *f* or *t* after the page number.

Symbols

A

B

C

D

O

P

Q

R

S

ART CREDITS

Chapter 1 Cover—Image credited to koya979. From Shutterstock.

Figure 1.1—Image credited to Grace Cary. From Getty Images. Modified from source.

Figure 1.26—Image credited to User: alphaspirit. From Shutterstock.

Chapter 2 Cover—Image credited to RTimages. From Shutterstock.

Figure 2.3—Image credited to User: Scott Ehardt. From Wikimedia Commons.

Figure 2.5—Image credited to User: Karelj. From Wikimedia Commons.

Figure 2.19—Image credited to User: Dnn87. From Wikimedia Commons. Copyright © 2008. Used under license: CC-BY-3.0.

Chapter 3 Cover—Image credited to Wire_man. From Shutterstock.

Chapter 4 Cover—Image credited to imagedb.com. From Shutterstock.

Figure 4.4—Image credited to User: Igor M Olekhnovitch. From Wikimedia Commons. Copyright © 2009. Used under license: CC-BY-3.0.

Figure 4.10—Image credited to User: butaiump. From Shutterstock.

Figure 4.14—Unless otherwise indicated, this information has been authored by an employee or employees of the University of California, operator of the Los Alamos National Laboratory under Contract No. W-7405-ENG-36 with the U.S. Department of Energy. The U.S. Government has rights to use, reproduce, and distribute this information. The public may copy and use this information without charge, provided that this Notice and any statement of authorship are reproduced on all copies. Neither the Government nor the University makes any warranty, express or implied, or assumes any liability or responsibility for the use of this information.

Figure 5.9—Image credited to User: DStrozzi. From Wikimedia Commons. Copyright © 2009. Used under license: CC-BY-2.5.

Chapter 6 Cover—Image credited to Kletr. From Shutterstock.

Chapter 7 Cover—Image credited to Michal Zduniak. From Shutterstock.

Chapter 10 Cover—Image credited to Shawn Hempel. From Shutterstock.

Chapter 12 Cover—Image credited to monticello. From Shutterstock.

Figure 12.5—Image credited to User: Synaptidude. From Wikimedia Commons. Copyright © 2011. Used under license: CC-BY-3.0.

Figure 12.7—Images credited to User: Riventree. From Wikimedia Commons. Copyright © 2011. Used under license: CC-BY-3.0.

Notes

Notes

Notes

Notes

Notes

Notes

Notes